Healthy Communities 2000: Model Standards

Steps for Putting Model Standards to Use

Activities for Implementation

- Assess and determine the role of one's health agency
- Assess the lead health agency's organizational capacity
- Develop an agency plan to build the necessary organizational capacity
- Assess the community's organizational and power structures
- Organize the community to build a stronger constituency for public health and establish a partnership for public health
- Assess the health needs and available community resources
- Determine local priorities
- Select outcome and process objectives that are compatible with local priorities and the *Healthy People 2000* Objectives
- Develop communitywide intervention strategies
- Develop and implement a plan of action
- Monitor and evaluate the effort on a continuing basis

Healthy Communities 2000: Model Standards. Guid
Year 2000 National Health Objectives. Washington, D
1991.

Nutrition
in the
Community
The Art of
Delivering Services

REVA T. FRANKLE, M.S., Ed.D., R.D.
Nutrition Consultant, Weight Watchers International, Inc., Jericho, New York;
President, Frankle Associates—Communications and the Media, Somers, New York;
Adjunct Associate Professor, Graduate School of Health Sciences, New York Medical College,
Valhalla, New York

ANITA L. OWEN, M.A., R.D.
President, Owen Associates—Consultants in Nutrition Education and Communications,
Evansville, Indiana and Scottsdale, Arizona;
Adjunct Associate Professor,
University of Hawaii, School of Public Health;
President, The American Dietetic Association, (1985-1986);
President, The American Dietetic Association Foundation (1989-1990)

Third Edition

with 110 illustrations

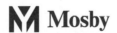 Mosby

St. Louis Baltimore Boston Chicago London Philadelphia Sydney Toronto

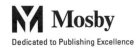

Mosby

Dedicated to Publishing Excellence

Editor-in-Chief: James Smith
Acquisitions Editor: Vicki Malinee
Developmental Editor: Loren M. Stevenson
Project Manager: Arofan Gregory
Designer: Dave Zielinski

THIRD EDITION

Printed in the United States of America

Mosby–Year Book, Inc.
11830 Westline Industrial Drive
St. Louis, Missouri 63146

ISBN 0-8016-6637-6

92 93 94 95 96 GW/PH/MV 9 8 7 6 5 4 3 2 1

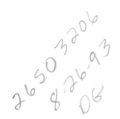

Preface

Through two editions, NUTRITION IN THE COMMUNITY has addressed the critical public health issues of the time. The first edition (1978) looked at the role of public health nutritionist, the art of program planning, community assessment programs, behavioral change, and evaluation. The second edition (1986) referred to as a "survival kit," was designed to guide students, teachers, and practitioners into the art of management with emphasis on managing both the internal and external environment to achieve health outcomes. The new third edition arrives at a time when there is scientific consensus on how people should eat to improve their chances for a healthy life. Presently, there is a trend toward recognition of the important role that diet plays in disease prevention, but surveys indicate that many people lack the knowledge, skills, and motivation to act effectively on this information.

In response, the third edition is a "strategic" approach designed for undergraduate and graduate students, nutritionists, dietitians, health educators, social workers, psychologists, community workers and others to understand the complexities of developing effective programs to improve dietary patterns for all segments of society.

Four important publications substantiate the importance of this new approach—The Future of Public Health (1989), Institute of Medicine; Healthy People 2000 (1990), the National Office of Health Promotion and Disease Prevention (ODPHP); Healthy Communities 2000—Model Standards, 3rd edition (1991), American Public Health Association; and Improving America's Diet and Health (1991), Institute of Medicine.

Hopefully, a new era beckons us. From the neglect of the early 1980s when our government went from the largest credit nation to the largest debt nation, the 1990s are fragile. With $260 billion in interest payments per year on our huge debt, human services have become downsized with the responsibility of health care delegated to local health departments. Health in the United States has become a fragmented patchwork of service.

Public health's promise for the future is inextricably related to efforts which maximize human potential and which realize the world's interdependence. Public health challenges are not only constant and complex, but are frequently surrounded by political issues.

Risk reduction through preventive and health promotion activities is the primary focus of public health but implementation is often dependent upon society's understanding the willingness-to-pay for such services—the consumer's frame of reference. In this environment, public health is empowered through its multidisciplinary approach. Americans must be concerned that there are adequate public health services in their community; they must voice their concern to their elected representatives; they must get involved in their own communities to address present health concerns, now and for the sake of future generations.

This text addresses the major health initiatives for the 1990s and beyond. It provides student, faculty member, and practitioner with guidelines for management and delivery of nutrition services.

NEW TO THIS EDITION

New to the third edition are six chapters that emphasize the approach of the text. Chapter 1, "The Changing Environment," focuses on how our environment has evolved over the past decade and the strategies that are needed to meet the challenges head on.

In recognition of the diversity of our society, the third edition includes a new chapter on how to deal with population groups with special needs (Chapter 2) and another on multi-cultural groups (Chapter 5). The new edition also looks at our food supply from development to consumption (Chapter 3) and guides us to work the communication process—getting the food to consumers (Chapter 4).

Also recognized in the third edition is the major role that the private sector (Chapter 11) plays in helping consumers select health promoting foods. We have finally realized that the private sector—from producer to retailer—greatly influences what people purchase and consume.

PEDAGOGY

Various learning aids are employed to enhance the usefulness of this text by students and faculty.

General Concept. Each chapter begins with a brief opening paragraph that provides an overview of the chapter.

Objectives. The major learning objectives for each chapter are stated to reinforce their significance for the student.

Chapter Opening Illustrations. All new illustrations open each chapter to help identify and reinforce the concepts covered in the chapter.

Figures and Tables. Strong visual materials are used in each chapter to illustrate important points.

Chapter Summaries. Each chapter ends with a brief summary that is particularly valuable for quick review of the subjects discussed in that chapter.

References. Each chapter provides current references to allow the reader to gain further information.

ACKNOWLEDGMENTS

Numerous persons have made significant contributions to this edition. Without their experience, guidance, and advice, this book would not have been completed. Receiving continual feedback from colleagues, practitioners, and students helped us create a truly teachable textbook. A special thanks and public acknowledgment should be made to the contributing authors, who provided materials, consultations, and their precious time:

Phyllis E. Bowen, Ph.D., R.D., Associate Professor, Department of Nutrition and Medical Dietetics, University of Illinois at Chicago, Chicago, Illinois.

J. Lynne Brown, Ph.D., R.D., Associate Professor, Department of Food Science, The Pennsylvania State University, University Park, Pennsylvania.

Judith E. Brown, Ph.D., M.P.H., R.D., Professor, Department of Human Development and Nutrition, School of Public Health, University of Minnesota, Minneapolis, Minnesota.

Catherine Cowell, Ph.D., Professor, Maternal and Child Health Program, Center for Population and Family Health, School of Public Health, Columbia University, New York, New York.

Johanna Dwyer, D.Sci., R.D., Professor, Department of Medicine and Nutrition, Tufts University Schools of Medicine; Senior Scientist, USDA Human Nutrition Research Center on Aging; Director, Frances Stern Nutrition Center.

Susan Finn, Ph.D., R.D., President, American Dietetic Association, Chicago, Illinois, 1992-1993; Director, Nutrition and Public Affairs, Ross Laboratories, Columbus, Ohio.

John R. Finnegan, Jr., Ph.D., Assistant Professor, Division of Epidemiology, School of Public Health, University of Minnesota, Minneapolis, Minnesota.

Karen Glanz, Ph.D., M.P.H., Professor, Department of Health Education, Temple University, Philadelphia, Pennsylvania.

James Hertog, Ph.D., Assistant Professor, School of Journalism, University of Kentucky, Lexington, Kentucky.

Penny Kris-Etherton, Ph.D., R.D., Professor, Nutrition Program, College of Human Development, The Pennsylvania State University, University Park, Pennsylvania.

Shiriki Kumanyika, Ph.D., Associate Professor, Center for Biostatistics and Epidemiology, The Pennsylvania State University College of Medicine, Hershey, Pennsylvania.

Sheryl L. Lee, M.P.H., R.D., Chief, Office of Nutrition Services, Arizona Department of Health Services, Phoenix, Arizona.

Christiaan B. Morssink, M.A., M.P.H., Doctoral Student, The Pennsylvania State University, University Park, Pennsylvania.

Lori Roth-Yousey, M.P.H., R.D., Consultant Dietitian, St. Paul, Minnesota.

Madeleine Sigman-Grant, Ph.D., R.D., Assistant Professor, Department of Food Services, The Pennsylvania State University, University Park, Pennsylvania.

Laura S. Sims, Ph.D., M.P.H., R.D., Professor, Department of Human Nutrition and Food Systems, University of Maryland, College Park, Maryland.

Patricia L. Splett, Ph.D., R.D., Assistant Professor, School of Public Health, University of Minnesota, Minneapolis, Minnesota.

Jacqueline M. Sullivan, M.S., Department of Nutrition and Medical Dietetics, University of Illinois at Chicago, Chicago, Illinois.

Donald B. Thompson, Ph.D., Associate Professor, Department of Food Service, The Pennsylvania State University, University Park, Pennsylvania.

Mosby–Year Book obtained an experienced ground of excellent reviewers. We appreciate their suggestions and criticisms which have had an influence on various aspects of this text. Our special thanks go to the following persons:

Garry Auld, Ph.D., R.D., Colorado State University
Jenell Ciak, Ph.D., Northwest Missouri State University
Michele W. Keane, Ph.D., Florida International University

A work of this kind involves the assistance and expertise of many organizations and individuals who contributed in various ways to its completion. Our heartfelt thanks to the following:

American Dietetic Association
Chicago, Illinois
Practice Group Chairmen
Teri Gargano M.B.A., M.S., L.D.
Coordinator, Position Development
Carol Flynn, R.D.
Assistant Executive Director

Association of State and Territorial Public Health Nutritionists
Washington, DC (202-546-6963)
Vernice Christian, M.P.H., R.D., L.N.

Association of Faculties of Graduate Program in Public Health Nutrition
Betsy Haughton, Ed.D., R.D.

Society for Nutrition Education
Darlene Lansing, Executive Director

Mary Ellen Collins, M.S., R.D.
Brigham and Women's Hospital, Boston, Massachusetts

Harold H. Fischer, A.B., J.D.
Regional Chief Administrative Law Judge, U.S. Department of Health & Human Services (Retired), Somers, New York

Jean H. Hankin, D.P.H., R.D.
University of Hawaii at Manoa, Cancer Research Center of Hawaii, Honolulu, Hawaii

Bruce Lafferty, J.D.
New York City, New York

Pamela R. McCarthy, M.S., R.D.
University of Minnesota School of Public Health, Minneapolis, Minnesota

Mosby–Year Book
Loren Stevenson, St. Louis, Missouri
Arofan Gregory, Philadelphia, Pennsylvania

Rebecca Mullis, Ph.D., R.D.
Division of Nutrition, CDC, Chronic Disease Prevention and Health Promotion, Atlanta, Georgia

George Owen, M.D.
Medical Director, Asia/Australasia, Bristol Myers Squibb Co., Evansville, Illinois

Lucille Rand
LR Services, Somers, New York

Wolf J. Rinke, Ph.D., R.D.
President, Wolf Rinke Associates Inc., Rockville, Maryland

Fay Wong, M.P.H., R.D.
Division of Cancer Prevention and Control Program, CDC, Atlanta, Georgia

Today's health issues are more visible and more complex. Health professionals have a role to play in forging the future. A new era beckons. Thus, the third edition is dedicated to the people—seeking their input, their participation, and their leadership.

Reva T. Frankle
Anita L. Owen

To
Harold H. Fischer and Joyce and Jonathon Yamaguchi
and grandchildren
Joshua and Jennifer

Reva T. Frankle

To
George, Gregory
and my mother
Evelyn Vangarelli

Anita L. Owen

Contents

PART

1

Forging the
Future:
Identification
of Problems

1

The Changing Environment: Nutrition Issues

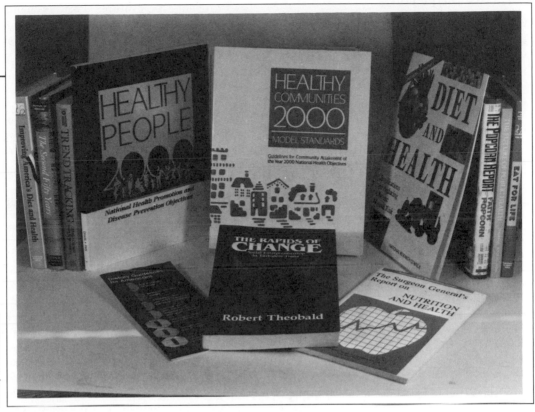

Courtesy of Laura Edwards

GENERAL CONCEPT

The external world surrounding community nutrition is important in stimulating change. The context for the nutrition educator is the milieu in which nutrition education and communication take place. It is also the environment in which our recommendations are interpreted and implemented by the people whose lives we wish to influence.

Consensus has developed about the role of diet in the etiology and prevention of chronic diseases. National documents provide authoritative reviews of the evidence relating dietary factors to health and disease and give us guidance for nutrition education programs. Preventive practices that can improve health, extend life, and reduce medical costs are already well known. The challenge is to apply them better.

Community nutrition is at a critical watershed, a turning point, as the economic and social environment has been changing. As time passes, the nature of the challenge changes. The dietitian-nutritionist, the change master, will envision a new reality and take a *leadership role* in the translation to the changing times, a departure from tradition.

OUTCOME OBJECTIVES

When you finish this Chapter, you should be able to:

- Describe context—environment in which the dietitian or nutritionist works and environment in which recommendations are interpreted and implemented—and how it differs from the past.
- List present-day health problems and societal concerns.
- Review and discuss national documents that have provided authoritative reviews of the evidence relating dietary factors to health and disease. These documents help shape nutrition education programs.
- Adopt the skills of change—the creation of new knowledge structures and communications with linkages between systems and new directions for innovation.
- Define the blueprint for the future—the role of the dietitian and nutritionist in creating and interpreting today's food and health environment.

THE CHANGING ENVIRONMENT

As change agents, or social entrepreneurs, as termed by Theobold,[24] we—the dietitians and nutritionists—will need to start with the skills that we have, use them as well as we can, watch the patterns that emerge, and then see where we can be most effective in terms of next steps. We need to dream and implement. Our messages will change to be current and meet the needs of society. We will need to encourage our constituency to listen to information that helps give meaning to their lives, even as it disrupts past thinking. Although we should maintain the old whenever we can to give people a sense of continuity, our ability to create the future will be based on a review of where we are and where we have been. People will learn they have the potential to change. People will experience personal empowerment, the capacity to define, analyze, and act on their own problems.[11] Empowered people believe that they are capable of achieving difficult goals and begin to take responsibility for their lives. Once personal improvement has occurred, people will be willing to strive

to change their futures. Positive change can happen only as we alter our visions of what we want to achieve and as we commit ourselves to creative activities. Human survival depends on this sense of personal responsibility.

CONTEXT CHANGE

- The American family has changed; we are a more heterogeneous society than ever before
- The population is aging and diverse in race, role, and culture, creating new opportunities for nutrition educators
- Hunger, homelessness, food scarcity, and a relatively high rate of unemployment are real issues in much of our country
- The food supply is dynamic and will continue to be as new technology appears at a rapid pace; *fast* and *convenient* are the watchwords of working parents
- Marketing of foods and new food products surrounds us

The values of the late 1990s are going to be different from the decade of the 1980s, known as the "Me-now-generation." The 1990s values are more like the values of the 1960s, only more pragmatic. People have more realistic economic expectations. They still want money, but they expect less. They want other things. They want rewarding work, free time, good health, satisfying relationships, and, above all, control over their lives. We see a greater sense of social responsibility and broader consensus on vital issues, because people from all age brackets, all socioeconomic levels, and all ethnic groups share concern for the future.[3]

As we move toward this value-based society, bureaucracies will inevitably be replaced by networks and linkages. These linkages will be made on the basis of competency and knowledge, with the most competent person having maximum influence on decision making.[24]

The Family

Families are the quintessential institution of our nation, providing both biological and social continuity, and are shaped by the larger society. Families are also the locus of consumption, savings, and some production activities that are vital to our overall economic well-being. They bear special responsibilities for nurturing and educating the nation's future work force, a critical function that is not well served by the deterioration of the nuclear family over the past 25 years or more.[32]

American families have changed in many ways as the population has adapted to evolving technologies, economic conditions, and social trends. Changes were particularly pronounced during the 1960s and 1970s as the baby-boom generation reached adulthood. Today there is no such thing as a "typical" family. In a nation as heterogeneous as the United States, the characteristics of families vary dramatically by race and ethnicity; education, age, and income of the adult members of the family; religious affiliation; region of the country; and by the interplay of these and other demographic, social, and economic factors. Relatively fewer of us are living in family households, and particularly in "traditional" nuclear families, than earlier in the twentieth century. The trend toward living in nonfamily households (usually alone) is associated with widowhood at older ages, the increased incidence of divorce among adults of all ages, and delayed marriage among young adults.

Women in the United States are bearing fewer children during their lives, and they are doing so later in their reproductive years. Consequently, the average size of families today is smaller than it has ever been before. The nation's total fertility rate—the number of children the average woman would be expected to bear in her lifetime—has been below the replacement level since 1972.[32]

Reflecting underlying changes in social attitudes and behavior, many more of today's new mothers are unmarried at the time their children are born than was the case in earlier generations. A basic problem of single parenthood is that children of single parents are much more likely than the children of intact marriages to be living in poverty. In 1988, for example, the poverty rate for married-couple families with children was 7.2%, but the rate for families maintained by women alone was 44.7%. In large part, this difference means more children in poverty, over 20% of all children—one of every five—were living in poverty during 1988, compared with 10.7% for persons 18 or more years of age.[1]

Those who live in family households—still a very substantial majority of the population—live in less stable, more heterogeneous families than did earlier generations. Kinship networks now often include former spouses and former in-laws, stepchildren, and, with increased life expectancy, more generations than were typical earlier in this century. Economic roles within the family have shifted significantly in the post–World War II years. In particular, regardless of the presence of children, including infants, women are now more likely to work outside the home than to work solely as homemakers.[32]

Aging Population

The aging of our population—the so-called graying of America—represents a major demographic shift with a powerful influence on this country's present and future course. The increase in the number of people living to old age has caused major shifts in the need for services for the elderly. The age of 65, used as the age of eligibility for Social Security and retirement benefits, is the cutoff point to classify individuals as *older adults, senior citizens,* or *elderly*. In 1900, persons over 65 made up less than 5% of the population. In 1980, more than 12% of the population were over 65, with a ratio of three women to every two men. In the year 2040, this age group is projected to reach 21% of the population as the baby boomers age.[31]

This aging of the U.S. population clearly brings with it many important social and economic implications. In 1984 the United States spent $387 billion on health care, which represented approximately 11% gross national product of the (GNP). Roughly one third of this amount went to care for the elderly. Per capita health expenditures for the elderly are 3.5 times those of the younger population.[22]

Health promotion activities for older people focus on six important areas where changes in behavior help older people reduce their risk of disabling disease and enable them to lead healthier, more productive lives. They are exercise, nutrition, safe use of medications, injury prevention, smoking cessation, and appropriate use of preventive services. There are many approaches to health promotion and disease prevention for the elderly. However, success should be measured not so much in terms of increasing longevity as in terms of improved health and quality of life. Our goals should be to foster the knowlege and skills necessary for an older individual to seek an independent and rewarding life in old age, not limited by any health problems that are within our capacity to control.[14]

Hunger and Food Security

Hunger is a priority issue for which definition and measurements are not currently available. *Hunger* has usually been defined by the dietitian or nutritionist as insufficient food to provide the calories and nutrients needed for activity, body function, and growth. A definition of *hunger* that has been suggested recently is lack of food security, food security being a condition in which people have access at all times to nutritionally adequate food from the customary food distributors, such as markets, gardens, restaurants, or fast-food outlets.[4] Food security includes both purchasing power and food availability. Another definition relates hunger to the federal poverty guidelines. Because these guidelines are linked to a family's ability to purchase a nutritionally adequate diet, households living on income below the poverty level index risk hunger. Families with incomes above the poverty level index may also risk hunger when high costs for housing, utilities, or excessive medical bills reduce the amount of money they have left to buy food.

The poverty rate is a controversial measure intended to reflect the percentage of Americans living below a threshold of minimal need, estimated at $13,359 for a family of four in 1990. It is not adjusted for regional variations in the cost of living. Many conservatives have said that the measurement, which includes noncash benefits like food stamps and health insurance, exaggerates the extent of poverty. In 1990 the poverty rate rose to 13.5% from 12.8% a year earlier. Median household income fell 1.7% to $29,943.

The poverty rate for children also rose to 20.6% in 1990 from 19.6% the previous year (in 1964 the poverty rate for children was 16.6%). Communities can work to achieve food security by encouraging eligible families to use federally funded food stamp, child nutrition, WIC, and elderly meal programs in combination with local food banks, soup kitchens, and food pantries. Although aggressive government actions are necessary to alleviate domestic hunger and to achieve food security for all citizens, local and community efforts are equally important in the fight against hunger.

Consumers and the Food Supply

The food habits of Americans are changing. These changes reflect such varied factors as declining birth rates, new methods of processing foods, concerns about health, and changing tastes and social patterns, such as eating out more frequently. Although 95% of Americans believe balance, variety, and moderation are the keys to healthy eating, many individuals fail to apply their nutritional knowledge when selecting foods, according to a national Gallup survey released at a news conference February 10, 1990.[5] The survey, commissioned by the International Food Information Council (IFIC) and the American Dietetic Association (ADA), reveals that more than two thirds of Americans choose foods based on "good" or "bad" perceptions, contrary to advice from nutrition and health experts. Although 83% recognized that what they ate may affect their future health, 35% were unsure if there was any difference between dietary cholesterol and blood cholesterol. Americans are surprisingly knowledgeable about nutrition and health, but when it comes to translating facts into food choices most people still opt for quick fixes and the latest health fads.

Many Americans report they do not find eating pleasurable because they worry about fat and cholesterol, 50% say they gain weight when they eat what they like, 45% say foods they like are not good for them, and 36% feel guilty about eating the foods they like. New foods have appeared in response to profound changes in American eating habits and technical innovations. The new emphasis on health and nutrition resulted in more than 200 oat bran products in 1989, and food companies predict that more than 2000 low-fat products will appear over the next several years.[17]

The market for ingredients that replace fat is currently less than $500 million. High-fat dairy products, like cheese and ice cream, are among the foods most frequently targeted for research. Livestock growers are trying to raise leaner strains of animals, and meat companies are looking for ways to strip the fat out of the final product. We are currently in a high-technology period for the red meat industry as these products, often using oat bran as a basis for new fat replacer, have the potential for once again increasing per capita meat consumption.[19]

New products clog the supermarket shelves. Although more than 12,000 products were introduced in 1989, more than 80% of all the new offerings failed because shoppers did not want or need them. Factors that have driven the product explosion include microwavable foods, single-serving portions, health foods, and fat-free selections.

About 60% of all supermarkets now have service delicatessens. The increased demand for prepared meals is behind this explosive growth in supermarket salad bars and delicatessens and places these stores in direct competition with take-out restaurants. Every year Americans spend 15% of their food dollars ($62 billion) on take-out meals. Another 19% goes to sit-down restaurants, and the rest is spent on home-prepared meals.[6]

In some communities farmers' markets are offering a low-cost source of foods. The use of food coupons has increased the buying power of low-income families, who are now joining regular customers. For example, under the 1991 New York State farmers' market coupon program, 66,000 low-income families enrolled in the Social Supplement Food Program for Women, Infants and Children receive $20 in coupons redeemable at the farmers' markets in the state. Because of this program, for the first time in 1991 an additional 5000 low-income elderly received $10 in coupons. Farmers are reim-

bursed for the coupons by market sponsors, using checks drawn on special bank accounts established with federal and state funds. Any farmer selling fresh fruits and vegetables at an authorized farmers' market may participate. Because there are no middlemen and transportation costs are low, consumers are able to get fresh fruits and vegetables at prices that are 5% to 20% lower than at retail stores.[18]

Among the forces that contribute to our changing environment is advanced technology in the food processing industry. Chapter 3 addresses the subject of food processing to help the nutrition educator effectively communicate the recommendations of national documents.

Influence of Marketing

Marketing—that is, satisfying the needs of the consumer through a product or service—includes everything associated with creating, delivering, and finally consuming the product. Marketing starts with the consumer's actual or perceived wants and needs.[12]

Social marketing—the design, implementation, and control of products calculated to influence the acceptability of social ideas—involves product planning, pricing, communication, and marketing research.[13] (See Chapter 4.) The dietitian or nutritionist will conduct social marketing when designing, implementing, and controlling programs to change eating behavior.

Today the consumer wants to know about the product's producer—what is being marketed by the producer in terms of environmental policy, stance on health care and child care, and the other brands in the company. Popcorn suggests four steps that companies can follow to find a "corporate soul" that will win the consumer's heart in the 1990s: acknowledgment, disclosure, accountability, and presentation.[21]

National Documents

Authoritative reviews of the evidence relating dietary factors to health and disease have led to a consensus among government, academic, and voluntary agencies. The Surgeon General, the National Research Council, the Centers for Disease Control, and the Institute of Medicine have agreed that preventive nutrition intervention can reduce the risk of diet-related chronic diseases. Eight of the ten leading causes of death—for example, heart diseases, strokes, atherosclerosis, cancers, and diabetes mellitus—are due largely to Americans' eating and drinking habits. Cirrhosis of the liver, unintentional injuries, and suicides have been associated with excessive alcohol intake. Provision of appropriate nutrition assessment, nutrition counseling, and nutrition support can change these statistics.

The nutrient intakes and nutritional status of the U.S. population are periodically documented by the National Health and Nutrition Examinations (NHANES) conducted by the National Center for Health Statistics (NCHS) of the Centers for Disease Control (CDC), the Nationwide Food Consumption Survey (NFCS), and the Continuing Surveys of Food Intakes by Individuals (CFSII) by the Human Nutrition Information Service (HNIS) of the U.S. Department of Agriculture (USDA). Further information about the nutrition and health status of specific subpopulations, consumer knowledge and behavior, and food and diet composition is provided by several other data sources, including the Pregnancy Nutrition and Pediatric Surveillance Surveys by the CDC, the National Health Interview Surveys (NHIS) by NCHS, the Diet and Health Knowledge Survey by HNIS, and the Total Diet and Diet and Health Surveys by the Food and Drug Administration (FDA). The National Institutes of Health and the Agricultural Research Service of USDA provide the primary research base for these nutrition monitoring activities. In the United States there have been a number of attempts to formulate a national nutrition policy and develop nutrition guidelines:

1969   The White House Conference on Food, Nutrition and Health

1977   The U.S. Senate Select Committee on Nutrition and Human Needs—*Dietary Goals for the United States*[30]

1979   *Healthy People: The Surgeon General's Report on Health Promotion and Disease Prevention*

1980   *Promoting Health/Preventing Disease: Objectives for the Nation* (Department of Health and Human Services [DHHS])[26]

1980   *Nutrition and Your Health: Dietary Guidelines for Americans*, 1st edition (USDA/DHHS) (2d edition 1985, 3d edition 1990)[25]

1988   *The Surgeon General's Report on Nutrition and Health* (DHHS)[27]

1989   *Diet and Health: Implications for Reducing Chronic Disease Risk* (Food and Nutrition Board/National Research Council/National Academy of Science)[16]

1990   *Healthy People 2000: National Health Promotion and Disease Prevention Objectives* (DHHS)[28]

1991   *Dietary Guidelines Implementation* (Food and Nutrition Board/National Research Council/National Academy of Science)[9]

1992   *Eat For Life* (Institute of Medicine/Food and Nutrition Board/National Research Council/National Academy of Science)[7a]

In addition, two other important reports have an impact on the implementation and delivery of nutrition programs:

1988   *The Future of Public Health* (Institute of Medicine/National Academy of Science)[8]

1991   *Healthy Communities: Model Standards. Guidelines for Community Attainment of the Year 2000 National Health Objectives*, 3d edition (American Public Health Association)[7]

Dietary Goals

The activities of the U.S. Senate Select Committee on Nutrition and Human Needs[30] served as a catalyst for federal legislation. The 1977 hearings, based on the then-current diet, gave rise to *Dietary Goals for the United States*, which made specific recommendations:

- To avoid overweight
- To increase complex carbohydrates from 28% of energy intake to about 48%
- Reduce consumption of refined and processed sugars to 10% of total energy intake
- Reduce saturated fat to 10% of total energy intake, and balance that with 10% each polyunsaturated and monounsaturated

- Reduce cholesterol consumption to about 300 mg/day
- Limit intake of sodium by reducing intake of salt to about 5 g/day

Dietary Guidelines (1980, 1985, 1990)

Interest in nutrition as a major component of disease prevention and health maintenance was further emphasized with the publication in 1980 of *Nutrition and Your Health: Dietary Guidelines for Americans*,[25] a USDA-DHHS joint project that became the basis for federal nutrition policies. Now in its third edition, these guidelines recommend that to stay healthy you should eat a variety of foods; maintain healthy weight; choose a diet low in fat, saturated fat, and cholesterol; choose a diet with plenty of vegetables, fruits, and grain products; use sugar, salt, and sodium only in moderation; and, if you drink alcoholic beverages, do so in moderation.

Healthy People: The Surgeon General's Report on Health Promotion and Disease Prevention[29]

This landmark document, in which the federal government explicitly recognized the importance of nutrition as a major influence on the nation's health, led to the 1990 document *Promoting Health/Preventing Disease: Objectives for the Nation*.[26]

The development of these objectives for the nation started in 1978, when public health workers from around the country met in Atlanta to see if agreement could be reached on health objectives for the United States for the year 1990. After 2 years of debate, the document was released. It presented 226 objectives in 15 broad categories, which were to be achieved by 1990. It had consequences for public health that were far more profound than the initiators could have imagined. Because it was a consensus document in public health, it became the guide for budget determinations in the 1980s at the federal, state, and local levels. Although the document had many shortcomings, it led to constructive debates, similar efforts at state and local levels, and attempts to develop better and more measurable objectives. It also provided protection from a collapse of public health programs in the

1980s, when budget cuts combined with the competition of the acquired immunodeficiency syndrome stressed the public health system of this country in ways not before seen. The final tally on the 1990 objectives shows that about 50% of the objectives were met, about one fourth were not met, and data are insufficient to judge the remainder. This achievement is remarkable for a first attempt.[26]

Healthy People 2000: National Health Promotion and Disease Prevention Objectives

These 1990 health objectives for the nation built on past experience to present an exciting vision of the health future of this country.[28] With about 300 specific objectives, this document provides one of the most important developments in the history of public health. The priority areas at a glance are shown in Figure 1-1. It includes input from all segments of the country, provides a road map for government budgeting, holds people accountable for outcomes, and provides a dynamic forum for debating priorities.

The objectives for the year 2000 derive from the 1990 objectives for nutrition. In addition, they have been guided by the *Surgeon General's Report on Nutrition and Health*,[27] the National Research Council's *Diet and Health*,[16] and oral and written comments from many nutrition experts. Four cornerstones are recognized as fundamental for achievement of these nutrition objectives: (1) the maintenance and improvement of a strong national program of basic and applied nutrition research, (2) further development of the scope and magnitude of the National Nutritional Monitoring System, (3) marked improvement in nutrition information and education programs for the general public, and (4) development of a sustained program to implement and evaluate these objectives.

Diet and Health: Implications for Reducing Chronic Disease Risk

This voluminous report reviews evidence regarding all major chronic public health conditions that diet is believed to influence.[16] It draws conclusions about the effects of nutrients, foods, and dietary

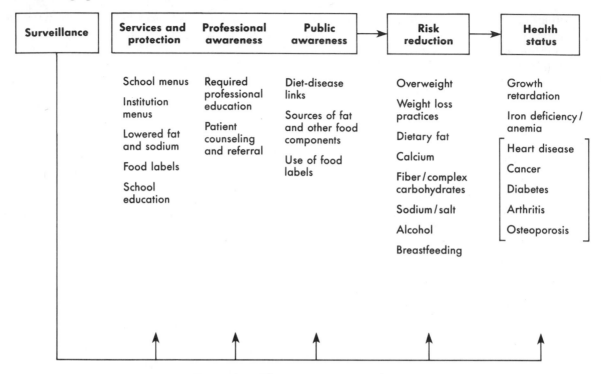

Figure 1-1. The priority area at a glance.

patterns on health; proposes dietary recommendations that have the potential for diminishing risk; and estimates their public health impact. This 749-page report became the background for recommendations to implement the dietary guidelines. The report complements the 1988 *Surgeon General's Report on Nutrition and Health*[27] and the 1985 *Nutrition and Your Health: Dietary Guidelines for Americans*.[25] However, it sheds new light on the process of arriving at dietary recommendations by documenting the considerations and logic that underlie the committee's recommendations to reduce the overall risk of diet-related chronic diseases.

The committee's recommendations pertain to total and specific fat intake; suggested daily servings of fruit, vegetables, starches, and other complex carbohydrates; protein intake; weight maintenance; alcohol consumption; salt intake; calcium intake; vitamin and mineral supplements; and fluoride intake.

Improving America's Diet and Health: From Recommendations to Action[9]

The Committee on Dietary Guidelines Implementation recognized that the main challenge no longer was to determine *what* eating patterns to recommend to the public but *how* to inform the public of ways to make changes for a healthier life. There has been an increasing recognition that simply issuing and disseminating recommendations is insufficient to produce change in most people's eating behavior. (See Chapter 10.) Many federal and state programs exist to implement the federal government's dietary guidelines. There are persistent efforts by the private sector to produce and publicize food products that help people meet various recommendations. However, there remains a clear need for comprehensive and coordinated actions to improve America's diet and health.

The Committee on Dietary Guidelines Implementation was convened in 1988 under the auspices of the Food and Nutrition Board (FNB) of the Institute of Medicine to address this widely felt need. In this report,[9] the committee promoted the recommendations of the 1989 *Diet and Health* report.[16] These recommendations are well suited for implementation because they are the most comprehensive evaluation of the scientific evidence linking nutrient intake, food intake, and dietary patterns with risks of developing many chronic degenerative diseases. In addition, the *Diet and Health* recommendations specify quantitative targets (e.g., limit fat intake to no more than 30% of calories) and are presented in a priority order that reflects their likely impact on public health. These recommendations will be reviewed regularly and revised as needed to incorporate new findings.

The primary issue facing the committee was determining how to mobilize the U.S. population to improve its habitual eating patterns in an effort to reduce the prevalence of diet-related chronic diseases in this country. It developed four overall goals for implementation:

- To enhance awareness, understanding, and acceptability of dietary recommendations
- To create legislative, regulatory, and educational environments supportive of the recommendations
- To improve the availability of foods and meals that facilitate implementation of the recommendations
- To increase the prevalence of eating patterns that conform to these recommendations

The tactics for accomplishing these goals were divided into three classes:

- *Altering the food supply* by subtraction (e.g., reducing the fat in red meat), addition (e.g., fortification of foods with vitamins, minerals, fiber), or substitution (e.g., replacing the fat in cheese with vegetable oil)
- *Altering the food acquisition environment* by providing information (e.g., more complete and easily understood product labeling), ad-

vice (e.g., tags noting a good nutrition buy at the supermarket or cafeteria), and greater opportunities for selecting health-promoting foods (e.g., better choices in vending machines)

- *Altering nutrition education* by changing the message mix (e.g., modifying advertisements for certain kinds of products or adding public service announcements) or by broadening exposure to both formal and informal nutrition education (e.g., mandating education on dietary recommendations in kindergarten through grade 6, in health care facilities, and in medical schools)

Although common sense suggests that desirable dietary changes are most likely to take place when all these components are structured to be mutually reinforcing, there is little research on the effectiveness of each or how they should be assembled into a package.

As stated earlier, two other important reports have an impact on the implementation and delivery of nutrition programs: the Institute of Medicine (IOM) report[8] and the American Public Health Association (APHA) report.[7]

The food guide pyramid replaces the four food groups, which have been used to teach nutrition in schools since the 1950s. This publication will affect the way young people learn about nutrition for years to come. The pyramid places the grain group at its base, vegetables and fruits, now two groups instead of one, just above it, and a narrow band for meat and dairy products near the top. At the apex are fats, oils, and sweets, which are not considered a food group, with the note to "use sparingly" (Fig. 1-2).

Eat for Life Food and Nutrition Boards's Guide to Reducing Your Risk of Chronic Disease[7a]

When the Food and Nutrition Board (FNB) began planning a study of what is known of diet and its relationship to chronic disease, three books were envisioned. The first, a comprehensive review and analysis of the scientific literature, *Diet and Health* (1989) has been discussed above. Also discussed

Food Guide Pyramid
A Guide to Daily Food Choices

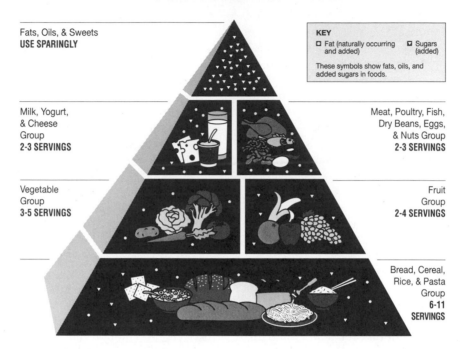

Figure 1-2. Food Guide Pyramid. (USDA, Food Guide Pyramid, April 28, 1992, Washington, DC.)

above is the second volume written to focus on implementing the dietary guidelines, *Improving America's Diet and Health: From Recommendations to Action* (1991). *Eat for Life* (1992), the final volume written for individuals interested in improving their health and incorporating the dietary guidelines into everyday health, offers nine dietary guidelines as shown in the box on p. 13.

The Future of Public Health

This landmark report recommended a renewal of efforts from all corners of society to address the mission of public health: "fulfilling society's interest in assuring conditions in which people can be healthy."[8] (See Appendix B.)

The report charged state public health agencies with establishing statewide health objectives, delegating power to localities as appropriate, and holding them accountable. The report reaffirmed local

public health agencies as "the final delivery point for all public health efforts" and called for policy development and leadership that foster local involvement and a sense of ownership, that emphasize local needs, and that advocate equitable distribution of public health resources and complementary private activities commensurate with community needs.

The federal government is essential to fulfilling this destiny. As most health issues affect the majority of Americans directly or indirectly, the federal government's involvement in national policy development is necessary. It has the obligation to take the initiative in bringing broad public health policy issues to the attention of the nation, to establish a framework within which interstate and national issues can be debated, and to set national health goals and standards of achievement. It is critically important to the achievement of *Healthy*

THE NINE DIETARY GUIDELINES

1. Reduce total fat intake to 30% or less of your total calorie consumption. Reduce saturated fatty acid intake to less than 10% of calories. Reduce cholesterol intake to less than 300 (mg) daily.
2. Eat five or more servings of a combination of vegetables and fruits daily, especially green and yellow vegetables and citrus fruits. Also, increase your intake of starches and other complex carbohydrates by eating six or more servings of a combination of breads, cereals, and legumes.
3. Eat a reasonable amount of protein, maintaining your protein consumption at moderate levels.
4. Balance the amount of food you eat with the amount of exercise you get to maintain appropriate body weight.
5. It is not recommended that you drink alcohol. If you do drink alcoholic beverages, limit the amount you drink in a single day to no more than two cans of beer, two small glasses of wine, or two average cocktails. Pregnant women should avoid alcoholic beverages.
6. Limit the amount of salt (sodium chloride) that you eat to 6 grams (g) (slightly more than 1 teaspoon of salt) per day or less. Limit the use of salt in cooking and avoid adding it to food at the table. Salty foods, including highly processed salty foods, salt-preserved foods, and salt-pickled foods, should be eaten sparingly, if at all.
7. Maintain adequate calcium intake.
8. Avoid taking dietary supplements in excess of the U.S. Recommended Daily Allowances in any one day.
9. Maintain an optimal level of fluoride in your diet and particularly in the diets of your children when their baby and adult teeth are forming.

From Institutes of Medicine. Eat for Life. Washington, DC: National Academy Press, 1992.

People 2000 objectives[28] that federal, state, and local health agencies take up this charge and use *Healthy Communities 2000: Model Standards*[7] in partnership with private sector organizations to fulfill their responsibilities in protecting the nation's health. The report is intended for a broad audience that includes selected public officials at all levels of government, voluntary health organizations, health care providers, educators in all health professions, and private citizens with interests in maintaining and improving community health.

Healthy Communities 2000: Model Standards*

This important document also pertains to the implementation of guidelines for community attainment of the year 2000 national health objectives.[7] (See Appendix A.) The model standards have been designed:

- To help individuals in the public health community to be both leaders and managers—those who do the right things and do them in the right way
- To encourage public health leaders in communities to engage a whole host of players in setting the health priorities for their locales and in implementing programs designed to achieve their health objectives
- To focus on the common good and to call for public health to be accountable for its shortfalls as well as its successes
- To provide comprehensive goals and objectives to encourage community leaders to work together to improve health, the environment, and quality of life in communities.

During the 1980s, national leaders recognized that improvements in health status required efforts targeted to people in communities where they live. Translating national objectives into achievable community health targets requires three elements:

1. An understandable set of health status and local process objectives that can be readily measured
2. The availability of strategies to achieve these objectives involving public, private, and voluntary sectors of the community
3. A coordinating process to help ensure that the community can work together

*In the late 1970s the CDC collaborated with the APHA and the national organizations of state and local health officials to develop model standards for community-oriented preventive health services. In local application, the standards take the form of quantifiable community-specific objectives for reducing present levels of preventable morbidity and mortality.

The Department of Health, Education, and Welfare (DHEW) secretary officially submitted the first volume of *Model Standards* to Congress in 1979. CDC has continued support for the model standards work group to test, refine, and expand the standards. A second edition was published by the APHA in 1985 and is now in use in scores of local and state agencies across the country. A third edition of the model standards, *Healthy Communities 2000*, was published in 1991 as the local implementation companion to *Healthy People 2000*.

This completely revised third edition of the *Model Standards*[7] reflects the years of field experience and testing on the standards. The development of the 520-page publication was funded by the CDC and housed at the APHA. It was a collaborative project with the APHA, the Association of Schools of Public Health, the Association of State and Territorial Health Officials, the National Association of County Health Officials, the United States Conference of Local Officials, and the CDC.

SKILLS OF CHANGE

It is in this combined context—the environment in which we work and the environment in which our recommendations are interpreted and implemented—that we need to develop and use the skills of change.

Kanter suggests that change can be exhilarating, refreshing—a chance to meet challenges, a chance to clean house.[10] It means excitement when it is considered normal, when people expect it routinely, a set of new messages, the unknown. Change brings opportunities when people have been planning for it, are ready for it, and have just the thing in mind to do when the new state comes into being. It provides a chance for social entrepreneurs to offer "change-management" services. Change is a fact of life. To proact is to anticipate the future and to act accordingly.

Creating New Knowledge Structures

These changing times require not only that we change our practices in our responses to situations but also that we change the way we think about what we do. Should we fail to understand the need for change or are inept in our ability to deal with change, we will fade or fall behind, if we survive at all.

Given the new publications from the federal government, including the *Dietary Guidelines for Americans*,[25] which incorporate not only the concept of nutritional adequacy but also health promotion, the dietitian or nutritionist needs to be ready to mount programs and empower communities.

To create new knowledge structures, we need to draw together information from a diversity of disciplines. To do this, a general systems approach is required. This approach demands that information be integrated from the various sectors of society. For nutrition intervention programs, this means examining the food marketplace, investigating the variety of nutrition message channels— mass media, health professionals, peers, books— incorporating information from the scientific community, and helping people understand how to apply the principles of selecting appropriate health and nutrition information, as well as how to integrate the information into their own lives.

It may mean that we provide indirect service through working with writers to help them to interpret scientific information in the language of the people. It may also mean interpreting nutrition science information in the language of the marketplace, that is, the grocery store or restaurant. This requires that we are familiar with the market system in order to interpret dietary guidelines in marketplace terms (see Chapters 3 and 12). It might also mean rethinking our educational materials, to adapt them to grocery store groups, where people select foods (see Chapter 10).

In order to incorporate the skills of change into our discipline, we must begin to redefine our role. In this context our role becomes that of a helper. We need to help people recognize and find information they want, at the time they want it, and in the language of their context. All too often, we give people what we think they need to know, when we are available to give it, and in our own context. Our information needs to be based on current science translated into current food products in today's marketplace. We must provide people with realistic choices they can easily make, given their life-style constraints. For example, we must help the busy mother trying to feed a young and active family by suggesting convenience foods as well as regular foods.

In order to meet people in their context, we must begin to link systems, as stated earlier. For example, we must begin to link the food system with the health care system; in clinical settings we need to make it easier for people to relate to the nutrition advice from the clinic and interpret it in the community at the grocery store, the restaurant, the worksite, the school, and wherever food choices are made. We also need to link market systems with health education systems.[15] We need to use the market system as a vehicle for education. We already see the demand for information about foods on the label, but the label is not a substitute for awareness. Labeling cannot provide the high-quality educational experience we know is necessary to change food behavior. In order to use market systems for educational purposes, we must be selective in the kinds of information we choose to share at the level of the marketplace. We must begin to link government with industry so that we have the consensus of science and industry working together to produce appropriate programs and products for people. It is our role as nutrition professionals to help create and maintain a demand for healthy food products. Industry's role is to respond to that demand by producing and marketing foods consistent with consensus health and nutrition messages.

It takes knowledge and information to make a difference. Those people with more information about matters at hand have an advantage over the others. (See Appendix 1-1.) We are living in a world that depends on information, information from reliable sources. Celente, a forecaster, relies most heavily on the daily newspaper—the *New York Times*, *USA Today*, the *Wall Street Journal*, and the *Washington Post*—as a primary source for information and tracking trends.[3] In the future the right to lead will be based on competence and knowledge rather than position. We are concerned with ideas, knowledge, and trends that will help us act to create a higher quality of life for our constituencies. A trend is a definite, predictable direction or segment of events, like the warming of the earth's climate. Tracking trends shows how we got here, where we are, and where we are going. Anticipating a new reality is the beginning of the process of creating it. Tracking trends is one way we anticipate new realities. Popcorn tracks some 300 newspapers and magazines and monitors the top 20 television shows, first-run movies, best-seller books, and hit music.[21] Major trends in a consumer-driven food system, demographics, disparate lifestyles, food economics, data sources, and special consumer groups such as the "forgotten poor" are all discussed by Senauer et al.[23]

What are the ideas, knowledge, and trends that will help the dietitian and nutritionist meet the needs of individuals and population groups now and into the twenty-first century? We need to start our thinking from the assumption that healthy human beings want to grow and help others to grow. We need to meet people in their context. What are their concerns?

Here the tools of market research may provide us with some guidance. Although market research is a tool and not a science, it has many goals that are similar to those in scientific research:

- To gather available information
- To assimilate that information in a meaningful manner
- To analyze the data
- To recommend action based on the results

Quantitative market research is designed to provide five important Ws: who, what, where, why, and when. For example:

Who in the population is most interested in reducing saturated fat intake?

What does a particular population know about cholesterol?

Where in the United States is dietary fat consumption the highest?

Why do individuals lose interest in low-fat diets?

When do individuals get serious about following a low-fat diet?

These kinds of questions that give insight into the needs of our clients can be answered by qualitative market research studies. Such data can identify and target high-risk populations, identify causes and motivational factors associated with dietary intervention programs, and identify highlights for designing preventive health programs.[20]

Another tool that can shed light on the needs of our consumers is the focus group. A focus group is a group discussion among a small number of individuals (up to 12 maximum) led by a professional moderator. The moderator asks questions of the group and keeps the discussion on target, usually with a prepared agenda. In a focus group a question can be discussed in great depth. Knowledge, attitudes, and practices can be freely explored. Often observers interested in the question view the focus group through a one-way mirror.

The social entrepreneur recognizes that social change requires that we either appeal to the existing self-interest of individuals and groups or help them gain different perspectives of their self-interest. For example, we need to convince the grocer of the benefits of stocking and actively marketing healthier food items, and we need to speak in grocers' terms—profit, community image, enhanced customer satisfaction, value, added service—and not just our terms of better nutrition information and healthier food choices.

Communication is the Key

Successful communication in the 1990s will rely on the forging of relationships with consumers. Consumers and communicators will have to look at one another as partners in solving problems and satisfying needs. To form a communication partnership and build relationships with consumers, three ingredients are required: trust, personal contact, and mutual understanding. Although it may appear obvious, the skill of communicating effectively is essential to our survival. (See Chapter 4.) The ability to communicate can be readily analyzed. The communicator should be able to relate to the individual or group on a short-term or long-term level. The subject matter should be simple and concise, and the communicator should be able to present an effective plan to support and implement any proposed action. To meet the challenges of the 1990s and beyond, the communication systems that transmit information are a key resource for all of us.

Creating Positive Directions

Health professionals share the awesome responsibility and the exciting challenge of improving the nation's health in this decade and the century ahead. We are the leaders. If we do not lead, who will? Leadership requires commitment. To strengthen our work force to deal with new challenges, another essential skill is leadership. In the past, leaders tried to mold events to achieve their personal reaction. Today our leadership task is to seek out and create opportunities for advocacy and to encourage and empower others to play their part—notably at the community level.[11] The di-

etitian and nutritionist can assume a leadership role alone or as a team member, setting forth the health agenda, building the necessary networks and alliances, mobilizing support, and calling on public and private resources for common health purposes (see Chapter 11). Individual and social behavior will only change if we provide opportunities for discussion and link people who can help each other. In the future the right to lead will be based on competence and knowledge rather than position. We need to work with each other rather than be controlled by hierarchical custody. The need for leadership is constant, but the required style of leadership changes with the times. The contemporary leader must understand reality well enough to work with others in the rapids of change, while creating support for a fundamentally changed, value-based future. Mistakes will be inevitable, but we will learn by our mistakes, and because we allow ourselves to make mistakes and learn, we are free to take risks.[24]

In this new mode of action, we need to begin with the skills we have, use them as well as we can, see what happens, and then determine where we can be most effective in terms of the next steps. We need to develop checks and balances if we are working with a public-private partnership to protect our credibility as nutrition educators. However, being a change agent or championing a new idea is not easy or necessarily popular. Facilitating change demands that we move beyond our own needs for ego satisfaction and learn to help people recognize the points at which they are ready to grow.

Our challenges as nutrition educators are consensus, consistency, and collaboration. We will need to work with nutrition scientists, health professionals, educators, policy makers, and others to reach a consensus. A priority is giving consistent messages. We will need collaborative programs that set and work toward the common goal of healthier eating for all people—which means adequate food as well as adequate information.

The Future

We have a very clear blueprint for the future. The process began back in 1969 with the White House

Conference on Food, Nutrition and Health, continued with *Dietary Goals*,[30] *Dietary Guidelines*,[25] and *Healthy People*[28] in the late 1970s, and proceeded through the delineation of the 1990 objectives, their monitoring throughout the 1980s, and our year 2000 objectives. These objectives have been developed by experts and consumers with very wide participation. They are precise, quantifiable, realistic, and demanding. They demand top performance and leadership. We cannot depend on the momentum of the 1980s to carry us forward. The architecture of change requires an awareness of foundations—a sense of where we have been. To know the past is to know the future. The scientific base of dietary recommendations of the past had led to the establishment of consensus. Conflicts disappear into consensus. For the current blueprints to have been established, we have had to design consensus conferences.

If the past few years have taught us anything, it has been the swiftness and power of change, particularly in the areas of politics and ecology. Those people and organizations who are adept at anticipating needs and of leading will succeed in productive change. The mastery of change comes through the ability to innovate. To embrace change is an opportunity to test limits. Innovation—the process of managing a new and useful idea from inception through successful introduction—requires a trust in the future but also a look at the past. What pieces of the past should be honored and preserved while we move toward a different future?[10]

Innovation is vital to our business. It allows us to prevail in the marketplace as an effective competitor, to exploit changes, and to enhance our reputation and image. Innovation strategy means that the leader in the field refuses to be content with the way things are and becomes a leader in new ideas and services.

Community nutrition is at a critical watershed, a turning point, as the economic and social environment has been changing. As time passes, the nature of challenge changes. If the art and science of community nutrition are to build on its past strengths and to secure a better future for itself, innovation and the risk of change that it implies are necessary to ensure survival. To continue to make the same once-successful response to the new challenge will stifle the future of community nutrition.

As our world becomes more precarious and complex, we find a greater need to understand what we may expect from the future. Whatever the future does hold for us, one thing is clear: the future, like the present, is double-edged, full of peril and promise. It will be shaped by the choices we make here and now.

SUMMARY

As change agents, or social entrepreneurs, dietitians and nutritionists will examine the external world and develop community nutrition services that are relevant to today's environment. Doing so means a review of the American family, the population segments (see Chapters 2 and 5), the food supply (see Chapter 3), and the influence of marketing. A review of the national documents that provide authoritative reviews and establish consensus of the evidence relating dietary factors to health promotion and disease prevention will give guidance for nutrition education programs.

In the combined context—the environment in which we work and the environment in which our recommendations are interpreted and implemented—the dietitian and nutritionist will develop and use the skills of change. New knowledge structures about working with people, linking systems, and the act of communication will give direction to leadership roles. Linking systems means linking people, population groups with special needs (Chapter 2), with the food supply (Chapter 3), and the communication system (Chapter 4). "What a marvelous moment in history to be a dietitian-nutritionist. It is like being an artist in the time of Michelangelo and Bernini, a Roman legionnaire in the Age of Caesar."[2]

REFERENCES

1. Bureau of Census: Money, income, poverty status, *Current Population Report Series* No. 166:60, 1989.
2. Califano JA Jr: America's health care revolution: health promotion and disease prevention, J Am Diet Assoc 87 (4):437, 1987.

3. Celente G: *Trend tracking*, New York, 1991, Warner Books.
4. Cohen BE: *Food security policy for the 1990s: elimination of hunger*, executive summary. Washington, DC, 1989, The Urban Institute (unpublished).
5. *Gallup survey of public opinion regarding diet and health*, Princeton, NJ, 1990. The Gallup Organization.
6. Hamel R: Food fight, *Am Demographics* March 1989, p 364.
7. *Healthy communities 2000: model standards. Guidelines for community attainment of the year 2000 national health objectives*, ed 3, Washington, DC, 1991, American Public Health Association.
7a. Institutes of Medicine: *Eat for life*, Washington, DC: National Academy Press, 1992.
8. Institute of Medicine: *The future of public health*, Washington DC, 1988, National Academy Press.
9. Institute of Medicine: *Improving America's diet and health: from recommendations to action*, Washington, DC, 1991, National Academy Press.
10. Kanter RM: *The change masters: innovation and entrepreneurship in the American corporation*, New York: Simon and Schuster, Inc., 1984.
11. Kent G: Nutrition education as an instrument of empowerment, *J Nutr Educ* 20:193, 1988.
12. Klug JR: *The basic book of business*, Boston 1977, Cahners.
13. Lotler P, Zaltman G: Social marketing: an approach to planned social change, *J Marketing* 35:5, 1971.
14. McGinnis JM: Nutrition and aging II, keynote address at health promotion and disease prevention in the elderly conference, Little Rock, Sept 10-11, 1986.
15. Mullis R, Shannon B: Building partnerships with the food marketing system: an expanding role for dieticians, *J Am Diet Assoc* 87(12):1631, 1990.
16. National Research Council: *Diet and health: implications for reducing chronic disease risk*. Washington, DC, 1989, National Academy Press.
17. *New York Times*, New foods, May 29, 1990, p 15.
18. *New York Times*, Coupon use expanding farmers market, Aug 25, 1991, p 12.
19. *New York Times*, Fat substitutes, Sept 29, 1991, p 5.
20. Owen A: Market research: a tool for scientists and health professionals, Oct 11, 1988, National Cholesterol Education Conference.
21. Popcorn F: *The Popcorn report*, New York, 1991, Bantam Doubleday Dell.
22. Rice DB, Estes CL: Health of the elderly: policy issues and challenges, *Health Aff (Millwood)* 3(4):26, 1984.
23. Senauer B, Asp E, Kinsey J: *Food trends and the changing consumer*, St. Paul, MN: Eagen Press, 1991.
24. Theobold R: *The rapids of change: social entrepreneurship in turbulent times*, Indianapolis, 1987, Knowledge Systems.
25. US Department of Agriculture, US Department of Health and Human Services: *Nutrition and your health: dietary guidelines for Americans*, 3 ed, Home and garden bulletin 232, Washington, DC, 1990, US Department of Agriculture and US Department of Health and Human Services.
26. US Department of Health and Human Services: *Promoting health/preventing disease: objectives for the nation*, Washington, DC, 1980, US Government Printing Office.
27. US Department of Health and Human Services: *The surgeon general's report on nutrition and health*, DHHS (PHS) Pub 88-50210. Washington, DC, 1988, US Government Printing Office.
28. US Department of Health and Human Services: *Healthy people 2000: national health promotion and disease prevention objectives*, Washington, DC, 1990, US Government Printing Office.
29. US Department of Health, Education, and Welfare: *Healthy people: The Surgeon General's report on health promotion and disease prevention*, Washington, DC: Superintendent of Documents, 1979.
30. US Senate Select Committee on Nutrition and Human Needs: *Dietary goals for the United States*, ed 2, Washington, DC, 1977, US Government Printing Office.
31. *Washington Post, Growing old in America*, Washington, DC, 1987, Washington Post Co.
32. Wetzel JR: American families: 75 years of change, *Monthly Labor Review*, March 1990, p 4.

APPENDIX 1-1

Information sources

Advertising Age. The International Newspaper of marketing news, and features on advertising, marketing and sales promotion.
Crain Communications Inc
740 N. Rush
Chicago, IL 60611
312-649-5200

American Consumer, The. Trends in attitudes, lifestyles and purchasing behavior of American consumer.
The American Consumer Consultants, Inc.
Box 255
Allendale, NY 07401
201-934-0990

American Demographics. Business magazine of demographic trends, sources and techniques.
American Demographics, Inc.
Box 6543
Syracuse, NY 13217
607-273-6343

Journal of Marketing. Serves as a bridge between marketing practitioners and educators.
American Marketing Association
250 S Wacker Drive, Ste 200
Chicago, IL 60606
312-648-0536

Family Factbook. History of the family, male/female roles, marriage, parenthood, midlife transition, widowhood, child development, health, work, income, housing, etc.
Marquis Who's Who, Inc.
200 E Ohio St
Chicago, IL 60611
312-787-2008

Health Values: Achieving High Level Wellness. Current trends in government, private and voluntary agencies relevant to preventive care, health promotion, health research, etc., to promote good health.
Charles B. Slack, Inc.
6900 Grove Rd
Thorofare, NJ 08086
609-848-1000

Journal Community Health. Devoted to original articles on practice, teaching and research in community health.
Hilman Sciences Press, Inc.
72 Fifth Ave
New York, NY 10011
212-243-6000

Public Health Reports. Delivery of health services, epidemiology, public health, and health economics.
Public Health Services
Dept of Health & Human Service
200 Independence Ave, SW
Washington, DC 20201

World Future Society: An Association for the Study of Alternative Futures. The World Future Society screens worldwide social and technological developments. The Society, an educational and scientific organization founded in 1966, has members in more than 80 countries and serves as a neutral clearinghouse for ideas and information about the future. Members receive *The Futurist*, a bimonthly journal of forecasts and trends; a resource catalog; a helpful book, *Careers Tomorrow*; special reports; and information on local groups and conferences.
World Future Society
4916 St Elmo Avenue
Bethesda, MD 20814
301-656-8274

2 Population Groups with Special Needs

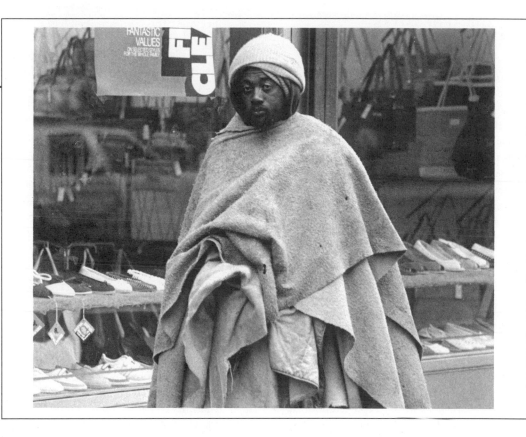

GENERAL CONCEPT

The current socioeconomic climate has created an emerging network of subgroups in the population which are vulnerable to nutrition-related problems. Although there have always been pockets of vulnerable groups such as the poor, those with handicapping conditions, those dependent on others for food, pregnant and lactating women, infants and children, and those in the drug culture, these growing subgroups—the homeless, the hungry, those with AIDS/HIV, and other target groups—present a serious challenge to dietitians and nutritionists.

OUTCOME OBJECTIVES

When you finish this chapter, you should be able to:

- Understand which population subgroups are vulnerable to health and nutrition-related problems.
- Identify factors that impact on the nutritional status of groups with special needs.
- Describe practical and appropriate nutrition assessment strategies to use with specific groups.
- Identify food assistance and nutrition resources available and accessible to groups with special needs.

BACKGROUND STATEMENT

Within any larger population there have always been subgroups or pockets of individuals who are considered at high risk for a range of health and nutrition problems. Historically these groups were so identified because the individuals who comprised the groups were nutritionally vulnerable for several reasons:

1. They consume an inadequate diet because they are poor or lack consistent access to the food supply or for other reasons.
2. They are unable to eat because of a handicapping condition.
3. Infants, young children, the elderly, and the mentally retarded are dependent on others for food.
4. They are unable to meet their need for increased nutrients and calories to support pregnancy, lactation, growth and development, and other physical conditions.

Population groups with special needs encompass individuals and groups at risk because of any one or more of these reasons. The concept of a balanced diet is based on consuming a variety of nourishing foods in proportion to essential nutrients and calories to support body growth and function. Malnutrition results when either deficiencies or excesses lead to imbalances of nutrients and energy. Undernutrition and overnutrition can be viewed as manifestations of malnutrition because both states result in an imbalance of nutrients and en-

ergy. At the community level malnutrition should be viewed in a comprehensive way because many interrelated factors contribute to this state. The health status, socioeconomic and education levels, and housing status of the population, along with the political climate, are some of the factors known to contribute to malnutrition. Poor nutrition reduces one's resistance to infection, which in turn aggravates malnutrition. Those vulnerable to malnutrition are placed into subgroups of the population as priorities for assessment, intervention, and evaluation to reduce the problems, promote healthy behaviors, and increase productivity. Each contributing factor is complex and must be viewed as such for developing health policies and strategies to address the basic needs of adequate amounts of nourishing foods, decent and affordable housing, employment, and quality education.

For this chapter, groups with special needs are divided into two groups as shown in Table 2-1. Those who are vulnerable include pregnant and lactating women and their infants and young children because of their need for increased nutrients and calories to support growth and development. Inability to eat or being totally dependent on others for food are some of the reasons that others are vulnerable. Individuals and families who move frequently from one community to another as migrants are subject to temporary and crowded housing conditions, poor sanitation, inadequate diets, and no or sporadic health care and are at high risk. Those living on reservations or in isolated rural

Table 2-1. Groups with special needs

Vulnerable groups	Emerging groups
Pregnant and lactating women	Poor (low socioeconomic status)
Infants	Hungry
Young children	Homeless
Older persons	AIDS/HIV-positive
Chronically ill or handicapping condition	Lead poisoning
Migrants	Tuberculosis (new drug-resistant strain)
Minorities	

communities are subject to some of the same negative factors and are groups with special needs. Increasingly, epidemiologists are showing that minority populations are at especially high risk of disabilities, diseases, and deaths.

HEALTHY PEOPLE 2000

The health needs of special population groups are addressed by *Healthy People 2000*.[25] This report notes that health disparities between the poor and those with higher incomes are almost universal for all health problems. The poor are rapidly growing in numbers. The downward trend of the national economy, loss of jobs, and low-paying jobs have all caused a significant increase in the number of poor, who are vulnerable to diseases and likely to have death rates twice those for people with higher incomes.

As the political, socioeconomic, and environmental climates changed over the last two decades, other subgroups with special needs began emerging and became targets for community food and nutrition resources and services. Beginning in the 1980s, states and local communities initiated surveys of their populations to obtain data to verify the extent of domestic hunger.[27] Community profiles of participants in federally funded food assistance and nutrition programs were developed, along with those of community-based initiatives such as food pantries, soup kitchens, food distribution sites, and food co-ops. These data provided information about the problems of hunger and often were a window on the homelessness in the communities around the country.

At the same time, there was growing visible evidence of the homeless. In some communities any attempt to determine the magnitude of the problem was difficult at best. Individuals and small groups often moved from one place to another several times during a day and most often had no central site or source for obtaining food on a consistent basis.

In the early 1980s those with acquired immunodeficiency syndrome (AIDS) and individuals infected with the human immunodeficiency virus (HIV) began to be reported to the Centers for Disease Control. Because the virus weakens and eventually destroys the immune system, persons with AIDS and those who are HIV-positive or have an AIDS-related complex (ARC) are high risk and vulnerable to a host of health and nutrition problems.

Other groups emerging with special needs are those with elevated blood levels of lead, especially young children living in old houses containing lead-based paint. Several urban communities are currently reporting increased cases of tuberculosis. This disease is caused by a new strain that is resistant to antibiotics. Over time other subgroups will emerge and require special concern from health and nutrition policy makers, providers, and advocates.

Some of the ecological factors that impact on groups with special needs are illustrated in Figure 2-1. The quality of life is influenced by the economy, income, housing, and education, along with availability and access to food to meet nutrient and caloric needs that is appropriate to disease state, cultural beliefs, and lifestyle behaviors. Depending on the severity, any one of these factors will determine the level of nutritional needs. The impact of one or more of these factors over a period increases the risk of chronic health and nutrition problems. Approximately 12 million American children and more than 400,000 pregnant women have no health insurance. Providing access to health care is a basic social obligation equivalent to providing access to education.

Assessing the health and nutrition status of groups with special needs is a basic component of community nutrition programs. Identification of and needs assessment of groups with special needs is the first step (Fig. 2-2). Based on a description or profile of the target group, policy and realistic intervention strategies can be developed to address specific needs that incorporate the cultural context and food behaviors of the group. Consistent ongoing monitoring will measure the impact of the intervention as well as indicate the need to modify the intervention strategy. When there are limited resources, including trained personnel, extra care in planning is essential to choose the most effective methods to monitor and evaluate community pro-

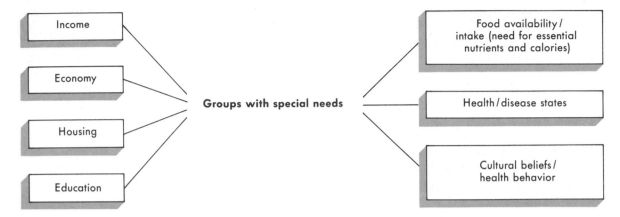

Figure 2-1. Ecological factors impacting on groups with special needs.

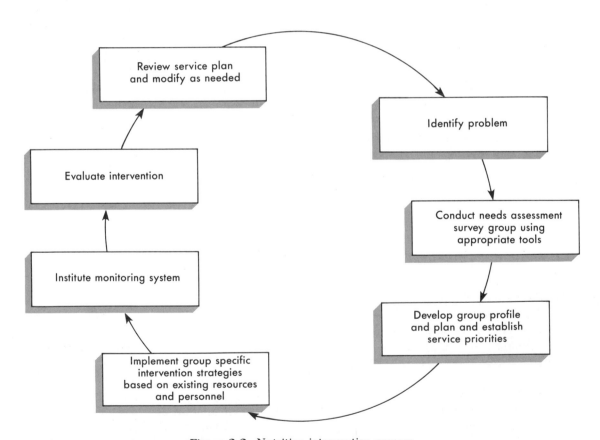

Figure 2-2. Nutrition intervention process.

grams, especially for groups with special needs who are the most vulnerable in the population.

This chapter is limited to the emerging subgroups of the population with special needs. Nutrition intervention in treatment and recovery from chemical dependency is addressed in the Position Paper of the American Dietetic Association (see Bibliography). Some of the other groups with special needs are covered in this textbook or in a wide range of other resources.

As subgroups with special needs have been identified, so have definitions. For this text, *groups with special needs* is broadly applied to those who are vulnerable and susceptible to a host of nutrition-related health problems. A description of each group is included in each section.

THE POOR

Who Are the Poor?

Those who are poor are:
- Low income (low socioeconomic status)
- At or below the poverty level*
- Working poor (poorly paying jobs).

Income is the common denominator of health disparities between those who are economically deprived and those with higher incomes.[35] In a report from the U.S. Census Bureau, the number of children under age 6 living in poverty grew by almost 100,000 between 1987 and 1989, to 5.1 million.[35] Currently, one in every four children under age 6 lives below the poverty line (Table 2-2).[11]

Children in Poverty

Young families with children have significantly less money than their counterparts did a generation ago and suffer from child poverty rates that are twice as high. Incomes in these families have dropped by 32% and the child poverty rate is now a sobering 40%.[19]

A Children's Defense Study attributed slightly more than half of the decline to demographic fac-

---

* Poverty level is a representative population sample for comparison of characteristics of poor and nonpoor, farm and nonfarm individuals and family units in terms of money income as developed by the Bureau of Census.

Table 2-2. 1989 poverty income guidelines*

Size of family	Poverty guideline ($)
1	5,980
2	8,020
3	10,060
4	12,100
5	14,140
6	16,180
7	18,220
8	20,260†

* Source: Federal Register, 1989. For all states, except Alaska and Hawaii.
† For family units with over eight persons, add $2,040 for each additional person.

tors, including the sharp rise in single-parent families. But even if family composition had not changed, the study said, almost half of the decline would have occurred, a result of eroded wages and declining government payments for welfare and unemployment.

The trends were most discouraging for young black and Hispanic families, and for those with little education, the study found. But young white families and those headed by high school graduates also saw their incomes fall and their poverty levels rise.

Marian Wright Edelman, the defense fund's president said the numbers presaged "more substance abuse, more crime, more violence, more school failures, more teen pregnancy, more racial tension, more envy, more despair and more cynicism—a long-term economic and social disaster."[19]

The reader/student who is unfamiliar with the extent of child poverty in America should examine photography in *Outside the Dream* depicting the plight of these children. *Outside the Dream* is a collection of over 50 black-and-white pictures that capture the truly desperate lifestyles of our youth. Many of the photographs document some of the social problems that co-exist with poverty—pictures of children fighting, using and selling drugs, and carrying or using handguns.[43]

The federal poverty guidelines are annually updated. This information is used to determine income eligibility for several federal food assistance

Table 2-3. Income eligibility guidelines (effective from July 1, 1991 to June 30, 1992)

Household size	Reduced-price meals: 185%			Federal poverty guidelines		
	Year	Month	Week	Year	Month	Week
48 Contiguous United States, District of Columbia, Guam, and territories						
1	12,247	1021	236	6620	552	128
2	16,428	1369	316	8880	740	171
3	20,609	1718	397	11,140	929	215
4	24,790	2066	477	13,400	1117	258
5	28,971	2415	558	15,660	1305	302
6	33,152	2763	638	17,920	1494	345
7	37,333	3112	718	20,180	1682	389
8	41,514	3460	799	22,440	1870	432
For each additional family member	+4,181	+349	+81	+2,260	+189	+44
Alaska						
1	15,337	1279	295	8290	691	160
2	20,554	1713	396	11,110	926	214
3	25,771	2148	496	13,930	1161	268
4	30,988	2583	596	16,750	1396	323
5	36,205	3018	697	19,570	1631	377
6	41,422	3452	797	22,390	1866	431
7	46,639	3887	897	25,210	2101	485
8	51,856	4322	998	28,030	2336	540
For each additional family member	+5,217	+435	+101	+2,820	+235	+55
Hawaii						
1	14,079	1174	271	7610	635	147
2	18,889	1575	364	10,210	851	197
3	23,699	1975	456	12,810	1068	247
4	28,509	2376	549	15,410	1285	297
5	33,319	2777	641	18,010	1501	347
6	38,129	3178	734	20,610	1718	397
7	42,939	3579	826	23,210	1935	447
8	47,749	3980	919	25,810	2151	497
For each additional family member	+4,810	+401	+93	+2,600	+217	+50

programs (Table 2-3). Income eligibility for school feeding programs (reduced-price meals) and basic guidelines for the Supplemental Foods for Women, Infants, and Children (WIC) use this standard.

Poor families are more likely to be unable to afford decent housing, buy nourishing food, purchase other basic goods and services, and have access to preventive health care. Usually these families live in poor neighborhoods that are medically underserved and are exposed to lead-based paint, asbestos, and other environmental pollutants. Compounding these problems are lifestyle behaviors that are not conducive to promoting health.[38] Since the 1970s it has been reported that those who

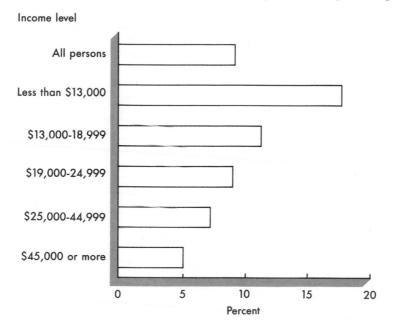

Income level

Figure 2-3. Percentage of people who experience limitation of major activity, by income level (1988, age-adjusted).
Source: National Health Interview Survey (CDC): *Healthy People 2000*.

live in poverty are disproportionately female. Moreover, more families are headed by single mothers. This trend was labeled the feminization of poverty by the sociologist Diana Pearce.[44]

Individuals working in low-paying jobs are called the *working poor* because their earnings are at or below the poverty level. Such persons are reported to have twice the death rates as those above the poverty level.[1] Families earning less than $13,000 a year (Fig. 2-3) are almost twice as likely as those earning $25,000 to $44,999 to experience limitation of major activities based on their health status.[25]

Infant mortality is the single strongest health indicator that connects poverty and poor health.[29,52] Infant mortality has been extensively used for decades as a measure of the health status of an area such as a city, county, state, or country. A close relationship between infant mortality rates and other measures of the quality of life in an area, including income levels, housing, educational levels, proportion of low birth weights, and quality

of and accessibility to medical care, has been documented. Low birth weight, prematurity, birth defects, and infant deaths are all associated with low socioeconomic status and poor life-style behaviors.

The effect of the poverty cycle leads to a poor outcome of pregnancy. Adverse social, behavioral, and biological factors all contribute to a poor nutritional status, which results in prematurity, low birth weight, and other poor outcomes of pregnancy. How these factors are interrelate is illustrated in Figure 2-4.

In spite of infant mortality dropping by 6% in the United States, the United States ranked twenty-fourth of 38 selected countries between 1982 and 1987, as shown in Table 2-4.[36]

Solutions to the problems of the poor are complex, requiring a continuum of public policies and strategies dealing with job training, affordable and safe housing, access to high-quality health care and education, and social service support systems. Access to clean, nutritious, and reasonably priced food

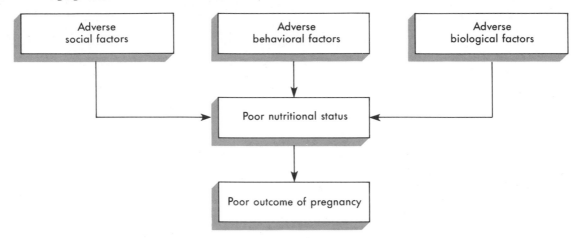

Figure 2-4. Effects of poverty cycle on outcome of pregnancy.

Table 2-4. U.S. infant mortality rate compared to other nations

Country*	1982† Infant deaths per 1,000 live births	1987‡	Average annual percent change	Country*	1982† Infant deaths per 1,000 live births	1987‡	Average annual percent change
Japan	6.6	5.0	−5.4	Belgium	11.1	9.7	−2.7
Sweden	6.9	5.7	−3.7	Austria	12.8	9.8	−5.2
Finland	6.8	6.2	−1.8	Italy	13.1	9.8	−5.6
Switzerland	7.7	6.9	−2.2	New Zealand	12.0	10.0	−3.6
Canada	9.1	7.3	−4.3	*United States*	*11.5*	*10.1*	−2.6
Singapore	10.7	7.3	−7.4	Israel	13.9	10.7	−5.1
Hong Kong	9.9	7.5	−5.4	Greece	15.1	12.6	−3.6
Netherlands	8.3	7.6	−1.7	Czechoslovakia	16.2	12.8	−4.6
France	9.5	7.8	−3.9	Cuba	17.3	13.3	−5.1
Ireland	10.5	7.9	−5.5	Puerto Rico	17.1	14.2	−3.6
Fed. Rep. of Germany	10.9	8.2	−5.5	Portugal	19.8	14.2	−6.4
Denmark	8.2	8.3	0.2	Bulgaria	18.2	14.8	−4.1
Norway	8.1	8.4	0.7	Kuwait‡	22.8	15.7	−8.9
Scotland	11.4	8.5	−5.7	Hungary	20.0	17.3	−2.9
Australia	10.3	8.7	−3.3	Costa Rica	19.4	17.4	−2.2
Northern Ireland	13.7	8.7	−8.7	Poland	20.2	17.5	−2.8
German Dem. Republic	11.4	8.8	−5.0	Chile	23.6	18.5	−4.8
Spain‡	11.3	9.0	−7.3	Romania	28.0	22.5	−4.3
England and Wales	10.8	9.2	−3.2	U.S.S.R.	25.1	25.4	0.3

From the National Center for Health Statistics

*Data based on reporting by countries.

†Data for the USSR are for 1983. From *Nation's Health*, Washington, DC, 1900, APHA.

‡Data for Kuwait are for 1986; data for Spain for 1985.

daily is a priority to prevent chronic consumption of poor diets that can result in costly nutrition-related diseases. In addition, the primary gate-keeper—the person responsible for food management and preparation—must be knowledgeable about meal planning, food shopping, and storage and preparation to ensure the family a variety of nourishing, attractive, and tasty food.

DOMESTIC HUNGER

"Hunger is more than simply an issue of comparison for those who do not have enough to eat. It is an issue of failed beginnings for millions of American children—the future of our country."

Mudd, 1992

The President's Task Force of Food Assistance in 1986 defined *hunger* as:

- Malnutrition as measured by anthropometric and clinical tests
- Inability to obtain an adequate amount of food even if the shortage is not prolonged enough to cause health problems[41]

History of Hunger

Fifteen years before, at the 1969 White House Conference on Food, Nutrition and Health, *hunger* was defined as a "biological phenomenon and is not in itself indicative of disease or of unsatisfactory nutritional status."[53] Twenty years later the problem of hunger was reviewed by Jean Mayer, the coordinator of the 1969 White House Conference, who reported it to have increased.[24]

Selected events in the history of federal policies to address hunger in the United States are reviewed in Table 12-2. The American Dietetic Association describes *hunger* as "discomfort, weakness, or pain caused by lack of food."[2] *Hunger* has been defined more recently by others such as the Physician's Task Force on Hunger in America,[39] the Association of State and Territorial Public Health Nutrition Directors,[6] and the House Select Committee on Hunger.[26]

It is important for community dietitians and nutritionists to distinguish hunger from undernutrition, which is a chronic caloric deficiency, and malnutrition, a disease caused by deficiency and an excess or imbalance of essential nutrients.

Food Security Versus Food Insecurity

The phenomenon loosely labelled *hunger* in the 1980s is now being discussed as *food security* or *insecurity*. Food security is defined as access by all people at all times to enough food for an active, healthy life, and at a minimum includes the following: (1) the ready availability of nutritionally adequate and safe foods, and (2) the assured ability to acquire personally acceptable foods in a socially acceptable way. Food insecurity exists whenever food security is limited or uncertain. The measurement of food insecurity at the household or individual level involves the measurement of those quantitative, qualitative, psychological, and social or normative constructs that are central to the experience of food insecurity, qualified by their involuntariness and periodicity. Risk factors for food insecurity include those that affect household resources and the proportion of those resources available for food acquisition.[9]

Potential consequences of food insecurity include hunger, malnutrition and (either directly or indirectly) negative effects on health and quality of life. The precise relationships between food insecurity and its risk factors and potential consequences need much more research now that there is an emerging consensus on the definition and measurement of food insecurity. Indicators of food security and insecurity are proposed as a necessary component of the core measures of the nutritional state of individuals, communities, or nations (see Chapter 12).[9] The problem of hunger is of national concern in spite of the lack of an accepted, standardized survey instrument to measure its magnitude in the population.[8,13] Tools to measure the extent of hunger encompass both direct and indirect methodologies. The direct method includes assessment of food intake and subsequently of nutritional status of an individual or group. Determining the number of persons eligible for food assistance and nutrition programs versus the actual numbers participating in these programs is an indirect method of measuring hunger. The United States Department of Agriculture notes significant jumps in individuals and families reaching out for help on food security. This is documented by increases in the number of participants in several food assistance programs like Food Stamps, Child Nutritional and WIC.[15]

Hunger in the 1980s has been variously portrayed as a result of government policies in the areas of housing, health, welfare, and food, or of household level changes in response to policy.[40] Two of the accepted indicators of hunger are socioeconomic status and calorie/nutrient intake. Others use such indicators as depressed quality of life, lack of variety of food, and lack of access to food on a daily basis.

A recent survey conducted by the Food Research and Action Center (FRAC) among low-income families in seven sites across the country, if applied to the best available national data, indicates an estimated 5.5 million children (one in eight) under age 12 are hungry.[23] The Community Childhood Hunger Identification Project (CCHIP) survey compared hungry children to nonhungry children. Their findings were that hungry children are more than 3 times as likely to suffer from unwanted weight loss; and more than 4 times as likely to suffer from fatigue, both of which impact on their health problems and school attendance.

For the purpose of the CCHIP survey, *hunger* is defined as "the mental and physical condition that comes from not eating enough food due to insufficient economic, family or community resources." A list of eight questions comprised the scale to measure hunger.[23] The scale (see the box at right) was used as a way to detect food insufficiency because of limited resources.

Community Childhood Hunger Identification Project

The Queens Community Childhood Hunger Identification Project was one of several studies on hunger commissioned across the country by the FRAC. The Queens study, which was sponsored in part by

---

CCHIP QUESTIONS TO MEASURE HUNGER

To measure hunger, a scale was formulated composed of eight questions—taken from the 105 questions in the survey—that indicate whether adults or children in the household experience food shortages, perceived food insufficiency, altered food intake due to resource limitations, or inadequate food resources. These key questions, each pertaining to the preceding 12 months, are:

- Does your household ever run out of money to buy food to make a meal?
- Do you or adult members of your household ever eat less than you feel you should because there is not enough money for food?
- Do you or adult members of your household ever cut the size of meals or skip meals because there is not enough money for food?
- Do your children ever eat less than you feel they should because there is not enough money for food?
- Do you ever cut the size of your children's meals or do they ever skip meals because there is not enough money for food?
- Do your children ever say they are hungry because there is not enough food in the house?
- Do you ever rely on a limited number of foods to feed your children because you are running out of money to buy food for a meal?
- Do any of your children ever go to bed hungry because there is not enough money to buy food?

---

the New York City Human Resources Administration, was based on a survey conducted of 389 low-income families in the borough in spring 1991.

Twenty percent of low-income families in Queens with at least one child under 12 years of age have at times gone hungry, in some cases because they were not aware that they qualified for government food assistance. Besides finding that one out of five of the families surveyed had experienced hunger, the report said that 47% of those families had at some point run out of money to buy food and that 20% of the families acknowledged reducing the size of a child's meal or skipping a meal altogether because there was not enough money to buy food.

Among Federal hunger initiatives, the report

found that almost 40% of the families who were eligible for the Food Stamps program or the Special Supplemental Food Program for Women, Infants and Children were not participating in those programs, in many cases because they did not know they were eligible or were too embarrassed to apply.

"Simply stated," the writers of the report concluded, "the key to eradicating hunger, if that is an acceptable goal in these dark fiscal times, requires that jobs be available for those who seek them and that the wages derived from those jobs should bring people out of poverty."[47]

Food Pantries and Soup Kitchens

Food pantries and soup kitchens have become symbols of hunger and poverty in the United States. Food drives are an accepted feature of life and the Emergency Feeding System (EFS), once regarded as a response to a temporary situation, has become institutionalized. As this occurs, government agencies, scholars, hunger activists, and emergency food providers have begun to question the advisability of expanding or even maintaining the system.

Requests for emergency food assistance through food banks has been increasing nationwide in recent years. Food banks and food pantries are private, community-based organizations that rely heavily on donations of food, money, and volunteer time to provide a few day's supply of groceries to people in need. These facilities are a temporary stop-gap measure for households without food and no other place to turn for help. A request for food assistance identifies a family in crisis.[45]

A study of 267 clients using the emergency food system in New York state documents the fact that incomes and benefits of low-income people are inadequate to provide sufficient shelter, food, and other necessities. Clients were surveyed personally in food pantries in three regions of the state to identify their sources and amounts of income, expenditures for foods, and use of food programs. The median income was 77% of the poverty levels, and median expenditures for housing and food were 52% and 24% of income, respectively. Food

stamps, school meal programs, and community foods were heavily used by respondents but senior meal programs were not. In an attempt to assist dietitians and nutritionists to better understand the causes of food insecurity, the authors provide background information and information on issues regarding the poverty level, housing, and food stamps. The study demonstrated that low income (even of working families), high housing costs, and other factors (e.g., cost of child care, and inadequate unemployment and health care benefits) are reasons for food insecurity in the United States.[12]

The Medford Declaration

Despite a decade of domestic hunger studies, there is as yet no single document spelling out how to end hunger in the United States, both in the short and long term. The Bellagio Declaration, a statement that spells out ways to address world hunger, was an outcome of a meeting of 23 experts who convened in Italy in November 1953. This statement spells out ways to cut world hunger in half by the year 2000. In 1990, at the Brown University World Hunger Conference, it was suggested that U.S. organizations concerned with domestic hunger needed a "domestic Bellagio." A drafting committee convened at Tufts University in Medford, Massachusetts and produced the Medford Declaration to End Hunger in the United States by 1995.[34]

The Medford Declaration will help to raise public awareness and promote debate about hunger in the nation. It is envisioned that Congressional hearings will be held to address pertinent issues and goals on both the national and local levels. The U.S. Senate Select Committee on Hunger has issued 14 criteria to be implemented to comprehensively address local hunger problems (see the box on p. 32).[51]

Student Projects

Many dietitians and nutritionists are distressed by the large numbers of people in their communities and states who have come to depend on emergency food assistance at food pantries and soup kitchens over the last decade.

HUNGER-FREE CRITERIA

"Hunger-free communities" must meet 14 criteria that should be implemented in order to comprehensively address local hunger problems:

1. Communities should develop a system for providing information on local food services and donors;
2. There should be coordinated efforts to collect information on the extent of food insecurity existing in the community;
3. A central group of residents should gather information detailing the needs of the community to help develop courses of action for responding to existing gaps in services;
4. Residents of the community should be educated about the different Federal food assistance programs and work with their local officials and potential private sponsors;
5. Steps should be taken to establish partnerships through which the public and private sectors work together to solve local food insecurity problems;
6. Communities should sponsor forums for educating residents about local food insecurity and encourage their involvement in activities to combat hunger;
7. Emergency food program sponsors should be familiar with support programs so that they can refer needy persons to broader and longer-term support;
8. Projects should be developed to improve the supply of low-cost, nutritious foods to residents of the community;
9. Efforts should be made to target services to those groups who are particularly vulnerable to food insecurity problems;
10. Steps should be taken to establish a reliable system for transporting food to programs that provide meals services for low-income households;
11. Communities should begin to establish food delivery at sites which are easily accessible by residents;
12. Communities should secure public transit routes to provide direct access to public assistance services and food outlets;
13. Nutrition education classes should be established to inform consumers about the relationship between diet and health to develop nutritious food-buying and preparation habits;
14. Communities should establish programs for collecting and channeling wholesome foods otherwise going to waste.

For more information, contact the Select Committee on Hunger, Room H2-505, Ford House Office Building; Washington, D.C. 20515-6408.

We have observed, documented and interacted with the increasing number of families who run out of food on a regular basis due to lack of money. We have heard the despair of single mothers, people who work but are still poor, and homeless families who worry regularly about where the next meal will come from.

Dodds, 1992

Nutrition students often lack experience working with low income groups including those who are homeless, the homebound elderly, and those needing emergency food assistance. Nutrition students are best served through hands-on community projects. The knowledge and experience gained at community programs can help students to develop the skills needed by dietitians and nutritionists in their expanding role in community nutrition. The competencies addressed include understanding the role of food and nutrition services in community programs, recognizing the impact of political, legislative, and economic factors on nutrition and dietetic practice, and serving as advocates for clients in need.

Eibe called for university-level nutrition curricula to recognize nutritional outcomes as products of and contributors to social and economic reality.[22] Though his call was not made explicit with respect to the teaching of hunger and related issues, Csetta advises that portraying nutritional status simply as a function of diet and disease without a broader social context does poor service to nutrition and dietetic students and, ultimately to the populations they will serve.[18] Future nutrition practitioners should be exposed to the varying circumstances by which a significant portion of the U.S. and world populations does not have access to adequate food.

Csetta's suggested some topics pertinent to nutrition students' understanding of the context of hunger problems[18]:

1. Hunger and population issues
2. Hunger and the environment
3. Hunger and the status of women
4. Hunger and budgetary and debt crises

The Hunger Project: Students in the Community

With the objective of providing students with a firsthand glimpse of hunger to heighten their sensitivity to the existence of the problem and to encourage social responsibility, nutrition educators at the University of Delaware designed a special assignment.[17]

Students were offered an opportunity to participate in a volunteer experience with Food Conservers, a branch of the Second Harvest Network, and one of its affiliated agencies. The project required 20 hours of volunteer time. The first 10 hours were spent at the food bank where students became familiar with program operations. Students learned about organizational structure, receiving and distributing procedures, eligibility requirements, and the process of program monitoring and evaluation. The remaining 10 hours were spent serving meals at soup kitchens. Students assisted with meal preparation and cleanup as well as meal service to participants.

Throughout the diversity of reported observations, one similarity emerged: the project was an eye-opening experience. Most of the students noted varying degrees of initial uneasiness about doing the project and admitted that they had no idea about what to expect but all noted it was a meaningful experience to venture outside of a secluded, sheltered lifestyle. The assignment provided a rich foundation for stimulating discussion on a variety of issues related to hunger including poverty, homelessness, value clarification, advocacy, and personal as well as professional social responsibility.

The Chancellor's Initiative on Poverty

To address the need of the dietitian or nutrition professional to understand the impact of food insecurity on individuals and families, a 3-week Community Services rotation was developed as part of an Approved Pre-Professional Practice (AP4) Program in Dietetics. This program is part of a university-wide Chancellor's Initiative on Poverty, and grows out of research that has been conducted by members of the nutrition faculty on the use of emergency food programs in New York State.

Each 3-week rotation included experience at a food bank, a home-delivered meals program, a food pantry, and one or more soup kitchens. At each community organization, students received an orientation to the program's goals, policies, services, and sources of funding. They assisted the staff and regular volunteers with day-to-day operations, including food preparation and service. Depending on the program, students were also able to assist with client interviews, develop and deliver short food and nutrition education sessions for client groups, assist with reporting for funding purposes, and complete special projects that used their nutrition expertise. Simple forms were developed for preceptors to comment on the students, and for the students to evaluate each placement.[46]

Next Steps for Nutrition Educators

Key contacts for hunger, poverty, and food assistance programs—a nutritionist's mini-directory of organizations and agencies—are listed in Appendix 2-1.

HOMELESSNESS

Homelessness is defined in this chapter as referring to persons who have been displaced and are unable to obtain replacement housing.[16] The reasons for a person being displaced are many and complex, including arrears in rent payments, fire or other disaster, conversion of housing into unaffordable rental units, demolition, walk-away landlord or owner, excessive building violations, landlord fines, and use of low rental subsidy to buy other basics. Runaway adolescents who may have been subject to abuse at home are represented among those who are homeless.

Although there have been national estimates of the number of homeless, the range is wide, and counting methods are unreliable because many homeless move from one site to the next on any given day or night.[16] What is known is that homelessness continues to grow significantly in urban and rural communities across the country.

The sites where homeless people live include such places as cars, boiler rooms, subway tunnels, railroad and bus stations, abandoned buildings, roofs and basements of buildings, corrugated makeshift houses, under highway structures, parks, and playgrounds. Others may live in a shelter or hotel/motel designated by community social service or housing agencies. Some of these sites are only available at night, so the homeless may spend the day walking around seeking other shelter.

The health status of the homeless is compromised by the lack of adequate, safe, and sanitary housing. Both the mental health and physical health of the homeless are aggravated by living on the streets. Lack of food can result in hunger, malnutrition accompanied by weight loss, increased susceptibility to upper respiratory infections, and a weakened immune system. In crowded shelters, tuberculosis, hepatitis, and AIDS are among the serious health conditions that providers may encounter.[14] Written policies developed in collaboration with local and state health departments should be used to protect the health of the homeless as well as that of the staff.

Homeless families with very young children have sharply increased and represent about 70% of the population.[7] These families are very vulnerable because their health and nutrition needs are critical to their children's growth and development. Family shelters such as hotel/motel or single room occupancy may or may not permit cooking in a room and may lack facilities for communal dining or food storage. Families often must resort to looking around the neighborhood for meals and snacks. The homeless have a limited access to an adequate diet, which is further aggravated by lack of money for food. Those dependent on community-based food resources are frequently restricted by policies regarding the availability of food on certain days of the week, hours of the day, distance to and from the distribution site, cost of public transportation, and the limited time the food is available. Sometimes the demand for food is such that individuals and families compete with one another for limited food supplies.

Over the past decade, private nonprofit groups have developed an impressive model on how to accommodate the homeless humanely and cost effectively. The model is called the "supported SRO," or single-room-occupancy residence. In the past 5 years, individuals and small private agencies have developed supported SROs for about 1,700 people in New York, 750 in Chicago, and 500 in San Francisco.

A supported SRO is a rooming house with caseworkers and facilities in which to meet with residents. The caseworkers, appearing daily, make sure the residents take medications, help them find substance abuse treatment and job training, and give other services.

Supported SROs in New York cost substantially less per resident than huge congregate shelters that offer no privacy and few services. SROs, unlike shelters, are able to qualify residents for Federal and state benefits that help to offset costs. Managers may organize tenants to help with maintenance and administration. Neighbors who react with horror to the idea of shelters near their homes find the smaller, better-managed SROs far less threatening.

Another program of services for mentally ill homeless people was embodied in the so-called Grand Central Initiative, one of several highly publicized "New York-New York Agreements" signed by Mayor Dinkins and Governor Cuomo in 1990 to coordinate city and state efforts to help the homeless.

A program that has provided treatment, counseling, and other services for mentally ill homeless people in the vicinity of Grand Central Terminal since 1990 under an unusual partnership of city, state, and private agencies may soon be expanded to the Pennsylvania Station area, according to city officials and providers of aid for the homeless.[32]

Arnstein and Alperstein report that problems of access to and use of health care facilities, coupled with the realistic difficulties of managing illness and disease are primary concerns to providers of housing and health care.[5] The Institute of Medicine, at the request of Congress, assigned a committee to study the delivery of in-patient and out-patient health care services to the homeless. The committee made site visits to evaluate various programs serving the homeless in 11 cities and met with public officials and service providers. The diversity of the homeless population includes urban and rural people, individual adults, females with children, youths, the elderly, Vietnam veterans, people with AIDS, the mentally ill, and even persons who are employed full or part-time. Health care services provided to this diverse population should be diverse enough to meet the needs of all, including adequate nutrition, mental health care, alcohol and drug abuse treatment and dental care.[28]

AIDS AND HIV

Since the first reported case of acquired immunodeficiency syndrome (AIDS) in 1981, there have been 179,136 AIDS cases among all age groups according to the Centers for Disease Control as of May 1991.[33] AIDS is the second leading cause of death among men 25 to 44 years of age and one of the five leading causes of death among women 15 to 44 years of age in the United States.[33]

Those who have AIDS or ARC or who are HIV-positive are vulnerable to a range of nutritionally debilitating problems. Weight loss accompanied by protein calorie malnutrition, esophagitis, oral lesions, and diarrhea are among some of the common nutritional problems observed.[42] Compounding these problems are those of the drugs and medi-cines used, which have nutritional implications such as the restriction of nutrient availability or utilization.

OTHER SPECIAL GROUPS

Tuberculosis

Tuberculosis (TB), once thought headed for elimination in the United States, has surged back in a new and more dangerous form. TBs return was accelerated by the spread of the AIDS virus, and the overlap in epidemics has greatly complicated efforts to control both diseases. New strains of tuberculosis resistant to multiple drugs have emerged in at least 17 states. A 1-month survey in New York City found 34% of all TB patients resistent to at least one drug, 19% resistant to the two main drugs, and some resistant to virtually all drugs. For them, there is little medicine can do.

The main reason that drug-resistant strains develop is that patients fail to complete full treatment. Organisms that survived the initial doses then proliferate in the body and in turn infect others. Such failures are understandable. TB patients must take three or four drugs daily or twice a week for 9 months or more, long after they have started feeling well and have little incentive to continue. It is hard enough for an educated, middle-class person; it is virtually impossible for the poor, the homeless, the mentally ill, and the drug addicts who comprise most of the infected population.

The tuberculosis problem has been exacerbated by the AIDS virus, which weakens the immune system. Roughly 25% to 50% of all tuberculosis victims in New York City are infected with the AIDS virus, and drug-resistant strains are heavily concentrated in the AIDS population. But many experts say tuberculosis and drug resistance would have increased even without the AIDS epidemic, though less sharply.[21]

As the number of cases reported increases, aggressive drug therapy and nutrition support is needed to contain the spread of this disease. Crowded housing, found in some correctional facilities, residential homes for children and adults, and shelters for the homeless, should be targets for treatment and health education campaigns. It is incumbent upon health providers to vigorously pursue treatment modalities and education about personal hygiene to halt the increase of tuberculosis.

Lead Toxicity

Elevated blood lead level is one outcome measure frequently used in monitoring child health services. Children at risk of lead poisoning are among those who are poor and living in old houses where there may be layer on layer of lead-based paint. Lead is a heavy metal that is ingested by some young children who eat paint chips, thereby increasing their risk of lead toxicity. Because lead has an affinity for bone and replaces calcium, nutrition guidance is indicated.

Recently the Centers for Disease Control (CDC) lowered the "threshold of concern" for blood lead levels in children.[10] The new threshold of 10 μg/deciliter of whole blood can still produce subtle effects in a child, such as developmental delays and reduced stature. Because approximately 3 to 4 million children in the United States under age 6 are estimated to have blood levels greater than 15 μg/deciliter, the Department of Health and Human Services (DHHS) developed a Strategies Plan to Eliminate Childhood Lead Poisoning, which outlines a 20-year plan to address this problem. Current intervention plans describe levels of action to specific blood lead levels found in children. Highest priority for intervention is given to those with the highest levels of blood lead.

COMMUNITY NUTRITION ASSESSMENT STRATEGIES

It is important to identify and know what some of the practical nutrition assessment strategies are and which group-specific tools exist. For example, there are several approaches to measuring the extent of hunger in a community.

USDA FOOD ASSISTANCE

Better nutrition means better health. Low-income families can get better nutrition by using the food programs listed below. To find out how you and your family can use these programs, contact the Food and Nutrition Service, USDA, Washington, DC 20250, or the offices listed here.

School lunch and breakfast programs	Offer free and reduced-price meals at school to children from low-income families Contact: Your local school principal
Child care food program	Offers meals and snacks to children in eligible day-care centers, family day-care homes, and outside-school-hours care centers Contact: Your state educational agency
Summer food program	Offers meals and snacks to children in needy areas during the summer Contact: Your state educational agency
Food program for women, infants, and children	Provides nutritious foods to add to the diets of pregnant and nursing women, infants, and children under 5 years of age Contact: Your local or state health department
Food stamp program	Helps low-income households buy the food they need for good health Contact: Your local social services or welfare department

The Department of Agriculture's food assistance programs are available to all eligible persons without regard to race, color, or national origin.
From: U.S. Department of Agriculture, Food and Nutrition Service, FNS-182, September 1979, U.S. Government Printing Office.

First, at the community level a standardized questionnaire can be used to interview providers and clients at emergency food sites or at income maintenance centers. Clients or providers are asked to complete a simple short list of questions. One way to encourage clients to participate is to format the questions with large print and ample open space. The same list of questions could be asked over the phone; however, a substantial number of clients would not be reached because they lack a phone.

A second method of assessing at the community level is to analyze eligibility and participation rates in programs like WIC, food stamps, and Child and Adult Care Feeding (see the box on p. 36). How many people are eligible for a specific food assistance program based on established eligibility criteria? Of that number, what number or percent actually participate? The difference between eligibility and participation levels describes the magnitude of those who are probably in great need. One outcome of this assessment is to determine the causes for not participating in a program. This could produce a prioritized list of barriers. These barriers can then be reviewed and strategies planned to increase participation levels.

Another approach is to use data generated and available from surveys conducted by the federal government. The U.S. Department of Agriculture conducts Nationwide Food Consumption Surveys (NFCS)[48] and the Department of Health and Human Services is responsible for National Health and Nutrition Examination Surveys (NHANES) and Hispanic HANES.[49] Although these surveys reflect a national sample and are not representative of the local community, they can be used to estimate the extent of the problem.

Regarding income as related to program participation, the Census Bureau issues periodic reports useful in making comparisons with findings at the local level. The cost of basic services and goods such as food, housing, clothing, health care, and related costs of essential services impact on family income and should be viewed in documenting the number of poor. The more a family spends on housing, utilities, transportation, medical care, cloth-ing, and school supplies, the less they have for food. What is left after other bills are paid is what usually is spent for food; thus some families are unable to provide adequate amounts of food for all in the household. Reports from the Bureau of Labor Statistics can also be used for comparison with community findings.

Other sources of data can be found at the state level. An example is the Hunger Watch initiative authorized by the governor of New York.[31] Results of the survey, which was designed to determine the scope and distribution of undernutrition among high-risk populations, led to the funding of the Supplemental Nutrition Assistance Program (SNAP). This program provided additional state dollars to WIC, emergency feeding, and meals for the elderly. Other states have formed coalitions and have conducted surveys, reported their findings, and made recommendations to address hunger and related issues.[37]

In addition, professionals should be knowledgeable about any previous surveys conducted in the community because data may already exist. An inventory of health and nutrition information available at the local level is useful in planning a community survey. A useful guide is *Model Standards: Guidelines for Community Attainment of the Year 2000 Objectives*.[4] Nutrition is among the health disciplines developed in the framework for organizing, carrying out, and evaluating services. One clue to conducting a community nutrition assessment is coalition building. Each community-based group or agency with an interest in the health and nutrition of a community is needed to conduct a comprehensive and representative survey of the population. Based on the purpose and resources available at the community level, federal, state, and local survey methodologies used in previous surveys can be modified or adapted to address local needs (see Chapters 1, 14, and 15).

Other assessment strategies might include or be in combination with dietary surveys, clinical surveys, surveys of food markets and food prices, data about the food and water supplies (enrichment, fortification, fluoridation, lead), vital statistics, child health records, and socioeconomic and demographic data. Special health and nutrition data are invaluable in developing strategies for a community nutrition assessment initiative.

After conducting nutrition assessment of hunger in a community, the next step is to describe and document the findings in a report that is widely disseminated in the community. Policy makers, health and nutrition and social service providers, consumers, and academics should be among those who collaborate not only in the survey but also in making recommendations for action to be taken. The American Dietetics Association outlines five such steps to address domestic hunger[3]:

1. Strengthen the infrastructure of governmental food programs
2. Devise new approaches aimed at developing permanent as well short-term programs to end hunger
3. Strengthen nutrition education aimed at health promotion and chronic disease prevention, including the educational components of food assistance programs
4. Monitor trends and evaluate the effects of intervention, including gaps in the safety net
5. Remove economic factors that place and keep citizens in poverty

BRIDGING THE GAP

The basic need for food assistance and nutrition resources of subgroups with special needs can be addressed by community nutrition sources. The sequential step in Figure 2-1 describes an approach that can be effectively used by nutritionists in collaboration with other members of the health care team and the consumers who represent the target subgroups. It is important for providers to be sensitive to the specific needs of each subgroup by producing culturally appropriate strategies, as described elsewhere in Chapter 5.

Among the dearth of information, nutritionists have what food assistance and nutrition resources exist, where they are located, and who is eligible as a participant (see Table 2-3). It is necessary to know not only what programs exist but also how

consumers can access these programs and what barriers are faced by participants.

The underlying issues of subgroups with special needs are basic social and economic problems such as employment, housing, education, and health; however, it is recognized that accessing food and nutrition programs helps these subgroups survive on a day-to-day basis. The long-range social and economic issues require complex solutions.

SUMMARY

The current socioeconomic climate has created an emerging network of subgroups in the population who are vulnerable to nutrition-related problems. Although there have always been pockets of vulnerable groups such as the poor, those with handicapping conditions, those dependent on others for food, and pregnant and lactating women and their infants and children, these newer subgroups present a serious challenge to community nutritionists. Today the poor are poorer and significantly growing in numbers because of continued downturn in the national economy, high unemployment, and high cost of living. Because of the lack of national economic growth, there are more hungry people. In addition, the crisis in housing has produced many homeless people at a time when diseases like AIDS and antibiotic-resistant tuberculosis have grown at alarming rates, thereby exacerbating the number of persons with special needs.

Dietitians and nutritionists have an important leadership role in community health and social programs. Defining and describing those with special needs and the magnitude of their food and nutrition problems can be articulated by the dietitian or nutritionist who first conducts a need assessment. Once this is accomplished, the dietitian or nutritionist, in collaboration with the multidisciplinary health care team, implements group-specific and culturally relevant nutrition intervention strategies. After monitoring the intervention, an evaluation of the impact of the intervention can be measured and, where needed, can be modified or changed.

REFERENCES

1. Ambler RW, Dull HB: *Closing the gap*, New York, 1987, Oxford University Press.
2. American Dietetic Association: Hunger: a worldwide problem. ADA timely statement, *J Am Diet Assoc* 86:1414, 1986.
3. American Dietetic Association: Position of the American Dietetic Association: domestic hunger and inadequate access to food. ADA reports, *J Am Diet Assoc* 90:1437, 1990.
4. American Public Health Association: *Model standards: guidelines for community attainment of the year 2000 objectives*, ed 3, Washington, DC, 1990, The Association.
5. Arnstein E, Alperstein G: Health care for the homeless, *Public Health Currents* 57:29, 1987.
6. Association of State and Territorial Public Health Nutrition Directors: *Position statement: adequate food for all*, March 1988, The Association.
7. Brickner PW: *Under the safety net*, New York, 1990, WW Norton.
8. Brown L, Allen D: Hunger in America, *Annu Rev Public Health* 9, 1988.
9. Campbell CA: Food Security: A nutritional outcome or a predictor variable? *J Nutr* 121:408, 1991.
10. Centers for Disease Control: *Preventing lead poisoning in young children*, Atlanta, 1991, CDC.
11. Children's Defense Fund: *Leave no child behind: An opinion maker's guide to children in election year 1992*, Washington, DC, 1991, CDF.
12. Clancy KL, Bowering J: The need for emergency food: poverty problems and policy responses. *J Nutr Educ* 24(1):128, 1992.
13. Cohen B: *Food security policy for the 1990s: Eliminating hunger, executive summary*, Washington, DC, 1989, The Urban Institute (unpublished).
14. Columbia University: *Working with homeless people*, Amy Haus, ed, rev, 1988, Columbia Press.
15. Community Nutrition Institute: Nutrition week: more Americans reach out for help on food security, *CNI* 21:6, 1991.
16. Community Service Society: *The making of America's homeless: from skid row to the poor, working paper in social poverty*, New York, 1984, CSS.
17. Cotugna N, Vickery CE: Nurturing social responsibility: nutrition students volunteer in hunger project, *J Am Diet Assoc* 92:297, 1992.
18. Csetta J: Hunger and the academy: Training nutritionists for the 1990s. *J Nutr Educ* 24(1) 1992.
19. DeParla J: Young families poorer. *New York Times* April 15, 1992.
20. Dodds J, Parker SL, Haines, PS: Hunger in the '80s and '90s: A challenge for nutrition educators. *J Nutr Educ* 24(1):25, 1992.
21. Editorial. The tuberculosis failure. *New York Times*, April 26, 1992.
22. Eide, WB. Training for nutritional wisdom: A challenge to academic education. *Food Nutr* 10(2):15, 1984.
23. Food Research and Action Center: *Community childhood hunger identification project*, Washington, DC, 1991. U.S. Gov't. Printing Office.
24. Goldberg J, Mayer J: The White House conference on food, nutrition and health: twenty years later; where are we now? *J Nutr Educ* 22:1, 1990.
25. *Healthy People 2000: national health promotion and disease prevention objectives*, Washington, DC, 1991, Department of Health and Human Services, Public Health Service.
26. House Select Committee on Hunger: *Food security in the United States: the measurement of hunger, issue brief*, Washington, DC, 1989.
27. Indiana State Board of Health: Hunger in Allen County, Indianapolis, 1986, State Board of Health.
28. Institute of Medicine. *Homelessness, health and human needs*, Washington, DC, 1988, National Academy Press.
29. Institute of Medicine: *Preventing low birthweight*, Washington, DC, 1985, National Academy Press.
30. Kerr NA: The evaluation of USDA surplus disposal programs. *Natl Food Rev* 11(3):25, 1988.
31. Lamphere JA: Hunger watch: New York state, *Natl Nutr Monitor* 4, 1984.
32. McFadden RD: Aid for midtown homeless may include Penn Station. *New York Times*, April 5, 1992.
33. Morbidity and Mortality Weekly Report: The HIV/AIDS epidemic: the first 10 years, MMWR 40:358, 1991.
34. National Activities to end Hunger: *J Nutr Educ* 24(1):895, 1992.
35. National Center for Children in Poverty: *Five million children, report summary*, New York, 1990, Columbia University School of Public health.
36. National Center for Health Statistics: *US infant mortality rate compared to other nations*, 1991.
37. Neuhauser L: Northern California hunger surveys: 1984-85, *Nat Nutr Monitor* 11, 1985.
38. Orshansky M: *Counting the poor: another look at the poverty profile*, US Department of Health, Education and Welfare. Social Security Administration. (Reprinted from *Social Security Bulletin*, January 1965.)
39. Physician's Task Force on Hunger in America: *Hunger reaches blue collar America*, Cambridge, 1987, Harvard University School of Public Health.
40. Physicians Task Force on Hunger in America: *The growing epidemic*. Middletown, CT: Wesleyan University Press, 1985.
41. President's Task Force on Food Assistance: *Summary of Findings*, Washington, DC, 1984, US Government Printing Office.
42. Rakower D: *Acquired immunodeficiency syndrome*. In *Practical nutrition, a quick reference for the health care practitioner*, Rockville, Md, 1989, Aspen.
43. Shames S: *Outside the dream: Child poverty in America*. Washington, DC, 1991, Aperture/Childrens Defense Fund.

44. Sidel R: *Women and children last: the plight of poor women in affluent America*, New York, 1986, Viking.
45. Smith PK, Holrr SL: Comparison of current food bank users, non-users and past users in a population of low income single mothers. *J Nutr Educ* 24(1):59S, 1992.
46. Snowman MK, Crockett EG: Caring for homeless, hungry, and homebound. *J Nutr Educ* 24(1), 1992.
47. Steinberg J: Report shows poor families going hungry. *New York Times* April 6,1992.
48. U.S. Department of Agriculture: *Nationwide food consumption surveys*, Washington, DC, 1982, U.S. Govt. Printing Office.
49. US Department of Health and Human Services and US Department of Agriculture: *Nutrition monitoring in the United States: an update on nutrition monitoring*, Hyattsville, Md, 1989, U.S. Govt. Printing Office.
50. U.S. Department of Health and Human Services. *The Surgeon General's report on nutrition and health*. DHHS (PHS) No 88-50210. Washington DC, 1988, U.S. Government Printing Office.
51. U.S. Senate Select Committee on Hunger. *Hunger-free criteria*. Washington, DC, 1992, Community Nutrition-News.
52. Wallace AM, Gold EM, Oglesby AC: *Maternal and child health practices: problems, resources and methods of delivery*, ed 2, New York, 1982, John Wiley & Sons.
53. White House Conference on Food, Nutrition and Health: US Department of Health, Education and Welfare. Washington DC, 1969.

BIBLIOGRAPHY

Alleviating hunger: progress and prospects. Hearing before the Select Committee on Hunger, House of Representatives, 98th Congress, second session, serial no 98-2, Washington, DC: 1984, US Government Printing Office.
American Dietetic Association: A position paper on chemical dependency, J Am Diet Assoc 90:1274, 1990.
Hunger emergency in America. Joint hearing before the Subcommittee on Domestic Marketing, Consumer Relations, and Nutrition of the Committee on Agriculture, and the Domestic Task Force of the Select Committee on Hunger, House of Representatives, 100th Congress, second session, serial no. 100-2, Washington, DC, 1988, US Government Printing Office.
Hunger in America. Hearing before the Subcommittee on Nutrition and Investigations of the Committee on Agriculture, Nutrition and Forestry, US Senate, 100th Congress, second session, Washington, DC, 1988, US Government Printing Office.
Mayer J: Social responsibilities of nutritionists, J Nutr 116:714, 1986.
SNE policy on the food and agricultural bill, Oakland, Calif, 1985, Society for Nutrition Education.
Waxman LD: *A status report on hunger and homelessness in America's cities, 1990: a 30-city survey*, Washington, DC, 1990, US Conference of Mayors.

APPENDIX 2-1

Next steps for nutrition educators: Key contacts for hunger, poverty, and food assistance programs—a nutritionist's mini-directory of organizations and agencies*

NON-PROFIT ORGANIZATIONS

American Association of Retired Persons
601 E Street, N.W.
Washington, DC 20049
(202) 434-2277

Bread for the World
802 Rhode Island Ave., N.E.
Washington, DC 20018
(202) 269-0200

Center on Budget and Policy Priorities
777 North Capitol Street, N.E., #705
Washington, DC 20002
(202) 408-1080

Center on Hunger, Poverty and Nutrition Policy
Tufts University School of Nutrition
126 Curtis Street
Medford, MA 02155
(617) 381-3223

*Reprinted with permission from *J Nutr Educ* 24(1):865, 1992.

Child Nutrition Forum
c/o FRAC
1875 Connecticut Ave., N.W., #540
Washington, DC 20009
(202) 986-2200

Children's Defense Fund
122 C Street, N.W.
Washington, DC 20001
(202) 628-8787

Coalition on Human Needs
1000 Wisconsin Ave., N.W.
Washington, DC 20007
(202) 342-0726

Community Nutrition Institute
2001 S Street, N.W.
Suite #530
Washington, DC 20009
(202) 462-4700

Food Research and Action Center
1875 Connecticut Ave., N.W. #540
Washington, DC 20009
(202) 986-2200

HandsNet (A Computer Network)
20195 Stevens Creek Blvd., Suite 120
Cupertino, CA 95104
(408) 257-4500

Interfaith Impact for Justice and Peace
110 Maryland Ave., N.E., Box #63
Washington, DC 20002
(202) 543-2800

National Council of Senior Citizens
1331 F Street, N.W.
Washington, DC 20004
(202) 347-8800

Public Voice For Food and Health Policy
1001 Connecticut Ave., N.W. #522
Washington, DC 20036
(202) 659-5930

Second Harvest
116 South Michigan Ave.
Suite #4
Chicago, IL 60603
(312) 263-2303

Urban Institute
2100 M Street, N.W.
5th Floor
Washington, DC 20037
(202) 833-7200

World Hunger Year
261 West 35th Street, #1402
New York, NY 10001
(212) 629-8850

U.S. DEPARTMENT OF AGRICULTURE

Office of Governmental Affairs and Public Information
Contact Person: Dick Thaxton
(703) 305-2039

Special Supplemental Food Program for Women, Infants and Children (WIC)
Contact Person: Ronald Vogel
(703) 305-2746

Child Nutrition Programs (School Lunch Program, School Breakfast, and Child Care Food Program, Summer Food Program)
Contact Person: Samuel Bauer
(703) 305-2590

Nutrition Education and Training Program (NET)
Contact Person: Pat Daniels
(703) 305-2554

Food Stamp Program
Contact Person: Tim O'Connor
(703) 305-2490

Temporary Emergency Food Assistance Program
Contact Person: Alberta Frost
(703) 305-2680

Expanded Food and Nutrition Education Program (EFNEP)
Contact Person: Wells Willis
(202) 720-7151

ADMINISTRATION ON AGING

Elderly Nutrition Programs
Contact Person: Fred Luman
(202) 619-2618

PROFESSIONAL ASSOCIATIONS

American Public Welfare Association
(Food Stamp Program Administrators)
810 First Street, N.E., #500
Washington, DC 20002
(202) 682-0100

American School Food Service Association
(Child Nutrition Program Personnel)
1600 Duke Street, 7th Floor
Alexandria, VA 22314
(703) 739-3900

Child Care Food Program Sponsors Forum
c/o Marge Langworthy
2440 Wild Blossom Drive
East Lansing, MI 48823
(517) 332-0226

National Association of WIC Directors
P.O. Box 53405
Washington, DC 20009
(202) 232-5492

U.S. Conference of Mayors
1620 I Street, N.W., 4th Floor
Washington, DC 20006
(202) 293-7330

U.S. CONGRESS

Select Committee on Children, Youth and Families
U.S. House of Representatives
385 House Annex #2
Washington, DC 20515
(202) 226-7660

Selection Committee On Hunger
U.S. House of Representatives
507 House Annex #2
Washington, DC 20515
(202) 226-5470

3

Perspectives on Food Processing and Technology: Defining Terminology for the Dietitian and Nutritionist and Consumer

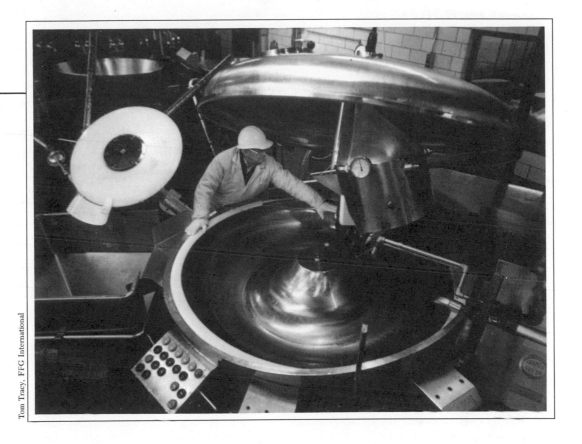

GENERAL CONCEPT

Among the forces that contribute to our changing environment are the advanced technologies in the food processing industry. The rapid developments in the food processing industry over the last 50 years have not been accompanied by consumer understanding of the changes. To understand the food industry and to develop a perspective on the subject the dietitian and nutritionist needs to perceive themes and commonalities of food manufacturing. A knowledge of food processing terminology helps the nutrition educator to communicate effectively with the consumer and those in the food industry about the Dietary Guidelines and other nutrition and health documents.

OUTCOME OBJECTIVES

When you finish this chapter, you should be able to:

- **Understand that *food processing* is a general term that includes food preservation, refinement, and preparation.**
- **Describe how food preservation and its various methods provide a benefit to the consumer.**
- **Give an example of food refinement processes that enhance area food supply.**
- **Discuss how food preparation treatment transforms the nature of the raw material, for example, wheat to bread and milk to yogurt.**
- **Prepare an explanation for the consumer that any risk incurred by food preservation techniques is accompanied by benefits with respect to food safety. Thus the consumer can make an informed evaluation of a preservation treatment by weighing the perceived benefit against the perceived risk.**

The strategies for obtaining raw materials and transforming them to food have been numerous and varied throughout history as well as across cultures. Historically, these two activities have demanded a large proportion of the time and energy resources of a society, and the strategies employed comprised an important part of that society's culture. In less technologically advanced societies, not only did individuals spend more time in obtaining raw materials and transforming them into food but the activities were less complex. Today, in the technologically advanced Western world, far fewer individuals are directly employed in obtaining raw materials (i.e., agricultural production) and transforming them to food. Although the efficiency of agricultural production has increased dramatically over the last 50 years, the paradigm for agricultural production has remained largely the same: farmers plant crops or raise livestock, and the commodities produced are sold. By contrast, the paradigm for transforming these commodities into food has changed profoundly. Industrial manufacture of convenient and appealing foods now represents the dominant strategy for transforming raw materials

into prepared food. For a particular food item, a detailed explanation of the method of transforming raw materials readily becomes mired in scientific and technological detail. To understand the food industry, one needs to perceive themes and commonalities of food manufacturing. Unfortunately, terminology in common use is vague and value-judgment laden (e.g., "processed food"); use of this imprecise terminology causes confusion rather than an understanding of industrial food manufacture. The objective of this chapter is to present food processing terminology that is sufficiently precise for a dietitian or nutritionist to use it to communicate effectively with the consumer and those in the food industry.

HISTORICAL BACKGROUND

Obtaining raw materials has always been of primary importance to a society. In some societies hunting and gathering gave way to an agriculture-based society almost 30,000 years ago, and in other (increasingly few) societies it is still the main method of obtaining food. Storing these raw materials and transforming them to food is secondary but no less important. The challenges associated with obtaining, storing, and transforming raw materials are interrelated, and a change in the circumstances related to any one of these three necessitates an altered response to the other two. For example, domestication of wheat for agricultural production made sense only if some means of grain storage was available and if some acceptable food could be made from the grain. Early agriculturalists could ensure a consistent food supply only if they could solve the problem of seasonal fluctuations related to the planting-harvest cycle. Simultaneous progress in obtaining raw materials, storing them, and transforming them led to change.

The problems of storage of agricultural materials and their transformation into food are intimately entwined. In some cases the two problems were dealt with in sequential fashion: grain was stored and later transformed into bread, for example. In other cases transformation facilitated storage: grapes were fermented to wine, which was then stored. It is important to recognize that the food (using these two examples) that became available regardless of the season was bread and wine, not wheat and grapes.

Production of raw materials and their conversion to food changed little from Roman times until the American Revolution.[7] Not coincidentally, during this period advances in the scientific understanding of the chemistry and physics of food were minimal. Preservation technology was limited to drying, salting, and fermentation, and no scientific foundation existed for these technologies. In the nineteenth century, advances in the scientific understanding of food preservation were limited to understanding the role of heat treatment. Thermal preservation was first successfully (and crudely) accomplished by Appert, who heat-treated food in champagne bottles in the first decade of the nineteenth century. At the time a scientific rationale for the success of his method was lacking. The rudiments of microbiology were developed by Pasteur in midcentury, and a quantitative scientific understanding of thermal preservation treatments was first established in the last decade of the century by H.L. Russell at the University of Wisconsin and by S.C. Prescott and W.L. Underwood at the Massachusetts Institute of Technology.[1] Commercial canning developed in the mid-nineteenth century (predating these scientific advances, a sequence not uncommon in food technology!) and became the most important method of food preservation until World War II. Before then, most preservation treatments involved raw materials that could later be transformed into food before consumption. Other than canning, the technology of preservation and transformation methods was based on centuries of experience with processes for which there was no scientific basis—they just worked.

Technological innovation in food processing was strongly stimulated during World War II by the critical need to supply food to troops under demanding conditions of distribution and storage.[11] The need might have been unfulfilled had not scientific developments in nutrition and the chemistry of nutrients taken place soon before. The objective at that time was to prove safe, nutritionally sound food; the taste and texture of some of these items

(dehydrated eggs, instant mashed potatoes, and dehydrated vegetables, for example) were suboptimal. Once the beachhead of safe and nutritional food was established in wartime, improvements in the sensory quality of these and other foods were steadily made in the subsequent years.

Since World War II, efforts to establish the scientific foundation of food processing have led to a relatively new field of applied science: food science, a degree program now available at most U.S. land grant institutions.[6] Food science involves the fundamentals of food process engineering, food microbiology, nutrition, and food chemistry.[16] The goal of a B.S. program is to transmit this multidisciplinary scientific foundation to the student, who will then be properly trained to take a responsible position in the food processing industry. The professionalization of the field has been further enhanced by the development of the Institute of Food Technologists (IFT, which originated in 1939). This organization has more than 20,000 members and is composed of food scientists and technologists from the industrial sector, government, and academia.

Today, the food processing industry has moved far beyond the stage of simply providing a safe and nutritious food supply. Success in this highly competitive industry is predicated upon keeping the consumer happy. Convenience, sensory qualities, and price determine consumer acceptance.

The rapid developments in the food processing industry over the last 50 years have not been accompanied by consumer understanding of the changes. As scientific advances have permitted efficient mass production of food, many of the traditional preservation (e.g., home drying or pickling) and transformation treatments (cooking from scratch) have been or are becoming lost. The supermarket now holds a dazzling array of appealing items manufactured by processes little understood by the average consumer (for example, extrusion cooking). Some of these items carry an impressively complex, even intimidating ingredient statement. An understanding of the manufacture of these complex new food products requires a technical background. Without this understanding, the technical jargon of the industry is difficult to follow and may lead to confusion and sometimes suspicion on the part of the consumer.

FOOD PROCESSING

Among consumers, the term *processed* is often used without precise meaning, sometimes in a perjorative sense, as in "I try to avoid highly processed foods." What specifically is the consumer's concern? Food technologists may respond to this consumer by pointing out the importance of food processing (preservation) in assuring a year-round supply of nutritious food, a response rooted in historical concerns. Such a response may miss the consumer concern entirely, at least partly because the consumer often cannot phrase a concern with sufficient precision. Both the food scientist and the consumer would be better served by more precise terminology.

The term *food processing* may be used to describe any physical, chemical, or microbiological treatment given a farm commodity, food ingredient, or food that transforms the starting material(s) into something of increased value. In the United States in 1850, much of home food processing could be or was performed on the multitude of small farms for consumption on those farms.[7] Salting of meats, drying of fruits, cheese production, various fermentations, and cold storage of root crops could be accomplished on such a small scale. Other ingredients, such as flour and sugar, were manufactured at locations away from the farm on which the raw commodities were produced. After purchase of the ingredient, final preparation of the food was done in the home. Although the processing treatments were not understood on a scientific basis, the farmer controlled a high proportion of the processing treatments in creation of food for the table.

Today most consumers still do not understand processing treatments on a scientific basis, even though the scientific basis is far better established; the scientific understanding is largely the province of food technologists. However, the consumer controls fewer and fewer of the treatments in creation of food for the table. Many consumers would not recognize the raw commodities or the treatments

given them, and now more and more of the preparation steps are done on an industrial scale. The consumer role is primarily that of evaluator of the finished product. He or she has delegated the responsibility for producing the agricultural commodities and for manufacturing food from them and must trust the integrity of these providers and of the government agencies that oversee the system. Many consumers are uneasy with the present situation, and a few are antagonistic. The term *food neophobia* has been coined to describe a consumer "fear or distrust of new practices, new chemicals, or new technologies," at least partially due to ignorance about these practices, chemicals, and technologies.[10] Well-educated dietitians, nutritionists, and consumers should be conversant with the terminology necessary to understand and describe the complexity of the modern food industry.

Food processing is a general term that may be broken down to include *food preservation, refinement,* and *food preparation*. A central theme of this chapter is that these more specific terms should be used in lieu of the more general one.

Food Preservation

Food preservation is any manipulation of the physical, chemical, or microbiological qualities of the food and its immediate surroundings to minimize undesirable changes in the food or food ingredient. These undesirable changes are generally either *microbial* or *chemical*. Preservation to minimize unwanted microbial activity leads to reduced microbial spoilage and reduced foodborne illness. Preservation methods include physical treatments such as applying heat (thermal processing), removing heat (refrigeration and freezing), removing water (dehydration), adjusting the gaseous environment (perhaps by removing oxygen), and irradiation; biological treatments such as fermentation; and chemical treatments such as the use of various antimicrobial agents.[16,19]

Thermal treatments may be geared toward killing specific undesirable disease-causing organisms. For example, in pasteurization of milk, numerous organisms survive the heat treatment. Although the shelf life of the pasteurized milk is extended by refrigeration, these nonpathogenic organisms ultimately multiply and cause the milk to sour.

Thermal treatments may also be designed to kill all vegetative microbial cells and specific types of microbial spores (especially the heat-resistant spores of *Clostridium botulinum*), as in commercial canning processes. The objective is to achieve "commercial sterilization," a condition in which surviving spores are unable to grow in the food. Rarely are thermal treatments designed to achieve complete microbial sterility because such harsh treatments are unnecessary from a safety perspective and the effect on the sensory qualities of the food is undesirable.

Refrigeration treatments are designed to slow microbial growth, whereas freezing effectively stops it. Killing microorganisms is not the goal of these treatments. Dehydration treatments likewise modify the environment such that microbial growth is eliminated, but the organisms and their spores may survive to grow if water is again present. The same is true for modification of the gaseous environment.

Irradiation treatment involves exposure of the food to high-energy radiation (either electromagnetic radiation, such as gamma rays, or high-energy electrons). This treatment is similar to thermal treatment in that the goal is to kill microorganisms (or insects, at much lower doses). By analogy to heat treatment, irradiation using moderate doses may be done to accomplish a pasteurization effect. At very high doses it may result in complete microbial sterilization. This sterilization treatment is given to a variety of foods by the U.S. military. For retail food items it is limited to prescribed materials (e.g., spices). Irradiation treatment causes chemical changes in the food and kills microorganisms by causing chemical changes in their cellular machinery. Similar effects result from thermal processing. Food irradiation treatments in use do not involve sufficient energy to cause the foods themselves to become radioactive.

Antimicrobial agents are selected on the basis of their toxicity to microorganisms and their si-

multaneous lack of toxicity to humans. For example, calcium propionate is often added to baked goods to retard mold growth. This chemical is the calcium salt of propionic acid. In solution, the acid and the salt forms are in equilibrium. Propionic acid is toxic to bread mold because the organism takes it up but is unable to metabolize it. Nevertheless, propionate (and propionic acid) occurs in normal human metabolism (by catabolism of branched-chain amino acids) and is therefore readily metabolized by the human. Understanding the details of the differing actions of the various other antimicrobial agents demands a thorough understanding of the differing metabolic capabilities of the human and of the target microorganisms. However, the general concept can be understood by consumers and should allay some fears and concerns.

Food preservation may also be done with the goal of minimizing undesirable chemical changes in the food. These chemical changes have more to do with sensory quality than with safety. Often a food label says "best when refrigerated," which indicates that sensory quality, not safety, is the concern. With regard to a specific product, there is often confusion in the consumer's mind on this point. For example, should prepared mustard be refrigerated? Most prepared mustards contain sufficient vinegar to accomplish microbial preservation and eliminate concerns about microbial food poisoning. However, at room temperature, chemical changes take place more rapidly, leading to undesirable flavors. Thus it is best to refrigerate mustard that will not be used rapidly.

One of the primary types of chemical change in foods is oxidation, which can cause undesirable changes in the sensory qualities. For example, unsaturated fats can combine with oxygen to form compounds contributing to a rancid flavor. Minute amounts of these compounds can make a food unpalatable (but probably still safe). Another oxidative change is browning. Antioxidant ingredients are commonly added to susceptible foods (recall that foods have been derived from living tissues). These chemicals may mimic the antioxidant action of ascorbic acid and tocopherols in living tissues. A recent trend is to use "natural" antioxidants, often in the form of spices or spice extracts. The active components of these ingredients are often the same or closely related to the action of purified chemicals used. Ironically, these "natural" ingredients also contain a wealth of other chemical species with unknown activities. To the consumer, an ingredient statement containing a particular spice may be more appealing than one with BHA (butylated hydroxyanisole, a common antioxidant), but the actual complexity of the spice-based food "additive" is much greater. The biological activity of some of these other minor spice components is unstudied.

In a quest for what are referred to as "minimally processed" foods, the manufacturer applies several preservation treatments to a food item; however, each treatment is applied less extensively than if it were the sole treatment. A prepared entrée may have been mildly heat-treated to reduce chemical changes due to food enzymes, antioxidants may have been added to reduce oxidative changes, antimicrobial compounds added to reduce microbial growth, nitrogen added to the package to retard growth of certain types of microorganism and reduce oxidation, and the entree may be distributed under refrigeration to reduce microbial growth. The main advantage of such a "minimally processed" food is the consumer perception of freshness that results. The application of preservation methods in addition to heating allows a diminished heat treatment, leading to improved sensory qualities. Thus the food is minimally processed with respect to *thermal* preservation treatment (even though the actual complexity of the preservation treatments may be great). Lund has termed this approach *invisible manufacturing*.[12] Considerable research is presently being done to determine synergistic interactions among preservation treatments, with the goal that the net preservation effect will be more than the sum of the individual treatments. One concern regarding these minimally processed food items is that the consumer may not understand the importance of the interrelatedness of the methods of preservation. For example, a food designed for distribution under refrigeration might become unsafe if stored at room temperature. Food manufacturers have placed great emphasis on developing fail-safe distribution systems and are working on indicators to show when mishandling of a package had occurred. To ensure food safety, consumer education is needed regarding the differences between minimally processed foods and traditionally processed foods.

Refinement

In modern food manufacturing, an ingredient is used to impart a particular desirable property to the finished food product. This property has been termed a *functional property* of the ingredient, implying that the ingredient serves that function in the overall food system. Traditional ingredients are complex materials made up of many chemical components. For example, egg yolk contains lipoproteins and a mixture of phospholipids (among other things). Isolated from the egg yolk, the phospholipid fraction may be used to provide certain functional properties as an ingredient in other foods. As the functionally important components of traditional food ingredients have become better understood, refinement has become increasingly important in food processing. Food *refinement* involves removal of some fraction of a raw material to make the composition of the remaining fraction more desirable, often for use as a food ingredient with a particular functional property. Refinement treatments were applied to wheat in the production of flour in early Egypt and in Roman times. The type of food that can be made from purified white flour differs dramatically in texture and color from food made from whole-wheat flour. For example, the textural properties of yeast-leavened bread are dependent on the concentration of the endosperm proteins, which form gluten and allow the dough to rise and form a light, pleasant texture. Diluted by the bran and germ present, a whole-wheat flour bread dough will not achieve the same light texture as a white flour bread dough, which is more concentrated in endosperm material and therefore in gluten. Consequently, the degree of refinement of the wheat is critical to the texture of the food product. Most commercially manufactured whole-wheat breads contain "vital wheat gluten" as an ingredient. This ingredient is purified gluten prepared from flour. The wheat gluten is added to the whole-wheat flour dough to provide a sufficient concentration of gluten to allow the desirable light texture to form. Thus even these whole-wheat breads rely on refinement technology.

Other common retail ingredients subjected to refinement are white sugar, refined primarily from sugarcane or sugar beets; and edible fats and oils, refined from animal products or tissues (butter, lard, and tallow) and plant sources (olive oil and "vegetable" oils, commonly derived from plant seeds).

The consumer is less aware of the refinement processes used to make specialty ingredients not available at the retail level but used by manufacturers of formulated foods. One example of such a product is lecithin, obtained as a by-product during the refinement of crude soybean oil to purified soybean oil. This material is a mixture of various types of phospholipids. Lecithin is used in a wide variety of formulated foods. For example, it is used as an emulsifier in spoonable salad dressing, in which it functions in much the same way as the phospholipid from egg yolk in mayonnaise. An increasing variety of refined edible oils has become available at retail. This variety is dwarfed by the variety of edible oil ingredients with different fatty acid composition available for use by food manufacturers, who may attempt to simultaneously meet nutritional and technological goals by the selection of the appropriate oil ingredient.

Many of the specific chemical entities on food labels are similarly obtained by refinement. The flavors and extracts industry is a major component of the food industry, functioning largely unnoticed by the typical consumer. A flavor extracted from a material is a highly complex mixture of chemicals that produces a specific flavor profile. An artificial flavor is created by analyzing the flavor extract to determine its components (a nontrivial task) and by formulating a reasonable copy from purified organic chemicals (which may have been either synthesized industrially or obtained by purification from some tissue) identical to those in the extract.

The major difference between the extract and the synthetic flavor is often the subtleties of the flavor profile, which can be extremely difficult to reproduce. However, the artificial flavor may be less expensive and more dependable (in the sense of availability and in the sense of being less subject to natural variation).

Use of many refinement technologies predates the understanding of the nutritional ramifications of the technology.[2] Production of white wheat flour on a mass scale became possible with the advent of steel roller milling in the second half of the nineteenth century. The air purifier was developed at about the same time, allowing efficient separation of the pure endosperm chunks produced by the new roller milling process. These endosperm chunks could then be reduced to flour-sized particles with a minimum of contamination by bran and germ. Reduction in vitamin content was not considered because the very concept of the class of nutrients called *vitamins* did not exist until the twentieth century. Nineteenth-century millers could have known nothing of the nutritional ramifications of reduced thiamin, riboflavin, and niacin caused by efficient removal of bran and germ. However, since 1942 these vitamins (along with iron) have been added at specified levels to make "enriched flour" and other enriched products in order to minimize the risks of vitamin deficiency in the population.

The larger question of the nutritional quality of white versus whole-wheat flour is not entirely straightforward. Certainly one can readily determine that removal of bran and germ leads to a lower concentration of vitamins and minerals in the flour as compared to the whole kernel. However, the refinement effect is complicated by enrichment with some vitamin and mineral components that had been removed. Furthermore, the removal of phytate and fiber (both of which reduce mineral bioavailability) in refinement to white flour improves the bioavailability of the minerals present. This nutritional benefit is countered by the loss of the bulk of the insoluble dietary fiber by refinement.

The 1985 USDA Dietary Guidelines suggested:

"Eat foods with adequate starch and fiber," specifically advising consumption of "whole-grain breads and cereals, fruits, and vegetables." The 1990 edition was revised in this respect to: "Choose a diet with plenty of vegetables, fruits, and grain products." Both editions advised: "Increase your fiber intake by eating more of those foods that contain fiber naturally." The meaning of the word *naturally* is rarely straightforward, but from the context it appears that the advice does not pertain to foods to which fiber has been added. The reason for this exclusion is that the evidence regarding a beneficial effect of fiber consumption is equivocal; in fact, nonfiber food components associated with fiber in unrefined items may be responsible for much of the putative benefit. Consequently, purified fiber should be considered a refined ingredient that might no longer contain the active properties of the intact material.

Preparation

Food preparation involves manipulation of foods or combinations of food ingredients by physical, chemical, or microbiological treatment to produce a food or food ingredient in a more nearly ready-to-consume state. Preparation of food before eating probably dates to the development of the ability to control fire, which allowed certain forms of cooking. Roasting meat on a spit represents a rudimentary form of preparation, not necessarily involving any other ingredients. Cooking grain products generally involved heat in the presence of another ingredient, water. Early gruels may have been the first *formulated foods* (that is, foods composed of more than one ingredient according to a formulation, elements of which are combined by physical treatments according to a recipe). Appropriate quantities of grain or meal were combined with an appropriate quantity of water and heated. The two-step process of grinding of grain followed by cooking is an example of an ingredient being manufactured before preparation of the food produced from it.

Some preparation treatments result in little change in the essential nature of the raw material. For example, a boiled potato differs from a raw potato in important ways, but it is nevertheless readily recognizable as a potato. By contrast, a preparation treatment may be a fundamental transformation of the nature of the raw material. Bread, for example, has little in common with wheat or even flour. An equally profound transformation occurs in the manufacture of cheese from milk and in the manufacture of a puffed corn snack from corn. The chemical changes underlying all these treatments have been investigated in depth. Although the problems might seem mundane because the foods are so familiar, the chemistry of food systems is often difficult to study because of the complexity of these systems.

THE MODERN FOOD INDUSTRY

The preceding discussion illustrated how food processing may be said to encompass three more specific treatments: preservation, refinement, and preparation. The interrelationship among these three types of treatment is sometimes complex. The potential complexity is illustrated in Figure 3-1, which is an attempt to show diagrammatically the components of the food industry before World War II and at the present. In these figures, the size of the rectangles indicates the relative importance of the operation as part of the overall scheme. Before World War II the major emphasis was on preserving raw food materials and subsequent final preparation in the home, the point of consumption. By contrast, at the present time preparation of formulated food products constitutes a major portion of the food industry effort. To accommodate this change, an extensive infrastructure of ingredient suppliers has emerged.[7] This portion of the industry is normally not visible to the consumer. However, one can readily obtain a glimpse of it from perusal of trade publications such as *Food Processing* and *Prepared Foods,* in which the advertising is often by ingredient suppliers and aimed at food manufacturers. A major food industry trade show of vast scope occurs each June organized by the IFT; the show is summarized in the IFT journal *Food Technology*. As the emphasis on convenience foods continues to increase, the importance of preparation in the home continues to decline in favor of formulated foods prepared industrially.

The scheme presented in Figure 3-1 may be

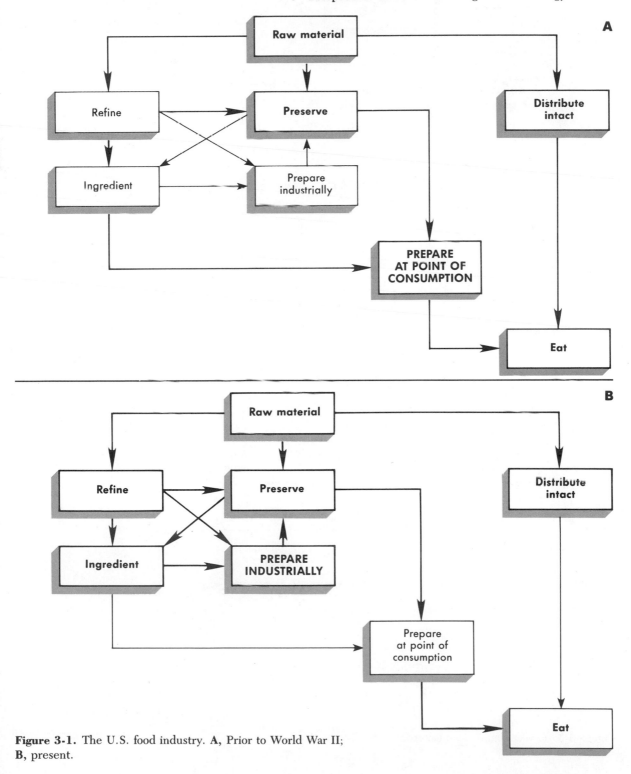

Figure 3-1. The U.S. food industry. **A,** Prior to World War II; **B,** present.

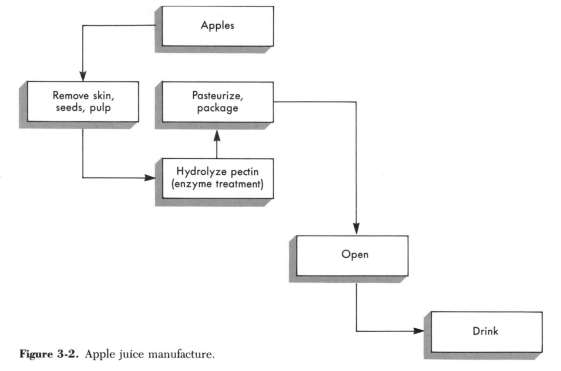

Figure 3-2. Apple juice manufacture.

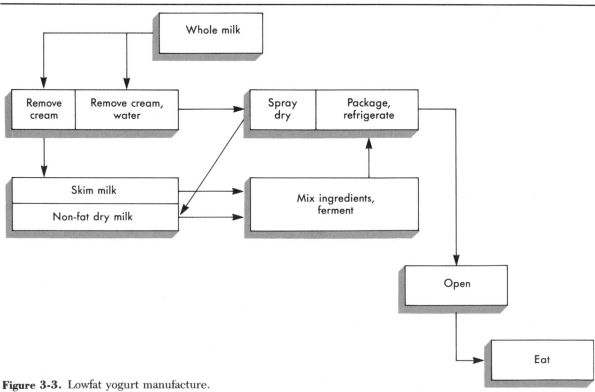

Figure 3-3. Lowfat yogurt manufacture.

used to describe the manufacture of some common retail foods. Apple juice production is illustrated in Figure 3-2. This ready-to-eat prepared food begins with a refinement step, when skin, seeds, and pulp are removed by pressing to yield a cloudy liquid. Treatment with the enzyme pectinase (obtained from a specialized ingredient supplier) represents a preparation treatment, done to clarify the juice. Preservation is accomplished by pasteurizing the juice and packaging it. Home preparation is essentially nil.

Manufacture of low-fat yogurt is more complex, as shown in Figure 3-3. Whole milk is subjected to refinement (by centrifugation) to remove the cream. Some of the skim milk is further refined (by removal of the water) to make nonfat dry milk. Appropriate proportions of skim milk and nonfat dry milk are mixed, and the starter culture (obtained from a specialized ingredient supplier) added in order to prepare the yogurt by fermen-

tation. To accomplish preservation, containers of fermented product are sealed, and they are stored and distributed under refrigeration. Once again, home preparation is essentially nil.

Manufacture of ready-to-eat pudding is even more complex, as shown in Figure 3-4. The main functional ingredient, starch, is obtained by refinement of dried common field corn, a multistep process that removes hull, germ, and protein. The starch so obtained is not chemically suitable for use in this product because the textural properties of the pudding would change with time in ways not desired by the consumer. The smooth texture would become increasingly firm, and the gel structure would shrink in volume, expressing liquid (the phenomenon of syneresis). The starch is altered by chemical modification in order to improve its physical behavior in the pudding. After this modification, the starch ingredient is preserved by dehydration and distributed to food manufacturers in

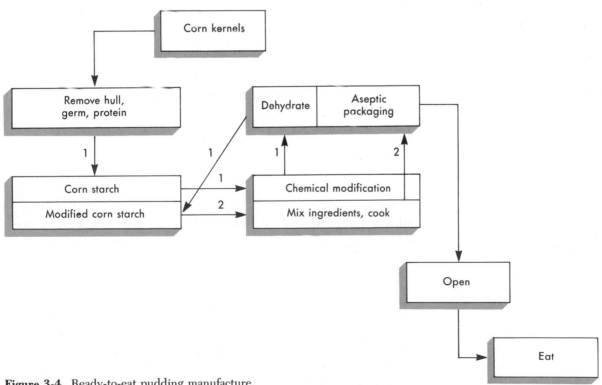

Figure 3-4. Ready-to-eat pudding manufacture.

the form of a dry powder. The modified starch is mixed with the other ingredients (commonly including milk, sugar, and flavoring), and the mixture is cooked outside the package to develop the pudding texture. The product is packaged hot in a sterile environment (a process termed *aseptic packaging*) to accomplish preservation. The product need not be refrigerated during storage and distribution because the cooking treatment and packaging are sufficient to eliminate undesirable microbial growth.

TRADITIONALLY PREPARED VERSUS ENGINEERED FOODS

Not all prepared foods are formulated, as, for example, when a raw commodity (e.g., meat or peanuts) is roasted. Those prepared foods that are formulated may be divided into two types: *traditionally prepared* foods, which could easily be prepared in the home if desired; and *engineered* foods, the manufacture of which requires special processing equipment or ingredients not readily available for home use. Traditionally prepared foods may be purchased to relieve or reduce the effort of traditional home preparation. At one level of convenience, one might purchase prepared spaghetti sauce and add it to freshly prepared spaghetti before consumption; increased convenience might result from purchase of "minimally processed" pasta in sauce that needs only to be heated or, at even less expense, from canned spaghetti with sauce. A hot dog is an example of an engineered food, in that the home preparation of a finely ground emulsion (before cooking the product in casings to form the familiar shape) would be difficult without special equipment. With many children, in-home preparation of a hot dog is limited to simply opening the package! Engineered foods might also result from a requirement for highly complex formulation composed of specialty ingredients not readily available to the consumer. Whipped nondairy topping would fit into this category. Another common example of an engineered food is chocolate, which is manufactured industrially by an intricate series of treatments that use highly specialized equipment.

Within each of the two subcategories of formulated foods (traditional and engineered), the complexity of the formulation may vary widely. Prepared foods might be classified according to the complexity of the formulation. In the same way, prepared foods may be classified according to the extent of preparation; foods more completely prepared would be more nearly ready to eat than foods less completely prepared. An increased appreciation for the variety of foods and food ingredients commercially available can result from a plot of the extent of preparation against the complexity of formulation, as shown in Figure 3-5. For example, oatmeal (more precisely, rolled oats) is made from a very simple formulation: oats and water (which is later removed). Nevertheless, some cooking and size reduction occurs in manufacture. This partial preparation means that only brief cooking is needed in the final preparation. The placement on the preparation scale reflects this partial preparation. Another example, a carbonated soda, is ready to consume upon opening, causing the food to be placed high on the preparation scale. The formulation complexity is low, the product being composed of about 90% water, 10% sugar, and minute quantities of flavor and coloring. A ready-to-eat product of high formulation complexity is refrigerated whipped topping. The ingredient statement for some whipped toppings can be impressively complex. This product is high on both the ingredient complexity and extent of preparation scales.

NUTRIENTS ADDED TO FORMULATED FOODS

The major ingredients in formulated foods have traditionally been chosen primarily on the basis of their functional properties. Minor ingredients added to other ingredients or added directly to formulated foods may be essential vitamins and minerals. These nutrients may be added to *restore* the nutrient levels to what was present before treatment, they may be added to *enrich* the levels of certain nutrients without regard to gains or losses due to prior treatment (e.g., thiamin, niacin, riboflavin, and iron added to white flour), or they may be added to *fortify* a food with a nutrient never present in the original food (e.g., vitamin D added

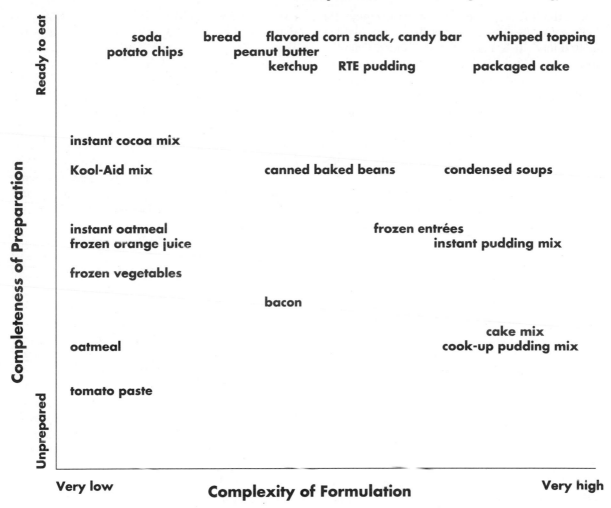

Figure 3-5. Prepared, formulated foods.

to milk or calcium added to orange juice). The Code of Federal Regulations (CFR) spells out the FDA policy regarding "rational addition of nutrients to foods" (CFR 104.20), as well as the standard of identity for certain "enriched" items.

The increasing importance of formulated foods in the Western diet provides an opportunity for nutritional improvement in ways other than manipulation of vitamin and mineral levels. For many individuals in the United States, preventing nutritional deficiency is less of a concern than minimizing the risk of chronic problems such as cancer

and coronary heart disease. Within the last few years, food manufacturers have begun to use nutrition as a marketing tool. The food manufacturer's choice of ingredients for a formulated product is increasingly made on the basis of consumer nutrition concerns. Reduction in fat and cholesterol and substitution of unsaturated fats for saturated fats are marketable goals. Accomplishing these goals and at the same time manufacturing a food with acceptable sensory qualities is a major technological challenge. Numerous ingredients are advertised to manufacturers as *fat substitutes*. This term implies that the ingredient has at least some of the functional properties of the fat in the original formulated food. It is a challenge for a food manufacturer to present the potential advantage of a product so formulated to consumers in a manner consistent with the CFR, which states that certain claims on the label mandate classification of that food as a drug and make the item subject to government seizure. Nevertheless, implicit (and sometimes not so implicit) health claims have proliferated in the last few years, and the concept of *nutraceuticals* (foods with a beneficial effect regarding a disease state) has emerged. The FDA is currently developing regulations to govern the use of health claims.

FOOD SAFETY

Most food scientists agree that the greatest food-related risk to health is microbial contamination of food, either through toxin production or infection.[10] Many consumers are aware of the potent bacterial toxin produced by *Clostridium botulinum*, at least to the extent that they know the term *botulism*. Some consumers are also aware that certain mold species produce toxins (mycotoxins) which are hazardous at extremely low concentrations, for example, the aflatoxin produced by *Aspergillus flavus*. In recent years, consumer perceptions of food-related risk have enlarged from concerns about food additives and agricultural chemical residues to include a concern about certain microbial infections. Bacterial infections due to *Salmonella* are responsible for thousands of reported cases per year in the United States, and many consumers are aware of the potential contamination of chicken and eggs with *Salmonella*. Consumers are less aware of other bacterial genera such as *Campylobacter* and *Listeria*, which cause infections that may also be acute and life-threatening. These microbial hazards may be addressed by food preservation techniques and proper food handling before consumption. Whatever risks may be incurred by the food preservation techniques are accompanied by benefits with respect to food safety.[15] In order to evaluate the desirability of using a process of preservative ingredient, one should first attempt to understand the

risks and benefits involved. A scientific estimate of risk is in the form of a statistical statement of the chance that some event will occur. Individual consumers often assess risk based on other factors as well, including the degree of familiarity, level of personal control, catastrophic potential, and equity in the ability to make informed decisions (e.g., children versus adults). Nutrition professionals should be sensitive to risk as perceived by the consumer. No consumer would willingly accept a risk without some justification, in the form of a benefit; a consumer who perceives no benefit prefers to be risk-free. Lack of awareness of the benefit of preservation treatment consequently leads to risk aversion. The evaluation of the benefit of a preservation treatment represents a value judgment on the part of the consumer and the food manufacturer, and these value judgments do not always agree. Nevertheless, the consumer can make an informed evaluation of a preservation treatment only by weighing the perceived benefit against the perceived risk.[8,18] The food and nutrition professional has an obligation to present this risk-benefit approach to the consumer and to encourage its use.

Agricultural practices can potentially influence food safety by the presence of residual agricultural chemicals. Some herbicides and pesticides are unquestionably toxic to humans at high doses. In fact, it has been argued that the best reason to minimize use of these chemicals is for the safety of the farmer rather than for that of the consumer. The chronic toxicity of agricultural chemicals at trace levels is a more difficult question, and there are unfortunately no clear answers. Even the meaning of *trace* changes with advances in analytical chemistry. The risk involved in these agricultural production practices may be to some extent balanced by the benefit of inexpensive food commodities. The judgment of what sort of balance is appropriate is open to debate. Unfortunately, both the risks and benefits are difficult to quantitate, and an appropriate balance is difficult to determine. The FDA is charged with enforcing standards in this regard to ensure a reasonably safe food supply.

Our concern with manufactured agricultural chemicals may blind us to a greater problem: naturally occurring chemicals in food. During evolution, plant and animal species have developed the ability to interact on a chemical level. Certain plants have developed the ability to manufacture secondary metabolites that are toxic to insect predators, for example. Other plants elaborate substances that inhibit growth of other plants nearby. These natural pesticides and herbicides are part of the communication network in complex ecosystems and are reasonably well understood in only a few cases. Other safety concerns include those chemical species that regulate growth and development of plants, chemicals with potent biological activity in the individual plant species. Regardless of the toxicity of manufactured agricultural chemicals, it is important to recognize that all raw agricultural commodities are composed of chemicals and that the biological activities of all of these chemicals are not well understood.

Table 3-1. Food additive categories according to the NAS-NRC

Processing additives	Final product additives
Aerating/foaming agents	Antimicrobial agents
Antifoam agents	Antioxidants
Catalysts	Appearance control agents
Clarifying/flocculating agents	Flavors and flavor modifiers
Color control agents	Moisture control agents
Freezing/cooling agents	Nutrients
Malting/fermenting aids	pH control agents
Material handling aids	Sequestrants
Oxidizing/reducing agents	Surface tension control agents
pH control/modification agents	Sweeteners
Release/antistick agents	Texture/consistency control agents (including emulsifiers, firming agents, leavening agents, and stabilizers and thickeners)
Sanitizing/fumigating agents	
Separation/filtration aids	Tracers
Solvents/carriers/encapsulating agents	
Washing/surface removal agents	

From Mathews RA, Stewart MR: Report summarizes data from additive surveys, *Food Tech* 38:53, 1984.

Although consumer concern with the safety of "food additives" is often quite real, the concern must be more precisely stated to carry specific meaning. For example, even the commonly used term *preservative* is used in at least two senses: an ingredient may preserve a food through its antimicrobial activity,[4] or it may preserve the sensory qualities of the food through its ability to slow undesirable chemical changes, as do antioxidants.[5] The National Academy of Sciences–National Research Council has sponsored gathering of detailed data on the chemicals used in food. To accomplish this task, it was necessary to establish more precise terminology. Table 3-1 shows how food additives were divided into processing additives and final product additives and then further divided according to their technical effect.[13] Note that the word *preservative* does not even appear on this list, as it is not sufficiently precise to be useful. Food use of specific additives is allowed only according to detailed regulations found in the CFR. Discussion of each subcategory is beyond the scope of this chapter.

THE ECONOMICS OF THE FOOD INDUSTRY

The food industry is immense. Based on the value of industry shipments, the food industry is the largest manufacturing industry in the United States.[3] Consequently, a large food manufacturing company can justify research into those areas of food processing related to the retail products it manufactures. Food manufacturers have acquired increasing sophistication regarding the scientific basis for the technological function of specific processes or ingredients[6,9]; by means of this increasing sophistication, they may gain a competitive market advantage. The need for individuals trained in the science and technology of food accounts for the industrial demand for those holding a Food Science undergraduate B.S. degree.

The successful food manufacturer strives to provide *value* to the consumer (i.e., a desirable balance between product price and its sensory and nutritional qualities). The level of quality (in the sense of high or low, good or bad) of a food product is a subjective judgment made by the consumer on the basis of sensory *qualities* and on the basis of the effect of marketing and advertising. Marketing and advertising can have a direct effect on the consumer's perception of the qualities or an indirect effect, by influencing the judgment of others whom the consumer respects. When the product is positioned, the manufacturer determines a product image and a relationship between *price* and sensory qualities, based on the manufacturer's perception of the consumer market. It then becomes critical to the manufacturer to deliver a product to the consumer with minimum variation in these sensory qualities. Nutritional qualities are not perceivable by the consumer, who must rely on the label for this information and on the government to ensure compliance with the label declaration. Consumer satisfaction with packaged, formulated food results from what might be considered the contract implied by the label on the package. Often the consumer has no way to perceive any of the sensory qualities of a packaged product until the item is purchased and the package is opened; the consumer does not like surprises. If the qualities do not consistently result in the expected value, repeat purchases are unlikely. Consequently, a great deal of effort is expended by the manufacturer to ensure that variation in the sensory (resulting from physical and chemical) qualities of a product is controlled within well-defined limits.[17] Whether this goal is achieved through what has been historically termed *quality control* or *quality assurance* or by newer approaches such as total quality management (TQM), the objective is not to improve the level of absolute quality but to fulfill the implict contract of the label. The level of absolute quality will be improved only if that new level can be generated in a consistent fashion (assuming either that production cost does not increase or that the consumer is willing to pay a higher price). It is ironic that an inconsistent improvement in quality is likely to be detrimental to achieving consumer satisfaction. A formulated food product for which the sensory and nutritional qualities cannot be controlled is unlikely to be successfully mass marketed.

From the manufacturer's perspective, one means of minimizing variation in the physical and chemical (resulting in sensory) qualities of a product is to minimize variation in the ingredient qualities that are responsible for product qualities. For example, a mass-production bakery must be able to ensure a consistent supply of flour with acceptable ingredient qualities. For baking bread, those qualities include protein content, moisture content, and color (for white bread). Agricultural production of raw commodities (in this case, hard wheat) with minimal variation in certain properties is a critical input to the mass manufacture of food. There is much interaction between the ingredient suppliers and the retail product manufacturers. In some cases the specifications for a particular ingredient are so precise as to justify the supplier making an ingredient on a custom basis for a major manufacturer.

The food manufacturing industry is highly competitive. Generally, profits are made based on the high-volume sales, each sale producing little profit by itself.[7] Even a minute increase in processing efficiency or savings in ingredient cost is financially important. The efficiency of this intricate system in producing mass-market foods is truly a marvel. One hidden cost to the consumer may be the lack of availability of items for which a mass market does not exist. Although great effort goes into discovering an unfulfilled market niche, the efficiency of the food system is based upon mass production and marketing, and there is a lower limit on the size of the niche that can be efficiently exploited. It is the marvelous efficiency of the mass production and marketing system that enables a cake to be made from a mix that can be purchased for less than the ingredients needed to bake a cake from scratch with retail ingredients. (Of course, the same cake will not result.) Another curiosity is the higher price of whole-wheat flour than that of white flour. The paradox is resolved when one realizes that the flour mills are designed to simultaneously grind and refine the kernel into its components, a process that is accomplished with great efficiency. To make whole-wheat flour, the separated components have to be mixed together again, an additional operation.

SUMMARY

Potential confusion arises from use of the term *food processing* and more specific terminology is presented in this chapter. Manufacture of a particular retail food product often involves a complex interplay of preservation, refinement, and preparation treatments. After a definition and general discussion of these three categories of processing treatments, several retail food examples illustrate how preservation, refinement, and preparation are involved in food manufacturing. In the context of food safety, potential confusion also arises from use of the term *preservatives;* again, more specific terminology is presented. In addition, a risk-benefit approach to food safety is described. The consumer-driven nature of the food industry provides support for the argument that improved consumer understanding of the complexity of the food industry is desirable for both consumers and manufacturers.

REFERENCES

1. Borgstrom G: *Food preservation in history*. In *Principles of food science, vol 1*, Toronto, 1968, Macmillan.
2. Chichester CO, Darby WJ: The historical relationship between food science and nutrition, *Food Tech* 29:38, 1975.
3. Connor JM: *Food processing: an industrial powerhouse in transition*, Lexington, Mass, 1988, Lexington Books.
4. Dziezak JD: Preservatives: antimicrobial agents, *Food Tech* 40:104, 1986.
5. Dziezak JD: Preservatives: antioxidants, *Food Tech* 40:94, 1986.
6. Goldblith SA: 50 years of progress in food science and technology: from art based on experience to technology based on science, *Food Tech* 43:88, 1989.
7. Hampe EC Jr, Wittenberg M: *The lifeline of America: development of the food industry*, New York, 1964, McGraw-Hill.
8. Institute of Food Technologists Expert Panel on Food Safety and Nutrition: The risk/benefit concept as applied to food, *Food Tech* 42:119, 1988.
9. Joslyn MA: Basic to food progress: developments in food science. *Food Tech* 18:54, 1964.
10. Lee K: Food neophobia: major causes and treatments, *Food Tech* 43:62, 1989.
11. Levine AS, Labuza TP, Morley JE: Food technology: a primer for physicians, *N Engl J Med* 312:628, 1985.
12. Lund D: Food processing: from art to engineering, *Food Tech* 43:242, 1989.
13. Mathews RA, Stewart MR: Report summarizes data from food additive surveys, *Food Tech* 38:53, 1984.
14. Morgan AF: Interactions of food technology with nutrition over the last twenty-five years, *Food Tech* 18:68, 1964.
15. Mossel DAA, Drake DM: Processing food for safety and reassuring the consumer, *Food Tech* 44:63, 1990.
16. Potter NN: *Food science*, ed 4, Westport, Conn, 1986, AVI Publishing.
17. Pyke M: *Technological eating, or where does the fish finger point?* London, 1972, Camelot Press.
18. Slovic P: Perception of risk, *Science* 236:280, 1987.
19. Stewart GF, Amerine MA: *Introduction to food science and technology*, ed 2, New York, 1982, Academic Press.

4 The Social Marketing Plan: A Campaign Approach to Communication with Consumers

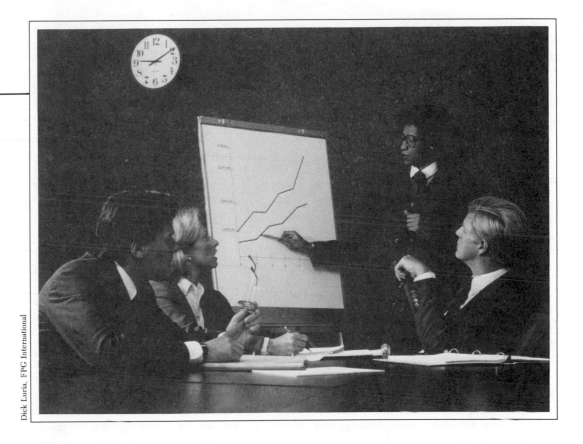

Dick Luria, FPG International

GENERAL CONCEPT

Dietary recommendations for population groups have been promulgated for almost a century. The main challenge no longer is to determine what eating patterns to recommend to the public but how to design a campaign to produce change in eating behavior. How do we design a social marketing plan? A public health campaign can focus mainly on changing the broad social environment, or it can focus on providing individuals with information and skills to make healthful behavior change.

OUTCOME OBJECTIVES

When you finish this chapter, you should be able to:

- Define strategies to use in a public health campaign and differentiate between individual and structural approaches.
- List characteristics of a successful public health campaign.
- Examine the framework for planning and managing a social market plan and the steps involved.
- Explain formative research methods and how they are used in planning the intervention.
- Determine the function of focus groups and the pros and cons involved.
- Plan a market survey at the community level and determine the target population, the data desired, and the methodology.

CONSUMERS AND THE FUTURE OF DIETARY CHANGE

What does the future hold for consumers and dietary change, and will there be a role for public health campaigns? A fleeting gaze into the crystal ball portends several emerging trends important to consumer dietary patterns in the United States. It also suggests directions and challenges for public health campaigns.

For example, the Food and Drug Administration's (FDA) proposed food labeling regulations (due in November 1992) promise that future visits to the grocery store will be somewhat less an exercise in sheer *caveat emptor* for the average American consumer than past visits. How much less remains unclear at this writing. Although such policy initiatives seek to compel some minimum of trustworthy nutritional information, labels alone do not make healthful diets. Consumers will still require skills to use labels effectively to guide food purchase, preparation, and consumption.

A second trend heralds greater clarification of the beneficial connections between food and health. Researchers have long studied the detrimental impact of the customary fat-rich American diet on health in the domains of heart disease and some kinds of cancer. More recently, researchers have been learning that our mothers were right: we should eat our fruits and vegetables and, for that matter, our beans, legumes, and grains.[5] Today evidence is rapidly accruing about their precise preventive characteristics, particularly those of plant foods. Evidence about their relationship to prevention of various adult chronic diseases likely will be further clarified through such projects as the National Cancer Institute's (NCI) Designer Food Program. Whether these will spawn innovative dietary supplements available to consumers also remains unclear at this writing. Presuming success, however, neither will these alone make healthful diets. No one is predicting dietary "magic bullets" or the imminent unhorsing of recommendations for population dietary and lifestyle change. Here, too, consumers still need skills to adopt healthful dietary patterns enhanced, perhaps, by engineered "designer foods."

A third trend is the apparently widening gap in health status between the haves and have-nots of U.S. society. Social class disparities in health risk behavior, prevalence of many diseases, and mortality and morbidity appear to be widening, despite more and better knowledge about prevention.[4,34] The continuing challenge to public health is to avoid "victim blaming" and to continue developing campaign strategies to reach especially lower socioeconomic and other underserved populations.

In brief, then, the crystal ball anticipates some fresh policy and even technological approaches that will potentially expand strategies to influence consumers toward more healthful diets. Just how well American consumers benefit may be bounded in part by social class disparities and the capacity of public health campaigns to reach all segments of the population. In this connection, a couple of decades of advances in public health campaigning have taught us a few lessons about what is a "good" public health campaign, but also include creative tensions about the emphasis campaigns should take.

PUBLIC HEALTH CAMPAIGN APPROACHES

Should public health campaigns focus mainly on changing the broader social environment for health (for example, using policy advocacy approaches to build public agendas), or should they focus on providing individuals with information and skills to make healthful behavior changes? Philosophically, the answer depends in part on whether one takes a structural or individual perspective regarding the sources of public health problems in the first place and the conditions that operate to maintain them as "problems."[15,17,30,31] Although these approaches are not mutually exclusive, an emphasis on one or the other may result in quite different applications.

For example, campaigns emphasizing voluntary adoption of healthful behavior changes by individuals might seek in part to use the mass media to communicate information about knowledge, skills, and motivation directly usable by individuals in making personal changes. Implicit in this approach is that solutions to the public health problem reside primarily in individuals and that they will recognize the need for personal changes and adopt them if they have sufficient information and motivation to do so. Public service announcements (PSAs), news features, and the like may serve as vehicles, along with other types of strategies.

By contrast, a campaign emphasizing the structural perspective likely would frame the behavior change problem in terms of the community environmental conditions that form and maintain it in populations. They may include entrenched institutional and marked conditions that permit, for example, widespread availability of certain products strongly tied to mortality and morbidity levels in certain populations. Policy approaches may be developed that are calculated to change these conditions (e.g., imposing restrictions that make some unsafe product less available for public consumption or elimination of restrictions that would make some product with preventive efficacy widely and conveniently available for public consumption). Such a campaign may also use the mass media, not to influence personal behavior per se, but to build a public agenda for change in broader social policy to affect the population prevalence of the problem in question.[31]

A concrete example of the difference in approach may be seen in efforts to discourage adolescent use of tobacco. In the individual behavior change approach, a campaign may seek to discourage young people from smoking by using mass media PSAs to emphasize the negative social consequences of tobacco use: bad breath, smelly clothes, yellow teeth, stained fingers, disapproval of friends.[1] In the structural approach, a campaign may seek to convince a legislative body to raise excise taxes on cigarettes or to restrict smoking in public places.[32] Both strategies are calculated to reduce the problem of adolescent smoking, but the focus and use of communication may be quite different. In the former case, the goal is to reduce adolescent smoking by directly educating and persuading adolescents with messages not to smoke. In the latter case, the goal is the same but is carried out by building a public agenda for policy restrictions calculated to discourage adolescent tobacco use. Here, the audience may be composed of several groups yet not explicitly include adolescents themselves: lawmakers, community leaders, and the general adult public.

Of course, the use of these approaches is not an either-or proposition; they are contrasted here to examine differences in the use of communication to achieve some public health outcome. Practically, the selection of strategies will depend on the nature of the public health problem. One or the other approach may be calculated to elicit the best results, and one or the other approach may be potentially or behaviorally inappropriate or simply unavailable. In addition, lessons learned over the past two decades suggest that in the application of approaches, one should do both where possible. That is to say, the idea of educating individuals about health—the mainstay of public health approaches for much of this century—has become part of the broader endeavor of health promotion.[13] Whether the object of a campaign is to build a public agenda for some public health policy change or to help individuals learn about personal lifestyle changes that they can make (or both), education and communication are central to the process.

CHARACTERISTICS OF SUCCESSFUL PUBLIC HEALTH CAMPAIGNS

Generally speaking, the most successful public health campaigns are community-based, multistrategy, and audience-centered.[2,26,28] *Community-based* means formation of partnerships with community institutions, organizations, and leaders to lay the groundwork for changing social environmental conditions that affect people's capacity to change.[2,7] This recognizes that individuals' behavior changes, especially in complex and important health aspects, do not occur in social isolation but are influenced for good or ill by social relations and the larger social environment. Community social environments can enhance individuals' capacity for change in two ways. Symbolically, organizations, institutions, and leaders can endow legitimacy on recommended health behavior changes as valuable, effective, and normative.[25] Tangibly, communities can provide concrete opportunities in various forms (e.g., through programs and policies) for people to act—to adopt recommended health behavior changes.

The multistrategy approach of successful public health campaigns is based on the recognition that a full range of health promotion techniques is generally necessary to propel adoption of healthful behavior changes through a population. The belief is that multiple strategies create a synergy that increases the likelihood of exposure to information and opportunities to act and therefore increases the likelihood of spreading change.[26]

Finally, the audience-centered approach includes systematic data-based planning, recognizing that individuals are heterogeneous with respect to making health behavior changes.[18] Different audience subgroups encounter varied conditions and possess varied motivations that may enhance or detract from change efforts or determine whether they seek to make changes in the first place.

These characteristics have been formulated into a global approach to planning and development of health promotion campaigns: the PRECEDE-PROCEED framework of Green and Kreuter.[14] The framework seeks in part to unite individual and structural approaches through separate diagnostic and development phases. Within this global approach, the authors emphasize the influence of social marketing as providing particularly a "consumer" orientation to health campaign planning that is driven by formative research.

PUBLIC HEALTH AND SOCIAL MARKETING

Social marketing emerged in the early 1970s as an effort to reformulate commercial marketing methods in situations involving the adoption of ideas and behaviors rather than the sale of products.[11,12,18] Like its commercial counterpart, social marketing recognizes that populations are not homogeneous but may be differentiated by their sociodemographic characteristics and by their needs, desires, lifestyles, and motivations to act. Moreover, they may be analyzed according to specific social environmental conditions that may influence different groups in varied fashion. These variables may be combined and analyzed to differentiate more homogeneous subgroups (target audiences) within the population. Informative and persuasive educational strategies may then be developed and tailored for each subgroup to enhance the potential for widespread adoption of ideas or behaviors. Moreover, other health promotion strategies may be developed to improve other social environmental ("market") conditions for the adoption of healthful behaviors.

Of course, a secondary purpose of defining target audiences in commercial marketing or general social marketing contexts is to permit effective use of scarce resources. That is, marketing strategists identify those subgroups most likely to purchase a product or adopt a new idea or behavior and then devote their resources to reaching those groups. Groups less likely to change are de-emphasized or ignored. In a public health context, however, campaign strategists seek health behavior change often within whole populations and consider it an ethical obligation to target even those groups for whom change may be more difficult. Although this does not preclude specifying target groups for better tailoring of messages and health promotional strategies, it often means that public health strategists must give special attention to difficult-to-reach groups and the individual and structural conditions and strategies that influence them.

Applied to public health situations, social marketing encompasses not so much a specific theoretical perspective as a framework for planning and

SOCIAL MARKETING FRAMEWORK

1. Consumer orientation: a focus on the needs and interests of the target population
2. Voluntary exchanges: the assumption that adoption of new ideas or practices involves the voluntary exchange of some resource (money, service, time) for a perceived benefit
3. Audience analysis and segmentation: the application of qualitative research methods to obtain information on the needs and special characteristics of the target population, which has been segmented to permit greater specificity of the message
4. Formative research: message design and pretesting of materials to be used in campaigns
5. Channel analysis: the identification of the various channels of communication including media outlets, community organizations, businesses, and "life-path points"
6. Marketing mix: the process of identifying the product, price, place, and promotion characteristics of intervention planning and implementation
7. Process tracking: a system to track the delivery of the program and to assess the utilization trends; a critical evaluation tool
8. Management: a commitment to a coordinated management system to assure quality of planning, implementation, and feedback functions

From Lefebvre CR and Flora JA: Social marketing and public health intervention. *Health Educ Q* 15:299, 1988. Copyright © 1988. Reprinted by permission of John Wiley & Sons, Inc.

management. The box above shows this framework as adapted to public health.[20]

These steps compose a recursive process of planning and management activities that encourage ongoing assessment of audience needs, strategy effectiveness, and program progress (measurement of exposure and contact reach and frequency; intermediate outcomes).

FORMATIVE ANALYSIS STRATEGIES AND A DIET CHANGE CAMPAIGN

In this context, public health campaign planners increasingly use formative analysis methods to improve the chances that health behavior change will spread among community populations.[7,8,23,33] Formative analysis includes a wide range of nonexperimental qualitative and quantitative research methods that permit campaign planners to differentiate potential target audiences, assess their health-related needs, construct informative and persuasive messages, synthesize and integrate multiple health education and promotion strategies, and deliver an integrated intervention through channel combinations likely to be used by and to influence different subgroups.[3,8,20]

The remainder of this chapter reviews the use of formative research methods in a diet-related cancer risk education campaign and how they were useful in planning the intervention. Entitled the Cancer and Diet Intervention Project (CANDI), the study overall sought to reduce diet-related cancer risk through multiple intervention strategies in an upper midwest community (population 20,000) compared to a matched reference community. The study design included 1 year devoted to formative analysis and strategy development, 1 year of intervention, and 1 year of follow-up evaluation.[24] Specifically, the project used three formative research methods consistent with our discussion thus far: focus groups, a cross-sectional market survey, and an analysis of community leadership.

Focus Groups

In commercial marketing, focus groups are a qualitative but systematic method long used for gathering information from individuals about the appeal of certain ideas, products, or programs. Applied to social marketing situations, they also have been used to assess social conditions and behavioral processes to provide insights for program development.[19] Public health campaign planners have begun to use focus groups as a first step in needs assessment and audience segmentation.[3,6,21,27]

A focus group typically is composed of seven to ten individuals usually selected as a convenience sample but roughly representative of community groups likely to participate in an intervention.[19] It should be clear that focus group results are not to be interpreted as empirically representative of communities. Their value is in process information about groups that may be useful in further empirical work and in developing strategies. A typical focus group is an open-ended discussion among people united by some common characteristic(s) deemed important to the campaign (e.g., gender, age, occupation, householder status) and is led by a trained moderator working from a schedule of questions. Focus groups typically take about 2 hours (longer is not recommended) and are taped, and a verbatim transcript is produced. The moderator must be trained in group process to assure that everyone speaks and no one is allowed to dominate the group or to impose opinions on others. The advantage of the technique is its open-ended approach: participants are allowed wide latitude in framing questions their own way, in exploring avenues not explicitly sanctioned by the moderator, and in reacting to the comments of others.

In processing the huge amount of information that focus groups generate, Krueger and other experts recommend independent analysis of transcripts by individuals who were not necessarily present at the group session.[19] Experts recommend that an independent analyst read the transcript(s) to note major themes and typical comments and also to debrief the moderator to better understand nonverbal contexts. These results are then compiled and interpreted in a narrative report.

There are several potential pitfalls in the use of focus groups. One is that focus group results can vary greatly depending on the quality of the moderator, time of day the session was conducted, the place, and other factors. Reliability is difficult to gage, although this may be offset by holding more than one focus group with the same types of individuals. Repeated thematic patterns emerging from groups of similar individuals provide some indication of reliability or at least that a full range of responses has been captured.[19] Second, it is often tempting to interpret focus group results as representative of communities, which they are not. Third, focus groups usually generate a wide enough range of opinion and ambiguous material that researchers are often tempted to overinterpret results. When the method is appropriately used, it can provide a fresh and interesting view of the topic of study, often from a viewpoint surprisingly different from that of investigators. It affords the opportunity to examine a topic from the bottom up (the consumer's perspective) and to rethink investigators' preconceptions about the topic.[3]

In the CANDI project, focus groups were used to examine social and behavioral conditions surrounding consumers' food purchase, preparation, and consumption decisions. Specifically, investigators sought to:

1. Develop a more detailed understanding of food behaviors
2. Improve our understanding of the roles of family members as they relate to food
3. Determine in greater depth the beliefs about relations between health and food choice and preparation
4. Find out what attempts at dietary change people had made and their relative success
5. Study the roles food plays in the social life of the community
6. Gain insight into previous community experience with health campaigns
7. Improve understanding of the social, political, and cultural life of the community

Three groups were assembled in the community in early 1988. We recruited single-gender groups, in part because experience suggested that men and women have quite different frameworks based on gender-differentiated roles in household food decision-making. One group was made up of female householders, one of males active in community civic affairs, and one of women involved in health issues because of their social or work roles.

Focus groups provided a richly detailed glimpse into the "food life" of families and the community itself. Major themes were as follows:

- Nutrition knowledge revolved around the "four food groups." Although increasing fruit and vegetable consumption was regarded as a strategy to improve diets, it was much less common for any of the groups to emphasize reduction of high-fat meats and dairy products. The male group agreed that a message encouraging people to reduce red meat consumption would be viewed as a threat to some local farmers and processors.
- Groups expressed little concern about the

health of their diets per se. Most considered their diets (and that of their families) to be relatively healthful but many mentioned snacking, fast foods, and missed meals as common problems. Participants expressed some concern for their children's diets. Homemakers were most concerned, agreeing that neither their children nor their spouses cared much about nutrition. They viewed the quality of their families' diets as primarily their responsibility; however, they also agreed that their ability to improve their families' diets was limited by working outside the home, "lifestyle," children's demands for convenience foods, fragmentation of meals, and the use of treats as rewards for good behavior. Some even told of strategies to hide vegetables under cheese or to refuse to identify a new dish before family members had tasted it.

- The female householder is the primary food gatekeeper, but the male householder has the greatest influence over menu selection. Despite increases in two-income families, the female head of household continues to remain the family gatekeeper for food and health. Women participants reported that when men "help out" in grocery shopping, they are given specific instructions about purchases. Many reported male householders "can't be trusted" to purchase healthful foods without guidance. Although women focus group members said they determined their families' diets in broad outline, they did not feel they controlled it completely or well enough. They reported that spouses had greatest say in the composition of the meals, especially dinner. Most wanted traditional farm-type meals: eggs and sausage or bacon for breakfast, and meat and potatoes for dinner.
- Focus group participants expressed little interest in major dietary change. Although many said they liked to try new foods, they also indicated difficulty in negotiating experimentation with other family members, especially children. Moreover, they reported avoiding preparation of new foods that posed skill difficulties or increased preparation time. Many

reported the need for "new ideas." Those who reported more extensive dietary change explained their reasons as improved health, a response to health problems, or boredom with the same old diet. Those expressing health reasons for dietary change were seldom specific, but a few mentioned decreased heart attack risk and weight loss.

- Of predominantly Scandinavian ethnic origins, the community regards food as intimately tied to the social life of the community. Participants reported frequent dining out and a cultural tradition of serving high-calorie desserts when visiting homes of friends or relatives. Most women reported having a special dish that they prepared for get-togethers. Women participants also reported that although some vegetable or fruit dishes were beginning to be common at many social gatherings, demonstration of culinary expertise continued to be with fancy desserts.
- Participants reported that involvement in community affairs was regarded as a value. Volunteer organizations and service groups— many involved in health issues—were mentioned, as well as a tradition of "pulling together" to solve community problems or to improve the community's quality of life. Many laid this tradition to the community's ethnic and agricultural traditions.
- Most also reported that the community's trust in and attachment to community leaders was strong. Key decision makers were characterized as a relatively small group of people who wield a great deal of influence and work rather quietly to shape the community agenda. Many stated that developing and implementing successful programs in the community would require acceptance by and even direct aid from at least a portion of this leadership group. Some also reported that an informal "coffee shop" communication network existed, helping to keep leaders and others up to date on various community activities.
- Participants reported that the community generally was oriented toward health as the principal community in the region and had sub-

stantial previous experience with health promotion efforts of various kinds, and that there was substantial information available in the community about nutrition and other health issues. Many also reported that supermarkets would likely be open to assisting nutrition interventions. Some mentioned that over the past several years, grocery stores had responded to consumer demands for a broader variety of produce.

Market Survey

To test the generalizability of some of the focus group findings and to examine other areas as well, investigators conducted a random-digit-dial cross-sectional survey in the intervention community between March and May 1988. Respondents were adults 25 to 69 years old, the project's target population. A total of 377 participated in the survey with a response rate of 92%. The same was composed of 45% males and 55% females with a mean age of 43 years. About 43% of the sample reported having a high school diploma or less; 23% reported a college or advanced degree. About 68% of respondents reported being married, and 48% of respondents reported having children under 21 years old living at home. Household income was bimodal: 37% reported annual household income of $10,000 to $25,000 and 29% reported annual household income greater than $35,000.

The survey sought to characterize the community on a number of diet-related dimensions useful in thinking about campaign strategy design:

1. General eating patterns
2. Level of interest in dietary change and salience of diet and health among different groups
3. Role and involvement of the men in food decisions
4. The relative importance of different food attributes (such as cost, convenience, health) in purchase and consumption
5. Level of knowledge concerning dietary improvement strategies
6. Sources of dietary information used by different groups
7. Experience with dietary change
8. Development of an approach to segmenting the audience for strategy development. Several highlights of the survey are summarized in the following pages.

Eating Patterns

Results showed that most respondents ate two or three meals a day with one or two snacks. Lunch and dinner were eaten away from home regularly. Respondents reported buying lunch several times a week; a majority also reported dining out for the evening meal at least once a week.

Dietary Change Interest

The majority of respondents strongly agreed that they liked to try new foods, but there was somewhat less agreement that their families were willing to try new foods, and overall dietary change was less appealing. When asked their personal interest in "changing what you eat," the mean of responses was 5.5 on a 0 to 10 scale from not very interested to very interested. However, nearly half said their interest in changing what they eat had increased over the past year. The personal importance of following a healthy diet was high (7.95 on a 0 to 10 scale). Most respondents felt their current diet was healthy (6.9 on a scale of 0 to 10 of not at all healthy to very healthy).

Roles in Decision-Making

Survey results confirmed focus group findings about the primary role of women in family nutrition. Some 68% of respondents reported that women performed all household shopping and cooking tasks. Only 5% of respondents reported that these tasks were equally shared by men and women.

Food Attributes

We asked survey respondents to rate a series of attributes about food that have been used especially by commercial marketers to understand consumer reasons for underlying food choices. Both open-ended and closed-ended methods were used. The results are shown in Table 4-1.

Table 4-1. Food attribute ranking

	Rank method	Open method
Health	1	1
Family preference	2	2
Taste	3	3
Cost	4	4
Convenience	5	8
Quality/Freshness	—	5
Advertising	—	6
Variety	—	7

The survey found a surprisingly high ranking of health as a reason for choosing different foods. In both closed-ended and open-ended methods, health ranked as the most important factor in the decision. Second most important was family preference, followed by taste. Cost was next, with convenience far behind. This was surprising in light of long-standing commercial research findings that price, taste, and convenience are the three most important factors in food purchases. We interpreted this finding with some caution, however, because interviewers identified themselves as associated with a school of public health.

Knowledge

We assessed knowledge of dietary change strategies by asking respondents in an open-ended question: If someone asked your advice about eating a more healthful diet, what would you tell them to do? The largest category of responses was to eat more vegetables, fruits, breads, and pastas (170 mentions). The next most common response was to reduce fat (90 mentions), followed closely by a general diet change including eating from the "four food groups" or eating balanced meals (88 mentions) and eating leaner meats (82 mentions). In general, some 44% of responses to this question were consistent with program-adopted dietary change guidelines.[9]

Sources of Nutrition Information

Respondents were asked to indicate what sources they would likely consult if they required information about healthy eating. Respondents men-

tioned doctors or health professionals most often (199 mentions), followed by libraries (144 mentions), magazines (92 mentions), local government agencies (76 mentions), books (61 mentions), and newspaper articles or advertisements (27 mentions).

Diet Change Experience

Sixty-eight percent of respondents said they had tried to make changes in their eating habits during the previous year. Those who attempted change felt that they were generally successful (mean score of 6.85). Specific changes mentioned included eating more vegetables, fruits, breads, or pastas (100 mentions); eating leaner meats (68 mentions); consuming fewer calories (63 mentions); reducing fat (38 mentions), snacks, junk food, or fast food (34 mentions); and reducing cholesterol (30 mentions).

Audience Segmentation

Finally, we used the survey to develop an audience segmentation scheme that would be useful in planning intervention strategies. Specifically, we developed scales to divide the audience into groups on the basis of their perceptions of the benefits of dietary change contrasted with their perceptions of the ease of making dietary changes. The scales were based on the constructs of benefits and barriers to health behavior change drawn from the Health Belief Model, but also have analogs in the contruct of self-efficacy drawn from Social Cognitive Theory.[16,29]

A median split on each scale was used to create a 2×2 typology (Fig. 4-1). Respondents were categorized as high or low on the horizontal dimension "ease of making changes" (the degree to which they believed they could make dietary changes with relative ease). Respondents also were categorized as high or low based on the degree to which they believed that dietary change could make a difference to one's health ("change makes a difference"). Finally, groups in each cell were further characterized by examining demographic variables and several additional attitudinal variables.

Respondents in the upper half of the figure be-

Ease of making changes

	High	Low
High	Female = 65% >HS = 64% Npay = 30% 35-44 = 31% No kids =57% Hi comm attach N = 98	Female = 64% Clerical = 37% Prof = 23% 25-34 = 38% Have kids = 56% Hi comm attach Salience + = 53% N = 110
Low	HS < = 57% Npay = 32% 35-44 = 27% 55-69 = 30% No kids = 63% Salience 0 = 63% N = 81	Male = 65% <Col degr = 80% Clerical = 48% 25-34 = 44% 35-44 = 30% Low comm attach Health of diet = lo N= 88

Change makes a difference (row label spanning High/Low)

Figure 4-1. Audience segmentation for a diet change campaign.
From Hertog J and others: Self-efficacy as a target population segmentation strategy in a diet and cancer risk reduction campaign, *Health Communications* (in press).

lieved more strongly than those in the lower half that dietary change makes a difference to one's health. The majority were women, possessed greater formal education, and generally were more involved in their community's civic and political affairs. Respondents in the upper left quadrant ("high" on both scales) in addition were somewhat older, with the majority reporting no children living at home. A significant percentage also reported not working outside the home ("Npay" = 30%). In terms of project goals and strategies, this group possessed very positive attitudes toward dietary changes and indicated relatively few barriers to making them.

Respondents in the upper right quadrant also believed strongly that dietary change makes a difference to one's health but perceived greater barriers to making dietary changes. This group generally was younger, the majority reported children living at home, and most held clerical or professional occupations. A further analysis of this group also showed a majority of two-income households.

Important barriers for this group included time constraints and food preferences of multiple family members. We reasoned that although this group possessed positive attitudes toward dietary change, it would be less likely to make them if strategies failed to encounter these constraints.

Respondents in the lower half of the figure generally believed that dietary change does not make much of a difference to one's health. In the lower left quadrant, however, respondents reported facing relatively few barriers to making dietary changes if they chose to do so. This group was about evenly split between genders, had somewhat less formal education, and was somewhat older. About 63% reported having no children living at home and also relatively unchanged salience for dietary change. Further examination of this group revealed that many were retired and living on fixed incomes ("Npay" = 32%). Although this group's interest in dietary change per se was low relative to the groups in the upper half of the figure, we reasoned that this group's food purchase decisions might be influenced by cost. Therefore, cost incentives including coupons, specials, and the like might be useful in place of an explicit health motivation for dietary change.

Finally, the group in the lower right quadrant scored relatively lower both on perceptions of dietary change benefits and the ease with which they could make them. This group was predominantly male, somewhat less formally educated, younger, and relatively less involved in community political and civic affairs. From the standpoint of project goals, this group appeared likely to be the most difficult to reach group at least directly. However, because the majority reported being married, we reasoned that this group might be indirectly reached through spouses who were more likely to have positive attitudes regarding the benefits of dietary change.

Strategy Development

The focus groups and market survey together confirmed several preliminary directions in developing intervention strategies and also clarified content and appeal issues. First, for about 55% of the survey sample, expectations of benefits from dietary change were positive, but about 53% of the sample overall perceived barriers to making changes. Conversely, 45% indicated less belief in dietary change benefits, whereas about 47% perceived few barriers to changing. This suggested overall a two-front approach: (1) efforts to improve perceptions of the benefits of dietary change and (2) efforts to provide concrete opportunities as well as skills for individuals to make changes but in the context of family, social, and time constraints. Moreover, investigators emphasized development of a relatively simple skills-oriented message about dietary change (see the box at right). This was based in part on survey and focus group results that suggested that community knowledge about healthful eating was generally good, but somewhat less on specifics of what to do.

Along these lines, investigators in conjunction with a community advisory board (described later) developed three main strategies to meet the overall intervention goals:

1. A grocery store–based program including product labeling to make it easier for consumers to identify and purchase products lower in fat, higher in fiber, or both; and in-store food demonstrations

2. A home-based learning program for those interested in more in-depth learning of diet change skills

3. A mass media news and advertising component to promote the grocery store and home-based programs but also to provide a continuing means to emphasize the benefits of dietary change.

The three strategies were designed to increase the likelihood of exposing all groups to the campaign, were integrated in such a way that they promoted one another and made available exposure of increasing intensity, provided evidence of the involvement of community leadership, provided opportunities for people to purchase more healthful foods and to learn other skills without major shifts

INTERVENTION EATING MESSAGE

High fiber

- Eat one or more servings of fruit at each meal; use fruits for snacks and desserts
- Eat one or more servings of vegetables at lunch and dinner
- Eat at least one serving of a high-fiber cereal every day
- Eat at least one of these foods at each meal: whole-grain bread, rice, pasta, or dried beans

Low-fat

- Choose fish, skinned chicken and turkey, and trimmed lean red meats, and keep the amount to 6 oz or less, cooked, per day. Three ounces is about the size of a deck of cards
- Choose low-fat dairy products, including skim, 1%, or 2% milk; low-fat yogurt; ice milk; low-fat frozen yogurt; and low-fat cheese
- If you eat baked goods, try to eat half your usual amount or choose low-fat baked goods such as angel food cake, bagels, or English muffins
- Use half the amount of fat and oil you normally use in cooking and at the table

in personal time, and provided incentives for those somewhat less interested in health per se (e.g., coupons, drawings for free groceries).[10,24]

Community Leadership Survey

The third formative analysis approach discussed here was actually conducted in the community first: a survey of community leaders. The main purpose of this analysis was to assist in the formation of a partnership with community organizations and leaders. Community analysis affords investigators systematic insight into the power and leadership structure of the community and how it may be best mobilized to benefit citizens' dietary change efforts. The purpose of this approach overall is, of course, not only to provide an entrée into communities for effective campaign planning and implementation but also to provide communities with direct experience in health promotion that may carry beyond demonstration projects themselves or into other health arenas.[2]

The approach we used was the "community reconnaissance" method suggested by Nix and Seerly[22] and also discussed in another health campaign context by Finnegan and associates.[7] In brief, principal leaders were identified first by community sector (government, business, education, health and medicine, mass media) and were interviewed about a variety of community issues, concerns, and characteristics. They also were asked to nominate others they regarded as community leaders either generally or in a specific community sector. In all, 15 such interviews were conducted. In addition to providing valuable insight into the community's leadership, decision-making structure, and social concerns, the survey generated a list of more than 120 people regarded as leaders generally or specifically. Of these, about 24 emerged as the most frequently mentioned. From this list, a community advisory board was formed and more formal relationships established with the county health department and extension agent. Finally, a task force of the leading grocers in the community was established to design and implement the in-store portion of the project.

SUMMARY

Formative analysis strategies ought to be central, especially in the early stages of conceptualizing, planning, and implementing public health campaigns. For diet change and other types of campaigns, formative analysis drives a consumer-centered perspective encouraging campaign planners to rethink their preconceptions about social, environmental, and behavioral processes affecting health. It also may provide insights for balancing individual and structural strategies and efforts to build communities' capacity for health promotion. This is particularly important in the area of diet change, where emerging scientific evidence and policy approaches in the near future may make available strategies in addition to traditional educational approaches.

REFERENCES

1. Bauman KE and others: The influence of three mass media campaigns on variables related to adolescent cigarette smoking: results of a field experiment, *Am J Public Health* 81:597, 1991.
2. Bracht N: *Introduction*. In Bracht N, editor: *Health promotion at the community level*, Newbury Park, Calif., 1990, Sage.
3. Brown JE and others: Development of a prenatal weight gain intervention using social marketing methods, *J Nutr Educ* 24:21, 1992.
4. Crawford P: The nutrition connection: why doesn't the public know? *Am J Public Health* 78:1147, 1988.
5. Department of Health and Human Services: *Healthy people 2000: national health promotion and disease prevention objectives*, Washington, DC, 1991, US Government Printing Office.
6. Erikkson CG: Focus groups and other methods for increased effectiveness of community interventions: a review, *Scand J Prim Health Care Suppl* 1:73–80, 1988.
7. Finnegan JR, Bracht N, Viswanath K: *Community power and leadership analysis in lifestyle campaigns*. In Salmon CT, editor: *Information campaigns: balancing social values and social change*, Newbury Park, Calif, 1989, Sage.
8. Finnegan JR, Murray DM, Kurth C, McCarthy P: Measuring and tracking education program implementation: the Minnesota Heart Health Program experience, *Health Educ Q* 16:77, 1989.
9. Finnegan JR and others: Predictors of knowledge about healthy eating in a rural midwestern US city, *Health Educ Res Theory Practice* 5:421, 1990.
10. Finnegan JR and others: Process evaluation of a home-based

program to reduce diet-related cancer risk: the "Win at Home" series, *Health Educ Q* 19(2):233, 1992.

11. Fox K, Kotler P: The marketing of social causes: the first ten years, *J Marketing* 44:34, 1980.

12. Frederiksen LW, Solomon LJ, Brehony KA: *Marketing health behavior: principles, techniques, and applications*, New York, 1984, Plenum Press.

13. Green LW: *Prevention and health education*. In Last JM, editor: *Public health and preventive medicine*, ed 12, New York, 1986, Appleton-Century-Crofts.

14. Green LW, Kreuter MW: *Applications of PRECEDE-PROCEED in community settings*. In Green LW, Kreuter MW, editors: *Health promotion planning: an educational and environmental approach*, ed 2, Mountain View, Calif, 1991, Mayfield.

15. Green LW, Raeburn J: *Communitywide change: theory and practice*. In Bracht N, editor: *Health promotion at the community level*, Newbury Park, Calif, 1990, Sage.

16. Hertog J and others: Self-efficacy as a target population segmentation strategy in a diet and cancer risk reduction campaign, *Health Communication* (in press).

17. Hornick RC: *Alternative models of behavior change* (working paper no 131), Philadelphia, 1990, Center for International, Health, and Development Communication, Annenberg School for Communication, University of Pennsylvania.

18. Kotler P: *Social marketing of health behavior*. In Frederiksen LW, Solomon LJ, Brehony KA, editors: *Marketing health behavior: principles, techniques, and applications*, New York, 1984, Plenum Press.

19. Krueger RA: *Focus groups: a practical guide for applied research*, Newbury Park, Calif, 1988, Sage.

20. Lefebvre CR, Flora JA: Social marketing and public health intervention, *Health Educ Q* 15:299, 1988.

21. Mullis RM, Lansing D: Using focus groups to plan worksite nutrition programs, *J Nutr Educ* 18:532, 1986.

22. Nix HL, Seerly NR: Community reconnaissance method: a synthesis of functions, *J Community Development Society* 2:62, 1971.

23. Novelli WD: *Developing marketing programs*. In Frederiksen LW, Solomon LJ, Brehony KA, editors: *Marketing health behavior: principles, techniques, and applications*, New York, 1984, Plenum Press.

24. Potter JD and others: The cancer and diet intervention project: a community-based intervention to reduce nutrition-related risk of cancer, *Health Educ Res Theory Practice* 5:489, 1990.

25. Rogers EM: *The diffusion of innovations*, New York, 1983, Free Press.

26. Rogers EM, Storey JD: *Communication campaigns*. In Berger CR, Chaffee SH, editors: *Handbook of communication science*, Beverly Hills, Calif, 1987, Sage.

27. Shepherd SK and others: Use of focus groups to explore consumers' preferences for content and graphic design of nutrition publications, *J Am Diet Assoc* 89:1612, 1989.

28. Stipp H, Weinman R: *The effects of mass media information and education campaigns to promote public health: a review of research*. In Blumenthal S, Eichler A, Weissman G, editors: *Women and AIDS: promoting healthy behaviors*, New York, 1989, American Psychiatric Press.

29. Trenkner LL and others: The development of a scale to measure benefits of and barriers to eating behavior change, *Health Educ Res Theory Practice* 5:479, 1990.

30. Wallack L: Social marketing as prevention: uncovering some critical assumptions, *Advances in Consumer Research* 11:682, 1984.

31. Wallack L: *Improving health promotion: media advocacy and social marketing approaches*. In Atkin C and Wallack L, editors: *Mass communication and public health: complexities and conflicts*, Newbury Park, Calif, 1990, Sage.

32. Wasserman J, Manning WG, Newhouse JP, Winkler JD: The effects of excise taxes and regulations on cigarette smoking, *J Health Economics* 10:43, 1991.

33. Windsor RA, Baranowski T, Clark N, Cutter G: *Evaluation of health promotion and education programs*, Palo Alto, Calif, 1984, Mayfield.

34. Winkleby M, Fortmann SP, Barrett DC: Social class disparities in risk factors for disease: eight-year prevalence patterns by level of education, *Prev Med* 19:1, 1988.

PART

2

Delivering Quality Nutrition Services

5

Working Effectively in Cross-Cultural and Multicultural Settings

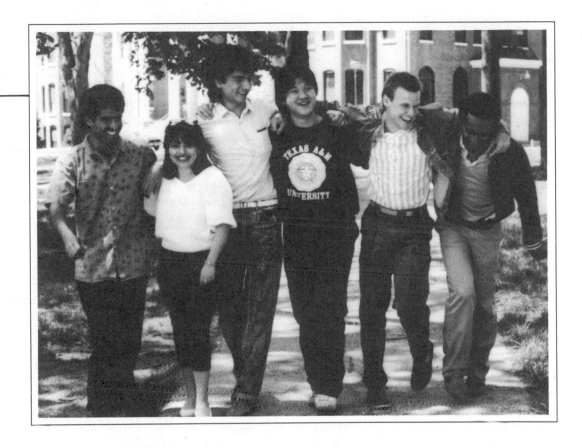

GENERAL CONCEPT

The ability to work effectively with persons from different cultures and in settings where several cultures coexist is of critical importance for dietitians and nutritionists planning to work either within or outside the United States. The cultural issues for community nutrition programming in the United States (or Great Britain) are defined primarily in conjunction with racial or ethnic minority groups and are influenced by the socioeconomic and health status of minority groups as well as the cultural and social climate regarding race relations.

79

OUTCOME OBJECTIVES

When you finish this chapter, you should be able to:

- Understand basic principles of cross-cultural relations.
- State the demographic profiles of U.S. racial and ethnic minority populations.
- Outline the health profiles of U.S. racial and ethnic minority populations.
- Identify steps to take for improving cross-cultural programming skills.
- Use programming approaches that are effective in U.S. minority communities.

The same principles of effective cross-cultural and multicultural programming apply to domestic and international settings, but the application of these principles can be very different in different contexts. This chapter focuses on cultural issues in community nutrition programming within the United States. In the context of this chapter, the term *cross-cultural* refers to situations in which the provider or the provider institution is from the mainstream U.S. culture (generally white, middle-class, of European ancestry) and the client or client population is from a racial or ethnic minority group. However, the issues and principles discussed can be applied more generally to any setting in which different cultural frames of reference are operating. To distinguish situations in which the client population is a relatively homogenous cultural group from those in which several cultural groups are represented, the term *multicultural* is reserved for the latter.

Working effectively with another cultural group requires an awareness of and ability to work around one's own cultural biases, a knowledge of the other culture, and skill in cross-cultural interaction. Cultural biases, as used here, include social class biases, which is relevant because many community nutrition services are delivered to low-income communities. Everyone has cultural biases to some degree. Knowledge of another culture includes assessment of facts not only about the relevant norms, values, world view, and practicalities of the other's everyday life but also about how the services pro-

vided and the providers are viewed by those others. Skill in cross-cultural programming constitutes the translation of this cultural self-awareness and knowledge of the other culture into effective ways of communicating (asking questions and hearing what is said as well as what is not said) and into the ability to think about program design, content, and logistics from a client- or community-centered perspective.

In this chapter we begin by clarifying some key concepts in cross-cultural relations and then discuss practical steps that can be taken to improve competence in cross-cultural relations. We subsequently provide and discuss some selected demographic and health indicators for U.S. racial and ethnic minority groups. The chapter concludes with a discussion of community nutrition programming strategies from a perspective of achieving optimum effectiveness in cross-cultural and multicultural settings.

CONCEPTS AND DEFINITIONS

The original concept of American society incorporates the idea of a mixture of *diverse cultural groups*, that is, groups who have different customs, beliefs about how society and the people within it should function, and, in some cases, languages and nonverbal communication styles. The founding fathers primarily had religion and language diversity in mind. Over time, the traditional view of American society became one of a *melting pot* in which cultures mix and blend through intermarriage, the economy, and education to produce a new culture[30] and, further, in which the norms and values of the Anglo-Saxon population segment would be the point of reference. In contrast with this older view, demographic and cultural realities have led to a new, more culturally pluralistic view of Amercian society in which the value to individuals and to society of preserving ethnic differences is recognized. This changing view of diversity in American society has profound implications for the way educucation and health services are delivered. Under the view of American society as a melting pot, the professional's role, even responsibility, would be to foster *cultural assimilation* (adoption of mainstream attitudes and behaviors), which translates into a scenario where the burden is on the minority client to move toward the mainstream. In W.M. Parker's words, the result is that service providers have a hidden agenda, "a plan to fix minority clients so that they begin to think, feel, and behave as white people do."[34] With a view of America as culturally pluralistic, the burden is on the professional to work with the client or community so that services are delivered in a manner compatible with the client's cultural and situational framework. The latter view is now clearly the dominant one, driven partly by a lack of *structural assimilation* (integration into the social structure) of minority populations and partly by the continuous influx of immigrants from other cultures, as well as by specific actions on the part of the federal government.

Numerous articles in the nutrition and health services literature of the 1980s and 1990s advocate increased attention to and respect for cultural differences.* Even if one is not motivated by a sense of equity, recognition of the powerful influence of culture on food- and health-related behaviors remains necessary on practical grounds. Programs that inadequately address cultural norms and values simply do not work.

Although harsh-sounding to Americans who pride themselves on being fair and unprejudiced, the concepts of *cultural imposition* and *ethnocentrism* are an essential part of the dialogue on cross-cultural programming.[28] In 1970, Leininger described cultural imposition—"the tendency for health personnel to impose their beliefs, practices, and values upon another culture because they believe that their ideas are superior to those of another person or group"—as one of the most serious continuing problems in the health field and one largely unrecognized by many health practitioners.[28] She refers to the deliberate cultural imposition associated with political domination (e.g., British or American colonization) and to the less clearly intentional cultural imposition that occurs when Western health practitioners attempt to introduce new ideas and services to people in developing countries without fully recognizing and accounting for indigenous, culturally embedded health care values and norms.

Ethnocentrism can be defined as "the universal tendency for any people to put its own culture and society in a central position of priority and worth"[20] or as the tendency for people "to see their own way of doing things as the only way of doing things."[1] Implicit in the concept of ethnocentrism is "the tendency to evaluate other cultures in terms of one's own and to conclude that the other cultures are inferior."[1] The current culturally pluralistic view of American society moves us away from the ethnocentric superiority implications of the Anglo-Saxon–oriented melting pot concept. Nevertheless, the context of community nutrition practice is very conducive to ethnocentric attitudes and practices on the part of the professionals involved, that is, attitudes that what is offered by the health care system is superior to and preferred over existing practices of the client or the community. Clients, in general, are at the powerless end of the hierarchy in the traditional service delivery model. When, as in most federally funded nutrition programs, eligibility for services is limited to persons with low incomes, negative attitudes about poor persons may contribute to the perceived inferiority of the client, and such perceptions can be aggravated when the poor person is also a member of a stigmatized minority group. The high value attached to objective scientific evidence in mainstream American culture also means that advice or prescriptions made "from a sound scientific perspective" will be viewed as superior to client beliefs and practices. Thus, dietitians and nutritionists and other health professionals who want to work effectively in cross-cultural settings must be vigilant in evaluating their own ethnocentrism and take deliberate steps to work around it.[28]

PRINCIPLES OF CULTURALLY SENSITIVE PROGRAMMING

Experts in cross-cultural training recognize that most people in helping professions and management positions, although not immune to ethnocentrism that affects all human beings, can be

*References 2, 3, 11, 14, 22, 23, 28, 36, 37, 44.

STEPS TOWARD INCREASING CROSS-CULTURAL COMPETENCE

Increasing personal readiness

- Cultural self-awareness
- Comfort level in cross-cultural situations
- Awareness of stereotypes and of your own stereotypic beliefs
- Willingness to learn from others
- Learning to value differences

Acquiring cultural knowledge

- Learning about other cultures
- Assessing how people in other cultures view you and your culture
- Sharing experiences with persons from other cultural groups
- Finding common ground with persons from other cultures

Developing cross-cultural interaction skills

- Verbal communication
- Nonverbal communication
- Flexibility
- Overcoming fears
- Obtaining feedback

Maintaining cross-cultural alertness

- Regular evaluation of your own feelings and reactions
- Continued assessment of overall climate for race relations
- Setting incremental goals toward increased appreciation of cultural differences
- Building cultural bridges extending beyond professional boundaries and into your personal sphere
- Remaining well informed about the client populations

Adapted from references 17, 22, 34, 35, 44.

helped to become more effective in cross-cultural interactions by progressing through three stages of development: increasing knowledge, increasing awareness, and increasing skill.[17,34,35] We have added a fourth stage, "maintaining cross-cultural alertness," and have given our interpretation of the steps at each stage (see box above) in the following paragraphs. The objective here is not to duplicate the cross-cultural training guidelines contained in manuals on the subject but rather to provide a sense that improving cultural competence is within everyone's reach, given the appropriate motivation and willingness to learn and to be challenged by new experiences.

Increasing Personal Readiness

Cultural Self-Awareness

Although there are overt aspects of culture (e.g., traditional clothing or rituals), a great deal of culture is subconscious and invisible to members of the cultural group. Checklists, such as the one given in the box on p. 83, can be helpful for learning to identify the more subtle aspects of one's cultural framework. Mithun used this checklist to compare Jewish-American, Chinese-American,

Black American, Puerto Rican, and Mexican-American cultures. Each culture was rated as being in "high," "some," or "low or little" agreement with the general U.S. pattern. Black American culture, for example, was scored as having low or little agreement with the mainstream (white Anglo-Saxon) culture on 12 of these 20 attitudinal factors, whereas Jewish culture was scored as being in high agreement with the general U.S. pattern on 15 of these factors. Recognizing that these attitudes are culturally driven is an important first step in increasing self-awareness of attitudes promoted by one's own culture and how they may differ from those of another. The temptation to consider one's own cultural attitudes to be the "correct" ones (e.g., placing a high value on punctuality or on thrifty) should become obvious once one begins this process.[31]

Comfort Level in Cross-Cultural Situations

Another step in the process of increasing self-awareness is for a person to determine how bound he or she is within a culturally ingrained way of perceiving things as opposed to being relatively comfortable in situations that permit or are domi-

A CHECKLIST FOR IDENTIFYING CULTURAL DIFFERENCES IN ATTITUDES

What are your attitudes toward . . . ?

Assess the attitudes of some of your relatives and colleagues. Take note of the difficulty you encounter.

Picture yourself in a meeting with representatives from the community. Do you have at least a rough idea of the types of attitudes you might encounter in relation to the issues listed below or as to whether these attitudes might be different from yours? How could you find this out? Is what you think you know based on knowledge or on stereotypes?

- Time
- Education
- Work
- Aggressive behavior
- Expression of emotion
- Competition
- Innovation
- Sexual behavior
- Self-reliance
- Self-sufficiency
- Individualism
- Industriousness
- Supernatural phenomena
- Status seeking
- Sobriety
- Thriftiness
- Authority
- Independence
- Intermarriage
- Children

Adapted from Mithun JS: *The role of the family in acculturation and assimilation in America: a psychocultural dimension*. In McCready WC, editor: *Culture, ethnicity, and identity: current issues in research*, New York, 1983, Academic Press.

nated by other cultural attitudes. Parker's "multicultural interaction index" for self-evaluation on a low, moderate, or high comfort level with ethnic differences includes items such as how comfortable a person would feel having an ethnically different person for a personal physician or a spouse or attending a religious service of a culturally different group.[34]

Awareness of Stereotypes

Stereotyping can be defined as "the categorization of individuals in ways that ignore their uniqueness and limit their potential."[34] It may be easier to practice identifying stereotypes used in your family or work about any group of people, for example, about old people or young people, Northerners or

Southerners, people from certain neighborhoods, rich versus middle-class persons, or men or women before trying to assess your own tendency to stereotype persons of other races. Analyze stereotypes in terms of their content and how rigidly or aggressively they are promulgated. Keep in mind that overly positive stereotypes can be as damaging as negative ones (for example, expecting all Asian-American students to be very smart in math can be as problematic as expecting all African-American students to be academically weak in this area). Develop a plan, not to rid yourself of stereotypes (which may be unrealistic), but to bring them out into the open. Also, listen carefully to see whether other groups have stereotypes about you. Find the unfairness and illogic in these stereotypes, try to neutralize them, and assess your reactions.

Learning to Value Differences

Practice seeing the positive side of diversity about things such as clothes, music, cars, architecture, hair designs, and foods—areas that are not as politically charged as race relations—and then try to think of human diversity in the same light. Think of people as "of many colors" rather than as "nonwhite." Recognize the inherent ethnocentricity in a term such as *nonwhite*, which implies that being white is the primary ethnicity from which others deviate.

Acquiring Cultural Knowledge
Learning About Other Cultures

Use the checklist of attitudes in the box at left to seek and catalog information about how these attitudes differ between your culture and another. This information can come from reading, observation, sharing experiences with persons from other cultures, and talking with others and can go a long way toward contradicting latent stereotypes and helping to anticipate issues that arise in cross-cultural interactions. See if you can list some alternative cultural values for each area listed in the box (e.g., competition versus cooperation; being emotionally expressive versus masking one's emotions). Focus on positive differences, not just on factors that might serve as barriers to the effectiveness of an intervention. Test your assumptions through discussions with others. Try to identify the more subtle cultural differences, such as body language, eye contact, and attitudes toward how the world is organized, rather than focusing only on the more obvious, external cultural expressions such as ethnic foods or language. An example used by Rody illustrates the point of differences in cultural values about competition: "When Micronesian children run a race, you may see the leaders looking back over their shoulders. They are not worried about someone catching up with them; they are making sure that they do not get too far ahead. To do so would be showing off. Social control of *individual* [emphasis added] achievements is strong."[40]

Recognize that what may appear to be small differences between otherwise similar persons sharing the same environment may actually represent significant variations in the way a particular interpersonal interaction or social transaction is viewed. For example, the cultural gap between black and white Americans can be described as "narrow but deep" in that language, eating patterns, and ways of living that overlap considerably may conceal deep-seated differences in underlying outlook, value systems, and change options.

Assessing How Other Cultures View You

There is usually a history between groups that affects how members from one cultural group view and interact with those from another. For example, are you seen as a do-gooder who derives satisfaction from seeing others' misery? In spite of any efforts on your part, are you viewed as an extension of an institution that has a bad reputation in the community, whether earned or not?

Finding Common Ground

Finding common ground does not mean finding aspects of other cultures that are like yours. We can create a false comfort level for ourselves by emphasizing to persons from other cultures how much they are "just like us," giving a message that the person can please us by suppressing differences. This closes off communication or throws it

out of balance. Finding common ground means establishing in your professional approach an access region in which the people are able to meet you on mutual terms. In practice this means developing ways of dealing with people in which elements of communication and behavior are evaluated as objectively as possible, suspending the value judgments that ordinarily take place in a cultural perspective, and freeing the practitioner to accept communications or behaviors at face value. For example, a person's interdependence with other family members might be viewed negatively as passivity or low self-esteem and rejected by a practitioner from a culture that places a high value on personal independence. However, when the professional and client meet in an access zone in which the professional is vigilant against the tendency to impose such value judgments, interdependence might be accepted without prejudice and recognized as an important factor in treatment.

Developing Cross-Cultural Interaction Skills
Verbal Communication

People born in the United States are generally monolingual, requiring that persons whose native language is not English speak English in order to communicate. Although the overall ethic of acculturation to an Anglo-Saxon orientation has softened, the view that persons living in the United States must ultimately learn to communicate in English is still firmly held. To some this may seem to obviate any need to be able to communicate with even very recent immigrants from non–English-speaking countries in their own language. However, as a practical matter, being able to communicate with people in their native tongue is indispensable for effective programming and does not necessarily deter people from learning English.

Cultural differences in language usage and connotations and in literacy level also affect communications among native English speakers. What is said may be misunderstood or not understood, even though the words used are familiar to both parties. Strategies to avoid communication problems include being informed about potential problems of this type, using the most widely understood terminology wherever possible, and using a communication style that builds in numerous opportunities to obtain direct feedback from the client as to what has been heard and understood.[9]

Nonverbal Communication

Nonverbal communications—messages communicated through silence, distance, eye contact, facial expressions, touching, or position of the body—can be as complicated and potentially damaging to effective cross-cultural relations as verbal communications.[44] Persons working in cross-cultural settings should be keenly aware of the nature of nonverbal communication and of the potential pitfalls of interpreting nonverbal behaviors outside one's known cultural context. A person from one culture may expect some periods of silence during a conversation, whereas a person from another culture may find silence awkward and search for something to fill the void as quickly as possible. A close seating arrangement in an office or a room may be uncomfortable for a client from a culture that prefers a greater physical distance between people. With respect to eye contact, looking directly at someone from a culture that finds it inappropriate may seem intimidating or rude. Not looking directly at someone who expects it may be interpreted as trying to conceal something or being uninterested. Different patterns of preferred eye contact among black, white, and Native Americans have been described. Informality such as addressing someone you have just met by their first name may be inappropriate in some cultures and therefore be interpreted as showing disrespect.

Being Flexible

Working with others requires sufficient flexibility to respond to them as things progress rather than only in ways that are predetermined from the outset. One way to promote flexibility is to have realistic expectations about what you can accomplish and to be able to modify those expectations when indicated. Also, it is necessary to respect people's rights to think and feel in unique ways in order to be willing to modify your approach in response to what is presented by the client. In addition, be-

cause people who are angry or upset tend to be rigid, it is important to ride out situations in which your emotions become aroused until things can be discussed in perspective. To anticipate such situations, make a list of things that upset you or your co-workers and evaluate them.

Overcoming Fears

Fears are among the primary factors predisposing to inflexibility. A person who is uncertain of his or her ability to be effective with another cultural group might be afraid to work with that group. A person who feels unable to overcome prejudice against members of a certain group may try to avoid working with this group for fear that this underlying prejudice will be revealed. These fears may affect the desire of people to work with clients of other ethnic backgrounds or the desire of middle-class professionals to work with persons from lower socioeconomic groups of the same or different ethnicity. Stereotypes or social conditions may cause a person to fear physical harm from members of a minority group or when working in certain communities. Professionals who are themselves members of minority groups may fear that they will lose status among their colleagues by working too closely with other minorities.

Practitioners should assess their apprehensions about working with clients from other cultures and should express these openly to elicit feedback and suggestions from co-workers about how they might be overcome. It will probably be possible to identify some aspect on which to focus as a first, manageable step. Self-acceptance of the natural tendency to be somewhat fearful in uncertain situations will help in taking things step by step and in avoiding the tendency to overreach by trying to conquer these apprehensions too quickly.

Obtaining Feedback

Always be open for feedback—before, during, and after cross-cultural encounters. View feedback as a way to obtain information about how you are perceived by others, how well you get your message across, and how well you listen. Solicit and attend to as many forms of feedback as possible, from both verbal and nonverbal communication and from both clients and co-workers. Realize that in many cultures open feedback may be considered rude, and critical feedback may reach you only after several meetings or through subtle messages.

Maintaining Cross-Cultural Alertness

The fourth set of steps toward increasing cross-cultural competence consists of strategies to reinforce those already listed as part of an ongoing process. Reevaluation of feelings and reactions is necessary because cultural biases are deeply ingrained and continually resurface and because growth in cross-cultural interaction skills must be incremental over time. Moreover, we are living in a dynamic situation in which cultures are continually interacting and changing and in which the environmental context for delivering programs is continually changing. Given that attitudinal change is a long-term process, the ongoing maintenance of cultural alertness is crucial to attaining effective cross-cultural programs. Also be aware that the process is one-sided in that the client population is not the

active agent here; clients have no professional drive for cross-cultural sensitivity. Their sensitivity is based on their vulnerability to actions and policies of majority individuals and institutions.

UNITED STATES MINORITY POPULATIONS

Demographic Profiles

Racial and ethnic minorities in the United States include persons designated as Black American, Hispanic American, Asian or Pacific Islander American, or Native American/Alaskan Natives in the U.S. census. Current estimates place the aggregate number of persons in these minority groups at 58.2 million, approximately 24% of the U.S. population.[32] The major subgroups in the Hispanic-American and Asian–Pacific Islander categories are shown in Figures 5-1 and 5-2, and selected demographic data for the four major minority groups are in Table 5-1. More than 500 American Indian groups are included in the category Native Americans as well as Eskimos, Aleuts, and Alaskan Indians.[38,45] Native Hawaiians are not usually listed as a separate census category but are grouped with either Native Americans or Asian/Pacific Islanders. Table 5-1 also shows that Asian/Pacific Islanders and Hispanic Americans are the fastest-growing minority populations and have high proportions of immigrants.

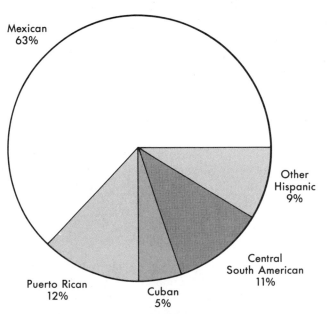

Figure 5-1. Hispanic subpopulations (percent of all Hispanics).

China	India
Japan	Pakistan
Korea	Bangladesh
	Sri Lanka
Philippines	Burma
Vietnam	
Cambodia	Hawaii
Laos	Guam
Thailand	Samoa
Malaysia	Tonga
Singapore	Fiji
Indonesia	Micronesia

Figure 5-2. Asian-Pacific Islander subpopulations in U.S. Census—country of origin.

Table 5-1. Demographic comparison of U.S. racial/ethnic groups

Indicator	White	Black	Hispanic	Asian/Pacific Islander	American Indian
Median age (yrs)	31.6	24.9	23.0	28.7	22.4
% Population growth 1970-1988	6	13	34	70	19
% U.S. born	5	3	29	68	100
% In poverty	12	36	30	13	28
% Of persons > age 25 with 0–8 yrs education	14.1	23.3	15.0	16.4	25.0
% Of persons > age 25 with ≥ 4 yrs of college	19.5	9.5	18.8	32.9	7.7
% Female-headed households	11	38	23	11	25
% Births to mothers < age 20 years	12	25	18	6	22
% Mothers with 4 or more children	9	14	16	11	17

Data are from 1980 or later but in some cases are not for the same year across ethnic groups; taken from references 29, 32, and 38.

Minority populations are generally younger than the majority white population. Therefore, comparisons within age categories or data that have been statistically adjusted to account for age differences are the most useful for comparing health indicators across groups. However, the absolute burden of a problem in a population is a function of the actual age distribution (e.g., a population with proportionately more women in their childbearing years needs more services for pregnant women and children).

The socioeconomic and health profiles of U.S. minorities are disadvantageous relative to those of the majority white population. Minority groups are therefore overrepresented in the service populations of programs targeted to low-income and high-risk groups. For example, although black and Hispanic persons are, respectively, 12% and 8% of the overall U.S. population, black and Hispanic persons comprised 47% (26% and 21%, respectively) of the population served by the Special Supplemental Food Program for Women, Infants, and Children (WIC) in 1988.[12] The proportions of households headed by females, of teenage pregnancies, and of mothers with four or more children

are higher among minority groups than among whites. Educational attainment tends to be lower in minority groups as a whole, although there are wide variations (Table 5-1).

Overall data for Asians and Pacific Islanders do not follow the pattern of socioeconomic disadvantage seen for the other minority groups. However, summary statistics for Asian/Pacific Islander Americans can be very misleading because this category includes population subgroups with markedly different socioeconomic and health profiles. Some subgroups of Asian/Pacific Islanders are better off than the majority population, whereas others are notably disadvantaged. For example, although the median income of the Asian/Pacific Islander population is higher than that of whites, the proportion of Asian Americans with very low incomes is similar to the proportion seen in other minorities and is twice that in whites.[29] This example of problems within certain subgroups being hidden in data for the larger group should be remembered as a general rule for interpreting minority health statistics, because the small numbers in some minority subgroups often result in "oversummarized" data across dissimilar groups.

Regional and community-level differences in the proportion of various minority groups in the population can greatly influence program perspectives. National data show that the composition of minority populations differs in different regions of the country.[38] More than half of black Americans live in the southern United States, fewer than 10% live in the west, and approximately 85% live in urban areas. These data mean that, although black Americans are a minority of the U.S. population overall, they constitute the majority of the population in certain areas (for example, black Americans constitute about 70% of the population of the District of Columbia) and can be approached as a majority population from a programmatic point of view. In other cities or localities throughout the country, different minority populations are in the majority or at least are a larger proportion of the population than in the national averages. In 1980 51% of American Indians lived in the West. The five states with the largest American Indian populations were California (0.23 million), Oklahoma (0.17 million), Arizona (0.15 million), New Mexico (0.11 million), and North Carolina (0.07 million), and American Indians made up 5% to 16% of the populations of Montana, Oklahoma, Arizona, South Dakota, New Mexico, and Alaska. In 1980 Asian/Pacific Islanders made up 61% of the population of Hawaii, 5.7% of the population of California, and 2% to 3% of the population of Washington, Nevada, and New York. Estimates for 1987 indicate that Hispanic Americans made up 37% of the population of New Mexico, 21% of Texas, 19% of California, 16% of Arizona, 12% of Colorado, and from 5% to 10% of Illinois, New Jersey, New York, and Florida.[35]

Health Profiles

One perspective on minority health comes from comparing health indicators among minorities and whites and noting whether minorities have higher or lower rates. This approach was taken by the Secretary's Task Force on Black and Minority Health that resulted in the identification of several nutrition-related health problems—cardiovascular diseases, cancers, diabetes, and infant mortality—

as four of the primary causes of "excess deaths"* among U.S. minority populations,[38] along with homicide, suicide, and cirrhosis of the liver, for which handgun activity or alcohol and drug use were viewed as the major modifiable risk factors.

In making such comparisons, one should keep in mind that the rates in whites may be higher than is desirable in an absolute sense and that bringing rates in minorities into line with those in whites is only an interim objective on the way to bringing overall rates down to acceptable levels. One should also be aware that cross-sectional comparisons of rates may be misleading as to relative group status if disease or risk factor trends are changing over time.[26] For example, during certain periods Black Americans appeared to have had relatively lower rates of deaths from colon cancer than whites, but after several years during which rates increased in blacks and decreased in whites, rates of colon cancer deaths in blacks were higher. Because of problems of low data availability on some groups, inaccuracies in racial and ethnic identification in health statistics (data that contribute to the numerator of disease rates) and the different set of problems in determining how many people are in the population base for calculating certain rates (data that make up the denominator for disease rates), no single data source should be taken as absolute evidence about the status of a minority group. Further, no impression given about the overall status of a minority group in national data should be applied directly as an indicator of the status of specific minority subgroups in a given locality. The importance of local needs assessment to support community-level programming cannot be overemphasized.[16]

With the increased attention to minority health issues as a critical subset of overall U.S. health care issues, national data are more frequently reported in a way that permits comparisons of minorities and

*Excess deaths were defined by comparing death rates in minority populations with those in whites within age and sex groups and calculating the actual number of deaths among minorities that would not have occurred if death rates were comparable to those of whites.

whites or across minority groups. Such data for several health indicators that have implications for nutrition programs (i.e., data relating to infant mortality, heart diseases, cancer, diabetes, tuberculosis, self-related health, and health insurance coverage) are shown in Appendix 5-1 (Tables 5-A through 5-H). Ratios in which rates in the minority population are divided by a comparable rate for whites have been calculated to provide an impression of whether rates in minorities are in "excess," as defined previously, or are equivalent to or below those of whites (either all whites or specifically non-Hispanic whites).

For example, among black Americans (Appendix Table 5-A), almost all health indicators are in the direction of higher risk or poorer health status than whites. Rates of infant mortality and related determinants are approximately twice those in whites. Rates of death from stroke are three times higher in blacks than in whites. Rates of tuberculosis are six times as high in blacks as in whites. Black Americans are 1.8 times more likely to be uninsured than white Americans. More black than white Americans report that they are in only fair or poor health, and this disparity is higher among persons with a high school education or more. The excess occurrence of diabetes, identified in blacks as well as in all other minority groups, is associated with a marked excess incidence of end-stage renal disease in minority populations (not shown in the tables).[43] For example, Teutsch and co-workers estimated that in 1983 to 1985, the rate of occurrence of new cases of end-stage renal disease was four times higher among blacks than whites and seven times higher among American Indians than whites.

Some data for Hispanic Americans are available for separate subgroups such as Mexican Americans, Puerto Ricans, and Cuban Americans (Appendix Tables 5-C to 5-E), but other indexes are reported only for Hispanics overall (Appendix Table 5-B). The consistent picture of a health status disadvantage seen for Black Americans is not observed in Hispanics. Heart disease and cancer death rates are lower among Hispanic than non-Hispanic whites. However, tuberculosis is four times as common among Hispanics than non-Hispanics, and being overweight and having diabetes are also notably more prevalent among Hispanic subgroups. Lower rates of health insurance coverage affect all three Hispanic subgroups.

As for Hispanics, some data for Asian/Pacific Islander Americans is subgroup specific (Appendix Table 5-G), and other data aggregate over the entire group (Appendix Table 5-F). Tuberculosis is a striking area of excess risk in this population, whereas for other indicators shown, this minority group is on par with whites or has a relatively better health status. However, the national data available do not reflect the high prevalence of diabetes in Asians and Pacific Islanders, the high prevalence of obesity in Pacific Islanders, the higher risks of hypertension in Filipinos as compared to some other Asian/Pacific Islander subgroups, or the high risks of cardiovascular diseases and cancers among Native Hawaiians.[8,10,24,38]

Data on Native Americans indicate excess risks in several areas, including infant mortality, diabetes, and tuberculosis (Appendix 5-1, Table 5-H). Diabetes and obesity are widespread problems among American Indians.[5,38] The issue of health insurance coverage is not applicable to Indians eligible for services through the Indian Health Service. However, Indians who do not live in Indian Health Service access areas and who have low incomes may have the same problems of noncoverage observed in other minority groups.

Nutrition priorities compete within the overall priorities in minority communities. Therefore, it is also useful to have a perspective on the relative importance of various health and social problems for minority groups versus the majority population. Ranking of causes of death, shown in Table 5-2, is a crude indicator of differences across population subgroups. The causes of death listed are those ranked 1 to 10 and 12 for white males, as published by the National Center for Health Statistics.[32] The rankings of these causes of death are also shown for white females and for black, American Indian, and Asian/Pacific Islander males and females. Diseases of the heart are the top-ranked cause of death

Table 5-2. Rank for selected causes of death by race and sex, U.S. population, 1988

Cause of death	White	Black	American Indian/ Alaska Native	Asian or Pacific Islander
Males				
Heart diseases	1	1	1	1
Cancers	2	2	3	2
Accidents and adverse effects	3	3	2	3
Strokes	4	5	7	4
Chronic obstructive pulmonary disease	5	9	10	6
Pneumonia and influenza	6	7	8	5
Suicide	7	14	5	7
Chronic liver disease and cirrhosis	8	11	4	11
Diabetes mellitus	9	10	9	9
HIV infection	10	6	15	14
Homicide and legal intervention	12*	4	6	8
Females				
Heart diseases	1	1	1	2
Cancers	2	2	2	1
Strokes	3	3	4	3
Pneumonia	4	6	7	5
Chronic obstructive pulmonary disease	5	11	8	7
Accidents and adverse effects	6	5	3	4
Diabetes mellitus	7	4	5	6
Chronic liver disease and cirrhosis	11	12	6	13
Suicide	12	20	14	10
Homicide and legal intervention	18	19	11	11
HIV infection	24	14	26	25

*The eleventh ranked cause of death in white males was not listed in the data source.
From National Center for Health Statistics: *Health United States, 1990*, DHHS publication (PHS) 91-1232, Hyattsville, Md, Public Health Service, 1991 (comparable data for Hispanics not in source).

for all groups except Asian/Pacific Islander females, for whom this cause ranks second. Among males the top three causes of death are heart diseases, cancers, and accidents, with strokes being among the major disease-related (i.e., as opposed to traumatic) causes of death in all groups. Among females, heart diseases, cancers, and stroke deaths are the top-ranked three causes for all groups shown, except among American Indian females, for whom stroke deaths are displaced to fourth place by "accidents and adverse events." Diabetes deaths are among the top ten causes of death for all groups shown and rank higher among black, American Indian, and Asian/Pacific Islander females than among white females. Other noteworthy differences include the relatively higher rank of deaths associated with chronic liver disease in American Indians and of suicide in American Indian males, the relatively higher rank of HIV infection among black males and females compared to the other groups, and the relatively higher rank of homicide and legal intervention among minority males. The relatively greater traumatic mortality among minority groups may substantially influence their relative risks of dying from chronic diseases. Persons who would ultimately be at risk for heart diseases, cancer, or strokes may die before these risks take effect.

Both the similarities and differences in the rankings should be noted. In regard to similarities, nutrition-related interventions for heart disease, cancer, stroke, and diabetes are of high priority for both men and women in all groups, even though the death rates in some groups are lower than in the white population. However, interventions that are not within the direct purview of nutrition programs, for example, to lower the rates of accidents, homicide, or HIV infection, are also of high priority for many minority communities and may be more immediate on a day-to-day basis. Being sensitive to the nonnutrition priorities that are of particular importance in certain racial and ethnic groups and, where possible, establishing programmatic links so that nutrition priorities are addressed in a comprehensive context will improve the cultural relevance of nutrition programs. Being sensitive to potential differences in disease rates and rankings across racial and ethnic groups and across genders improves the cultural specificity of nutrition programs in multicultural communities. For example, priorities may be different between black and Puerto Rican or between Mexican-American and Filipino-American communities within the same locale or between native-born Asian Americans versus recent immigrants.

ACHIEVING CULTURALLY SENSITIVE AND CULTURALLY SPECIFIC NUTRITION PROGRAMS

It is useful to define both *cultural sensitivity* and *cultural specificity* as two important but somewhat different dimensions of the effectiveness of community nutrition programs. *Cultural sensitivity* can be defined as a characteristic of the service provider: an awareness of cultural factors relevant to interventions in a given population and a willingness to incorporate these factors into program design and implementation. *Cultural specificity* can be defined as a characteristic of an intervention program that results from cultural sensitivity on the part of the provider: the extent to which the program design, content, and delivery strategies incorporate and reflect the specific norms, values, and situational context of the population served by the program. This distinction helps to clarify that the ultimate goal in cross-cultural programming is cultural specificity. Cultural sensitivity is a means to achieving this goal. A key principle to remember in thinking about culturally sensitive and specific programming is that everyone operates within a cultural framework. Approaches for improving the effectiveness of programs involving easily identifiable cultural subgroups are also useful for improving effectiveness within cultural contexts that are less visible. Insights into ways to increase effectiveness with minority groups can lead to general insights about improving community nutrition skills. In one sense the comments that follow simply represent the application of sound community nutrition programming principles in situations where very different cultural frameworks may be operating.

Needs Assessment

Culturally sensitive needs assessment requires knowing what to measure as well as being aware of cultural variables that influence the validity of assessments made. Consistent with approaches described elsewhere in this book, the entire spectrum of factors that potentially influence the effectiveness of nutrition interventions should be assessed in relation to a proposed program (see the box on p. 92). The environmental factors and provider and program variables would be assessed at the institutional or locality level and the client variables through surveys, reference to medical or program records, and specialized techniques such as focus group interviews or discussions with key infor-

FACTORS RELATED TO THE EFFECTIVENESS OF NUTRITION INTERVENTIONS IN MINORITY COMMUNITIES

Environmental variables

- Health care system
- Other health and social problems
- Extant media campaigns
- Risk factors
- Cultural changes in general population

Provider and program variables

- Nature of services offered
- Intervention approach
- Credibility, legitimacy in community
- Structural and cultural accessibility

Client variables

- Family history
- Health problems
- Health insurance coverage
- Income, occupation, education
- Household composition
- Social orientation
- Generation
- Worldview
- Religious beliefs
- Literacy level
- Skill in cross-cultural communication
- Alienation from government
- Health care–seeking practices
- Food preferences and dietary practices
- Food ideology and folk beliefs
- Other health-related attitudes and practices
- Experience with prior programs

Adapted from references 7, 19, 33.

mants like community leaders or client advocates. Environmental and provider variables are intentionally listed before client variables in the box to counteract the tendency toward "victim blaming," in which client behaviors or circumstance are viewed as barriers that make clients seem hard to reach with the approaches that may be the most convenient for or familiar to service providers.[14]

The needs assessment variables in the box are highlighted here because they vary systematically by race or ethnicity and social class. Therefore, it cannot be assumed that these variables are homogeneous among racial or ethnic or socioeconomic status groups within the same locality or that, within the same racial or ethnic or socioeconomic status group, they are similar across localities. Each item in the box is worthy of detailed consideration that is beyond the scope of this chapter. Appendix 5-2 lists resource materials that elaborate further on these variables.

Deciding on the Type of Intervention

The continuum of intervention possibilities extends from a totally provider-centered approach at one extreme to a totally client-centered approach at the other extreme. The most client-centered approaches are oriented towards *empowerment*. Kent defines empowerment "as the capacity to define, analyze, and act on your own problems."[21] Empowerment-oriented interventions are not viewed as necessarily working within existing environmental constraints but rather as challenging these constraints and attempt to remove them. From a culturally sensitive perspective, programs that focus on empowerment are the ideal.

The classical model for empowerment approaches is that of Paulo Freire.[15] A program in a Micronesian community is often cited as an empowerment approach applied in the community. In this program, community residents were helped to understand the system behind the promotion of a commercial soft drink. The resulting motivation to gain more control on this issue led to identification of locally produced coconut milk as a more profitable and nutritious alternative to soft drinks that could be promoted by community residents to the advantage of both merchants and consumers.[40]

Having institutional policies that are culturally sensitive and genuinely oriented toward the goal of improved nutritional status and that take a long- rather than short-term view is critical to the ability to design and implement effective cross-cultural programs. Intervention programs that attempt to empower clients to develop their own analysis and problem-solving approaches generally require more effort, time, and resources as well as an institutional tolerance for decentralized programming, lower cost-efficiency, client-centered attitudes among staff, and a possible apparent lack of results in the short term.[40] Urban gardening programs are another example of programs that attempt to improve dietary intake by helping people to take control of their food resources at the production level.[4]

A review of the literature on programs for "special populations," as minority groups are sometimes termed, provides many useful examples of the effective use of community-based programming strategies. Such strategies can help to achieve programs that, although less ambitious than some that would reach the empowerment ideal, do incorporate the concepts of forming partnerships with the community, seeking solutions from the community, planning *with* rather than *for* the community, and permitting the pace and nature of efforts to achieve the goal to be shaped in the relevant cultural framework.* A clear advantage of such approaches is that they build in legitimacy and credibility and can lead to mechanisms for reaching those who are in the community but currently outside the usual health care delivery system. (See reference 16, Gonzalez et al. Three appendixes list organizations serving diverse cultural communities, activities for training in cultural sensitivity and awareness, and types of community contact.)

Two other important characteristics of effective programs in minority communities are the use of multiple strategies—recognizing that there is not one best strategy for reaching everyone—and integrating or linking programs that address multiple outcomes. Fragmentation of services that results from categorical programming approaches in which separate and often duplicate systems are established to meet different nutrition program objectives is legendary in the United States health and welfare system. Such approaches place a large burden on members of the client group to access all of the different service components they need. The health profiles of minority and low-income populations indicate a coexistence of multiple problems.

*References 6, 7, 13, 18, 19, 25, 27, 39, 41.

Client-centered approaches that reduce artificial divisions and competition among an individual's health problems or among the needs of members of the same family can reduce the burden on the individual or family who needs to access those services.

SUMMARY

Cultural variables potentially apply to all programmatic settings. Within the United States, cultural factors that influence the effectiveness of programs for racial or ethnic minority groups are of particular interest because the health and socioeconomic profiles of these groups are disadvantageous relative to majority population. Health indicators for which rates are higher in Black Americans than in white Americans include infant mortality, deaths from cardiovascular and cerebrovascular diseases and cancer, obesity, diabetes, and other cardiovascular risk factors. Diabetes and, with the exception of some Asian-American populations, obesity are more prevalent in all U.S. minority groups than in whites. End-stage renal disease and tuberculosis are other conditions that disproportionately affect minority populations. Except for those American Indians who have access to services provided by the Indian Health Service, minority populations are less likely than whites to have health insurance.

The now heightened *awareness* of the need to be effective with minority populations reflect the changing demographics of the United States in which minority populations now constitute nearly one fourth of the population overall and the majority of the population in some areas. *Acceptance* of the need to be effective with minority populations reflects the changing image of American society and the realization that the melting pot concept in which ethnic groups acculturate toward an Anglo-Saxon reference culture will probably never take place but, more important, *should* never take place. There is recognition that the suppression of ethnic diversity, largely motivated by ethnocentric devaluing of other cultures, deprives both minority group members and the population as a whole of the richness of a multicultural environment.

The steps toward improving cultural sensitivity

are much easier to outline than to accomplish. A process including cultural consciousness-raising, self-evaluation, unlearning of stereotypes, and relaxation of professional style is needed. Given the willingness to think carefully about and respect cultural differences, the requirements for achieving culturally specific programs include facilitative institutional policies, willingness to extend oneself—psychologically and physically—to the client population, and the willingness and ability to approach program design and implementation in a client-centered and goal-oriented manner.

Maintaining cultural sensitivity and implementing culturally relevant programs will be among the greatest challenges faced by dietitians and nutritionists in the next century. The sociopolitical context for race relations in America and in the world will determine how members of different cultural groups view each other. Competition for resources will determine how far an agency can extend itself by using approaches in which the practitioner's role is to help members of the community identify the problems and develop the solutions. Changing demographics may redefine which cultural groups are in the minority. Changing health patterns among economically advancing minority populations may result in even greater health disparities than are now seen.

REFERENCES

1. Bassis MS, Gelles RG, Levine A: *Sociology: an introduction*, ed 2, New York, 1984, Random House.
2. Berg J, Berg BL: Compliance, diet, and cultural factors among black Americans with end-stage renal disease, *J Natl Black Nurses Assoc* 3:16, 1989.
3. Bertorelli A: Nutrition counseling: meeting the needs of ethnic clients with diabetes, *Diabetes Educ* 16:285, 1990.
4. Blair D, Giesecke CC, Sherman S: A dietary, social and economic evaluation of the Philadelphia Urban Gardening Project, *J Nutr Educ* 23:161, 1991.
5. Broussard BA and others: Prevalence of obesity in American Indians and Alaska Natives, *Am J Clin Nutr* 53:1535S, 1991.
6. Bruerd B, Kinney MB, Bothwell E: Preventing baby bottle tooth decay in American Indian and Alaska Native communities: a model for planning, *Public Health Rep* 104:631, 1989.
7. Burrell-Roberson N: *Outreach programs: community networking.* In *Proceedings of the fourth national conference on cancer nursing*, Atlanta, 1983, American Cancer Society.

8. Curb JD and others: Cardiovascular risk factor levels in ethnic Hawaiians, *Am J Public Health* 81:164, 1991.
9. Doak C, Doak LE, Root JH: *Teaching patients with low literacy skills*, Philadelphia, 1985, JB Lippincott Co.
10. Ernst ND, Harlan WR: Obesity and cardiovascular disease in minority populations: proceedings of conference held in Bethesda Md, August 28-30, 1990, *Am J Clin Nutr* 53(Suppl):1507, 1991.
11. Fleming J: Meeting the challenge of culturally diverse populations, *Pediatr Nurs* 15:566;648, 1989.
12. Food and Nutrition Service, Office of Analysis and Evaluation, United States Department of Agriculture: *Study of WIC participant and program characteristics, 1988, final report, vol 2, detailed tables*, Report prepared by Research Triangle Institute, Contract No 53-3198-7-57, April 10, 1990.
13. Foreyt JP, Ramirez AG, Cousins JH: Cuidando el Corazon: a weight reduction intervention for Mexican Americans, *Am J Clin Nutr* 53:1639S, 1991.
14. Freimuth VS, Mettger W: Is there a hard-to-reach audience? *Public Health Rep* 105:232, 1990.
15. Freire P: *Pedagogy of the oppressed*, New York, 1970, Seabury.
16. Gonzalez VM and others: Health promotion in diverse cultural communities. Palo Alto, Calif, 1991, Health Promotion Resource Center.
17. Harris PR, Moran RT: *Managing cultural differences*, ed 2, Houston, 1990, Gulf Publishing Co.
18. Heath GW and others: Community-based exercise and weight control: diabetes risk reduction and glycemic control in Zuni Indians, *Am J Clin Nutr* 53:1642S, 1991.
19. Hutchins V, Walch C: Meeting minority health needs through special MCH projects, *Public Health Rep* 104:621, 1989.
20. Keesing FM: *Cultural anthropology: the science of custom*, New York, 1965, Holt, Reinhart, and Winston.
21. Kent G: Nutrition education as an instrument of empowerment, *J Nutri Educ* 20:193, 1988.
22. Kittler PG, Sucher KP: Diet counseling in a multicultural society, *Diabetes Educ* 16:127, 1990.
23. Kuhnlein HV: Culture and ecology in dietetics and nutrition, *J Am Diet Assoc* 89:1059, 1989.
24. Kumanyika S: Diet and chronic disease issues for minority populations, *J Nutr Educ* 22:89, 1990.
25. Kumanyika SK, Charleston JB: Lose weight and win: a church-based program for weight and high blood pressure control among black women, *Patient Educ Counseling* 19:19, 1992.
26. Kumanyika SK, Golden PM: Cross-sectional differences in health status in U.S. racial/ethnic minority groups: potential influence of temporal changes, diseases, and life-style transitions, *Ethnicity Dis* 1:50, 1991.
27. Lasco RA and others: Participation rates, weight loss, and blood pressure changes among obese women in a nutrition-exercise program, *Public Health Rep* 104:640, 1989.

28. Leininger M: Becoming aware of types of health practitioners and cultural imposition, *J Transcult Nurs* 2:32, 1991.

29. Lin-Fu JS: Population characteristics and health care needs of Asian Pacific Americans, *Public Health Rep* 103:18, 1988.

30. Luhman R, Gilman S: *Race and ethnic relations: the social and political experience of minority groups*, Belmont, Calif, 1980, Wadsworth.

31. Mithun JS: *The role of the family in acculturation and assimilation in America: a psychocultural dimension*. In McCready WC, editor: *Culture, ethnicity, and identity: current issues in research*, New York, 1983, Academic Press.

32. National Center for Health Statistics: *Health United States, 1990*, DHHS publication (PHS) 91-1232, Hyattsville, Md, 1991, Public Health Service.

33. Nickens HW: Health promotion and disease prevention among minorities, *Health Aff (Millwood)* 9:133, 1990.

34. Parker WM: *Consciousness-raising: a primer for multicultural counseling*, Springfield, Ill, 1988, Charles C Thomas.

35. Pedersen P: *A handbook for developing multicultural awareness*, Alexandria, Va, 1988, American Association for Counseling and Development.

36. Perkin J, McCann SF: *Food for ethnic Americans: is the government trying to turn the melting pot into a one-dish dinner?* In Brown LK, Mussel K, editors: *Ethnic and regional foodways in the U.S.: The performance of group identity*. Knoxville, 1984, Univ. of Tennessee Press.

37. Report of the Expert Panel on Populations Strategies for Blood Cholesterol Reduction: A statement from the National Cholesterol Education Program, National Heart, Lung, and Blood Institute, and National Institutes of Health, *Circulation* 83:2154, 1991.

38. *Report of the Secretary's task force on black and minority health, executive summary, vols 1 and 2, Crosscutting issues in minority health*, US Department of Health and Human Services, August 1985.

39. Robbins K: Heart, body, and soul: the gospel of good health, *Hopkins Med News*, Spring 1991.

40. Rody N: Empowerment as organizational policy in nutrition intervention program: a case study from the Pacific island, *J Nutr Educ* 20:133, 1988.

41. Shintani TT and others: Obesity and cardiovascular risk intervention through the ad libitum feeding of traditional Hawaiian diet, *Am J Clin Nutr* 53:1647S, 1991.

42. Snider DE, Salinas L, Kelly GD: Tuberculosis: an increasing problem among minorities in the United States, *Public Health Rep* 104:646, 1989.

43. Teutsch S, Newman H, Eggers P: The problem of diabetic renal failure in the United States, *Am J Kidney Dis* 13:11, 1989.

44. United States Department of Agriculture: *Cross-cultural counseling: a guide for nutrition and health counselors*, FNS-20, September 1986.

45. United States Department of Commerce, Bureau of the Census: *We, the first Americans*, SuDoc No C3.2:AM 3/9, Washington DC, nd, US Government Printing Office.

APPENDIX 5-1

Selected health indicators in Black and white Americans

Appendix Table 5-A. Selected health indicators in Black and white Americans

Annual indicator	Population subgroup	Rate in Blacks	Rate in whites	Ratio
Infant mortality and determinants				
Beginning prenatal care after first trimester (%)	Pregnant women	39.3	20.7	1.9
Beginning prenatal care in third trimester or no prenatal care (%)	Pregnant women	10.9	5.0	2.2
Live births weighing < 1,500 g (%)	Infants < 1 year old	2.9	0.9	3.2
Live births weighing 1500-2499 g (%)	Infants < 1 year old	10.4	4.7	2.2
Neonatal deaths per 1000 live births	Infants < 28 days old	12.2	5.9	2.1
Postneonatal deaths per 1000 live births	Infants 28 days to 1 year old	6.4	3.1	2.1
Chronic diseases and related risk factors				
Deaths per 100,000 due to heart diseases	Adults 45-64 years old	426	244	1.7
Deaths per 100,000 due to cancer	Adults 45-64 years old	401	289	1.4
Deaths per 100,000 due to strokes	Adults 45-64 years old	86	29	3.0
Undiagnosed diabetes (%)	Adults 45-74 years old	9.3	6.1	1.5
Diagnosed diabetes (%)	Adults 45-74 years old	10.1	5.9	1.7
Overweight (%)	Males 20-74 years old	26.0	24.2	1.1
	Females 20-74 years old	44.0	23.9	1.8
Hypertension (%)	Males 20-74 years old	41.6	33.8	1.2
	Females 20-74 years old	43.8	25.1	1.7
High blood cholesterol (%)	Males 20-74 years old	24.1	24.7	1.0
	Females 20-74 years old	25.0	28.3	0.9
Smokers (%)	Males 18 years and older	39.4	30.9	1.3
	Females 18 years and older	29.1	28.6	1.0

Adapted from National Center for Health Statistics: *Health United States, 1990*, DHHS publication (PHS) 91-1232, Hyattsville, Md, 1991, Public Health Service; and Snider DE, Salinas L, Kelly GD: Tuberculosis: an increasing problem among minorities in the United States, *Public Health Rep* 104:646, 1989.

Appendix Table 5-A. Selected health indicators in Black and white Americans—cont'd

Annual indicator	Population subgroup	Rate in Blacks	Rate in whites	Ratio
Other indexes				
No health insurance (%)	Persons < 65 years old	21.7	12.3	1.8
Poor or fair self-rated health (%)	Adults 45-64 years old with < 12 years education	44.4	31.1	1.4
	With > 12 years education	21.6	10.8	2.0
Tuberculosis case rate per 100,000	All ages	27.6	4.3	6.4

Appendix Table 5-B. Selected health indicators in Hispanic and white Americans

Annual indicator	Population subgroup	Rate in Hispanic Americans	Rate in whites	Ratio
Chronic diseases				
Deaths per 100,000 due to heart diseases	Adults 45-64 years old	166	244	0.7
Deaths per 100,000 due to cancers	Adults 45-64 years old	152	289	0.5
Deaths per 100,000 due to strokes	Adults 45-64 years old	31	29	1.1
Other index				
Tuberculosis case rate per 100,000	All ages	18.7	4.3	4.3

Adapted from National Center for Health Statistics: *Health United States, 1990,* DHHS publication (PHS) 91-1232, Hyattsville, Md, 1991, Public Health Service; and Snider DE, Salinas L, Kelly GD: Tuberculosis: an increasing problem among minorities in the United States, *Public Health Rep* 104:646, 1989.

Appendix Table 5-C. Selected health indicators in Mexican-Americans and white Americans

Annual indicator	Population subgroup	Rate in Mexican Americans	Rate in whites	Ratio
Infant mortality and determinants				
Beginning prenatal care after first trimester (%)	Pregnant women	41.7	20.7	2.0
Live births weighing < 1500 g (%)	Infants < 1 year old	0.9	0.9	1.0
Live births weighing 1500-2499 g (%)	Infants < 1 year old	4.7	4.7	1.0
Neonatal deaths per 1000 live births	Infants < 28 days old	5.7	5.9	1.0
Postneonatal deaths per 1000 live births	Infants 28 days to 1 year old	3.2	3.1	1.0
Cardiovascular risk factors and diabetes				
Undiagnosed diabetes (%)	Adults 45-74 years old	9.6	6.1	1.6
Diagnosed diabetes (%)	Adults 45-74 years old	14.3	5.9	2.4
Overweight (%)	Males 20-74 years old	30.9	24.2	1.3
	Females 20-74 years old	41.6	23.9	1.7
Hypertension (%)	Males 20-74 years old	23.9	33.8	0.7
	Females 20-74 years old	20.3	25.1	0.8
High blood cholesterol (%)	Males 20-74 years old	18.8	24.7	0.8
	Females 20-74 years old	20.0	28.3	0.7
Smokers (%)	Males 18 years and older	30.3	30.9	1.0
	Females 18 years and older	15.5	28.6	0.5
Other indexes				
No health insurance (%)	Persons < 65 years old	34.9	12.3	2.8
Poor or fair self-rated health (%)	Adults 45-64 years old with < 12 years education	31.0	31.1	1.0
	With ≥ 12 years education	14.4	10.8	1.3

Adapted from National Center for Health Statistics: *Health United States, 1990*, DHHS publication (PHS) 91-1232, Hyattsville, Md, 1991, Public Health Service.

Appendix Table 5-D. Selected health indicators in Puerto Rican and white Americans

Annual indicator	Population subgroup	Rate in Puerto Ricans	Rate in whites	Ratio
Infant mortality and determinants				
Beginning prenatal care after first trimester (%)	Pregnant women	36.7	20.7	1.7
Live births weighing < 1500 g (%)	Infants < 1 year old	1.6	0.9	1.8
Live births weighing 1500-2499 g (%)	Infants < 1 year old	7.8	4.7	1.7
Neonatal deaths per 1000 live births	Infants < 28 days old	8.3	5.9	1.4
Postneonatal deaths per 1000 live births	Infants 28 days to 1 year old	4.0	3.1	1.3
Cardiovascular risk factors and diabetes				
Undiagnosed diabetes (%)	Adults 45-74 years old	11.8	6.1	1.9
Diagnosed diabetes (%)	Adults 45-74 years old	14.3	5.9	2.4
Overweight (%)	Males 20-74 years old	25.6	24.2	1.1
	Females 20-74 years old	40.2	23.9	1.7
Hypertension (%)	Males 20-74 years old	21.4	33.8	0.6
	Females 20-74 years old	19.2	25.1	0.8
High blood cholesterol (%)	Males 20-74 years old	17.7	24.7	0.7
	Females 20-74 years old	22.7	28.3	0.8
Smokers (%)	Males 18 years and older	36.7	30.9	1.2
	Females 18 years and older	23.4	28.6	0.8
Other indexes				
No health insurance (%)	Persons < 65 years old	21.4	12.3	1.7
Poor or fair self-rated health (%)	Adults 45-64 years old with < 12 years education	41.4	31.1	1.3
	With ≥ 12 years education	17.3	10.8	1.6

Adapted from National Center for Health Statistics: *Health United States, 1990*, DHHS publication (PHS) 91-1232, Hyattsville, Md, 1991, Public Health Service.

Appendix Table 5-E. Selected health indicators in Cuban and white Americans

Annual indicator	Population subgroup	Rate in Cubans	Rate in whites	Ratio
Infant mortality and determinants				
Beginning prenatal care after first trimester (%)	Pregnant women	16.6	20.7	0.8
Live births weighing < 1500 g (%)	Infants < 1 year old	1.2	0.9	1.3
Live births weighing 1500-2499 g (%)	Infants < 1 year old	4.8	4.7	1.0
Neonatal deaths per 1000 live births	Infants < 28 days old	5.9	5.9	1.0
Postneonatal deaths per 1000 live births	Infants 28 days to 1 year old	2.2	3.1	0.7
Cardiovascular risk factors and diabetes				
Undiagnosed diabetes (%)	Adults 45-74 years old	9.9	6.1	1.6
Diagnosed diabetes (%)	Adults 45-74 years old	5.9	5.9	1.0
Overweight (%)	Males 20-74 years old	27.6	24.2	1.1
	Females 20-74 years old	31.6	23.9	1.3
Hypertension (%)	Males 20-74 years old	20.7	33.8	0.6
	Females 20-74 years old	14.4	25.1	0.6
High blood cholesterol (%)	Males 20-74 years old	16.1	24.7	0.7
	Females 20-74 years old	16.9	28.3	0.6
Smokers (%)	Males 18 years and older	24.0	30.9	0.6
	Females 18 years and older	20.2	28.6	0.7
Other indexes				
No health insurance (%)	Persons < 65 years old	23.3	12.3	1.9
Poor or fair self-rated health	Adults 45-64 years old with < 12 years education	23.1	31.1	0.7
	With ≥ 12 years education	13.1	10.8	1.2

Adapted from National Center for Health Statistics: *Health United States, 1990*, DHHS publication (PHS) 91-1232, Hyattsville, Md, 1991, Public Health Service.

Appendix Table 5-F. Selected health indicators in Asian and white Americans

Annual indicator	Population subgroup	Rate in Asian Americans	Rate in whites	Ratio
Chronic diseases				
Deaths per 100,000 due to heart disease	Adults 45-64 years old	99	244	0.4
Deaths per 100,000 due to cancers	Adults 45-64 years old	159	289	0.5
Deaths per 100,000 due to strokes	Adults 45-64 years old	29	29	1.0
Smoking				
Smokers (%)	Males 18 years and older	24.9	30.9	0.8
	Females 18 years and older	11.9	28.6	0.4
Other indicators				
No health insurance (%)	Persons < 65 years old	16.3	12.3	1.3
Poor or fair self-rated health (%)	Adults 45-64 years old with < 12 years education	23.2	31.1	0.7
	With ≥ 12 years education	8.9	10.8	0.8
Tuberculosis case rate per 100,000	All ages	48.1	4.3	11.2

Adapted from National Center for Health Statistics: *Health United States, 1990*, DHHS publication (PHS) 91-1232, Hyattsville, Md, 1991, Public Health Service; and Snider DE, Salinas L, Kelly GD: Tuberculosis: an increasing problem among minorities in the United States, *Public Health Rep* 104:646, 1989.

Appendix Table 5-G. Selected health indicators in Japanese, Chinese, Filipino, and white Americans

Annual indicator	Population subgroup	Rate in Japanese Americans	Rate in Chinese Americans	Rate in Filipino Americans	Rate in whites	Ratio
Beginning prenatal care after first trimester (%)	Pregnant women	13.7	17.6	21.6	20.7	0.7
Live births weighing < 1500 g (%)	Infants < 1 yr old	0.9	0.6	0.9	0.9	1.0
Live births weighing 1500-2499 g (%)	Infants < 1 year old	5.8	4.1	6.2	4.7	1.2
Neonatal deaths per 1000 live births	Infants < 28 days old	3.4	4.3	5.3	5.9	0.6
Postneonatal deaths per 1000 live births	Infants 28 days to 1 year old	2.6	3.1	2.9	3.1	0.8

Adapted from National Center for Health Statistics: *Health United States, 1990*, DHHS publication (PHS) 91-1232, Hyattsville, Md, 1991, Public Health Service.

Appendix Table 5-H. Selected health indicators in American Indians/Alaska Natives and white Americans

Annual indicator	Population subgroup	Rate in American Indians/ Alaskan Natives	Rate in whites	Ratio
Infant mortality and determinants				
Beginning prenatal care after first trimester (%)	Pregnant women	41.9	20.7	2.0
Beginning prenatal care in third trimester or no pre-natal care (%)	Pregnant women	12.0	5.0	2.4
Live births weighing < 1500 g (%)	Infants < 1 year old	1.0	0.9	1.0
Live births weighing 1500-2499 g (%)	Infants < 1 year old	5.0	4.7	1.0
Neonatal deaths per 1000 live births	Infants < 28 days old	6.7	5.9	1.1
Postneonatal deaths per 1000 live births	Infants 28 days to 1 year old	7.2	3.1	2.3
Chronic disease mortality				
Deaths per 100,000 due to heart diseases	Adults 45-64 years old	224	244	0.9
Deaths per 100,000 due to cancer	Adults 45-64 years old	183	289	0.6
Deaths per 100,000 due to strokes	Adults 45-64 years old	31	29	1.1
Deaths per 100,000 due to diabetes	All ages	25.8	10.1*	2.6
Smoking				
Smokers (%)	Males 18 years and older	36.5	30.9	1.2
	Females 18 years and older	30.6	28.6	1.1
Other Indexes				
% with poor or fair self-rated health	Adults 45-64 years old with < 12 years education	39.6	31.1	1.3
	With ≥ 12 years edu-cation	18.7	10.8	1.7
Tuberculosis case rate per 100,000	All ages	20.0	4.3	4.7

*Rate for United States, all races.
Adapted from Trends in Indian Health, 1991; National Center for Health Statistics: *Health United States, 1990*, DHHS publication (PHS) 91-1232, Hyattsville, Md, 1991, Public Health Service; and Snider DE, Salinas L, Kelly GD: Tuberculosis: an increasing problem among minorities in the United States, *Public Health Rep* 104:646, 1989.

APPENDIX 5-2

Resources for in-depth information on variables and issues of special relevance to interventions in U.S. minority or low socioeconomic status groups

American Association for Retired Persons Minority Affairs Institute: *A portrait of older minorities*, Washington, DC, 1988, American Association for Retired Persons.

American Heart Association: Special report on cardiovascular diseases and stroke in African-Americans and other racial minorities in the United States: a statement for health professionals, American Heart Association medical/scientific statement, *Circulation* 83:1463, 1991.

Axelson ML: The impact of culture on food-related behavior, Ann Rev Nutr 6:345, 1986.

Brown LK, Mussell K, editors: *Ethnic and regional foodways in the United States*. In *The performance of group identity*, Knoxville, 1984, University of Tennessee Press.

CDC Minority Health Office: Social epidemiology, JAMA 263:2565, 1990.

Coreil J, Mull JD: *Anthropology and primary health care*, Boulder, Colo, 1990, Westview Press.

Freimuth VS, Mettger W: Is there a hard-to-reach audience? *Public Health Rep* 105:232, 1990.

Gillick MR: Common-sense models of health and disease, *N Engl J Med* 313:700, 1985.

Health education approaches to culturally diverse populations. In *Proceedings of the 1980 forum on hypertension in minority populations*. Washington, DC, 1980, Department of Health and Human Services, National High Blood Pressure Education Program, National Heart, Lung, and Blood Institute, and National Institutes of Health.

Helman CF: *Culture, health, and illness: an introduction for health professionals*, Boston, 1990, Wright.

Indian Women's Health Issues: *Final report of a roundtable conference sponsored by the Indian Health Service Offices of Planning, Evaluation, and Legislation and of Health Program Research and Development*, Washington, DC, 1991, Kaufman and Associates.

Kittler PG, Sucher K: *Food and culture in America*, New York, 1989, Van Nostrand Reinhold.

Matthews HF: Rootwork: description of an ethnomedical system in the American South, *South Med J* 80:885, 1987.

Nickens HW: Health promotion and disease prevention among minorities, *Health Aff (Millwood)* 9:133, 1990.

Payne KW, Ugarte CA: The Office of Minority Health Resource Center: impacting on health-related disparities among minority populations, *Health Educ* 20:6, 1989.

Snow LF: Folk medical beliefs and their implications for the care of patients, *Ann Intern Med* 81:82, 1974.

Thomas SB: Community health advocacy for racial and ethnic minorities in the United States: issues and challenges for health education, *Health Educ Q* 17:13, 1990.

"To what extent is lactose intolerance a significant problem among different ethnic groups, e.g., Asians, Hispanics, American Indians, and Alaskan Natives?" Technical paper No 11, in Guthrie HA, Kumanyika SK, Picciano MF, Smiciklas-Wright H, editors: *Review of WIC food packages*, prepared for the Food and Nutrition Service, U.S. Department of Agriculture, under cooperative agreement No 58-3198-1-006, 1991.

United States Department of Agriculture: *Cross-cultural counseling: a guide for nutrition and health counselors*, FNS-20, Sept 1986.

White SL, Maloney SK: Promoting health diets and active lives to hard-to-reach groups: market research study, *Public Health Rep* 105:224, 1990.

Maternal Nutrition

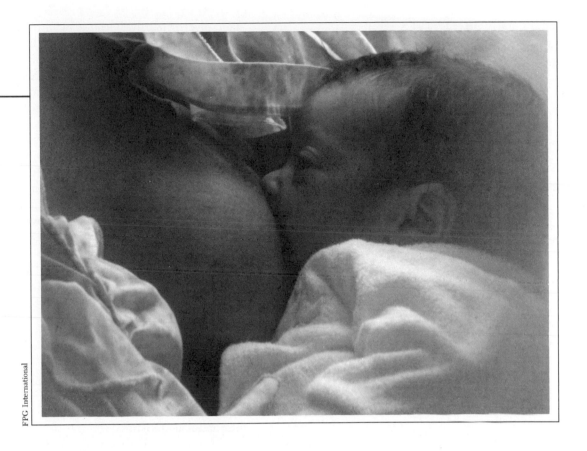

GENERAL CONCEPT

Nutrition has a broad influence on reproduction. The nutritional status of women affects fertility, the course of pregnancy, and fetal growth and development. The importance of nutrition extends to the period of lactation, when the composition of human milk and the duration of breastfeeding depend, in part, on maternal nutritional status.

Presented in this chapter is an overview of the status of outcomes of pregnancy in the United States. Relationships between maternal nutritional status, the course and outcome of pregnancy, and nutrition and lactation are summarized. Nutritional needs of women during and after pregnancy are highlighted. Risk factors for reproductive problems and specific recommendations for patient management are included in this chapter. Health policies and guidelines related to maternal nutrition are summarized, and model programs for service delivery described.

OUTCOME OBJECTIVES

When you finish this chapter you should be able to:

* Comprehend the importance of nutrition during reproduction.
* Know the key nutritional factors that influence pregnancy and lactation.
* Understand nutritional guidelines and recommendations for women during and after pregnancy.
* Identify public policy goals and guidelines that bear directly on the development and delivery of maternal nutrition services.
* Review the effectiveness of existing maternal nutrition programs and services and improve the effectiveness of nutrition services in the future.

PREGNANCY OUTCOMES IN THE UNITED STATES

A large part of the rationale for improving the nutritional health of women before and during pregnancy stems from data that link maternal nutrition to infant outcome. The importance of optimizing maternal nutrition is demonstrated by the relatively high proportion of poor infant outcomes in the United States.

The Status of Infant Health in the United States

*Infant mortality is the most
sensitive index we possess of
social welfare and sanitary
administration.*

Newsholme, 1910

Infant mortality rates (the number of liveborn infants who die within the first year of life per 1000 births) have long been used as an indicator of the health status and quality of life of populations. They are also used as a measure of the nutritional status of populations and population subgroups. Infant mortality rates tend to decline within a population as quality of life—reflected in standards of housing and health care, sanitation, nutritional health, income, and education—improves. Between 1900 and 1950, infant mortality rates in the United States and other industrialized countries dropped sub-

stantially, primarily because of improvements in the quality of life. In approximately 1970, declines achieved in the rate of infant mortality in the United States began to reflect advances in neonatal intensive care and the saving of infants who would have had little chance for survival in previous years. Rather than sustain efforts to decrease infant mortality through further improvements in quality of life, as was done by a number of European countries, Japan, and Canada, U.S. health care policy directed resources toward medical care of ill newborns. Although the decline in infant mortality in the United States attributed to advances in medical care averaged 4% per year between 1970 and 1982, the rate achieved was less than that of countries such as Sweden, France, Japan, and Canada.

The rate of decline in infant mortality in the United States began to flatten in 1981 and corresponded to reductions in funding for several public health programs for women and infants.[13] The relatively low rate of decline in infant mortality has placed the United States in twenty-first place in the World Health Organization's ranking of infant mortality rates by country (Table 6-1). Ten years earlier, the United States ranked sixteenth in the international statistics.

The underlying reason for the relatively poor infant mortality rates in the United States has been attributed to the proportion of U.S. infants born with low birth weights.

Birth Weight and Health

Birth weight is by far the strongest predictor of infant well-being and is related to death and illness through the early childhood years. Minimum infant mortality occurs among infants who weigh 3500 to 4000 g at birth (Figure 6-1), a range that does not contain the median birth weight of U.S. newborns. Infants born small are at far greater risk of death and disorders than infants born large. The problem in the United States is that too many infants are born small. Their smallness is mainly due to fetal growth retardation, prematurity (delivery before 37 weeks of gestation), or a combination of both. In 1987, 6.9% of U.S. infants were born with low birth weights, that is, weighed less than 2500 g (5.5 lb),

Table 6-1. Births and infant mortality rates in 28 countries with populations greater than 2,500,000 and infant mortality rates less than 15 in 1988

Country (listed in order of 1988 infant mortality rate)	Births*		Infant mortality rate	
	No.	Rate	1989†	1988
Japan	1,243,000	10.1	4.4	4.8
Sweden	115,900	13.6	6.0	5.8
Finland	63,388	12.8	5.8	6.1
Switzerland	81,200	12.2	6.8	6.8
Singapore	52,822	20.0		7.0
Canada	375,743	14.5		7.2
Hong Kong	75,625	13.3	7.4	7.4
Netherlands	188,999	12.7	6.8	7.5
German Federal Republic	677,407	10.9		7.5
Denmark	59,196	11.5	8.4	7.6
France	770,690	13.8		7.7
Austria	87,930	11.5	8.3	8.1
German Democratic Republic	198,922	12.0	8.6	8.1
Norway	59,227	14.0		8.4
United Kingdom	777,300	13.6	8.4	9.0
Belgium	117,402	11.9		9.1
Spain	434,490	11.2		(1986) 9.2
Ireland	51,659	14.7	7.7	9.2
Australia	250,926	14.9		9.2
Italy	568,291	9.9		9.5
United States	4,021,000	16.2	9.7	10.0
Israel	100,500	22.3	10.0	10.0
New Zealand	58,091	17.5	10.2	10.7
Greece	107,668	10.8		11.0
Cuba	184,892	17.6	11.3	11.9
Czechoslovakia	208,552	13.3	11.3	11.9
Portugal	122,121	11.9		13.1
Bulgaria	117,440	13.1		13.6

From Wegman ME: Annual summary of vital statistics: 1989, *Pediatrics* 86:835, 1990.
Data from United Nations Statistical Office. Birth rate per 1000 population; infant mortality rate per 1000 live births.
* Data for 1989 or latest available year.
† Provisional.

and 10.2% were premature. More than half of all infants born in the United States weigh less than 3500 g. Since 1980, rates of prematurity have trended upward while rates of low-birth-weight infants have stabilized. The slight improvement in birth weights of U.S. infants over the past decade has been hidden by increasing rates of prematurity.[1]

Any presentation about the health status of U.S. infants would be incomplete if it failed to address the disparities between American black and white infants (Table 6-2). Average birth weights of black infants are 240 g less than white infants. Twice as many black infants are born weighing 1500 to 2499 g, and three times more black infants weigh less than 1500 g than white infants. Rates of infant mortality, prematurity, and low birth weight are more than twice as high in American blacks than in whites, and the rate of low birth weight among black infants is increasing.[12]

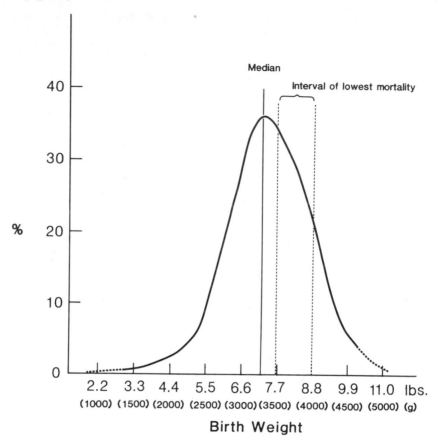

Figure 6-1. Distribution of infant birth weights with the median U.S. birth weight and range of birth weights associated with lowest infant mortality shown.
(From Brown, 1991, personal communication.)

Table 6-2. Differences in infant outcomes by ethnicity

Infant outcomes	American blacks	American whites	United States overall
Percent prematurity	18.0	8.5	10.2
Percent low birth weight	12.4	5.6	6.9
Mean birth weight (g)	3180	3420	3370
Infant mortality rate (deaths per 1000 live births in the first year)	12.7	5.7	9.9

Data from Wegman M: Annual summary of vital statistics: 1988, *Pediatrics* 84:943, 1989; and the National Center for Health Statistics, 1989.

Maternal nutrition is considered to be a major factor influencing infant outcomes in the United States. Key relationships between maternal nutrition and infant health are considered next.

NUTRITION-RELATED HEALTH PROBLEMS OF PREGNANT WOMEN

The nutritional status of women before and during pregnancy exert important influences on maternal health and fetal growth and development. The severity of the impact largely depends on the timing, duration, and intensity of nutritional insults. Of the potential relationships among measures of nutritional status and fetal growth and development, the effects of prepregnancy weight status, prenatal weight gain, and usual dietary intake levels of calories, protein, zinc, iron, and folacin have received the most attention. Knowledge of the effects of dietary intake on the course and outcome of pregnancy is cursory, however. Studies required to test hypotheses related to maternal intakes of a variety of specific nutrients and pregnancy outcome have yet to be undertaken. This situation exists because it is very difficult and expensive to accurately access dietary intake throughout the whole pregnancy. Given this situation and the proportion of pregnancy outcomes that are poor, the reasonable course of action is to promote adequate intakes of all essential nutrients by women before and during pregnancy.

Prepregnancy Weight Status and Prenatal Weight Gain

Low weight prior to pregnancy, low rates of weight gain in the second and third trimesters, and low total weight gains during pregnancy are factors strongly associated with infant birth weight. Entering pregnancy underweight clearly increases the risk that infants will be born small. (See Table 6-3 for weight-for-height values for underweight, nor-

Table 6-3. Healthy infant outcome project: table for identifying prepregnancy weight status

Height (no shoes)		Weight status category			
		A Under	B Normal	C Over	D Obese
Feet	Inches	Weight in pounds (light indoor clothing)			
4	9	92 or less	93-113	114-134	135 or more
4	10	94 or less	95-117	118-138	139 or more
4	11	97 or less	98-120	121-142	143 or more
5	0	100 or less	101-123	124-146	147 or more
5	1	103 or less	104-127	128-150	151 or more
5	2	106 or less	107-131	132-155	156 or more
5	3	109 or less	110-134	135-159	160 or more
5	4	113 or less	114-140	141-165	166 or more
5	5	117 or less	118-144	145-170	171 or more
5	6	121 or less	122-149	150-176	177 or more
5	7	124 or less	125-153	154-181	182 or more
5	8	128 or less	129-157	158-186	187 or more
5	9	131 or less	132-162	163-191	192 or more
5	10	135 or less	136-166	167-196	197 or more
5	11	139 or less	140-171	172-202	203 or more
6	0	142 or less	143-175	176-207	208 or more

From Brown JE: Personal communication, Minneapolis, 1991.
Technical notes: Weight for height ranges are calculated from the 1959 Metropolitan Height and Weight Tables for Women over the age of 25 years. A midpoint value was determined from the range of weight for height for women of "medium frame." The cutpoint for underweight women is designated as a weight for height that is more than 10% below the midpoint. The normal weight range is calculated as plus or minus 10% of the midpoint for each height. The overweight range is calculated as greater than 10% through 30% above the midpoint of weight for height. The cutpoint in weight for the obese category is calculated as a weight for height that is more than 30% above the midpoint of weight for height.

Table 6-4. Recommended prenatal weight gains by prepregnancy weight status and twin pregnancy

Prepregnancy weight status	Recommended total gain	
	(lb)	(kg)
Underweight	28-40	12.5-18
Normal weight	25-35	11.5-16
Overweight	15-25	7-11.5
Obese*	15	6.8
Twin pregnancy	35-45	16-20.5

Adapted from National Academy of Sciences (Institute of Medicine): *Nutrition During Pregnancy*, Washington, DC, 1990, National Academy Press.

*Represents minimum weight gain. Consumption of nutritious foods and positive rate of gain should be emphasized during counseling with obese clients.

Table 6-5. Estimate of components of weight gain during pregnancy based on full-term 8-lb infant

Component	lb
Fetus	8
Uterus	2
Placenta	1.5
Blood	3
Amniotic fluid	2
Breast tissue	1
Other fluid	6
Fat stores	8.5
Total weight gain	32

Adapted from Hytten FE, Leitch I: *The physiology of human pregnancy*, Philadelphia, 1963, FA Davis Co.

mal, overweight, and obese.) This risk approximately doubles if combined with a low weight gain (less than 20 lb) during pregnancy. Approximately one half of infants born to low-income, underweight women who gain less than 20 lb during pregnancy are at risk of being born with low birth weight. Dietary and weight gain restriction during pregnancy reduces maternal tissue accumulation and fetal growth and have not been found to benefit maternal health. Low rates of weight gain (less than 1 lb/week) during the second half of pregnancy are associated with retarded fetal growth and development and preterm delivery.

For women entering pregnancy at normal weight, a gradual gain in weight that totals 25 to 35 lb appears to be consistent with optimal fetal growth and development. Recommended weight gains based on fetal growth and development for women who enter pregnancy underweight are higher (28 to 40 lb) and lower (15 to 25 lb) for women who enter pregnancy overweight.[14] Women who enter pregnancy obese should gain at least 15 lb and those carrying twins, 35 to 45 lb. These recommended prenatal weight gains are summarized in Table 6-4. Above-average weight gains during pregnancy have been noted to counteract partially the negative effect of cigarette smoking on fetal growth.

Earlier in this century it was thought that women do not need to gain much more than what

an infant weighs at birth, about 7 lb. It was assumed that the only tissue that grew during pregnancy was the fetus. However, fetal growth is accompanied by marked increases in maternal blood volume, fat stores, and breast and uterus size. The accumulation of amniotic fluid (the water that surrounds the fetus in the uterus), the increase in the volume of fluid that exists outside the cells, and the placenta also account for weight gain during pregnancy. Broken down into individual components, a gain of 32 lb during pregnancy would be distributed approximately as shown in Table 6-5. At full term, an 8-lb infant accounts for about a fourth of the mother's total weight gain.

Weight Loss After Pregnancy

It does not appear that women whose weight gains are close to the recommended levels are more likely to become obese or to experience complications of pregnancy than are women who gain less. On average, a new mother loses 15 lb within the first week and 28 lb on average by 4 months. Although the subject of controversy, it does not appear that breastfeeding enhances weight loss after pregnancy for most women.

Nutrient Intake During Pregnancy

To a large extent, the raw materials needed to support the growth and development of a fetus are supplied by a woman's diet during pregnancy.

Many women enter pregnancy with reserves of fat that can be used to meet a portion of the energy needs of the fetus, and many women enter pregnancy with stores of certain vitamins and minerals such as vitamins A and B_{12} that can be used to nourish the fetus. Because of low maternal storage levels of protein and most vitamins and minerals, however, the growth and development of the fetus largely depend on the quality and quantity of food consumed by women throughout pregnancy. If a woman fails to consume sufficient calories, protein, vitamins, and minerals to maintain her own health and nutrient stores, the fetus cannot receive the level of nutrients needed for optimal growth and development. This biological fact stands in contrast to the common belief that the fetus is a parasite that obtains needed nutrients regardless of what the mother consumes in her diet. The fetus is not a parasite; it would make no sense in terms of survival of the species, and the notion cannot be supported experimentally. Moreover, women have not been shown to have "maternal instincts" that draw them to select an optimal diet for pregnancy.

Low intake of calories and protein and low and high intakes of specific vitamins and minerals have been associated with abnormal fetal growth and development.

Calories

Diets that provide fewer than about 1800 calories/day are considered "low calorie" during pregnancy. Such diets can present several problems for a growing fetus. The first has to do with the availability of protein for fetal growth and tissue formation. Without enough calories to meet a pregnant woman's need for energy, dietary protein is diverted from use in tissue construction to use in energy formation. The requirement for energy is the body's first priority; only when the mother's energy needs are met can dietary protein be used for the mother's and the baby's tissue growth and maintenance needs. This principle applies throughout all phases of life but is particularly relevant to pregnancy, when protein tissue formation is extensive. The second problem is that low-calorie diets do not supply enough energy to meet the needs for normal

fetal growth. This shortage increases the probability of low birth weight. Third, diets that fail to supply enough calories generally provide inadequate amounts of essential nutrients as well. This situation can leave the fetus with a short supply of vitamins and minerals and interfere with normal growth and development.

The ill effects of low-calorie diets during pregnancy on fetal growth and development are most pronounced when the restriction continues throughout pregnancy. Infants born under this circumstance may be permanently delayed in growth and intellectual development. If low-calorie intakes are the exception rather than the routine, permanent damage to the infant is not likely to result; adaptive mechanisms help the fetus withstand fluctuations in maternal food intake. Ideally, pregnant women should eat regular meals and snacks and avoid even short periods of fasting and weight loss.

Protein

Protein intakes below 74 g/day on average have been associated with the birth of smaller-than-average infants. A number of studies have shown that infants born to women who consumed about 90 g of protein daily during pregnancy from foods in their diets tend to be healthier than infants born to women who have consumed less. Whether pregnant women in the United States should be encouraged to consume 90 g of protein per day is a matter of controversy. Most women in the United States consume between 70 and 90 g of protein per day during pregnancy.

Folacin

Deficiencies of folacin around the time of conception have been associated with neural tube defects such as spina bifida. Folacin deficiency during pregnancy causes megaloblastic anemia in women and reduces fetal growth. As many as 15% of low-income women in the United States develop a deficiency of folacin during pregnancy.

Iron

Iron deficiency is the most common nutrient deficiency in pregnant women in the United States.

It develops when a woman enters pregnancy with low iron stores and fails to consume enough iron during her pregnancy. Iron deficiency anemia during pregnancy is defined as a hemoglobin level of less than 11 g/dl in the first, less than 10.5 g/dl in the second, and less than 11 g/dl in the third trimester of pregnancy.[14]

Women who develop iron deficiency anemia are more likely to deliver infants who are small and at risk of developing iron deficiency in their first year than are women who do not become anemic.

Concern about iron deficiency in the United States has led to the use of excessive levels of iron supplements during pregnancy, and that use has created a separate problem. Large amounts of iron interfere with zinc absorption. The use of supplements containing 100 mg of iron per day have been associated with low maternal levels of zinc and decreased fetal growth.

Zinc

Marginal deficiencies of zinc among women may be quite common during pregnancy. Zinc deficiency during pregnancy has been associated with abnormally long labor and with the delivery of small infants. High-dose iron supplements may contribute to the development of zinc deficiency.

Alcohol and Pregnancy

As early as the 1800s, maternal consumption of alcohol during pregnancy was said to cause the birth of "sickly" infants. The ill effects of alcohol on babies were not fully acknowledged until the 1970s, when several research reports described a condition called *fetal alcohol syndrome*. Women who drink heavily or frequently binge on alcohol during pregnancy are at high risk of delivering infants with specific malformities and retarded physical and mental development. The effect of maternal alcohol intake on the fetus worsens with increasing alcohol intake. Heavy drinking in the first half of pregnancy is closely associated with the birth of malformed, small, mentally impaired infants. When excessive drinking occurs only in the second half of pregnancy, infants are less likely to be malformed, but they are still likely to be small and to suffer ab-

normal mental development. These conditions are lasting; they cannot be fully corrected with special treatment, and the child does not outgrow them.

No amount of alcohol has been found to be absolutely safe during pregnancy. When only an occasional drink is consumed, however, the adverse effects of alcohol on fetal development appear to be small and rare.

Overdose Reactions to Vitamin and Mineral Supplements

Overdose reactions have been observed in pregnant women and newborns to six vitamins and three minerals: vitamins B_{12}, C, B_6, A, D, and E and iron, zinc, and iodine. Amounts that have been associated with harmful effects start at two to three times the Recommended Dietary Allowance (RDA). A fetus is generally much more susceptible to the ill effects of vitamin and mineral overdoses than is a pregnant woman, primarily because of the small size and rapid growth and development of the fetus. Overdoses of vitamin and mineral supplements produce the most serious threats to infant health when they occur early in pregnancy, when the fetus's organs are developing.

Vitamins

"Rebound" deficiencies have been observed in infants whose mothers have taken excessive amounts of vitamins B_{12}, C, and B_6 in pregnancy. The excretion mechanisms that rid the fetus of the high levels of these vitamins appear to continue after birth, even though large amounts of the vitamins are no longer being received. Consequently, the newborns excrete too much of the vitamins and develop deficiencies within a few days after birth. Infants can be protected from the effects of rebound vitamin deficiencies if they are supplemented with the particular vitamin and then gradually weaned from it.

As little as 25,000 IU of vitamin A taken daily in the early months of pregnancy has been associated with central nervous system and bone abnormalities in newborns. The increasingly popular use of vitamin A-like compounds for the treatment of acne, wrinkles, and other skin conditions has lead to new warnings about their use by women who are or may become pregnant.

Daily doses of supplemental vitamin D at levels five times the RDA (2000 IU) have been associated with the birth of infants who are mentally retarded and have heart abnormalities. There is also evidence to indicate that megadoses of vitamin E may result in spontaneous abortion.

Minerals

Iron, zinc, and iodine supplements during pregnancy can also be hazardous. Iron overdose primarily affects the pregnant woman by causing gastrointestinal upset. The fetus does not receive excessive levels of iron because high amounts are not usually absorbed by the mother's intestinal tract. Zinc supplements that deliver in the neighborhood of 100 mg/day provide excessive levels of zinc to the fetus. Zinc overdoses in pregnancy have been shown to be related to preterm delivery. The consequences of iodine overdose in pregnancy include the development of goiter and mental retardation in infants.

The ingestion of high amounts of supplemental vitamins and minerals by healthy pregnant women has never been found to improve maternal or infant health. Problems resulting from overdose could be prevented if women took no more than the RDA levels for vitamins and minerals during pregnancy. With the exception of iron, pregnant women can— and should—get the nutrients they need from a balanced diet.

Fiber

Constipation is a problem for many women during pregnancy. It appears to result from hormonal changes. It can be alleviated to some extent by including 10 additional g of dietary fiber in the daily diet, for a total of about 30 g. Fluid intake should increase along with the increased dietary fiber.

Pica

Pica is defined as the regular consumption of nonfood substances. It is not uncommon for pregnant women (and children) to habitually consume such things as clay or laundry starch. Scientists know very little about the reason for this practice. Some evidence suggests that it may be related to iron deficiency, but the evidence is far from solid—and the substances typically consumed do not provide the body with iron.

The regular ingestion of clay or laundry starch can cause problems. Clay may contain bacteria and other harmful substances, and it may reduce the amount of minerals absorbed from foods. Also, it may cause intestinal obstructions that must be surgically removed. Laundry starch may contain contaminants because it is not manufactured for consumption as a food. The body digests and absorbs laundry starch just as it does other sources of starch. Laundry starch can become a significant source of empty calories.

Shifts in Food Preferences

An interesting and common effect of pregnancy is changing food preferences. Food preferences have been noted to change in about three fourths of pregnant women. Foods such as fish, beef, fried foods, alcoholic beverages, diet soft drinks, and coffee are often reported to taste or smell unpleasant during pregnancy, whereas ice cream, chocolate, salty snacks, milk, and fruit are reported to taste better. Pregnant women are less sensitive to the taste of salt; they prefer stronger salt solutions than they do after pregnancy.[3]

Present evidence indicates that shifts in salt preference may be related to changes in estrogen levels that occur during pregnancy. Nonpregnant monkeys that are given estrogen have been found to develop a preference for stronger salt solutions. The increased preference observed among pregnant women for nutritious foods such as milk and fruit may be related to their desire to eat well during pregnancy.

Results of Dietary Intake Studies in the United States

Results of 13 studies that quantitated caloric level and intakes of up to 16 nutrients of U.S. women during pregnancy were summarized in the National Academy of Science's *Nutrition During Pregnancy*.[14] Mean caloric levels and mean intakes of

Table 6-6. Adequacy of nutrient intake during pregnancy

Less than 77% RDA	More than 77% RDA
Calories	Protein
Vitamin D*	Vitamin A
Vitamin E	Thiamin
Vitamin B$_6$	Riboflavin
Folate*	Niacin
Iron*	Vitamin B$_{12}$
Zinc*	Vitamin C
Magnesium	

Summarized from National Academy of Sciences (Institute of Medicine): *Nutrition during pregnancy*, Washington, DC, 1990, National Academy Press.
*Less than 65% of RDA.

vitamins D, E, and B$_6$, and folacin, iron, zinc, calcium, and magnesium were less than the 1989 RDAs for pregnant women in nearly all studies. Mean intakes of protein, vitamins A, B$_{12}$, and C and thiamin, riboflavin, and niacin tended to exceed the RDAs in these studies (Table 6-6).

It is generally asserted that intake levels below 100% of the RDAs do not constitute sufficient evidence of dietary inadequacy. However, the likelihood of true dietary inadequacy increases as nutrient intakes fall below the margin of safety built into the RDAs. The margin of safetly included in the RDAs for most nutrients no longer exists when usual intake levels are less than 80% of the RDAs. The likelihood that dietary inadequacy exists is approximately 50% within a population when less than 77% of the RDA is consumed. The probability that nutrient intake is inadequate increases to 83% when less than 65% of the RDA is consumed.[7] Mean caloric levels and intakes of folate, vitamin B$_6$, iron, zinc, and magnesium were below 77% of the RDA in the majority of the studies summarized in the report. Furthermore, when the more stringent cut point of less than 65% of the RDA is applied, mean intake of vitamin D, folate, iron, and zinc fell below this level for the majority of studies.

Although results from the diverse studies may not apply to women in the United States in general, they do raise concern about the quality of diets consumed during pregnancy. They also highlight the need for criteria for defining inadequate dietary intake. In the absence of more objective measures of nutrient status, defining inadequate dietary intakes as those that meet less than 77% of the RDA appears reasonable for practical applications. Because a margin of safety is not built into the RDA for calories and because caloric need varies widely, use of this criterion to evaluate caloric adequacy would be inappropriate.

HEALTHY PEOPLE 2000: OBJECTIVES RELATED TO MATERNAL NUTRITION

Priority health problems in the United States and objectives intended to facilitate their resolution are delineated in a major public health policy document *Healthy People 2000: National Health Promotion and Disease Prevention Objectives*.[8] (See Chapter 1.) Objectives related to maternal nutrition are listed in the Nutrition and the Maternal and Child Health sections of the document. These objectives are summarized in the box on p. 115. As happened after the first set of health objectives for the nation were published 10 years earlier, the objectives will be used by many state and local health agencies in the development and refinement of maternal nutrition programs and services.

PHYSIOLOGICAL CHANGES IN PREGNANCY

Several physiological changes occur during the course of pregnancy, including the following.

Increase in the Amount of Blood (Blood Volume)

Blood volume increases by almost 50% so that enough oxygen can be available to support the growing fetal and maternal tissues. Thus there is an increase in the need for those nutrients most important for making blood: protein, iron (hemoglobin is a protein with iron in it), folacin, and vitamin B$_6$. If a woman has sufficient dietary intake and stores of these nutrients before and during pregnancy, she will make this adjustment with little problem; otherwise, anemia may result. To help the body receive more oxygen, other changes occur in addition to blood volume (e.g., breathing becomes faster and deeper, and the heart pumps more blood in a given amount of time).

HEALTHY PEOPLE 2000: NATIONAL HEALTH PROMOTION AND DISEASE PREVENTION OBJECTIVES

National health objectives related to maternal nutrition

* Reduce the infant mortality rate to no more than 7 per 1000 live births
  (Baseline: 10.1 per 1000 live births in 1987)
* Reduce low birth weight to an incidence of no more than 5% of live births
  (Baseline: 6.9% in 1987)
* Increase to at least 85% the proportion of mothers who achieve the minimum recommended weight gain during their pregnancies
  (Baseline: 67% of married women in 1980)
* Reduce the incidence of fetal alcohol syndrome to no more than 0.12 per 1000 live births
  (Baseline: 0.22 per 1000 live births in 1987)
* Increase calcium intake so at least 50% of pregnant and lactating women consume three or more servings daily of foods rich in calcium

(Baseline: 24% of pregnant and lactating women in 1985-86)
* Reduce iron deficiency to less than 3% among women of childbearing age
  (Baseline: 5% for women aged 20 to 44 years in 1976-80)
* Reduce iron deficiency to 20% among low-income, pregnant, black women
  (Baseline: 41% in 1983-85)
* Increase to at least 75% the proportion of mothers who breastfeed their babies in the early postpartum period and to at least 50% the proportion who continue breastfeeding until their babies are 5 to 6 months old.
  (Baseline: 54% at discharge and 21% at 5 to 6 months in 1988)

From *Healthy people 2000: national health promotion and disease promotion objectives*, DHHS publication (PHS) 91-50212, Washington, DC, 1991, Department of Health and Human Services.

Changes in the Gastrointestinal Tract

Food moves through the gastrointestinal tract more slowly, allowing the mother to digest food more completely, which in turn helps her absorb more nutrients from food. Thus absorption of nutrients such as calcium and iron is increased during pregnancy; however, this slower movement of food may lead to constipation.

Changes Affecting Fluid Needs

More fluid is needed by the woman's body because of:
1. Increased blood volume for the mother and development of blood for the fetus
2. Amniotic fluid, which surrounds the fetus in the uterus and protects it from trauma or shock
3. Increased urine output because the woman is now getting rid of waste products for both herself *and* her baby

For this reason, a woman needs to drink more fluids during pregnancy: at least eight glasses per day, including water, fruit and vegetable juices, and milk. The pregnant woman should try to avoid caffeine and not drink alcohol-containing beverages and low nutrient beverages such as soft drinks.

Increase in Breast Tissue and Fat Stores

The mammary glands in the breast begin to enlarge during pregnancy to allow the milk ducts to prepare for lactation. Fat stores increase in preparation for breastfeeding.

Changes in Weight

The woman gains weight as both her tissues and the tissues of the fetus increase and develop. Additional nutrients are required to build this new tissue and to maintain them. Some of the more striking increases in nutrient need are those for protein, folacin, vitamins C and B_6, and iron. Satisfactory progress with regard to weight gain is essential to the well-being of the developing fetus. It also serves as a major indicator to the health care provider that the pregnancy is proceeding normally.

NUTRITIONAL NEEDS OF PREGNANT WOMEN

Pregnancy represents a period of high nutrient needs, and the diet of a pregnant woman should provide the vast majority of her nutrient needs.[2]

Regardless of the pregnant woman's age and whether she is a vegetarian or not, her diet should contain:

1. Sufficient calories for adequate weight gain
2. A variety of foods from each food group
3. Regular meals and snacks
4. Sufficient dietary fiber (about 30 g/day)
5. Eight or more cups of fluid each day
6. Salt to taste
7. No alcoholic beverages

Planning the diet around the basic food groups is the most straightforward approach to meeting nutrient needs for pregnancy (Table 6-7). Compared to nonpregnant adult women, pregnant women should consume an additional serving of milk or milk product and an additional serving of meat or meat alternate. Consuming only the minimum number of servings from each food group does not provide the needed calories. Additional servings of foods within the groups and from the miscellaneous category are needed for the calories they provide.

Table 6-7. Food group recommendations for pregnant women

Food group	Minimum number of servings per day
Breads and cereals	6
Vegetables and fruits	(4)
Vitamin A rich	1
Vitamin C rich	1
Other	2
Milk and milk products	3
Meats or alternates	3
Miscellaneous	based on caloric need

Modified from National Research Council: *Diet and health: implications for reducing chronic disease risk*. Washington, DC, 1989, National Academy Press.

Nutrient Needs

According to the 1989 RDAs shown in Table 6-8, healthy pregnant women need approximately 300 more calories per day than before pregnancy during the second and third trimesters of pregnancy. This figure is an average. Women entering pregnancy underweight need more calories, and those entering overweight need fewer. In addition, physically active pregnant women require higher caloric intakes than these averages. It is generally easier and more accurate to monitor the adequacy of caloric intake by tracking weight gain than by counting calories.

The protein content of a woman's body increases by about 2 lb during pregnancy. About half of this increase is in the buildup of the mother's uterus, breasts, and blood supply; the other half is deposited in fetal tissues.

With the exception of vitamins A and D, calcium, and phosphorus (nutrients that do not have higher RDAs for pregnancy), nutrient allowances for healthy pregnany women are 10% to 100% higher than for nonpregnant women who are healthy. The relatively high requirements for many nutrients mean that pregnant women should increase their intake of nutrient-dense foods more than they increse their consumption of calorie-rich foods.

Water

Water requirements increase substantially during pregnancy. It is generally advised that women stay well hydrated during pregnancy and that women living in hot climates pay special attention to fluid intake. For most women, a daily intake of 8 to 10 cups of fluids is sufficient.

Vitamin and Mineral Supplements

Current recommendations for prenatal supplements call for the routine use of iron only during pregnancy. Specifically, the National Academy of Sciences *Nutrition During Pregnancy*[14] recommends that pregnant women receive 30 mg ferrous iron daily beginning at about week 12 of gestation. As identified in the report, the use of other supplements should be restricted to women identified

Table 6-8. Recommended dietary allowances

Energy and nutrients	Women 19-24 years	Pregnant	Lactating (first 6 months)
Energy (kcal)*	2200	2500	2700
Protein (g)	46	60	65
Vitamin A (µg RE)	800	800	1300
Vitamin D (µg)	10	10	10
Vitamin E (mg α-TE)	8	10	12
Vitamin K (µg)	60	65	65
Vitamin C (mg)	60	70	95
Thiamin (mg)	1.1	1.5	1.6
Riboflavin (mg)	1.3	1.6	1.8
Niacin (mg NE)	15	17	20
Vitamin B_6 (mg)	1.6	2.2	2.1
Folate (µg)	180	400	280
Vitamin B_{12} (µg)	2	2.2	2.6
Calcium (mg)	1200	1200	1200
Phosphorus (mg)	1200	1200	1200
Magnesium (mg)	280	320	355
Iron (mg)	15	30	15
Zinc (mg)	12	15	19
Iodine (µg)	150	175	200
Selenium (µg)	55	65	75

Developed from RDAs, Washington, DC, 1989, Food and Nutrition Board, National Academy of Science, National Research Council.
*Value for pregnant women is for the second and third trimester. Energy need during pregnancy varies, based on prepregnancy weight and activity level.
RE, Retinal equivalents.
TE, Tocopherol equivalents.
NE, Niacin equivalents.

as having or as being at risk of sustaining low nutrient intakes. (See the box on p. 118 for a summary of the recommendations regarding supplements made in *Nutrition During Pregnancy*.) Supplements should be employed only when dietary counseling fails to lead to the needed improvements in diet. If a multivitamin and mineral supplement is indicated, the one described in Table 6-9 should be provided.

Which Pregnant Women Are at Nutritional Risk?

Nutrition During Pregnancy[14] cites a number of predictors for poor pregnancy outcomes and a set of circumstances that place women at nutritional risk (see boxes on p. 119). The categories of women at "nutritional risk" probably include the

Table 6-9. Composition of multivitamin and mineral supplement recommended for nutritionally at-risk pregnant women

Nutrient	Amount	% of 1989 RDA for pregnant women
Iron	30 mg	100
Zinc	15 mg	100
Copper	2 mg	no RDA
Calcium	250 mg	21
Vitamin B_6	2 mg	91
Folate	300 µg	75
Vitamin C	50 mg	71
Vitamin D	5 µg	50

Adapted from National Academy of Sciences (Institute of Medicine): *Nutrition during pregnancy*, Washington, DC, 1990, National Academy Press.

SUMMARY OF RECOMMENDATIONS FOR MATERNAL NUTRITION

- Routine assessment of dietary practices is recommended for all pregnant women in the United States to allow evaluation of the need for improved diet or vitamin or mineral supplements.
- Where possible, poor dietary practices should be improved by nutrition education, counseling, and referral to food assistance programs. If, in the judgment of the clinician, such interventions are likely to be or have been unsuccessful, then recommendation of a multivitamin-mineral supplement may be the only practical strategy to improve nutrient intake.
- To prevent iron deficiency, the subcommittee recommends the routine use of 30 mg of ferrous iron per day beginning at about week 12 of gestation, in conjunction with a well-balanced diet that contains enhancers of iron absorption (ascorbic acid, meat).
- Zinc supplementation is recommended when less than 30 mg of supplemental iron is administered per day.
- If a zinc supplement is administered, however, the subcommittee recommends that a 2-mg copper supplement also be given.
- Younger women [less than 25 years] with low calcium intakes [less than 600 mg/day] should either increase their intake of food sources of calcium, such as milk or cheese or, less preferably, add a supplement that provides 600 mg of calcium per day.
- When dietary sources [of water-soluble vitamins] are inadequate, daily supplementation with 300 mg of folate, 2 mg of vitamin B_6, and 50 mg of vitamin C is recommended.
- Pending further research, the subcommittee considers it prudent to supplement the diet with low amounts of folate if there is any question of adequacy of intake of this nutrient.
- For women at high risk for inadequate nutrient [vitamin B_6] intake, e.g., substance abusers, pregnancy adolescents, and women bearing multiple fetuses, the subcommittee recommends a daily multivitamin supplement containing 2 mg of vitamin B_6.
- For women at risk of deficiency [users of street drugs and cigarettes, heavy users of alcohol, long-term users of oral contraceptives, regular users of aspirin and salicylates, and women bearing more than one fetus], an ascorbic acid supplement of 50 mg/day is recommended if increased consumption of fruits and vegetables is unlikely.
- For complete vegetarians, a daily vitamin B_{12} supplement of 2 mg is recommended.

From National Academy of Sciences (Institute of Medicine): *Nutrition during pregnancy*, Washington, DC, 1990, National Academy Press.

majority of pregnant women in the United States. Approximately one third of women in the United States smoke cigarettes before pregnancy (about one third of smokers quit for a portion of the pregnancy), illicit drugs are used by between 6% and 25% of women, and 70% to 75% of African-American and 5% to 20% of white Americans are intolerant of lactose. Teen pregnancies represent 12% of all pregnancies in the United States.

The precentage of pregnant women with poor nutrition knowledge or who have insufficient money to buy food is not known. However, results of recent surveys indicate that the level of general nutrition knowledge of U.S. adults is poor. A random survey of 500 women and 500 men in the United States, conducted by Nutri/Systems in 1989,[5] showed that 41% of adults thought ketchup was a vegetable and 61% categorized asparagus, broccoli, and green beans as legumes. Results of a 1990 Gallup Poll,[6] commissioned in part by the American Dietetic Association, indicated that 72% of adults could not name the four food groups. In this survey, 53% of women responded that they had eliminated red meat and 36% eliminated dairy products to help improve their diet. The Gallup Poll found that only 3% of adults listed registered dietitians as a source of nutrition information. Yet, information and advice received from dietitians was perceived as being more useful than that obtained from any other source.

Weight Gain Recommendations for Pregnancy

No specific amount of weight gain during pregnancy is right for everyone. How much a woman should gain depends on her weight before pregnancy (see Table 6-4).

MATERNAL PREDICTORS OF POOR PREGNANCY OUTCOME

Poverty
Limited education
Substance abuse (cocaine, heroin, alcohol, tobacco)
Young age (less than 16 years)
Obesity, gestational diabetes, low pregnancy weight gain, suboptimal nutrition, anemia
Underweight
Poor or no prenatal care
Clinical complications (placenta previa, abruptio placentae, pregnancy-induced hypertension)
Chronic and acute diseases and disorders (hypertension, diabetes, infection)

Summarized from National Academy of Sciences (Institute of Medicine): *Nutrition during pregnancy*, Washington, DC, 1990, National Academy Press.

WOMEN DEFINED AS NUTRITIONALLY AT RISK DURING PREGNANCY

* Women who do not ordinarily consume an adequate diet
* Women carrying more than one fetus
* Women who use cigarettes, alcohol, or illicit drugs
* Women with lactose intolerance
* Women who are underweight or overweight at conception or who gain inadequate or excessive weight during pregnancy
* Adolescents
* Women with poor knowledge about nutrition or who have insufficient financial resources to purchase adequate food

National Academy of Sciences (Institute of Medicine): *Nutrition during pregnancy*, Washington, DC, 1990, National Academy Press.

Two other factors are important to consider within this topic: the rate of weight gain and the quality of the diet that produces the weight gain. Weight gain should be gradual and continue in an upward direction, even for woman who enter pregnancy overweight or obese. All guidelines assume that weight gain is achieved by eating high-quality diets.

Hunger and food intake fluctuate widely during pregnancy, and increases in food intake usually do not produce the smooth rate of maternal weight gain shown in the weight gain graphs. There are spurts in food intake and in weight gain.

Hunger, food intake, and weight gain generally are greatest in the second trimester. The calorie and nutrient stores that develop as a result of the increased food intake are used to support the high rate of fetal growth that occurs in the last trimester. Thus peak hunger, food intake, and rate of weight gain precede the time of the largest gains in fetal weight.

Teen Pregnancy

Each day about 1300 babies are born to teenagers in the United States. The major problems related to teen pregnancy are the high incidence of health problems in the babies and the impact of the pregnancy and parenthood on the mother's educational

and economic future. Few teenagers are psychologically and economically prepared to succeed in securing a healthy future for themselves while being the primary source of support for one or more children.

It was once thought that the greater number of complications accompanying teenage pregnancies and the higher rates of low birth weight, illness, and death for babies born to teenage mothers were due to the mothers' biologic immaturity. It was thought that these problems stemmed from the fact that the mother had not completed her growth and was thus not biologically prepared for pregnancy. It now appears that the most important factor is the day-to-day health practices of the mother. Regardless of their age, teenage mothers who have healthy lifestyles—those who generally consume balanced diets, gain the recommended amount of weight during pregnancy (young teens may need to gain weight at the high end of the recommended weight gain ranges), and do not smoke or use drugs—tend to be healthier and to remain healthier during pregnancy than other teenage mothers. The infants of healthy teenage girls also tend to be healthy. Poor nutritional practices—including frequent dieting, meal skipping, imbalanced diets, and inadequate weight gain during pregnancy—are more strongly associated with complications during pregnancy and poor infant outcomes than is the mother's age. (See Appendix 6-1 for Position of the American Dietetic Association: Nutrition Management of Adolescent Pregnancy.)

LACTATION

Food is the first enjoyment of life.

Lin Yü-t'ang

Breastfeeding represents a fascinating process that provides complete nutrition plus regular doses of preventive medicine. Women who breastfeed need an adequate and balanced diet in order to replenish their nutrition stores, maintain their health, and produce sufficient milk for their infants.

Breastfeeding is undergoing a resurgence of popularity in the United States. Before 1900, nearly every mother breastfed her infant. By 1920, however, evaporated milk and commercial infant formulas had become widely available, and for a time they were considered to be better for infants than breast milk. Rates of breastfeeding fell sharply from 1920 to 1955 but then rose sharply when the post–World War II baby boomers began having families. Many of the breastfeeding mothers of the 1970s felt a bit like pioneers, not having been breastfed as infants or having seen a relative or other role model breastfeed. Indeed, they were the leaders of a return to breastfeeding. In 1985 it was estimated that 60% of women were breastfeeding their infants after delivery. Because of the increasing proportion of new mothers who are employed outside the home, the incidence of breastfeeding had declined to approximately 52% by 1989 (Table 6-10).[17]

"Preventive Medicine" Components of Breast Milk

Breast milk "immunizes" infants against certain infectious diseases, and it may confer some protection against the development of cancer of the lymph system and of insulin-dependent diabetes during childhood. Protection against infectious diseases is particularly important in developing countries, where the purchase of formula represents a financial hardship and where refrigeration and medical

Table 6-10. Breastfeeding prevalence

	1982	1989
Overall United States (at hospital discharge)	61%	52%
By employment status	Full-time	Not employed
Hospital	54.5%	54.5%
6 months	10.0%	24.3%
By WIC status, 1989	WIC	Non-WIC
Hospital	34.2%	62.9%
5-6 months	9.2%	25.7%

Adapted from National Academy of Sciences (Institute of Medicine): *Nutrition during lactation*, Washington, DC, 1991, National Academy Press.

care are lacking. The quality of water used to dilute infant formulas is also a problem in some locales. These infants are exposed to a high level of disease-causing agents and at the same time are more vulnerable to disease because they do not receive the infection-protective substances of breast milk.

Breastfed infants tend to get sick less often than do bottle-fed infants. There is an even larger margin of safety associated with breastfeeding in developing countries than elsewhere.

Antibodies in breast milk can confer protection against disease such as polio, the "flu," respiratory tract infections, ear infections, meningitis, and gastrointestinal tract infections. Antibodies secreted into breast milk have been concentrated and effectively used to prevent diarrhea in infants and adults exposed to a strain of bacteria that causes diarrhea. Infants continue to receive immunity against a number of infectious diseases as long as breastfeeding continues.

Breastfed infants are far less likely than formula-fed infants to develop allergies. Up to 7% of infants may be allergic to cow's milk formula, whereas allergic reactions to breast milk are very rare—probably less than 1%. Once an infant develops an allergy to cow's milk, he or she is at high risk of becoming allergic to other types of foods and may also experience other illnesses more often than do infants who do not have food allergies.

Infants born to parents who experienced food allergies early in life are at risk of developing allergies, too. Breastfeeding these infants holds a particular advantage in that it may prevent or postpone the development of food allergies. Although breastfeeding does not protect all infants from developing allergies, it may be the ounce of prevention that is worth a pound of cure.

Most infants outgrow food allergies by the time they are 2 years old. By then, their gastrointestinal tracts have matured sufficiently to prevent allergic reactions to offending substances in foods.

Advantages of Breastfeeding

Breastfeeding offers advantages to mothers as well as to infants. Breastfeeding causes the release of oxytocin, a hormone that stimulates the muscles of the uterus to contract. Contraction of the uterus helps stop the bleeding caused by the detachment of the placenta from the wall of the uterus during delivery. (This effect of breastfeeding is quite noticeable. During the first few days after delivery, women can feel their uterus contract while they are breastfeeding.)

Another advantage of breastfeeding is a reduced risk of developing breast cancer later in life. The longer a woman breastfeeds, the less likely she is to develop breast cancer. The risk of developing breast cancer decreases as the number of infants breastfed increases.

Disadvantages of Breastfeeding

Breastfeeding is not best for everyone. Although at least 96% of women are biologically capable of breastfeeding, not all women are psychologically able to do it successfully. Many women who feel socially pressured into breastfeeding, for example, find that their attempts fail. Breastfeeding can fail if the mother does not receive social and emotional support for her decision to breastfeed. Women who are exposed to high levels of stress and women who suffer depression or other psychological disorders also may be unable to breastfeed successfully. Infant growth and development can be delayed or permanently retarded if breastfeeding is continued when it does not go well and infants fail to get enough to eat.

Although breastfeeding is a very natural process, problems are not unusual, and generally they can be overcome with supportive guidance. The importance of the early establishment of successful breastfeeding has led to the policy in many European countries of not allowing mothers to leave the hospital with their babies until breastfeeding is going well. The usual practice in some African countries is to relieve a breastfeeding mother's work load so that she can devote nearly full time to feeding and caring for her young infant. A relative may move in with the family and take over household chores, or the mother and baby may live with her parents for a time. As a cultural practice, supporting new mothers by relieving them of family and household responsibilities does not appear to be nearly as common in the United States as in other parts of the world.

Breastfeeding limits the participation of fathers in feeding their infants and intensifies the mother's responsibility and commitment. Because most infants eat every 3 or 4 hours around the clock during the first month or so, breastfeeding mothers can become exhausted. These disadvantages can be overcome to an extent if the mother *expresses* her milk, that is, releases it from the breast by hand or with the aid of a special pump—and stores it for later use. This practice allows the father or babysitter to give the baby feedings of expressed milk from a bottle.

How expressed breast milk is stored is important. It should be placed in a clean, airtight container and either frozen or refrigerated. Breast milk stays fresh for at least a month if it is solidly frozen, and it holds up well in a refrigerator for 2 days. The antiinfection components of breast milk help it stay fresh when stored. Bacteria that enter breast milk after it is released from the breast multiply much more slowly than bacteria that have entered infant formulas.

The Process of Lactation

The mother's body prepares for breastfeeding during pregnancy. Fat is deposited in breast tissue, and networks of blood vessels and nerves infiltrate the breasts. Ducts that will channel milk from the milk-producing cells forward to the nipple—the milk-collection ducts—also mature.

Hormonal changes that occur at delivery signal milk production to begin. Because delivery and not length of pregnancy initiates milk production, breast milk is available for infants born prematurely.

The breast milk produced during the first 3 days or so after delivery is different from the milk produced later. Called *colostrum*, this early milk contains higher levels of protein, minerals, and antibodies than does "mature" milk. The extra infection-fighting antibodies help newborns remain healthy during the transition from a germ-free environment to a germ-filled one.

Milk is present in the breasts as "fore milk" and "hind milk." Before a feeding, fore milk is present in the milk-collection ducts that lead from the milk-producing cells to the nipple. It is readily available to the infant. Fore milk contains less fat and protein—and therefore fewer calories—than hind milk. Hind milk is produced and stored in the milk-producing cells and is not initially available to the infant. It is released (let down) by oxytocin, the

hormone that also signals the uterus to contract after delivery (see Fig. 6-2). Oxytocin causes the milk-producing cells to contract and thereby release the hind milk. This process is commonly referred to as the *letdown reflex*, and it is so powerful that milk is actually ejected from the breast. The letdown reflex gives the infant access to the calorically dense milk stored in the milk-producing cells. If the hind milk is not released, the infant does not receive sufficient nourishment and is soon hungry again. If this continues, the infant will be hungry most of the time and may grow and develop poorly. These consequences are discussed because a number of conditions can interfere with the release of oxytocin during breastfeeding. The failure of the letdown reflex is a major cause of breastfeeding failure.

The Letdown Reflex

The letdown reflex is unique as a physiologic process in that it can be initiated by either physical or psychological stimuli. Normally, the letdown reflex

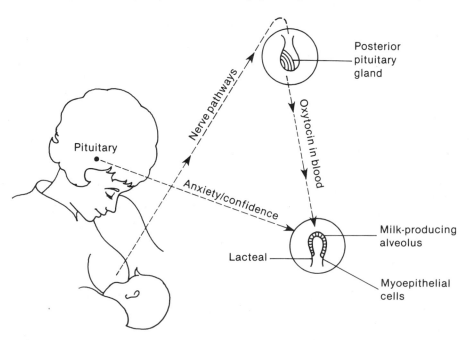

Figure 6-2. The letdown reflex simplified.
(Redrawn from Jelliffe DB, Jelliffe EFP: Psychophysiology of lactation: human milk in the modern world, Oxford, England, 1978, Oxford University Press.)

is triggered when the mother feels the infant sucking at her nipple. It can also occur when the mother hears her infant cry in hunger or when the thought occurs to her that it is time for a feeding. The physical or psychological stimulus signals a part of the mother's brain to release oxytocin into the bloodstream. When the oxytocin reaches the milk-producing cells, they contract and let down milk. Oxytocin is normally released within a minute after breastfeeding starts. During the first few weeks of breastfeeding and sometimes longer, the mother may feel the letdown reflex as a tingling sensation in the nipples.

Certain physical and psychological stimuli can prevent the letdown reflex from occurring. Stress, pain, anxiety, and other distractions can block the release of oxytocin. If the mother is distracted by pain or pressured for time, for example, the letdown reflex may not occur, and the infant will not get enough to eat. If this happens often enough, the mother may think she does not have enough milk for her baby and may decide to switch to bottle-feeding. Oxytocin inhalers are sometimes used to turn on the letdown reflex.

The Rooting Reflex

Humans, like other mammals, are born with a rooting reflex. When an infant's face touches the mother's breast, he or she instinctively "roots around" for the nipple. Once the nipple is felt, the hungry infant places her or his mouth around it and begins to suck vigorously. If the flow of milk is not limited, the infant feeds until full and then loses interest in eating. A hungry infant feeds with enormous intensity. (It has been said that minor surgery could be performed painlessly on an actively breastfeeding infant.)

Infants demonstrate that they are hungry in a number of ways: they move their head toward a breast if they are being held, they act irritable, and they cry. They also demonstrate it by the way they start to feed. Hungry infants start to feed with intensity and with their fists tightly clenched. They gradually loosen their fists as their hunger is satisfied, and their hands are fully relaxed and open when they have had enough to eat.

Breast Milk Production

While consuming one meal, an infant is "ordering" the next one. The pressure produced inside the breast by the infant's sucking and the emptying of the breasts during a feeding causes the hormone prolactin to be released from special cells in the brain. Prolactin stimulates the production of milk so that as much milk is produced for the next feeding as the infant consumes. It generally takes about 2 hours for the milk-producing cells to produce sufficient milk for the next feeding. An important exception occurs when an infant enters a growth spurt.

Like children and adolescents, infants grow in spurts, not at a constant rate. In preparation for a growth spurt, hunger increases and the demand for milk may double. The increased food intake causes a gain in weight, which in turn is followed by an increase in height.

Growth spurts occur frequently between an infant's third and seventh week of life, but less often after that. The initial increase in hunger associated with a growth spurt makes producing a refill in milk supply take longer. Instead of 2 hours, up to 24 hours may be needed for the supply of breast milk to catch up with the infant's increased need for it, and for about a day the infant wants to feed often and may not be completely satisfied. Although the mother may spend much of her day (and night) breastfeeding an infant who is entering a growth spurt, she may feel that she does not have enough milk to satisfy the baby and may give the baby a bottle. Because breast milk production is determined by how much and how often an infant feeds, supplementary bottle feedings lead to a decrease in milk production. With less breast milk available, the mother's feeling that she has too little breast milk is strengthened. Some women stop breastfeeding because of these longer-than-usual delays in producing enough milk to satisfy their growing infants' need for food.

It is very rare that a breastfeeding woman cannot produce enough milk. As long as an infant is allowed to breastfeed as often as desired, the mother's production will catch up with the baby's need for milk.

MATERNAL NUTRITIONAL NEEDS DURING LACTATION

The RDA for calories is about 25% higher for breastfeeding women than for nonpregnant women who are not breastfeeding (see Table 6-8). The actual increase in caloric need is higher than the RDA, around 40%. Energy supplied from fat stores that normally accumulate during pregnancy contributes to meeting energy needs during breastfeeding, so not all of the calories must come from the mother's diet. The RDA calls for increasing caloric intake by 500 calories/day. An additional 300 calories are needed to support breastfeeding, but this energy is assumed to be provided by maternal fat stores.

The average increases in nutrient allowances for breastfeeding are generally higher than the increases for pregnancy. As during pregnancy, proportionately higher amounts of nutrients than calories are required, which indicates the need for a nutrient-dense diet. As can be seen in Table 6-8, the RDAs for nutrients for breastfeeding women increase to varying extents.

Concern has been expressed about the possibility that breastfeeding may weaken a woman's bones if she fails to get enough calcium and other bone-building minerals in her diet, and this concern appears to have some basis in fact. Breastfeeding women, especially those younger than 30 years of age who have not achieved peak bone density, may lose minerals from their bones if they consume a low-calcium diet during breastfeeding. Breastfeeding four or more children while consuming a low-calcium diet may increase the risk that a woman will develop osteoporosis later in life.

The RDA for iron is not increased because of the savings in iron that occur with breastfeeding. A woman who breastfeeds generally does not resume menstrual periods until the infant consumes most of his or her calories from foods other than breast milk. The resulting iron savings reduce the breastfeeding woman's need for dietary iron.

Dietary Recommendations for Lactation

The calories and nutrients needed by the breastfeeding woman can be obtained from a varied diet

Table 6-11. Food group recommendations for lactating women

Food group	Minimum number of servings per day
Breads and cereals	6
Vegetables and fruits	(5)
Vitamin A rich	1
Vitamin C rich	2
Other	2
Milk and milk products	4
Meats or alternates	3
Miscellaneous	Based on caloric need

From Brown JE, personal communication, Minneapolis, 1991. Used with permission.

that includes foods from each of the basic food groups. The recommended numbers of servings from each food group are shown in Table 6-11. Compared with the recommendations for pregnancy, breastfeeding women are advised to consume an additional serving of a vitamin C–rich fruit or vegetable and an additional serving of milk or a milk product.

Increases in hunger and food intake that accompany breastfeeding generally take care of meeting caloric needs. If the diet includes at least the recommended minimal number of servings from each food group and sufficient calories, the breastfeeding woman is helping to assure an adequate diet for herself and her infant. Failure to consume enough calories from food can decrease milk production. Weight loss that exceeds 1½ lb/week— even in women with a good supply of fat stores— can reduce the amount of milk produced.

Maternal Diet and Breast Milk Composition

Milk-producing cells in the breast are supplied with the raw materials they need to manufacture milk from the mother's blood. For a number of substances, what ends up in the mother's blood reflects what she has consumed; therefore, the composition of breast milk varies with the maternal diet. For other substances, the amount that enters breast milk is regulated within the milk-producing cells; the levels of these substances remain fairly constant regardless of maternal diet.

Milk-producing cells enforce "quality control" processes on the amount of carbohydrate, protein, fat, and minerals (including calcium, sodium, potassium, iron, and fluoride) in breast milk. They also regulate the amount of milk produced when the maternal calorie intake is low. Rather than the energy content of milk being diluted in response to a low-calorie diet, the volume of milk is decreased.

The amount of carbohydrate, protein, and fat in breast milk varies only slightly in response to maternal diet, but the type of fat present can vary substantially. If a woman consumes more vegetable oils than animal fats, her breast milk contains a high proportion of unsaturated fats. If she fasts, her milk contains the type of fat present in her fat stores.

The vitamin content of breast milk corresponds more closely to maternal intake than is the case for the energy nutrients. The amounts of thiamin and vitamins C and B_{12} in breast milk, for example, vary with the types of food and supplements that the mother ingests. Thiamin deficiency (beriberi) and vitamin B_{12} deficiency (pernicious anemia) have been diagnosed in infants breastfed by deficient mothers.

The amount of several minerals in breast milk also are influenced by what the mother eats. The zinc and iodine content of breast milk reflects the mother's diet. Infants who fail to get sufficient zinc and iodine grow and develop slowly.

Nonnutrient Substances in Breast Milk

Foods contain many substances in addition to nutrients, and other substances enter the body through drugs, medications, and other ingested nonfood substances. All of these substances may end up in breast milk.

When a breastfeeding woman drinks coffee, her infant receives a small dose of caffeine. Breastfed infants of women who are heavy coffee drinkers (ten or more cups per day) may develop "caffeine jitters." Alcohol also is transferred from a woman's body to breast milk, and therefore alcohol consumption during breastfeeding should be restricted.

Nearly any drug or toxin that enters the mother's blood ends up in her breast milk. Environmental contaminants such as DDT, chlordane, PCB, and PBBs, for example, are transferred into breast milk. Many environmental contaminants are fat-soluble, and if they are ingested they may be stored in a woman's fat tissues. When the fat stores are later broken down for use in breast milk, the contaminants stored in the fat may enter her milk. The ingestion of fish from contaminated waters in Lake Ontario and Lake Michigan has been directly linked to abnormally high levels of PCB in breast milk. Infants exposed to PCB can develop rashes, digestive upsets, and nervous system problems.

Infants are much smaller than women, and a smaller dose of caffeine, alcohol, drugs, or environmental contaminants has an effect on them. Whereas breastfeeding mothers may show no adverse effects from these substances, their infants may.

Maternal Diet and Infant Distress

Some infants may be sensitive to components of certain foods a mother consumes that are transferred into breast milk. Peanut butter, chocolate, egg whites, and nuts contain substances that enter breast milk and cause some infants to develop a rash, wheezing, or a runny nose. Onions and foods from the cabbage family such as cabbage, broccoli, and brussels sprouts also are suspected to cause adverse reactions in some breastfed infants. Although causing no distress to mothers, these foods give some infants pronounced gas and cramps.

Why some infants are sensitive to certain components of the foods in their mothers' diets is not known, and many of the conclusions drawn about the relationships are based on hearsay because the appropriate studies have not been done. The general advice for breastfeeding women is to experiment with small amounts of the potentially offending foods to see if the infant is sensitive. If the infant does not appear to be, these foods do not need to be omitted from the diet.

GUIDELINES FOR PATIENT MANAGEMENT

The National Academy of Science published *Nutrition During Lactation* in 1991[14] and the *Surgeon*

RECOMMENDATIONS FOR NUTRITION DURING LACTATION

1. Breastfeeding is recommended for all infants in the United States under ordinary circumstances.
   A. Exclusive breastfeeding for normal, full-term infants from birth to age 4 to 6 months
   B. Breastfeeding plus appropriate foods for remainder of first year; continue breastfeeding beyond first year if desired
2. If breastfeeding is not possible, appropriate formula feeding is an acceptable alternative.
3. Lactating women should be encouraged to obtain their nutrients from a well-balanced, varied diet rather than from vitamin and mineral supplements.
   A. Routine supplements *not* recommended, need for supplements should be individually established
   B. Fluids should be consumed to meet thirst
   C. Remove foods suspected of causing adverse reactions in infants (e.g., dairy products) only if oral elimination-challenge tests prove positive
4. Health care should include screening for nutritional problems and provide dietary guidance.
5. Breastfeeding guidance should be provided prenatally, after delivery in hospital, and during the early postpartum period.
6. Provide anticipatory guidance on weight loss with lactation.

   A. Average loss 2 lb/month from 1 to 6 months
   B. Approximately 20% of women do not lose weight
   C. Rapid loss (≥4.5 lb/month) after first month *not* recommended
   D. Caloric intakes less than 1500 Kcal *not* recommended
7. Use of illicit drugs should be actively discouraged.
   A. No evidence that alcohol-containing beverages improve lactation performance
   B. Limit alcohol to no more than 0.5 g/kg body weight/day (e.g., 60-kg (130-lb) women = 2 drinks/day)
   C. Limit coffee to 1 to 2 cups/day
8. Infant nutrition:
   A. Give 0.5- to 1-mg injection, or 1- to 2-mg oral dose vitamin K after birth.
   B. Give 5 to 7.5 µg vitamin D/day if exposure to sunlight is low.
   C. Give 0.25 mg fluoride/day if content of household drinking water is less than 0.3 ppm.
   D. Give low-dose iron supplement by 6 months or bioavailable source of iron.

From National Academy of Sciences (Institute of Medicine): *Nutrition during lactation*, Washington, DC, 1991, National Academy Press.

General's Followup Report on Breast Feeding and Human Lactation.[17] *Nutrition During Lactation* describes the scientific basis of nutritional needs during lactation and gives recommendations (see the box above). The *Breast Feeding and Human Lactation* report describes breastfeeding promotion efforts throughout the nation. This document also serves as a resource for health professionals working to improve breastfeeding promotion and support. Appendixes in this report include valuable references such as guidelines for breastfeeding promotion in the WIC program and WHO-UNICEF's *Ten Steps to Successful Breastfeeding*.

Results of surveys on the quality of diets consumed by pregnant women and the high proportion of women who are nutritionally at risk for various reasons establish the importance of developing programs and services that enable women to consume adequate diets before and during pregnancy. If maternal nutritional status is to reach desired levels, accepted standards for the delivery of nutrition services to women before and during pregnancy need to be broadly implemented. An overview of components of preconceptual and prenatal nutrition services that may guide the delivery of high-quality care are overviewed in the box on p. 127. The components outlined take into account the recommendations of *Nutrition During Pregnancy*[14] but are not exclusively based on them.

PUBLIC FOOD AND NUTRITION PROGRAMS

The major food and nutrition education program for low-income pregnant women in the United States is the Supplemental Food Program for

SELECTED COMPONENTS OF PRECONCEPTUAL AND PRENATAL NUTRITION SERVICES

Preconceptual nutrition services

I. Patient History
  A. Oral contraceptive use (risk of folate, vitamin C and B_6 deficiency)
  B. Closely spaced pregnancy
  C. Course and outcome of previous pregnancies
    1. Clinical complications with dietary implications (e.g., allergies, iron deficiency, pregnancy-induced hypertension, gestational diabetes)
    2. Pregnancy weight gains (inadequate or excessive)
    3. Infants' birth weights, gestational ages
    4. Infants' physical and developmental status (e.g., congenital abnormalities such as neural tube defects, growth retardation, developmental delays)
    5. Infant feeding (breast or bottle)
II. Current Status
  A. Assessment of weight status (body mass index [BMI], weight for height)
  B. Estimation of body fat content (skinfold thicknesses)
  C. Determination of iron status (hemoglobin, serum ferritin)
  D. Utilization of modified or therapeutic diets (e.g., for diabetes, hypertension, gastrointestinal disorders)
  E. Assessment of dietary intake
    1. Recording of usual diet (food frequency questionnaire, diet history, 4 or more days of food intake records)
    2. Analysis of dietary intake (computerized, on-site, rapid turnaround)
    3. Comparison of energy (kcal) and nutrient levels to RDAs
  F. Dietary practices and patterns
    1. Food availability and resources (adequacy of cooking facilities, food storage and preparation techniques, transportation, etc.)
    2. Review of typical meal pattern (e.g., skipped meals, snacks, fast foods)
    3. Weight control practices, disordered eating behaviors

4. Food restrictions, aversions, intolerances, allergies, and misnomers
    5. Adherence to vegetarian diets
    6. Cultural, ethnic, or religious diet-related practices
  G. Review of personal habits
    1. Usual physical activity level
    2. Alcohol, cigarette, and drug use
    3. Stress levels and social support
  H. Assessment of supplement use
    1. Usual intake of vitamin, mineral, and other nutrient supplements
    2. Comparison of supplement intake levels with RDAs and results of dietary analysis (supplements should not exceed 100% of the RDA unless indicated)
  I. Discussion of client's concerns and questions regarding foods, diet supplements, and the like
    1. Recommendation of quality resources of additional information
  J. Nutrition counseling based on results of assessments
    1. Discuss results of assessments (e.g., nutrient intake levels <77% of the RDA, need for increased physical activity)
    2. Present and discuss options for meeting desired changes while maintaining assets
    3. Develop care plan based on client's decisions
    4. Supplement recommendations (if indicated, e.g., folate)
  K. Arrange for follow-up prior to conception (if needed)
  L. Referral to food assistance programs (if eligible)

Prenatal nutrition services

I. First Visit
  A. Undertake or update history and current status assessments and actions outlined under preconceptual nutrition services. If it is an update, follow up and revise care plan. Enroll in or refer to WIC, if eligible, and other food assistance programs (food stamps), if needed.

From Brown JE, Personal communication, Minneapolis, 1991. Used with permission.   *Continued.*

SELECTED COMPONENTS OF PRECONCEPTUAL AND PRENATAL NUTRITION SERVICES—cont'd

Prenatal nutrition services—cont'd

B. Prenatal weight gain
1. Identification of prenatal weight gain range based on prepregnancy weight status
2. Measure weight; plot results on weight gain grid
3. Provide client a weight gain grid; explain how to use it
4. Discuss components of prenatal weight gain
5. Discuss desired rate of weight gain
6. Discuss dietary aids for nausea and vomiting (if present)
7. Discuss the link between food intake and weight gain to fetal growth and development
C. Supplement recommendations
1. Iron: 30 mg elemental iron per day if iron status normal (Hgb $\geq$ 11 g/dl during first trimester); employ 60 to 120 mg/day if iron status is poor (serum ferritin < 12 mg/dl). Give 15 mg zinc and 2 mg copper if iron dose exceeds 30 mg per day.

2. Folate: diets should be supplemented with 300 μg folate per day if there is any question of dietary inadequacy
3. Others: as indicated by severity of dietary inadequacy and potential for improving nutrient intakes through dietary modifications
   a. Drug abusers, heavy users of cigarettes, pregnant adolescents, and women bearing multiple fetuses should receive daily the multivitamin and mineral supplement recommended in the 1990 report *Nutrition During Pregnancy* (Table 6-9).
   b. Vegans should receive 2 μg vitamin B_{12} daily.

II. Follow-up Visits
A. Repeat dietary assessments on at-risk clients
B. Monitor weight gain progress
C. Monitor implementation of care plan
D. Revise care plan as needed

Women, Infants, and Children, better known as WIC. In addition, the Food Stamp Program and the Commodity Distribution Program are also available.

The WIC Program

The WIC program was enacted in 1974 to help reduce the incidence of low birth weight and to improve maternal and child health by providing nutrition education and food supplements. The program has proven to be effective and has grown in funding each year.

Pregnant women and children up to the age of 5 who live in poverty and are assessed as being at risk of poor nutrition are generally eligible for the program. *Poor nutrition* is defined as the presence of a condition such as underweight, iron deficiency, or inadequate diet. Once enrolled in WIC, pregnant and breastfeeding women and their children receive an assessment of their nutritional status, nutrition education, and coupons for foods to sup-

plement their existing diets. Only such nutrient-dense foods as milk, infant formula, eggs, beans, cheese, peanut butter, and fruit juices are provided by the WIC program.

WIC works. Women who enroll in WIC during pregnancy are less likely to deliver low-birth-weight infants and to experience iron deficiency than are women who are eligible but do not participate. Participation in WIC has also been shown to improve diet quality and to prevent iron deficiency in infants and young children.

The WIC program is administered by state health departments. The Center on Budget and Policy Priorities has estimated that approximately half of women, infants, and children eligible for WIC actually participate.

INNOVATIVE MODELS OF MATERNAL NUTRITION SERVICE DELIVERY

A number of problem-oriented, client need–based nutrition intervention programs aimed at improv-

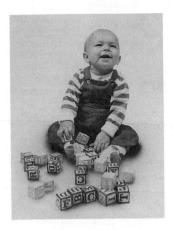

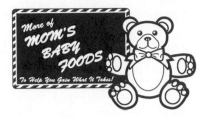

To help you gain the right amount of weight during your pregnancy, choose ____ foods from this list to eat *in addition* to the foods you're already eating each day.*

For example, if you've been eating three meals and one snack each day, try eating this extra food as another snack.

*Helpful Hints

1) ☑ Check the boxes next to the foods you like, to make it easier to choose your extra foods each day.

2) *Half* the amounts of *two* foods on the single-food list add up to one choice. For example, half a bagel plus about a tablespoon of peanut butter counts as one choice. Make up your own combinations!

3) Take this list with you when you go shopping, or add the foods you have selected to your grocery list.

Produced by the
Healthy Infant Outcome Project (HIOP)
University of Minnesota

Supported in part by project #MCJ 276008 from the Maternal and Child Health program (Title V, Social Security Act), Health Resources and Services Administration, Department of Health and Human Services.

Single foods that count as ONE choice

High-Calcium Foods
- ☐ 1 cup whole milk **or** 1 ¹/₂ cups skim milk
- ☐ 1 cup regular yogurt
- ☐ 1 ¹/₂ ounces cheese (1 ¹/₂ slices)
- ☐ ¹/₂ cup pudding
- ☐ ³/₄ cup ice milk
- ☐ 1 frozen yogurt **or** soft-serve cone

High-Carbohydrate-and-Fiber Foods
- ☐ 2 slices bread
- ☐ 2 dinner rolls
- ☐ 1 large hamburger bun or hot dog bun
- ☐ 1 ¹/₂ flour tortillas or corn tortillas
- ☐ 1 large muffin
- ☐ 1 large bagel
- ☐ 1 English muffin
- ☐ 1 cup hot cereal
- ☐ 1 ¹/₂ cups cold cereal
- ☐ 12 to 15 small crackers
- ☐ 5 graham crackers (2-inch squares)
- ☐ 1 small waffle
- ☐ 2 medium pancakes
- ☐ ³/₄ cup cooked rice
- ☐ 1 cup cooked spaghetti, noodles, or macaroni
- ☐ 1 large baked potato or ³/₄ cup potatoes
- ☐ 1 slice pizza (¹/₈ of a 12-inch pizza)

High-Protein Foods
- ☐ 3 ounces fish
- ☐ 2 ounces lean beef
- ☐ 2 ounces lean pork
- ☐ 3 ounces chicken or ¹/₂ chicken breast
- ☐ 2 eggs
- ☐ 1 cup cooked dried beans, dried peas, or lentils
- ☐ ²/₃ cup chili with meat and beans
- ☐ 1 ¹/₂ tablespoons peanut butter

High-Vitamin-and-Mineral Foods
- ☐ 2 medium oranges
- ☐ 2 medium apples
- ☐ 1 ¹/₂ cups applesauce (unsweetened)
- ☐ 2 small bananas
- ☐ 2 medium pears
- ☐ 1 ¹/₂ cups grapes
- ☐ 1 cup canned pineapple ("lite" or juice-packed)
- ☐ 1 ¹/₂ cups canned peaches ("lite" or juice-packed)
- ☐ 1 ¹/₄ cups canned pears ("lite" or juice-packed)
- ☐ ¹/₃ cup raisins or 2 snack boxes
- ☐ 1 ¹/₂ cups orange juice, grapefruit juice, or apple juice
- ☐ 1 cup grape juice or pineapple juice
- ☐ 1 small sweet potato or ¹/₂ cup sweet potato
- ☐ 1 ¹/₂ cups winter squash
- ☐ 1 cup corn
- ☐ 1 cup peas

Combination foods that count as ONE choice

- ☐ ¹/₂ sandwich (meat, cheese, peanut butter, tuna salad **or** chicken salad)
- ☐ ¹/₂ cup hotdish or mixed dish
- ☐ ¹/₂ cup chow mein or chop suey with ¹/₄ cup rice or chow mein noodles
- ☐ 1 to 1 ¹/₂ cups chicken noodle, turkey noodle, chicken vegetable, beef noodle, vegetable beef or tomato soup with 5 soda crackers (2 inch squares)
- ☐ ²/₃ to 1 cup cream-style soup
- ☐ 1 cup split-pea soup or bean soup
- ☐ ¹/₂ cup tuna macaroni salad or chicken macaroni salad

Fast-food items that count as TWO choices

- ☐ 1 regular roast beef sandwich
- ☐ 1 tostada
- ☐ 1 bean burrito
- ☐ 1 serving frijoles with cheese
- ☐ 1 regular hamburger
- ☐ 1 serving chili con carne
- ☐ 1 serving fresh vegetables from the salad bar **or** 1 side or specialty salad **with** 1 to 2 tablespoons dressing
- ☐ 1 small shake
- ☐ 1 large frozen yogurt or soft-serve cone

Figure 6-3. Healthy Infant Outcome Project (HIOP), at The University of Minnesota.

Your Weight-Gain Chart

Weigh yourself on the same day every week during your pregnancy. Each time you weigh yourself, look on this chart and find the total number of pounds you've gained, line it up with the number of weeks you've been pregnant, and make a dot where the two lines meet on the chart. Your goal is to keep your dots inside the shaded area for your category. Don't worry if the line isn't smooth – small peaks and valleys are normal!

Name: _____   Weight-Gain Range: _____

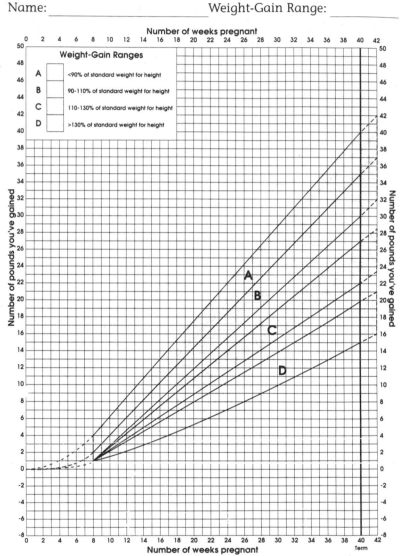

Supported in part by project #MCJ 276008 from the Maternal and Child Health program (Title V, Social Security Act), Health Resources and Services Administration, Department of Health and Human Services.

© Regents of the University of Minnesota, 1988

Figure 6-4. Weight gain chart.

ing maternal health and infant outcomes have been developed, including the Montreal Diet Dispensary program, the Virginia State Health Department program, and the Healthy Infant Outcome Project (HIOP).

The Montreal Diet Dispensary Program

The Montreal Diet Dispensary Program (MDD) has existed in Montreal since 1898. During the mid-1900s, under the leadership of Agnes Higgins, the dispensary developed an innovative nutrition assessment, counseling, and food distribution program for low-income pregnant women. The Higgins program utilizes an in-depth dietary history approach to nutrition counseling and specifies particular at risk diagnoses, depending on the results of the assessment. Each diagnosis corresponds to a particular nutrition protocol and food supplement package. Specific information on the Higgins method is available in her publications.[9,10] Infants of women participating in the MDD program experience a 50% lower rate of low birth weight, weighed an average of 107 g more, and had lower rates of intrauterine growth retardation than infants born to women prior to their participation in the program.[10]

Based on the MDD model, Clements at the Virginia Health Department instituted a large nutrition intervention project aimed at reducing the rate of low-birth-weight deliveries among underweight women served in public health clinics.[4] Women who gained the recommended amount of weight were rewarded by significantly fewer low-birth-weight deliveries than women who gained less than the amounts recommended.

Health Infant Outcome Project

The Health Infant Outcome Project was a weight gain and diet intervention program conducted by Brown, McKay, and Tharp in Minnesota. Based on the results of social marketing research conducted with prospective low-income clients, this project developed nutrition intervention materials (audiovisual tape, magazine, posters) and a nutrition protocol. (Fig. 6-3 displays *Mom's Baby Foods*, a pamphlet that is part of the nutritional protocol.)

The intervention materials and protocols were aimed at enhancing dietary behavior and weight gain during pregnancy. The prenatal weight gain recommendations for this project were developed by an expert panel and based on weight gains associated with the delivery of infants of optimal health in terms of birth weight (Brown JE, et al, unpublished data, Minneapolis, 1991). The prenatal weight gain grid used in the intervention project is displayed in Figure 6-4. Preliminary results indicate that the intervention project reduced low birth weight significantly (by approximately 50%) but did not affect rates of preterm delivery (Brown JE, unpublished data, Minneapolis, 1991).

SUMMARY

Infant outcomes in the United States are poorer than expected, given the resources of this nation. Improvements in maternal and infant health will, in part, depend on our ability to enhance the nutritional status of women before and during pregnancy. For this challenge to be met, scientifically based and uniform standards for the delivery of nutrition services, as well as supporting activities such as assurance that adequate diets and knowledge about them are available to all pregnant women, must become a reality. Whether efforts to improve maternal nutrition and infant outcomes are successful will largely depend on the ability of individual professionals within local agencies to deliver effective services to women during their pregnancies.

REFERENCES

1. *Advance report of final natality statistics, 1987*, Monthly vital statistics report 38, No 3, 1989. DHHS publication (PHS) 89-1120, Hyattsville, Md, 1989, National Center for Health Statistics.
2. Brown JE: Nutrition services for pregnant women, infants, children and adolescents, *Clin Nutr* 3:100, 1984.
3. Brown JE, Tomas RB: Taste changes during pregnancy, *Am J Clin Nutr* 43:414, 1986.
4. Clements DF: The nutrition intervention project for underweight pregnant women, *Clin Nutr* 7:205, 1988.
5. Flynn MM, Sade S: National results: Nutri/Systems nutrition literacy survey, Willow Grove, Pa, 1989, Nutri/Systems, Inc.
6. *Gallup survey of public opinion regarding diet and health,*

January 1990, Princeton, NJ, 1990, The Gallup Organization, Inc.

7. Guthrie HA, Scheer JC: Nutritional adequacy of self-selected diets that satisfy the Four Food Groups Guide, *J Nutr Educ* 13:46, 1981.

8. *Healthy people 2000: national health promotion and disease prevention objectives*, DHHS publication (PHS) 91-50212, Washington, DC, 1991, Department of Health and Human Services.

9. Higgins AC, Crampton EW, Moxley JE: *Nutrition and the outcome of pregnancy*. In: *Proceedings of the fourth international congress of endocrinology*, International Congress Series No 273, Washington, DC, 1972, Excerpta Medica.

10. Higgins AC and others: Impact of the Higgins Nutrition Intervention Program on birth weight: a within-mother analysis, *J Am Diet Assoc* 89:1097, 1989.

11. Hytten FE, Leitch I: *The physiology of human pregnancy*, Philadelphia, 1963, FA Davis Co.

12. Joyce T: The dramatic increase in the rate of low birthweight in New York City: an aggregate time-series analysis, *Am J Public Health* 80:682, 1990.

13. Miller CA: Infant mortality in the U.S., *Sci Am* 253:31, 1985.

14. National Academy of Sciences (Institute of Medicine): *Nutrition during pregnancy*. I. Weight gain. II. Nutrient supplements. Washington, DC, 1990, National Academy Press.

15. National Academy of Sciences (Institute of Medicine): *Nutrition during lactation*, Washington, DC, 1991, National Academy Press.

16. Newsholme A: *Report by the medical officer on child mortality*, supplement to the 30th annual report of the Local Government Board, London, 1910.

17. Second Followup Report: The Surgeon General's Workshop of Breast Feeding and Human Lactation. Washington, DC, 1991, National Center for Education in Maternal and Child Health.

APPENDIX 6-1

Position of the American Dietetic Association: Nutrition management of adolescent pregnancy*

Any pregnant adolescent is at nutritional risk because her own needs for growth and development are compromised by the extra demands on her system from the growth and development needs of the fetus. Low income, leading to an inadequate diet and limited access to appropriate medical care, may contribute significantly to nutritional risk. Early nutrition intervention is essential and can substantially change the course of events and improve pregnancy outcome.

*Reprinted with permission from J Am Diet Assoc 1989, 89:104. Approved by the House of Delegates on August 26, 1988, to be in effect until August 1993, unless it is reaffirmed or withdrawn as directed in the position development procedures of the House of Delgates. The American Dietetic Association authorizes republication of this position, in its entirety, provided full and proper credit is given.

It is the position of The American Dietetic Association that pregnant adolescents as a group are nutritionally at risk and require nutrition intervention early and throughout the duration of their pregnancies.

Adolescent pregnancy continues to be a major public health problem in the United States.[1] Infant mortality and low birth weight (LBW) remain high in this population, particularly when maternal age is less than 15 years.[2] The cost of infant mortality to society is difficult to quantitate in monetary terms. The financial cost of short-term and long-term morbidity related to low–birth-weight delivery and its numerous associated risks is very high ($13,616 per LBW infant for postpartum care in the neonatal intensive care unit, 1983 dollars).[3] The impact on individual families and society in general of caring for mentally and/or physically handicapped offspring of probalematic teen pregnancies is unmeasurable but clearly very great. High priority should be given to the prevention of low birth weight and its associated mortality and morbidity, especially in this high-risk population.

Although many biological and environmental variables have an impact on pregnancy outcome in the adolescent population, nutritional status is one of the more important modifiable variables affecting the health of the teenage mother and her fetus. Teenagers are more likely than their older counterparts to be underweight at the beginning of pregnancy and to gain less than 16 lb during pregnancy. Nineteen percent of infants born to teenagers weigh less than 2,500 g (<5.2 lb). Early nutrition intervention can substantially change the course of events. Increased weight gain during pregnancy can lower the risk of low–birth-weight outcome. When teenagers gain 21 to 25 lb, the incidence of LBW drops to 7.4% and to 6.3% when weight gain increases to 26 to 35 lb. Improved weight gain may also decrease fetal mortality. When weight gain during teen pregnancy increases from 16 to 26 to 35 lb, fetal mortality declines 50%, from 8.0 to 3.9 deaths per 1,000 live births. The NIH Consensus Conferences on Access to Prenatal Care and Low Birthweight defined the seven most effective components of prenatal care to improve pregnancy outcome; nutrition counseling is high on the list of important interventions.

To assure maintenance of health in the pregnant teen and optimum growth and development of her fetus, nutrition assessment and counseling should begin in early pregnancy and continue as an ongoing focus of prenatal care. In reality, this means that all adolescent or prenatal health clinics should provide nutrition assessment for their clients. Ideally, the assessment should be made by a dietitian/public health nutritionist trained to counsel adolescent clients and skilled at functioning on an interdisciplinary team. When pregnancy has been recognized, dietary patterns, laboratory data, and weight gain should be closely monitored; specific changes should be recommended when necessary. When there are concerns about access to food and nutritional risk, arrangements for participation in the Special Supplemental Food Program for Women, Infants, and Children (WIC) and other food assistance programs should be made.[4] Food budgeting should be examined, and assistance should be provided when necessary. Great effort should be made to enlist the support of the teen's partner, a friend, or a relative to encourage the establishment and maintenance of a healthful lifestyle during and after the pregnancy.

REFERENCES

1. National Center for Health Statistics. Advance report of final natality statistics, 1985. *Monthly Vital Statistics Report* 36, No. 4, July 17, 1987.
2. Mott, FL. The pace of repeated childbearing among young American mothers. *Fam Plann Perspect* 18:5, 1986.
3. Institute of Medicine. Preventing Low Birthweight. Washington, DC: National Academy Press, 1985.
4. Food Research and Action Center. WIC: A Success Story. Rev. ed. Washington, DC: Food Research and Action Center, 1988.

7 Infants, Children, and Adolescents

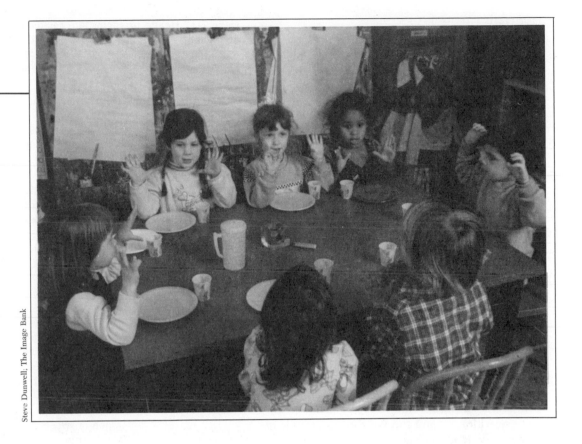

GENERAL CONCEPT

Nutrition is an important component of health care for infants, children, and adolescents. Infants grow rapidly and have requirements for protein, energy, and other essential nutrients that are higher per unit of body weight than at any other time in childhood. Thus the infants' increase in size is among the most dramatic developmental changes during the first year of life. A young child's growth rate slows considerably after the first year of life. Preschoolers' rate of growth is also slow. As a result, toddlers and preschoolers require less food because their appetites decrease. Adolescence is a time of emotional, physical, social, biological, and educational transitions. The adolescent's health and nutritional needs should be viewed in the context of children seeking to establish their identity in a changing adult world. There are infants, children, and adolescents who are described as "children with special health care needs" because of a variety of disabilities, handicaps, and chronic illnesses and conditions. Their complex needs require particular attention to enable them to achieve their maximum potential.

OUTCOME OBJECTIVES

When you finish this chapter, you should be able to:

- Understand the psychological and developmental maturation of infants, children, and adolescents and its influences on nutrient requirements of these age groups.
- Understand the role of major nutrients needed in each age group.
- Describe the health consequences of infants, children, and adolescents at nutritional risk.
- Understand and implement guidelines for patient management, including nutritional assessment, nutrition intervention, and referral.
- Describe nutrition services for children requiring special health care.

Nutrition plays a vital role in the growth and development of infants, children, and adolescents and its a major component in promoting health and preventing disease. Since the 1900s, publicly funded nutrition services have blossomed, wilted, and reblossomed, depending on economic conditions and political climates. However, our society continues to strongly value the importance of adequate nutrition during the vulnerable periods of infancy, childhood, and adolescence.[3]

NUTRITION-RELATED HEALTH PROBLEMS OF INFANTS, CHILDREN, AND ADOLESCENTS

The U.S. Department of Health and Human Services has identified several nutrition problems that affect infants and children: iron deficiency anemia in high-risk groups, suboptimum mental and physical development associated with inadequate nutrition, dental caries, and decreased resistance to infection in children.[33] Table 7-1 describes additional health-related problems of infants, children, and adolescents.

In the national goal to prevent unnecessary disease and disability and to achieve a better quality of life for all Americans, specific actions are needed for infants, children, and adolescents. These actions were first identified in 1979 in the health strategy published in the *Healthy People: The Sur-*

Table 7-1. Health problems and related nutritional risk factors

Health problems	Related nutritional risk factors
Infants and children	
Growth retardation, underweight	Dietary inadequacies
Elevated serum cholesterol	Excessive total fat, saturated fat, and cholesterol intake
Dental caries	Excessive, frequent consumption of sweets, lack of fluoride, baby bottle tooth decay
Iron deficiency anemia	Malnutrition, inadequate dietary iron intake
Infection	Malnutrition
Obesity	Caloric consumption exceeds caloric need
Constipation	Low fiber intake
Adolescents	
Hypertension	Overweight, excessive sodium intake, low potassium intake
Underweight	Undernutrition, anorexia nervosa, bulimia nervosa
Obesity	Caloric consumption exceeds caloric need
Dental caries	Excessive, frequent consumption of sweets
Infections	Malnutrition
Iron deficiency anemia	Early introduction of cow's milk, malnutrition, inadequate dietary iron intake
Elevated serum cholesterol	Excessive total fat, saturated fat, and cholesterol intake

Adapted from Brown JE: *Clin Nutr* 3:104, 1984.

geon General's Report on Health Promotion and Disease Prevention and expanded in 1980 in *Promoting Health/Preventing Disease: Objectives for the Nation*, which set a 10-year agenda to 1990. To continue the progress toward a healthier society, specific objectives for the next decade are noted in the *Healthy People 2000: National Health Promotion and Disease Prevention Objectives*, issued in 1991.[34] Specific nutrition objectives to be accomplished by 2000 relating to infants, children, and adolescents follow.

Infants and Children

By 2000 growth retardation among low-income children aged 5 and younger should be reduced to less than 10%. Up to 16% of low-income children, depending on age and race or ethnicity, were identified in 1988 to have growth retardation that most likely reflects the inadequacy of the child's diet. By 2000 the proportion of mothers who breastfeed their babies in the early postpartum period should be increased to 75%; those who continue breast-feeding until their babies are 5 to 6 months old should be increased to 50%. In 1988 the proportions were 54% at discharge from birth site and 21% at 5 to 6 months. By 2000 the proportion of parents and caregivers who use feeding practices that prevent baby bottle tooth decay should be increased to at least 75%. The prevalence has been estimated at 53% among American Indians and Alaska Native Head Start children and in urban populations from 1 to 11%. By 2000 iron deficiency should be reduced to less than 3% among children aged 1 through 4 and among women of childbearing age. Between 1976 and 1980 iron deficiency was 9% for children aged 1 through 2, 4% for children 3 to 4, and 5% for women aged 20 through 44. By 2000 the proportion of primary care providers who provide nutrition assessment and counseling and/or referral to qualified nutritionists or dietitians should be increased to at least 75%. In 1988, physicians provided diet counseling for an estimated 40 to 50% of patients but failed to refer many of the patients to qualified nutritionists and dietitians.

Adolescents

By 2000 overweight should be reduced to a prevalence of no more than 15% among adolescents aged 12 through 19. Between 1976 and 1980 it was estimated that 15% of adolescents ages 12 through 19 years were overweight.

IDENTIFYING PROBLEMS IN THE COMMUNITY: PEDIATRIC NUTRITION SURVEILLANCE SYSTEM

Conditions Related to Deficiencies

The Centers for Disease Control (CDC) Pediatric Nutrition Surveillance system identified that iron deficiency anemia was prevalent in high-risk groups, including young children. The national prevalence of low hematocrit was 15.4% and low hemoglobin 22.6% in 1990. Low-income children, ages 2 to 4 years, and in particular black children, had a higher prevalence of low hemoglobin and hematocrit levels. The risk for anemia decreased for children older than 3 years of age. Data from nutrition surveillance for the period 1980 to 1990 suggests that there has been a generalized improvement in the 1980s in child iron status among white, black, and Hispanic children participating in public health programs.[4]

Growth Stunting

The national prevalence of short stature, a measure of chronic undernutrition, was 9.4% in low-income children in 1990. Infants less than age 1 year and in particular black infants had the highest prevalence of low height for age. This is perhaps a reflection of their increased rate of low-birth weight.

In contrast to results for infants, black children in the CDC Pediatric Surveillance System had the lowest prevalence of short stature by ages 2 to 4 years, reflecting a more rapid rate of growth in early childhood (Fig. 7-1). Growth stunting increased in prevalence with age among Hispanic and Native American children. In the period from 1980 to 1990 trends from surveillance suggested that the prevalence of growth stunting among children has remained relatively stable except among the Asians, who have continued to decrease their rate.[4]

Dietary Deficiencies

In 1985 the Continuing Survey of Food Intakes by Individuals (CSFII) was conducted on women 19 to 50 years of age and children 1 to 5 years old. CSFII had basic features similar to the individual intake component of the Nationwide Food Consumption Survey (NFCS) conducted in 1977 and 1978. In NFCS potentially low intakes were documented for nutrients such as iron, calcium, vitamin B_6, and magnesium.[13] The highest-risk group includes females from adolescence through old age; this group had deficient intakes of all four of these nutrients. People on weight-reduction diets, par-

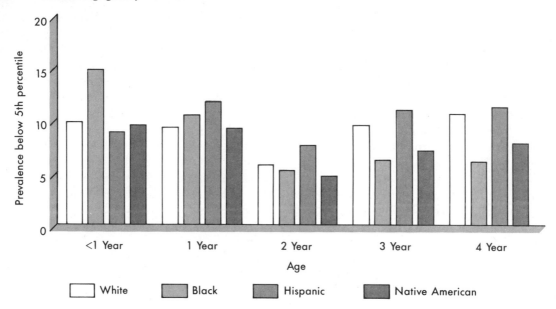

Figure 7-1. Prevalence of short stature (low height for age) among children screened in selected states, CDC Pediatric Nutrition Surveillance System, 1990.
Redrawn from unpublished data.

ticularly if they were dieting for extended periods of time, comprised another high-risk group for inadequate nutrient intake. Low income was also associated with poor intakes of some nutrients.

Young children continued to show deficient intakes of iron in the 1965 and 1977 NFCSs and in the 1985 CSFII. In the NFCSs the iron intake of children ages 1 to 2 years was less than half of that of children under 1 year of age. For infants, there was a threefold increase in iron intake between the 1965 and 1977 surveys. This factor was attributed to the higher consumption of iron-fortified formulas and cereals. A similar finding of low iron intake in young children was observed in the first National Health and Nutrition Examination Survey (NHANES I).[30] Children's intakes of food energy and nutrients expressed as percentages of 1980 RDA were higher in CSFII than in NFCS except for iron and zinc, which did not meet RDA but were significantly higher than the 1977 intake (zinc was not measured in 1977).

Conditions Related to Excesses or Imbalances

In the CDC Pediatric Nutrition Surveillance System 1990 findings, overweight among children increased to its highest rate, 9.5%, since 1980. Hispanic and Native American children had higher overall prevalences of obesity than other ethnic groups, especially at age 1 year (Fig. 7-2). Childhood obesity may persist into adult years, with long-term success for treatment for obesity being poor.

INFANTS

Physical Growth

The infant's increase in size is among the most obvious developmental changes occurring during the first year of life. Following birth, the newborn progresses from a weight of 1 to 4 kg (2 to 8 lb) to a mature weight of approximately 70 kg (154 lb). Average weight gain in the first year is 7 kg (15 lb), about half of which occurs in the first 4 months of life. Approximately 61,000 kcal are required to

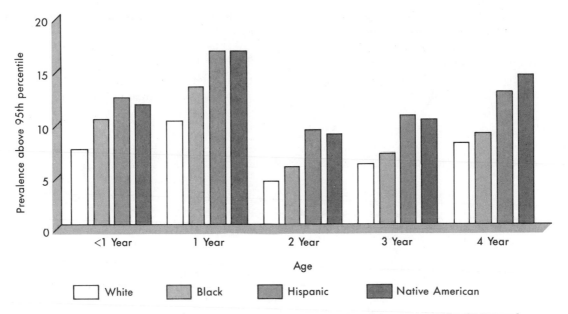

Figure 7-2. Prevalence of overweight (high weight for height) among children screened in selected states, CDC Pediatric Nutrition Surveillance System, 1990. Redrawn from unpublished data.

achieve the 3.5 kg (7 lb) growth between birth and 4 months of age.[25] Infants approximately triple or quadruple their birth weight in the first year.

Approximately 33% of calories consumed are used for growth during the first 4 months. This rapid growth in the healthy term infant during the first 4 months of life requires more energy, protein, and other essential nutrients per unit body weight than at any other time in infancy or childhood. These needs can be met completely with human milk, formula, or both.

At about 5 months of age, the infant enters a transitional period characterized by a decreased rate of growth and an increased level of caloric expenditure for physical activity, developmental readiness, and physiological capacity. Although total nutrient requirements continue to increase as a result of growth, the decreasing requirement for energy and protein pertinent to body weight reflects the progressive decrease in rate of growth.

By age 8 or 9 months, solid foods provide sig-

nificant source of energy and other nutrients to supplement the basic intake from human milk or formula. Infants usually increase in length by 50% by 1 year of age, double by 4 years of age, and triple in length by 13 years of age.

Physiology of Infant Nutrition

The enormously complex, yet efficient, gastrointestinal mechanism required for the absorption of nutrients and maintenance of health are well developed at birth, but not mature. All the secretions of the digestive tract contain enzymes especially suited to the digestion of human milk.

The ability to handle foods other than milk depends on the physiological development of the infant. The capacities for salivary, gastric, pancreatic, and intestinal digestion increase with age, indicating what may be a natural pattern for introduction of various sources of solid foods. During the first 3 months, salivary fluids seem to play a limited role in the digestion of milk. They become more important when solid foods are added to the diet. Table 7-2 describes the process, functions, and effects of digestion from birth to 6 months. The major changes in digestive capacity that occur at 4 to 6 months involve salivary and intestinal functions. Gastric capacities are usually adequate soon after birth and do not change significantly during this period.

Psychosocial Development

The mother's feeding practices from the infant's birth determine the infant's exposure to tactile

Table 7-2. Digestion in infancy

Location	Function	Effect on feeding
Birth to 3 months*		
Salivary	Lactose not produced in salivary secretions; amylase not available in significant quantities	Salivary enzymes play no role in digestion of milk
Gastric	Hydrochloric acid and pepsin precipitate casein into curds separate and acidify whey protein	Beginning of protein digestion; carbohydrate digestion partly begins; fat indigested in the stomach
Intestinal	Pancreatic and intestinal enzymes digest proteins into amino acids, reduce carbohydrates to monosaccharides, and split fatty acids from triglycerides in the small intestine	Protein from human milk is 95% digested, and a similar percentage of protein is digested from commercial formulas, which are heat-treated and sufficiently dilute to produce a soft curd
	Disaccharidases are present in the border of the intestinal mucosa	Human milk and commercial formulas; carbohydrate digested here
	Pancreatic amylase is present in small quantities	Complex carbohydrates poorly utilized
	Pancreatic lipase is present in sufficient quantity	Eighty percent of human milk fat is digested at birth, and almost 95% is digested by 1 month
	Lipase is naturally found in human milk, which is activated by bile salts	Digestion of fats from commercial formulas equals that of human milk
		Fat from other sources (butterfat) is poorly digested
4 to 6 months†		
Salivary	Ptyalin aids digestion to starch	As solid foods are added to the diet, ptyalin plays a role in the digestion of starches
Gastric	Functions already mature (occurs soon after birth with hydrochloric acid and pepsin for digestion of milk and nonmilk foods)	Aids in digestion of milk and nonmilk foods
Intestinal	Enzymes previously lacking are produced in larger quantities and digest nonmilk food substances; more putrefactive bacteria occur in intestinal flora as solid foods increase amount of protein in lower gastrointestinal tract	Amylase production increases and provides better utilization of starch-containing foods; increased production of amylase coincides with observed increase in infant's utilization of iron from cereals and nonmilk foods

From Willis NH: *Infant nutrition, birth to 6 months, a syllabus*, Philadelphia, 1971, JB Lippincott Co.
*The capacities for salivary, gastric, pancreatic, and intestinal digestion increase with age, indicating what may be a natural pattern for the introduction of various sources of solid foods.
†The major changes in digestive capacity that occur at 4 to 6 months involve principally salivary and intestinal functions. Gastric capacities are usually adequate soon after birth and do not change significantly after the third month of life.

stimulation, which is essential to the infant's physical and emotional growth. Appendix 7-1 describes the neuromuscular and psychosocial development of the infant (up to 12 months) with implications for feeding.

Nutrient Requirements

Requirements for infants younger than 6 months of age usually are based on the nutrients consumed by healthy, thriving infants who are breastfed by healthy, well-nourished mothers.[25] In Table 7-3 minimum requirements, advisable intakes, and recommended dietary allowances (RDAs) for selected nutrients are summarized. The minimum requirement is the smallest amount of a nutrient needed to protect the individual from undernutrition attributable to deficiency. The term *advisable intake* applies to levels of intake somewhat in excess of the estimated requirement.[8] The RDAs for most nutrients represent a value well above the average estimated requirement and encompasses the range of variability observed in individual requirement estimates.

RDAs for infants up to 6 months old are based primarily on the amount provided by human milk (750 ml), but in some cases the allowances may exceed those levels to provide for infants receiving formula.[10] RDAs for infants 6 months to 1 year of age are based on consumption of formula (600 ml) and increasing amounts of solid foods. In contrast to the allowances for specific nutrients, the allowance for energy is based on average needs of the

Table 7-3. Minimum requirements, advisable intakes, and recommended allowances of selected nutrients for infants: birth to 6 months and 6 to 12 months

Nutrient	Minimum requirements		Advisable intake		Recommended allowance*	
	0-6 months	6-12 months	0-6 months	6-12 months	0-6 months	6-12 months
Protein (g/100 kcal)	1.6	1.4	1.9	1.7	1.9	1.5
Protein (g/kg)	1.8	1.5	2.2	1.8	2.2	1.6
Vitamins						
A (RE)	75	75	150	150	375	375
D (μg cholecalciferol)	2.5	5	10	10	7.5	10
E (mg α-TE)	2	2	3	3	3	4
K (μg)	5	5	15	15	5	10
C (mg)	10	10	20	20	30	35
B$_1$ (mg)	0.1	0.1	0.2	0.2	0.3	0.4
B$_2$ (mg)	0.1	0.4	0.4	0.4	0.4	0.5
Niacin (mg NE)	2.0	4.5	5	5	5	6
B$_6$ (mg)	0.1	0.2	0.4	0.4	0.3	0.6
Folacin (μg)	50	50	50	50	25	35
Minerals						
Sodium (mEq)	2.5	2.1	8	6	12	9
Chloride (mEq)	2.3	2.1	7	6		
Potassium (mEq)	2.4	2.0	7	6		
Calcium (mg)	388	289	450	350	400	600
Phosphorus (mg)	132	110	160	130	300	500
Magnesium (mg)	16.5	13.5	25	20	40	60
Iron (mg)	7	7	7	7	6	10

From Owen GM, Paige DM: *Infancy*. In Paige DM, editor: *Manual of clinical nutrition*, St Louis, 1983, The CV Mosby Co.
*Food and Nutrition Board, National Research Council, National Academy of Sciences: *Recommended dietary allowances*, ed 10, Washington DC, 1989, National Academy Press.

population groups under consideration, and no adjustment is made for individual variability.

For the infant up to 6 months of age, average energy needs are met at an intake of 108 kcal/kg per day, and for the 6- to 12-month-old infant, 98 kcal/kg per day. The protein allowances for infants up to 6 months of age is 2.2 g/kg per day, and for 6- to 12-month-old infants, 1.6 g/kg per day.

Sources of Nutrients

Ranges of nutrient intakes for healthy infants who are exclusively breastfed or bottle-fed during the early months of life are shown in Table 7-4.[25] Breastfed infants at the lower end of the energy intake distribution consumed several nutrients in amounts very close to the estimated requirements. Nutrients in human milk tend to be more bioavailable than the same nutrients in formula, cow's milk, or solid foods.

Human milk. Levels of some nutrients secreted in human milk vary with maternal diet, stages of lactation, duration of lactation, and individual biochemical variability among women.[16] Caloric density and relative proportions of protein, fat, and carbohydrate in colostrum, transitional milk, and mature human milk vary considerably. Recent research has shown that neither maternal diet nor nutritional status has much effect on relative proportions of protein, fat, and carbohydrate in mature human milk. The malnourished woman may be able to produce milk of acceptable quality, although the quantity may be limited. In the healthy, well-nourished mother, the fatty acid composition of milk fat is determined primarily by the diet.

There is a 30% decrease in protein content of human milk between the first and sixth months of lactation.[21] During the same time lactose content does not change; concentrations of calcium, phosphorus, zinc, iron, sodium, potassium, and chloride all decrease 10% to 20%.[8] Studies of mineral content of milk from women 1 to 31 months postpartum showed that levels of some trace metals, particularly zinc, declined substantially over time. Levels of iron and copper decreased only moderately after the first 6 months.

Vitamin D and iron appear to be deficient in human milk. In the United States vitamin and mineral supplements are used widely during pregnancy and postpartum, especially during lactation. Thus variations in maternal diet appear to have a limited effect on levels of fat-soluble vitamins (A, D, E, K) in human milk. Variations in maternal intake of water-soluble vitamins (B vitamins and ascorbic acid) are reflected in levels of these vitamins in human milk. Vitamin B_{12} deficiency has been reported in a 6-month-old infant breastfed by his vegan mother.

Immunological benefits of breastfeeding. In the past decade there has been considerable research on the nonnutritional aspects of human milk, especially its immunological and other protective constituents. Three mechanisms are proposed by which human milk constituents protect infants. Two are based on immunological factors in milk and the third on its high nutrient value. The mechanism that has the strongest interaction evidence is the immunological mechanism, in which specific human milk constituents interact with the infant's epithelial surfaces or with specific nutrients or potential pathogens in the gastrointestinal lumen during digestion and absorption.[11]

Secretory immunoglobulin A (IgA) in mammary glands and human milk is largely derived from maternal gut associated with lymphoid tissue. Secretory IgA resists the proleolytic action of the infant's gastroenteric secretions to diminish antigen contact with the intestinal mucosa until the infant's own antibody responses develop. Lysozymes, lactoperoxidases, and lactoferrin are protein macromolecules in human milk that may be important host resistance factors for the infant. The importance of these immunological, cellular, and enzymatic components of human milk to the infant are indisputable where circumstances preclude preparation, storage, and feeding of a nutritionally adequate and hygienically safe formula.

Other non-nutrient components of human milk. Drugs taken by the lactating woman may reach her infant through the milk she produces. The amount of drug secreted into human milk depends on the lipid solubility of the medication, mechanisms of transport, degree of ionization, and

Table 7-4. Ranges of daily intakes of nutrients by 3-month-old infants exclusively breast- or formula-fed

Nutrient*	Breastfed		Formula-fed†	
	10th Percentile	90th Percentile	10th Percentile	90th Percentile
Protein (g/kg)	1.4	2.0	2.0	3.2
Vitamins				
A (RE)	380	600	455	715
D (μg)	0.4	0.6	7	11
E (mg α-TE)	1	1.5	7	11
K (μg)	10	16	22	34
C (mg)	30	45	35	65
B_1 (mg)	0.1	0.2	0.4	0.6
B_2 (mg)	0.3	0.4	0.6	0.9
Niacin (mg NE)	1	1.5	5.5	8.5
B_6 (mg)	0.05	0.08	0.3	0.4
Folacin (μg)	35	56	56	87
Minerals				
Sodium (mEq)	4.5	7.2	10.5	16.7
Chloride (mEq)	7.5	12	13.1	20.7
Potassium (mEq)	8.5	13.5	15.7	24.6
Calcium (mg)	225	360	415	650
Phosphorus (mg)	95	150	323	509
Magnesium (mg)	27	42	32	50
Iron (mg)	0.4	0.6	9	14

From Owen GM, Paige DM: *Infancy*. In Paige DM, editor: *Manual of clinical nutrition*, St Louis, 1983, The CV Mosby Co.
*Estimates of levels of intakes of various nutrients are based on average composition (amount of nutrients) of human milk and formulas in relation to the 10th and 90th percentiles of energy intakes of infants involved in a longitudinal growth study.
†Iron-fortified Enfamil or Similac.

changes in plasma pH. The higher the lipid solubility, the greater the concentration in human milk. The American Academy of Pediatrics in 1989 revised its statement on the transfer of drugs and other chemicals into human milk because certain drugs taken by breastfeeding women can have an effect in either the infant or on breastfeeding.

Prepared formula. The majority of infants who are bottlefed receive formulas composed of cow's milk protein, vegetable oils, and added carbohydrates. These products meet the infant's nutritional needs during the first 6 months of life (Table 7-5).

Cow's milk. The major difference between cow's milk and human milk is the greater concentration of protein and minerals and lower concentration of lactose in cow's milk. The higher ratio of whey proteins (lactalbumin and lactoglobulin) to casein in human milk versus cow's milk has not been shown to be of nutritional significance for the infant.[25]

Butterfat in cow's milk is less well digested and absorbed by the infant than is human milk fat. Cow's milk or evaporated milk meets the infant's needs for most of the B vitamins and for vitamins A and K. Most cow's milk is fortified with vitamin D, but it contains inadequate amounts of vitamins C and E, iron, and copper to serve as the only source of nutrition for the infant. In addition to the nutritional inadequacies of whole cow's milk or evaporated milk, there are problems related to curd formation (relatively high casein content), digestibility of fat, and potential excess renal solute

Table 7-5. Nutrient composition of human milk and proprietary infant formulas and recommended levels for full term and low-birth-weight infants (per 100 calories)

Nutrient	Minimum level recommended	Human milk	Enfamil (Mead-Johnson)	Similac (Ross)	SMA (Wyeth)	Enfamil premature formula	Similac PM (60/40) (Ross)
Protein, g	1.8[a]	1.3-1.6	2.2	2.22	2.2	3	2.34
Fat, g	3.3	5	5.6	5.37	5.3	5.1	5.56
Carbohydrate, g	—	10.3	10.3	10.7	10.6	11.1	10.2
Ash, g	—	0.28	0.45	0.61	0.4	0.64	—
Vitamin A, IU	250	250	310	300	300	1200	300
Vitamin D, IU	40	3	63	60	60	270	60
Vitamin E, IU	0.5	0.3	3.1	3	1.4	4.6	3
Vitamin K, μg	4	2	8.6	8	8	13	8
Vitamin C, mg	8	7.8	8.1	9	8.5	8.5	9
Thiamin, μg	40	25	78	100	100	35	100
Riboflavin, μg	60	60	156	150	150	350	150
Niacin, μg	250	250	1250	1050	750	4000	1050
Vitamin B_6, μg	35[b]	15	63	60	62.5	250	60
Folic acid, μg	4	4	15.6	15	7.5	0.3	15
Pantothenic acid, μg	300	300	470	450	315	1200	450
Vitamin B_{12}, μg	0.15	0.15	0.23	0.25	0.2	0.2	0.25
Biotin, μg	1.5	1.0	2.3	4.4	2.2	2	4.5
Inositol, mg	4	20	4.7	4.7	—	4.7	24
Choline, mg	7	13	15.6	16	15	7.6	12
Calcium, mg	60	50	69	75	63	165	56
Phosphorus, mg	30[c,d]	25	47	58	42	83	28
Magnesium, mg	6	6	7.8	6	7	7.6	6
Iron, mg	1g (0.15)	0.1	1.88	1.8	1.8	1.88	2.2
Iodine, μg	5	4-9	6	15	9	7.9	6
Copper, μg	60	60	94	90	70	130	90
Zinc, mg	0.5	0.5	0.78	0.75	0.8	1.56	0.75
Manganese, μg	5	1.5	15.6	5	22	13	5
Sodium, mg	20[d]	24	27	28	22	39	24
Potassium, mg	80	81	108	108	83	103	86
Chloride, mg	55	55	63	66	55.5	85	59
Renal solute load, mOsm	—	11.3[e]	20.0	14.7	91.2	21	14.3

Modified from American Academy of Pediatrics: *Pediatric Nutrition Handbook*, Evanston, Ill, 1985, American Academy of Pediatrics.

[a]Protein quality not less than 70% of casein. Lesser quality requires proportionately greater minimum amount of protein.

[b]At least 15 μg of Vitamin B_6 per gram of protein.

[c]Calcium/phosphorus ratio not less than 1:1, not more than 2:1.

[d]Some evidence of higher requirement for low-birth-weight infant.

[e]Calculated by method of Ziegler and Fomon.

load because of the relatively high levels of protein (urea) and minerals (sodium, potassium, chloride, phosphorus) excreted in the urine.

Solid food (Beikost). To meet the special needs of infants, the Academy of Pediatrics recommends breast milk or formula up to age 1 year, with a gradual addition of appropriate foods starting at 6 months. The introduction of solid foods should be delayed until the infant is approximately 5 months old. By this age, the healthy youngster will have developed fine, gross, and oral motor skills, be able to sit with some support and control the head, and show some hand-eye coordination to consume semisolid foods. During the next 6 or 7 months, as solid foods are introduced, human milk or formula provides a progressively smaller share of total calories; by age 9 to 12 months approximately one third and one half of the calories, respectively, will be supplied by solid foods.[1] Solid foods supply nearly half the total protein and iron intake, even though the infant receives an iron-fortified formula. If an isocaloric amount of human milk is substituted for the iron-fortified formula, approximate total intakes of protein, iron, and calcium are 20 g, 10.5 mg, and 550 mg, respectively, and solid foods account for half the calcium, two thirds of the protein, and essentially all the iron in the infant's diet.[25]

Recent Trends in Infant Feeding Practices

From the 1970s through the 1980s, important changes have occurred in patterns of infant feeding. From 1971 to 1983, the incidence of breastfeeding increased from 25% to 61% nationally, with considerable variation among socioeconomic groups. Breastfeeding rates continue to be the highest among women who are older, better educated, more affluent, or living in the western United States and lowest among those who are younger, less educated, lower income, black, or living in southeastern United States (Table 7-6). In the 1980s the incidence of initiating breastfeeding declined 16% from a high of 62% in 1982 to 52.2% in 1989, and the duration rate of breastfeeding declined 33% at 6 months of age, from 27% in 1983 to 18.1% in 1989 (Fig. 7-3). About 90% of the women who use bottle formula are using commercial formulas.

It appears that 65% to 75% of infants receive supplemental vitamins and minerals during the first year of life.[1] In general, the use of vitamin supplements increases with socioeconomic status.

A detailed review of the effects of breastfeeding on the mother's health, effects of the mother's nutrition on milk quality and quantity, and other breastfeeding issues are described in the report of *Nutrition during Lactation*.[15] (See Chapter 6.)

Table 7-6. Breastfeeding of infants born to ever-married mothers 15 to 44 years of age, according to selected characteristics of mother*: United States, 1981-1987

	Percent breastfeed at all		Percent breastfeed 3 months or more	
	1981-83	1984-87	1981-83	1984-87
Total	58.2	59	39	33.8
Race				
White	62	62.1	41.9	35.7
Black	30.3	30.2	17.7	16.2
Education				
Less than 12 years	30.1	30.7	12	16
12 years	54	50.9	31.9	25.7
13 years more	71.5	73.3	54.6	45.2
Geographic region				
Northeast	65.7	70.5	51.1	44.5
Northcentral	58.1	53.7	38.5	28.3
South	47.4	47.9	26.9	25.1
West	73.1	77.2	51.7	48.3

From National Center for Health Statistics, Centers for Disease Control: *National survey of family growth*, Hyattsville, Md, 1988, National Center for Health Statistics.

*Characteristics of mothers are reported as of the interview date in 1988. From Garza C, Cowell C: *Infant nutrition*. In Sharbaugh CO, editor: *Call to action: better nutrition for mothers, children, and families*, Washington, DC, 1991, National Center for Education in Maternal and Child Health.

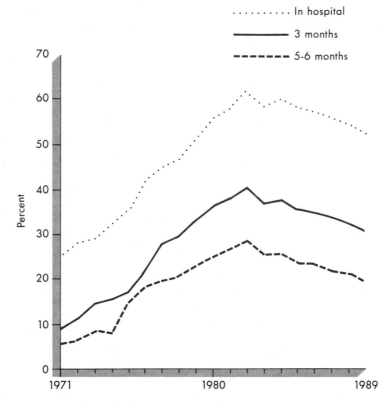

Figure 7-3. Percent breastfeeding: 1971-1989 all races
Redrawn from Office of Maternal and Child Health, Public Health Service, US Department of Health and Human Services; *Child health USA '89,* Washington, DC, 1989, US Department of Health and Human Services.

Health Consequences of Infants at Nutritional Risk

Iron Deficiency

Iron deficiency is one of the most common nutritional deficiencies in North America. Although signs of anemia appear after 12 months of age, they have their genesis in inadequate iron nutrition during the first year of life. Prolonged iron deficiency eventually results in iron deficiency anemia. In healthy full-term infants, iron deficiency anemia is uncommon before 4 to 6 months because of iron stores. In infants 6 to 24 months of age, *anemia* is defined as hemoglobin concentration less than 11 g/dl.

Obesity

Infantile obesity has been defined by some as weight above the 95th percentile in relation to height, age, sex, and body build. Infantile obesity is commonly secondary to excessive intake of food. Poor infant feeding practices and misuse of solid foods, such as introducing them too early, can readily contribute to overfeeding.

Atherosclerosis

Evidence exists that the atherosclerotic process begins in childhood and progresses slowly into adulthood. The National Cholesterol Education Program published in 1991, *Report of the Expert Panel on Blood Cholesterol Levels in Children and Adolescents,*[36] reviewed the evidence that atherosclerosis or its precursors begin in young people and made nutrient recommendations intended for all healthy children and adolescents over the age of about 2 years. A safe guide is to pattern dietary intake in the early months of life on the nutrients found in human milk. For any infant, either healthy or with familial lipid disorder, there would appear to be no particular advantage in consuming solid food before the first 5 to 6 months of life and no particular advantage in the use of foods high in saturated fats or cholesterol during the second 6 months of life.

Guidelines for Patient Management

The expected outcomes of care for a normal infant include the following:[19]

- Infants maintain acceptable weight and length between the 5th and 95th percentile when plotted on the National Center for Health Statistics (NCHS) growth grid.
- Infants do not deviate more than 25 percentile points from the established pattern of growth (height and weight).
- Infants' hemoglobin levels are equal to or greater than 11 g or hematocrit levels are equal to or greater than 33%.
- Infants are breastfed or consume human milk up to 1 year of age. If this is not feasible, iron-fortified formula should be used throughout the first year.
- Infants consume solid food in accordance with stages of neuromuscular readiness and growth.
- Infants' food intake is nutritionally adequate for age or stage of development.

Nutrition Screening and Assessment

Nutritional Disorders of Children: Prevention, Screening and Follow-Up[9] is a useful guide to assist community dietitians and nutritionists and other health care providers to perform nutritional assessments of infants and children. Nutritional assessment and intervention guidelines for infants and children are presented in Table 7-7. Screening for blood lead has been included based on the 1991 CDC recommendations on lead screening and consequences of lead poisoning in children.[35]

Anthropometric Assessment

Anthropometric measurements recommended for neonates and infants include weight, recumbent length (crown-heel), head circumference, triceps skinfold, and upper arm circumference.

Appraisal of body size and pattern of growth is a fundamental part of pediatric care. Abnormal size and growth are commonly associated with malnutrition or disease. Evaluation of growth helps in the detection and diagnosis of disorders of infancy and childhood. Discussion of an infant's growth is often the starting point for effective dialogue with that child's parent or caretaker.

In 1975 the National Center for Health Statistics (NCHS) compiled data and prepared a series of percentile curves reflecting the growth of comtemporary infants, children, and youth in the United States.[30] These charts should be effective in facilitating uniformity in the clinical appraisal of growth and nutritional status and should help to simplify comparative interpretation of growth data. Figures 7-4 and 7-5 are examples of growth charts for boys and girls, prepubescent and 2 to 18 years.

Tables 7-8 and 7-9 include the NCHS percentiles for length, weight, and head circumference for boys and girls up to 36 months of age (Table 7-10).

Weight. Body weight should be measured to the nearest 10 g (½ oz) for infants or 100 g (¼ lb) for children. A beam balance scale should be used. The infant's clothes should be removed before he or she is weighed. The infant should be placed in the center of the weighing surface. Zero should be checked before every session and when the scale is moved. The scales should be calibrated at least every few months against reference weights.

Length. Recumbent length is measured for children younger than 24 months or for children between 24 and 36 months of age who cannot stand unassisted.[22] The measurement should be made on an examining table with a length-measuring device with a headboard and a movable front board that are perpendicular to the table surface. Length is

Text continued on p. 152.

Table 7-7. Nutrition assessment and intervention guidelines for population groups in community nutrition

Nutritional assessment components	Methods	Risks and problems indicated	Intervention guidelines	Referral sources
Infants and children				
Anthropometric Height for weight Height for age Weight for age Head circumference (to age 2 years) Skinfold thickness	Beam balance scale (nude or lightly dressed), measuring board and nonstretch tape: status using National Center for Health Statistics (NCHS) growth grids; skinfold calipers using standardized technique and validated predictive equation or nomogram	Undernutrition, malnutrition; stunting; failure to thrive (height for age <5th percentile); severe malnutrition (above plus head circumference <5th percentile or a significant drop in range on growth grid); overweight, obesity (weight for height >95th percentile), percent body fat >95th percentile	Refer and report cases of child abuse; refer children and families to food assistance programs; adjust dietary intake to increase weight gain, or stabilize intake until overweight is compensated by increases in height; adjust activity level	Private physicians-primary care: WIC Program; Children and Youth Programs; Services for Children with Special Health Care Needs; Regional Center for High-Risk Newborns; Title XIX; Head Start; Child abuse and neglect centers; Food Stamps; Commodity Supplemental Food Program
Biochemical Hemoglobin Hematocrit Serum cholesterol* Lead†	Standard technique	Malnutrition; anemia; elevated serum cholesterol (>170 mg/dl); blood lead (≥10.0 μg/dl)	Improve iron intake, supplement with iron; reduce total fat and cholesterol intake, apply additional serum cholesterol lowering methods as indicated; environmental intervention for lead	
Clinical Birth weight for gestational age	Beam balance scale, digital scale, reference standard	Intrauterine growth retardation, large for gestational age	Adjust feeding to meet nutritional needs based on gestational age and catch-up group potential; rule out hypoglycemia in small and large newborns	
Blood pressure	Monitor in children over 3 years of age	"High normal" blood pressure	Weight management; reduction of dietary salt intake if excessive	

Dietary
  Dietary quantity and quality
  Feeding development
	Interview or questionnaire on food groups, food recall, or record analysis	Malnutrition, underweight, overweight risk; abnormal development of feeding and motor skills	Adjust dietary intake to meet nutrient needs; progress toward normal feeding developmental milestones	Prenatal care; WIC Program; Maternal and Infant Care Programs; Commodity Supplemental Food Program; physical fitness program and recreational facilities

Adolescents				

Anthropometric
  Height
  Weight
  Skinfold thickness
	Beam balance scales, nonstretch tape, calipers; NCHS growth grids for boys and girls 3 to 18 years of age; assess weight status using weight-for-height grid; assess percentage body fat using a reference standard; assess growth velocity using reference standard	Short stature; underweight, overweight	Adjust dietary intake and activity level	

Biochemical
  Hemoglobin
  Hematocrit
  Serum cholesterol*
	Standard techniques	Malnutrition; anemia; elevated cholesterol	Adjust diet, iron supplementation as indicated	Physician, psychologist, or guidance center

Clinical
  Blood pressure
  Dental disease
	Standard techniques	"High normal" blood pressure; dental caries	Weight management; salt reduction; reduction of sticky sweets consumption	Drug treatment centers; Alcoholics Anonymous; neighborhood health center

Dietary: dietary quantity and quality	3-day food record, diet history (computerized nutrient analysis)	Malnutrition	Adjust diet to meet requirements	Adolescent clinics; nontraditional alternative health centers

Update of Brown JE: *Clin Nutri* 3:105, 1984.

*Children ages ≥2 years with family history of premature cardiovascular disease or at least one parent with high blood cholesterol. US Department of Health and Human Services, Public Health Services, National Institutes of Health: National Cholesterol Education Program: *Report of the expert panel on blood cholesterol in children and adolescents*, Pub (NIH) 91-2732, Washington, DC, 1991, US Government Printing Office.

†US Department of Health and Human Services, Public Health Services, Centers for Disease Control: *Preventing lead poisoning in young children*, Atlanta, 1991, US Government Printing Office.

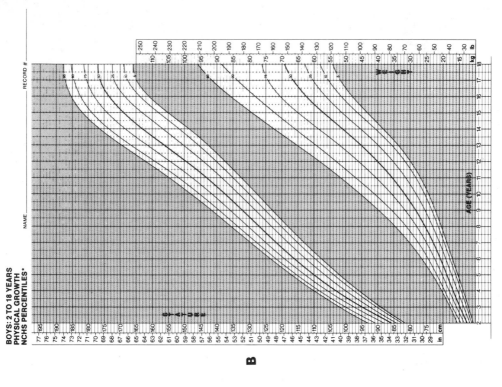

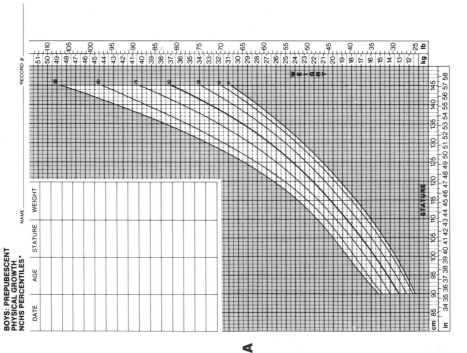

Figure 7-4. A, Physical growth NCHS percentiles in prepubescent boys. **B,** Physical growth NCHS percentiles in boys ages 2 to 18 years. From Ross Laboratories, Inc., Columbus, Ohio.

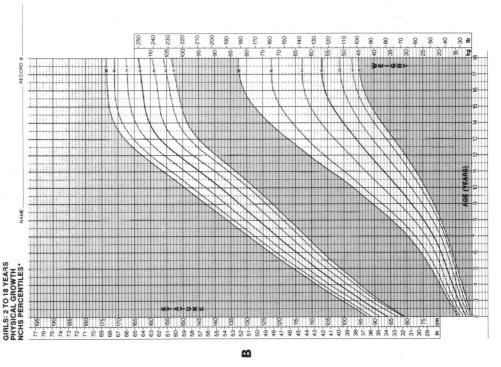

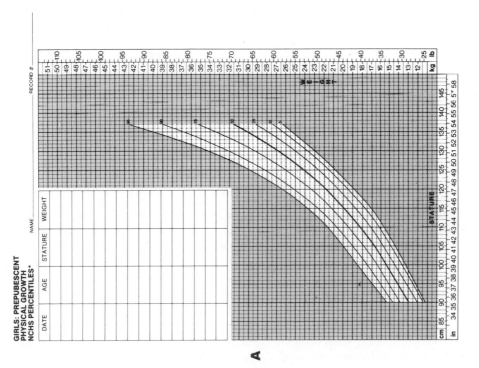

Figure 7-5. **A,** Physical growth NCHS percentiles in prepubescent girls. **B,** Physical growth NCHS percentiles in girls ages 2 to 18 years. From Ross Laboratories, Inc., Columbus, Ohio.

Table 7-8. NCHS percentiles for length, weight, and head circumference for age: boys, birth to 36 months

Age (months)	Percentile							Measurement
	5th	10th	25th	50th	75th	90th	95th	
Birth	46.4	47.5	49	50.5	51.8	53.5	54.4	Length (cm)
	18¼	18¾	19¼	20	20½	21	21½	Length (in)
	2.54	2.78	3	3.27	3.64	3.82	4.15	Weight (kg)
	5½	6¼	6¼	7¼	8	8½	9¼	Weight (lb)
	32.6	33	33.9	34.8	35.6	36.6	37.2	Head C (cm)
	12¾	13	13¼	13¾	14	14½	14¾	Head C (in)
1	50.4	51.3	53	54.6	56.2	57.7	58.6	Length (cm)
	19¾	20¼	20¾	21½	22¼	22¾	23	Length (in)
	3.16	3.43	3.82	4.29	4.75	5.14	5.38	Weight (kg)
	7	7½	8½	9½	10½	11¼	11¾	Weight (lb)
	34.9	35.4	36.2	37.2	38.1	39	39.6	Head C (cm)
	13¾	14	14¼	14¾	15	15¼	15½	Head C (in)
3	56.7	57.7	59.4	61.1	63	64.5	65.4	Length (cm)
	22¼	22¾	23½	24	24¾	25½	25¾	Length (in)
	4.43	4.78	5.32	5.98	6.56	7.14	7.37	Weight (kg)
	9¾	10½	11¾	13¼	14½	15¾	16¼	Weight (lb)
	38.4	38.9	39.7	40.6	41.7	42.5	43.1	Head C (cm)
	15	15¼	15¾	16	16½	16¾	17	Head C (in)
6	63.4	64.4	66.1	67.8	69.7	71.3	72.3	Length (cm)
	25	25¼	26	26¾	27½	28	28½	Length (in)
	6.2	6.61	7.2	7.85	8.49	9.1	9.46	Weight (kg)
	13¾	14½	15¾	17¼	18¾	20	20¾	Weight (lb)
	41.5	42	42.8	43.8	44.7	45.6	46.2	Head C (cm)
	16¼	16½	16¾	17¼	17½	18	18¼	Head C (in)
9	68	69.1	70.6	72.3	74	75.9	77.1	Length (cm)
	26¾	27¼	27¾	28½	29¼	30	30¼	Length (in)
	7.52	7.95	8.56	9.18	9.88	10.49	10.93	Weight (kg)
	16½	17½	18¾	20¼	21¾	23¼	24	Weight (lb)
	43.5	44	44.8	45.8	46.6	47.5	48.1	Head C (cm)
	17¼	17¼	17¾	18	18¼	18¾	19	Head C (in)

recorded as the distance between the headboard and frontboard when the infant has been positioned properly. Two people are required for measuring an infant's length. Length should be recorded to the nearest 0.1 cm (⅛ inch).

Head circumference. An insertion tape provides adequate positioning and fixation of the tape around the head. Springy hair should be compressed. A hair layer 0.6 cm (1.4 in) thick around one half of the head will theoretically increase head

circumference by almost 2.5 cm (1 inch). Increments in head circumference at various age levels are shown in Tables 7-8 and 7-9.

Skinfold thickness. Skinfold thickness has been proposed as a useful index of relative fatness of the body because subcutaneous adipose tissue is a major component of body fat.[24] The thickness of the skin and subcutaneous fat can be measured with calipers. In 1968 the Committee on Nutrition of the American Academy of Pediatrics suggested that

Table 7-8. NCHS percentiles for length, weight, and head circumference for age: boys, birth to 36 months— cont'd

Age (months)	Percentile							Measurement
	5th	10th	25th	50th	75th	90th	95th	
12	71.7	72.8	74.3	76.1	77.7	79.8	81.2	Length (cm)
	28¼	28¾	29¼	30	30½	31½	32	Length (in)
	8.43	8.84	9.49	10.15	10.91	11.54	11.99	Weight (kg)
	18½	19½	21	22½	24	25½	26½	Weight (lb)
	44.8	45.3	46.1	47	47.9	48.8	49.3	Head C (cm)
	17¾	17¾	18¼	18½	18¾	19¼	19½	Head C (in)
18	77.5	78.7	80.5	82.4	84.3	86.6	88.1	Length (cm)
	30½	31	31¾	32½	33¼	34	34¾	Length (in)
	9.59	9.92	10.67	11.47	12.31	13.05	13.44	Weight (kg)
	21¼	21¾	23¼	25¼	27¼	28¾	29½	Weight (lb)
	46.3	47.7	47.4	48.4	49.3	50.1	50.6	Head C (cm)
	18¼	18½	18¾	19	19½	19¾	20	Head C (in)
24	82.3	83.5	85.6	87.6	89.9	92.2	93.8	Length (cm)
	32½	32¾	33¾	34½	35½	36¼	37	Length (in)
	10.54	10.85	11.65	12.59	13.44	14.29	14.7	Weight (kg)
	23¼	24	25¾	27¾	29¾	31½	32½	Weight (lb)
	47.3	47.7	48.3	49.2	50.2	51	51.4	Head C (cm)
	18½	18¾	19	19¼	19¾	20	20¼	Head C (in)
30	87	88.2	90.1	92.3	94.6	97	98.7	Length (cm)
	34¼	34¾	35½	36¼	37¼	38¼	38¾	Length (in)
	11.44	11.8	12.63	13.67	14.51	15.47	15.97	Weight (kg)
	25¼	26	27¾	30¼	32	34	35¼	Weight (lb)
	48	48.4	49.1	49.9	51	51.7	52.2	Head C (cm)
	19	19	19¼	19¾	20	20¼	20½	Head C (in)
36	91.2	92.4	94.2	96.5	98.9	101.4	103.1	Length (cm)
	36	36½	37	38	39	40	40½	Length (in)
	12.26	12.69	13.58	14.69	15.59	16.66	17.28	Weight (kg)
	27	28	30	32½	34¼	36¾	38	Weight (lb)
	48.6	49	49.7	50.5	51.5	52.3	52.8	Head C (cm)
	19¼	19¼	19½	20	20¼	20½	20¾	Head C (in)

before techniques of measuring skinfold thickness were promulgated as a practical clinical tool for assessing relative fatness of individual children, basic reference data should be collected.[5] Between 1963 and 1974, NCHS pooled skinfold thickness and upper arm girth measurements of about 20,000 children ages 1 to 17 years in the United States and developed smoothed percentiles to serve as reference data.

In a report of a small conference convened to discuss the data pooled by the NCHS, it was emphasized that the percentiles described the skinfold thicknesses of American children and adolescents and should not be considered "norms" or "standards."[24] The NCHS skinfold thickness percentiles are based on data from National Health Examination Surveys (NHES) Cycle II and III and NHANES I.[17] It is considered inappropriate to conclude that a skinfold thickness above or below some arbitrary percentile is unacceptable because avail-

Table 7-9. NCHS percentiles for length, weight, and head circumference for age: girls, birth to 36 months

Age (months)	Percentile							Measurement
	5th	10th	25th	50th	75th	90th	95th	
Birth	45.4	46.5	48.2	49.9	51	52	52.9	Length (cm)
	17¾	18¼	19	19¾	20	20½	20¾	Length (in)
	2.36	2.58	2.93	3.23	3.52	3.64	3.81	Weight (kg)
	5¼	5¾	6½	7	7¾	8	8½	Weight (lb)
	32.1	32.9	33.5	34.3	34.8	35.5	35.9	Head C (cm)
	12¾	13	13¼	13½	13¾	14	14¼	Head C (in)
1	49.2	50.2	51.9	53.5	54.9	56.1	56.9	Length (cm)
	19¼	19¾	20½	21	21½	22	22½	Length (in)
	2.97	3.22	3.59	3.98	4.36	4.65	4.92	Weight (kg)
	6½	7	8	8¾	9½	10¼	10¾	Weight (lb)
	34.2	34.8	35.6	36.4	37.1	37.8	38.3	Head C (cm)
	13½	13¾	14	14¼	14½	15	15	Head C (in)
3	55.4	56.2	57.8	59.5	61.2	62.7	63.4	Length (cm)
	21¾	22¼	22¾	23½	24	24¾	25	Length (in)
	4.18	4.47	4.88	5.4	5.9	6.39	6.74	Weight (kg)
	9¼	9¾	10¾	12	13	14	14¾	Weight (lb)
	37.3	37.8	38.7	39.5	40.4	41.2	41.7	Head C (cm)
	14¾	15	15¼	15½	16	16¼	16½	Head C (in)
6	61.8	62.6	64.2	65.9	67.8	69.4	70.2	Length (cm)
	24¼	24¾	25¼	26	26¾	27¼	27¾	Length (in)
	5.79	6.12	6.6	7.21	7.83	8.38	8.73	Weight (kg)
	12¾	13½	14½	16	17¼	18½	19¼	Weight (lb)
	40.3	40.9	41.6	42.4	43.3	44.1	44.6	Head C (cm)
	15¾	16	16½	16¾	17	17¼	17½	Head C (in)
9	66.1	67	68.7	70.4	72.4	74	75	Length (cm)
	26	26½	27	27¾	28½	29¼	29½	Length (in)
	7	7.34	7.89	8.56	9.24	9.83	10.17	Weight (kg)
	15½	16¼	17½	18¾	20¼	21¾	22½	Weight (lb)
	42.3	42.8	43.5	44.3	45.1	46	46.4	Head C (cm)
	16¾	16¾	17¼	17½	17¾	18	18¼	Head C (in)

Modified from National Center for Health Statistics, Health Resources Administration, U.S. Department of Health and Human Services, Hyattsville, Md, 1978, US Government Printing Office. Reprinted with permission of Ross Laboratories, Columbus, OH 43216, from *Pediatric Anthropometry*, © 1982 Ross Laboratories.

able information is inadequate to define risks of relative fatness. Finally, it was suggested that skinfold thickness should probably not be used as a routine screening measurement in well child care. However, it is operationally reasonable to limit measurements of skinfolds during infancy and childhood to individuals whose weight for stature is greater than the 90th percentile or less than the 10th percentile. Skinfold measurements are useful in follow-up and monitoring of individual children who are identified as having a potential or real problem of obesity.[24]

Methods of measuring triceps skinfold thickness. Tricep skinfold thickness is a measurement of a double layer of skin and subcutaneous fat on the back of the upper arm. It is a convenient-to-measure, useful index of body fat. Measurement of triceps skinfold thickness requires a flexible, nonstretchable tape measure and a skinfold caliper. A Lange, Harpenden, or Holtain caliper is suitable.

Triceps skinfold thickness is measured on the back of the left arm midway between the shoulder and elbow. This measurement may be difficult to obtain in infants, and much patience is required.

Table 7-9. NCHS percentiles for length, weight, and head circumference for age: girls, birth to 36 months—cont'd

Age (months)	Percentile							Measurement
	5th	10th	25th	50th	75th	90th	95th	
12	69.8	70.8	72.4	74.3	76.3	78	79.1	Length (cm)
	27½	27¾	28½	29¼	30	30¾	31¼	Length (in)
	7.84	8.19	8.81	9.53	10.23	10.87	11.24	Weight (kg)
	17¼	18	19½	21	22½	24	24¾	Weight (lb)
	43.5	44.1	44.8	45.6	46.4	47.2	47.6	Head C (cm)
	17¼	17¼	17¾	18	18¼	18½	18¾	Head C (in)
18	76	77.2	78.8	80.9	83	85	86.1	Length (cm)
	30	30½	31	31¾	32¾	33½	34	Length (in)
	8.92	9.3	10.04	10.82	11.55	12.3	12.76	Weight (kg)
	19¾	20½	22¼	23¾	25½	27	28¼	Weight (lb)
	45	45.6	46.3	47.1	47.9	48.6	49.1	Head C (cm)
	17¾	18	18¼	18½	18¾	19¼	19¼	Head C (in)
24	81.3	82.5	84.2	86.5	88.7	90.8	92	Length (cm)
	32	32½	33¼	34	35	35¾	36¼	Length (in)
	9.87	10.26	11.1	11.9	12.74	13.57	14.08	Weight (kg)
	21¾	22½	24½	26¼	28	30	31	Weight (lb)
	46.1	46.5	47.3	48.1	48.8	49.6	50.1	Head C (cm)
	18¼	18¼	18½	19	19¼	19½	19¾	Head C (in)
30	86	87	88.9	91.3	93.7	95.6	96.9	Length (cm)
	33¾	34¼	35	36	37	37¾	38¼	Length (in)
	10.78	11.21	12.11	12.93	13.93	14.81	15.35	Weight (kg)
	23¾	24¾	26¾	28½	30¾	32¾	33¾	Weight (lb)
	47	47.3	48	48.8	49.4	50.3	50.8	Head C (cm)
	18½	18½	19	19¼	19½	19¾	20	Head C (in)
36	90	91	93.1	95.6	98.1	100	101.5	Length (cm)
	35½	35¾	36¾	37¾	38½	39¼	40	Length (in)
	11.6	12.07	12.99	13.93	15.03	15.97	16.54	Weight (kg)
	25½	26½	28¾	30¾	33¼	35¼	36½	Weight (lb)
	47.6	47.9	48.5	49.3	50	50.8	51.4	Head C (cm)
	18¾	18¾	19	19½	19¾	20	20¼	Head C (in)

The infant should be held in a semiupright position on the lap of the mother or an attendant. The infant's right side should be adjacent to the mother's body, with the infant's head erect. The infant's left hand should be gently restrained, with the elbow flexed 90 degrees and the forearm pressed gently against the infant's abdomen. The tape should be used to locate the midpoint between the left shoulder and elbow placement of the caliper jaws.

At a level about 1 cm above the midpoint, a vertical fold of skin and subcutaneous tissue is grasped between the thumb and index finger. The long axis of the skinfold should be parallel to the long axis of the arm. The skinfold should be pulled gently away from the underlying muscle and held while the jaws of the caliper are placed over it at the previously marked midpoint. Variability of repeated triceps skinfold measurements will be large if they are made at different sites (e.g., above, below, to the right of, or to the left of the marked point). To avoid reading error caused by parallax, the person making the measurement should look directly down on the caliper, which is held horizontally.

Table 7-10. CDC NCHS fifth and third percentiles weight for height for age: girls, 2 years of age and older

Height		Weight/height				Height		Weight/height				Height		Weight/height			
		5th PCTL		3rd PCTL				5th PCTL		3rd PCTL				5th PCTL		3rd PCTL	
in	8ths	lb	¼ lb	lb	¼ lb	in	8ths	lb	¼ lb	lb	¼ lb	in	8ths	lb	¼ lb	lb	¼ lb
29	0	17	1	16	2	34	0	22	3	22	1	39	0	28	2	27	3
29	1	17	1	16	3	34	1	23	0	22	1	39	1	28	3	28	0
29	2	17	2	17	0	34	2	23	0	22	2	39	2	28	3	28	0
29	3	17	2	17	0	34	3	23	1	22	3	39	3	29	0	28	1
29	4	17	3	17	1	34	4	23	1	22	3	39	4	29	0	28	2
29	5	18	0	17	1	34	5	23	2	23	0	39	5	29	1	28	2
29	6	18	0	17	2	34	6	23	3	23	0	39	6	29	2	28	3
29	7	18	1	17	3	34	7	23	3	23	1	39	7	29	2	28	3
30	0	18	1	17	3	35	0	24	0	23	1	40	0	29	3	29	0
30	1	18	2	18	0	35	1	24	0	23	2	40	1	30	0	29	1
30	2	18	2	18	0	35	2	24	1	23	2	40	2	30	0	29	1
30	3	18	3	18	1	35	3	24	1	23	3	40	3	30	1	29	2
30	4	19	0	18	1	35	4	24	2	23	3	40	4	30	2	29	3
30	5	19	0	18	2	35	5	24	2	24	0	40	5	30	2	29	3
30	6	19	1	18	3	35	6	24	3	24	1	40	6	30	3	30	0
30	7	19	1	18	3	35	7	24	3	24	1	40	7	31	0	30	1
31	0	19	2	19	0	36	0	25	0	24	2	41	0	31	0	30	1
31	1	19	2	19	0	36	1	25	1	24	2	41	1	31	1	30	2
31	2	19	3	19	1	36	2	25	1	24	3	41	2	31	2	30	3
31	3	20	0	19	1	36	3	25	2	24	3	41	3	31	2	30	3
31	4	20	0	19	2	36	4	25	2	25	0	41	4	31	3	31	0
31	5	20	1	19	3	36	5	25	3	25	0	41	5	32	0	31	1
31	6	20	1	19	3	36	6	25	3	25	1	41	6	32	0	31	1
31	7	20	2	20	0	36	7	26	0	25	1	41	7	32	1	31	2
32	0	20	2	20	0	37	0	26	1	25	2	42	0	32	2	31	3
32	1	20	3	20	1	37	1	26	1	25	3	42	1	32	3	31	3
32	2	20	3	20	1	37	2	26	2	25	3	42	2	32	3	32	0
32	3	21	0	20	2	37	3	26	2	26	0	42	3	33	0	32	1
32	4	21	1	20	2	37	4	26	3	26	0	42	4	33	1	32	2
32	5	21	1	20	3	37	5	26	3	26	1	42	5	33	2	32	2
32	6	21	2	20	3	37	6	27	0	26	1	42	6	33	2	32	3
32	7	21	2	21	0	37	7	27	1	26	2	42	7	33	3	33	0
33	0	21	3	21	1	38	0	27	1	26	3	43	0	34	0	33	0
33	1	21	3	21	1	38	1	27	2	26	3	43	1	34	1	33	1
33	2	22	0	21	2	38	2	27	2	27	0	43	2	34	1	33	2
33	3	22	0	21	2	38	3	27	3	27	0	43	3	34	2	33	3
33	4	22	1	21	3	38	4	28	0	27	1	43	4	34	3	34	0
33	5	22	2	21	3	38	5	28	0	27	1	43	5	35	0	34	0
33	6	22	2	22	0	38	6	28	1	27	2	43	6	35	0	34	1
33	7	22	3	22	0	38	7	28	1	27	3	43	7	35	1	34	2

From Centers for Disease Control: *NCHS/CDC/WHO normalized reference data*, Centers for Disease Control, Atlanta, 1988.

Table 7-10. CDC NCHS fifth and third percentiles weight for height for age: girls, 2 years of age and older—cont'd

Height		Weight/height				Height		Weight/height			
		5th PCTL		3rd PCTL				5th PCTL		3rd PCTL	
in	8ths	lb	¼ lb	lb	¼ lb	in	8ths	lb	¼ lb	lb	¼ lb
44	0	35	2	34	3	49	0	45	0	44	0
44	1	35	3	34	3	49	1	45	1	44	1
44	2	36	0	35	0	49	2	45	2	44	2
44	3	36	1	35	1	49	3	45	3	44	3
44	4	36	1	35	2	49	4	46	0	45	0
44	5	36	2	35	3	49	5	46	2	45	1
44	6	36	3	36	0	49	6	46	3	45	2
44	7	37	0	36	0	49	7	47	0	45	3
45	0	37	1	36	1	50	0	47	1	46	0
45	1	37	2	36	2	50	1	47	2	46	1
45	2	37	2	36	3	50	2	47	3	46	3
45	3	37	3	37	0	50	3	48	1	47	0
45	4	38	0	37	1	50	4	48	2	47	1
45	5	38	1	37	2	50	5	48	3	47	2
45	6	38	2	37	2	50	6	49	0	47	3
45	7	38	3	37	3	50	7	49	1	48	0
46	0	39	0	38	0	51	0	49	3	48	2
46	1	39	1	38	1	51	1	50	0	48	3
46	2	39	2	38	2	51	2	50	1	49	0
46	3	39	3	38	3	51	3	50	2	49	1
46	4	40	0	39	0	51	4	51	0	49	2
46	5	40	1	39	1	51	5	51	1	50	0
46	6	40	1	39	2	51	6	51	2	50	1
46	7	40	2	39	3	51	7	52	0	50	2
47	0	40	3	40	0						
47	1	41	0	40	1						
47	2	41	1	40	1						
47	3	41	2	40	2						
47	4	41	3	40	3						
47	5	42	0	41	0						
47	6	42	1	41	1						
47	7	42	2	41	2						
48	0	42	3	41	3						
48	1	43	0	42	0						
48	2	43	2	42	1						
48	3	43	3	42	2						
48	4	44	0	42	3						
48	5	44	1	43	0						
48	6	44	2	43	2						
48	7	44	3	43	3						

Table 7-11. Laboratory indicators of current dietary intake and nutritional status of the young child

Dietary component	Current intake	Nutritional status	Comments
Protein	Serum or urine urea nitrogen	Serum albumin	Urea nitrogen in serum or urine correlates reasonably well with current net intake of protein if renal function is normal. Creatinine values in serum <6 mg/dl or in urine <8 mg/g suggest low recent intake of protein. Serum albumin is a rather insensitive and nonspecific indicator of protein status, but values <3.2 gm/dl suggest a poor protein nutritional status.
Iron	Transferrin saturation	Hemoglobin, hematocrit, cell indices	Levels of transferrin saturation (iron/total iron-building capacity × 100) <16% suggest iron deficiency even when the concentration of hemoglobin is <10.5 g/dl. Hemoglobin concentration >10.5 g/dl (hematocrit 32%) is suggested as lower limit of normal for 6-year-old child. A mean corpuscular hemoglobin concentration (MCHC) <30 g/dl of packed erythrocytes suggests iron deficiency.
Vitamin A	Serum carotene	Serum vitamin A	Approximately one half of total vitamin A intake from foods is supplied by fruits, vegetables, and cereal grains in the form of carotene. A level of serum carotene <40 μg/dl suggests low net intake of carotene. A level of serum vitamin A <20 μg/dl suggests low stores in vitamin A or may indicate failure of transport of retinol out of liver into blood.
Ascorbic acid	Serum ascorbate or whole blood ascorbate	Leukocyte ascorbate	At usual levels of intake of ascorbic acid from foods there is good correlation between intake and serum ascorbate; levels in serum <0.3 mg/dl suggest that recent intake has been low. Whole blood ascorbate levels <0.3 mg/dl indicate low intake and reduction in body pool of ascorbic acid. Leukocyte ascorbic acid levels <20 mg/100 g suggests poor nutritional status.
Riboflavin	Urinary riboflavin	Erythrocyte glutathione reductase	There is a reasonably good correlation between intake and urinary excretion of riboflavin. Excretion of <250 μg/g creatinine suggests low recent intake of riboflavin. Glutathione reductase-FAD (flavin-adenine dinucleotide) effect expressed as a ratio >1.2 suggests poor nutritional status.
Thiamin	Urinary thiamin	Erythrocyte transketolase	Excretion of <125 μg/g creatinine suggests low intake of thiamin. Transketolase-TPP (thiamin pyrophosphate) effect expressed as a ratio >15 suggests poor nutritional status.
Folacin	Serum folacin	Erythrocyte folacin, formiminoglutamic acid (FIGLU)	Level of serum folacin <6 μg/dl suggests low intake. Levels of erythrocyte folacin <20 μg/dl or increased excretion of FIGLU in urine following a histidine load suggests poor nutritional status.
Iodine	Urinary iodine	Protein-bound iodine (PBI)	Urinary excretion of <50 μg/g creatinine suggests low recent intake of iodine. PBI <3 μg/dl suggests poor nutritional status.

From Owen GM, Lippman G: Nutritional status of infants and young children: U.S.A., *Pediatr Clin North Am* 24:211, 1977.

Biochemical Assessment

Laboratory indicators of current dietary intake and of the nutritional status of young children are presented in Table 7-11.

Dietary Assessment

Fomon's questionnaire on infants up to 1 year of age is designed to identify infants who may be at nutritional risk because of unusual eating habits. Fomon's questionnaire covers a range of points: whether the baby is breastfed or drinks milk or formula, the type of milk or formula, consumption of other foods (eggs; dried beans or peas; meat; bread, rice, potatoes, etc.), the frequency of consumption, and the kinds of fruits and vegetables consumed. Other questions cover the access of the infant's care provider to basic kitchen necessities, use of iron drops as a supplement, any special diet the infant is on and who recommended the diet, consumption of clay, paint chips, or other non-food items, and whether or not the respondent thinks the infant has a feeding problem.[8a]

The questions are designed to select from among a large group of infants those few (perhaps 5% or 10%) receiving a diet most likely to be deficient or excessive in one or more nutrients and who are in need of further dietary evaluation and counseling. The dietitian or nutritionist will review all completed questionnaires and decide which children are likely to profit from an interview with the community dietitian or nutritionist. It is important to note that the questions are not meant to determine the child's recent intake of calories, protein, iron, or specific vitamins.

Clinical Assessment

The physical examination may reveal signs of a host of other diseases that merit diagnosis and treatment. Table 7-12 indicates the physical signs indicative of suggested malnutrition.

Table 7-12. Physical signs of value in clinical assessment of malnutrition

Organ system	Group 1	Group 2
Hair	Lack of luster, thin, sparse, dyspigmentation, easily plucked	
Face	Diffuse depigmentation, nasolabial dyssebacia	
Eyes	Pale conjunctiva, conjunctival xerosis, Bitot's spots, corneal xerosis, keratomalacia	Corneal vascularization, conjunctival injection, conjunctival and scleral pigmentation
Lips	Angular stomatitis, angular scars, cheilosis	
Tongue	Edema, scarlet color, purple color, atrophy of filiform papillae	Hypertrophy of papillae, fissures, geographical tongue
Gums	Spongy, bleeding	Recession
Glands	Thyroid enlargement, parathyroid enlargement	
Skin	Xerosis, follicular hyperkeratosis, petechiae, pellagrous dermatosis, flaky paint dermatosis, edema (subcutaneous)	
Nails	Koilonychia	Transverse ridging
Musculoskeletal	Muscle wasting, craniotabes, frontal or parietal bossing, epiphyseal enlargement, beading of ribs	
Gastroenteric	Hepatomegaly	
Nervous	Psychomotor changes, mental confusion	
Cardiovascular	Cardiac enlargement	

From Owen GM: *Physical examination as an assessment tool.* In Simko M, Cowell C, Gilbride J, editors: *Nutrition assessment: a comprehensive guide for planning intervention*, Rockville, Md, 1984, Aspen Systems Corp. Reprinted with permission of Aspen Systems Corporation.

Nutrition Intervention and Counseling

Guidelines for Feeding the Normal Infant

Based on current knowledge there is an optimum feeding schedule to match the special nutritional needs and unique physiological characteristics of the infant during the first year of life. The consensus of current research from most sources covered previously in the chapter indicates the need for providing guidelines regarding feeding practices. Two basic principles should be used in guiding the feeding process: necessary nutrients are required, not any specific food; and food is the basis for early learning, both personal development and cultural needs.

The first 6 months. Human milk should be used as the sole source of food for the first 6 months. The breastfed infant should receive the following supplements:

Iron	7 mg daily from ferrous sulfate or other preparations of high bioavailability after 4 to 6 months of age
Vitamin D	400 IU daily if sunlight exposure is less than 2 hours/week
Fluoride	0.25 mg daily if water supply is less than 0.3 ppm

Infants fed commercially prepared iron-fortified formula do not require supplements except fluoride (depending on the fluoride content in local drinking water). Infant formula manufacturers now make their products with defluoridated water so that the fluoride content is less than 0.3 ppm. Infants receiving evaporated milk formulas should receive vitamin C (20 mg) and iron (7 mg) daily.

Solid foods should not be introduced before 5 to 6 months of age.

After 6 months. Human milk should be used up to 1 year. If breastfeeding is not possible, an iron-fortified commercial formula should be used throughout the first year.

Between 5 and 6 months of age, solids should be introduced. Iron-fortified dry cereal commercially prepared for infants should be introduced first and fed daily until 18 months of age to assure adequate iron intake. Other foods such as fruit and vegetables prepared commerically or at home should then be introduced singly, and no more than two new foods in the same week.

If breastfeeding is continued beyond age 5 to 6 months, some foods that are relatively rich in protein should be included. Milks of reduced fat content are not recommended.

Supplements

Iron. Full-term infants born to well-nourished mothers have a 4- to 6-month iron store in the liver. These infants can maintain satisfactory hemoglobin levels from human milk during the first 3 months of life. Individuals from birth to 3 years of age who are not breastfed should have an iron intake of 1 mg/kg per day. The low birth weight (1000 to 2500 g) infant requires iron supplementation of 2 mg/kg per day starting at 2 months of age. The RDA for an infant 6 months to 10 years of age is 10 mg/day.

The American Academy of Pediatrics states that, in the normal infant, the addition of iron-fortified cereal at 6 months of age will supply adequate amounts of iron to prevent iron deficiency anemia. Three tablespoons of iron-fortified infant cereal mixed with formula, breast milk, or water provides 7 mg of iron, the suggested level of supplementation per day. This iron supplement also can be in the form of iron drops prescribed by a physician. Foods can contribute the additional nutrients needed by the infant.

Fluoride. The usual source of fluoride is the water supply. Because breast milk contains very small amounts of fluoride and breastfed infants consume little fluoridated water, there is a need for adding fluoride to the diets of these infants. Breastfed infants should be referred to the pediatrician for a prescription.

Referral

The food assistance programs available to infants includes the Special Supplemental Food Program for Women, Infants and Children (WIC) and Commodity Supplemental Food Program (CSFP). The WIC program is described in Chapters 6 and 12. Table 7-13 describes the food programs available to infants and children. Other areas for referral include the private physician, Early and Periodic Screening, Diagnosis, and Treatment (EPSDT)

Table 7-13. Federally sponsored food assistance programs for infants, children, and adolescents

Program offered	Purpose of program	Administering agencies
Special Supplemental Food Program for Women, Infants, and Children (WIC)	Assist pregnant, lactating, and postpartum women and children up to 5 years of age in obtaining specified nutritious foods and nutrition education	US Department of Agriculture, Food and Nutrition Services (FNS) and state and tribal health agencies
Commodity Supplemental Food Program (CSFP)	Provides pregnant, lactating, and postpartum women and children up to 6 years of age with supplemental foods and nutrition education	FNS and state agencies or Indian tribes
School Lunch Program	Provides nutritious lunch to all children (some at free or at reduced prices) attending participating schools; safeguard the health and well-being of the nation's children and educate children about nutritious food habits	FNS and state educational agencies
School Breakfast Program	Provide a nutritious breakfast to all children (some at free or at reduced prices) attending participating schools	FNS and state educational agencies
Child Care Food Program	Provides cash reimbursements and/or commodities for nonresidential child care institutions	FNS and state educational agencies and public or private not-for-profit day-care centers
Summer Food Service Program	Provides nutritious meals for preschool and schoolaged children in participating schools, recreation centers, or camps during the summertime	FNS and state educational agencies; governmental entities; and public or private not-for-profit residential summer camps
Food Stamp Program	Assist families in providing nutritious meals	FNS and state welfare agencies

Modified from Owen AL, Owen GM, Lanna G: *Health and nutritional benefits of federal food assessment program* In *Cost and Benefits of Nutritional Care Phase 1*, Chicago, 1979, American Dietetic Association. Copyright The American Dietetic Association. Reprinted by permission; and Budget of the U.S. Government, 1984 (appendix), Executive Office of the President.

programs, Head Start, and child abuse and neglect centers.

Assuring Quality of Health and Nutrition Care for Infants

Quality assurance standards have been developed for the normal infant (Table 7-14). These standards provide a basis for evaluating the quality of care.

CHILDREN

A young child's growth rate slows considerably from the first year of age. Toddlers (1 and 2 years old) gain only from 2 to 4 kg (5 to 10 lb) each year. Preschoolers (3 through 4 years old) have even a slower rate of growth, averaging from 1 to 2 kg (3 to 5 lb) each year. As a result of this significant slowing down in growth, the toddler and the preschooler require less food and their appetites decrease. This often is mistaken as poor appetite.

Between ages 1 and 2, children learn to feed themselves independently. They progress from eating with their hands to using utensils. Messiness and spilling are the rule during the first half of the second year, but by age 2 hand-to-mouth coordination has noticeably improved. Children should be allowed to try new skills over and over again.

Hallmark characteristics of a toddler are curiosity and independence. Explanation of the envi-

Table 7-14. Model criteria for quality assurance in ambulatory care of normal infant*

Criteria			
Identify outcome (O) and process (P)	Critical time	Exceptions†	References
1. Infant maintains acceptable weight for length between the 5th and 95th percentile on NCHS growth chart (O)	Birth to 12 months		NCHS growth charts, 1976, *Monthly Vital Statistics Rep* 25:3, 1976
2. Infant does not deviate more than 25 percentile points from his or her established pattern of growth (weight for height) on NCHS growth charts (O)	Birth to 12 months		Fomon SJ: *Nutritional disorders of children*, DHEW Pub (HSA) 77-5104, Rockville, Md, 1977, US Government Printing Office
3. Infant's hemoglobin is equal to or greater than:	4 to 12 months	Higher altitudes	Centers for Disease Control: *Ten-state nutrition survey, 1968-1970, IV. biochemical*, DHEW Pub (HSM) 72-8132, Atlanta, 1980, CDC

Hemoglobin   **Hematocrit**
    10 g   31%
        or
    11 g   33%
			Centers for Disease Control: *Nutrition surveillance, annual summary, 1978*, Atlanta, 1980, CDC.
			Fomon SJ: *Nutritional disorders of children*, DHEW Pub (HSA) 77-5014, Rockville, Md, 1977, US Government Printing Office
			In CDC Criteria for anemia in children and childbearing-aged women, *MMRW* 38:400, 1989

Updated from Kaufman M, editor: *Guide to quality assurance in ambulatory nutrition care*, Chicago, 1983, The American Dietetic Association.
*Birth to age 12 months; weight/length from 5th up to and including the 95th percentile; no medical complications (physical handicaps, mental retardation, or other syndromes).
† Lost to follow-up applies to all criteria.

ronment is enabled by the child's increasing mobility, manipulation, and attempts at various skills.

During the preschool years (ages 3 to 5) there is a greater increase in height relative to weight; the chubby toddler becomes a leaner preschooler. Each child will grow at his or her own rate as determined by heredity, state of health, and nutritional adequacy of the diet.[7]

The mid-childhood years (from ages 6 to the onset of puberty) are relatively stable, compared to the preschool and adolescent periods, with regard to growth rate and behavior. Height and weight vary greatly among children because of genetic and environmental influences, but for an individual child growth is usually slow and steady. In spite of a relatively slow growth rate, nutrition still plays an important role by (1) furnishing the energy needed for the vigorous activities of this age group, (2) helping to maintain resistance to infection, (3) providing building materials for growth, and (4) providing adequate nutrient stores to assist in adolescent growth.

Nutritional Requirements
Energy
Energy requirements in a child must allow for basal metabolism, specific dynamic action of food, losses in excreta, muscular activity, and growth.[26] The average energy requirement for basal metabolism during the first 12 to 18 months of life is 55 kcal/kg body weight. Thereafter the requirement on a weight-specific basis declines to an adult level of 25 to 30 kcal/kg. As children grow older, the level of calories increases because of the larger body size,

Table 7-15. Recommended dietary allowances for children

	1-3 years	4-6 years	7-10 years
Weight (kg)	13	20	28
Energy (kcal)	1300	1800	2000
Protein (g)	16	24	28
Vitamin A (μg RE)	400	500	700
Vitamin D (μg)	10	10	10
Vitamin E (mg TE)	6	7	7
Vitamin C (mg)	40	45	45
Folate (μg)	50	75	100
Niacin (mg)	9	12	13
Riboflavin (mg)	0.8	1.1	1.4
Thiamin (mg)	0.7	0.9	1.0
Vitamin B_6 (mg)	1.0	1.1	1.4
Vitamin B_{12} (μg)	0.7	1.0	1.4
Calcium (mg)	800	800	800
Phosphorus (mg)	800	800	800
Iodine (μg)	70	90	120
Iron (mg)	10	10	10
Magnesium (mg)	80	120	170
Zinc (mg)	10	10	10

From Food and Nutrition Board, National Research Council, National Academy of Sciences: *Recommended dietary allowances*, ed 10, Washington, DC, 1989, National Academy Press.

but the need for energy per unit size actually decreases. The contribution of physical activity to total energy expenditures varies daily and between each child. Energy needs of individual children of the same age, size, and sex varies with the reasons undetermined. The adequacy of an infant or child's energy intake is best evaluated by the adequacy and comparison of their weight and length growth rates. The recommended energy requirements for children are 102 kcal/kg (1300 to 1500 kcal) for 1 to 3 years of age, 90 kcal/kg (1800 kcal) for 4 to 6 years, and 70 kcal/kg (2000 kcal) for 7 to 10 years (Table 7-15).[10]

Protein

Protein needs for growth decrease as the rates of growth decline. On a weight-specific basis, protein requirements decrease from the first month of life through childhood and adolescence. The decrease is most precipitous during the first 6 months of life. Fifty percent of protein requirement is used for growth in the first 2 months of life. This declines to 11% at 2 to 3 years of age and gradually to 0 after the completion of the final adolescent growth spurt. Safe levels of protein intake, assuming an adequate intake of energy, are approximately 2.2 g/kg per day below age 6 months; 1.6 g/kg per day at 6 to 11 months; 1.2 g/kg per day at 1 to 3 years; 1.1 g/kg per day at 4 to 6 years; and 1.0 g/kg per day at 7 to 10 years.[10]

Lipids

During the early months of life, fat provides nearly one half of the calories in the infant diet. This is especially true during the period of exclusive breastfeeding. Generally after the nursing period about one third of calories should be from fat. An essential nutrient for children and adults is the polyunsaturated fatty acid linoleic acid. The requirement for linoleic acid is a minimum of 1% to a maximum of 4% to 5% of the calories consumed. It is not clear whether, in children without a family history of hyperlipidemia, diets low in saturated fats reduce the likelihood of adult atherosclerosis. The population dietary approach is that total fat consumption should be an average of no more than 30% and that saturated fatty acids should be less than 10% of total calories.

Minerals

During childhood there is a progressive increase in mineral content of the body. The three major groups of minerals include (1) sodium, potassium, calcium, and magnesium; (2) chlorine, phosphorus, and sulfur; and (3) iron, iodine, and trace elements. Sodium and potassium requirements for growing children are met easily because most foods contain an abundant supply. Calcium required during growth is estimated to be 50 mg to 70 mg/kg per day. The recommended allowance for calcium in children 1 to 10 years of age is 800 mg per day. Exact magnesium requirements are not known for young children. Almost 16% of ingested magnesium is retained with 50% deposited in bone. The usual diet is assumed to contain an adequate amount of magnesium. A requirement has been set at 6 mg/kg per day.

Iron

The importance of this mineral in the diets of infants and children has long been recognized. Up to 4 to 6 months of age, the full-term infant's iron stores, which were deposited in fetal life, are generally adequate for body needs (e.g., the production of hemoglobin). After that age, body stores must be resupplied by the diet to ensure prompt blood formation. The usual hemoglobin level at birth is high, 16 to 18 g/dl of blood, and falls normally to a level of 10 to 11 g/dl at 3 to 4 months of age. The hemoglobin level should be 11 g/dl or more thereafter. Because children need iron to maintain hemoglobin concentrations and total iron mass for periods of growth, the allowance of 10 mg/day is recommended for children 1 to 10 years of age.[10]

Nutrition-Related Problems

The most common manifestation of nutrition problems in this age group include anemia, obesity, and dental caries. Also included are hyperlipidemia and prevention of atherosclerosis.

Anemia

Iron deficiency anemia is the most common cause of anemia among children today. It is most common between the ages of 6 months to 3 years. The lack of dietary iron is seen most often among children in lower socioeconomic and minority groupings, although there has been an increased iron intake among infants and children across all socioeconomic groups as supported by the CSFII.[14] The lack of dietary iron may be the result of parental ignorance of the importance and sources of iron, poverty that restricts the amount and variety of foods available, or the difficulty of providing recommended levels of iron in the diet under the best of circumstances. A few instances are recorded of anemia resulting from the exclusive use of a milk diet, which is low in iron, after the first 6 months of life.

Treatment of anemia of childhood usually involves the therapeutic use of iron salts at levels providing from 30 to 100 mg of iron a day, often in conjunction with ascorbic acid, until hemoglobin levels have been restored to normal levels. This regimen is followed by the use of a diet high in iron-rich foods such as meat, green leafy vegetables, and enriched cereals. The child who suffers from anemia is usually lethargic, tires easily, is irritable, has a short attention span and decreased ability to concentrate, and is highly susceptible to infection. Anemic children do poorly on vocabulary, reading, mathematics, problem-solving, and psychological tests.

Obesity

Overnutrition represents excesses, the other end of the spectrum. Childhood- or juvenile-onset obesity is one of the most prevalent nutrition problems among children. There is no single common definition of obesity; therefore, the prevalence estimate ranges from 10% to 30%. Obesity is generally defined in the relation to standardized growth charts. Obesity can either be weight for height greater than 90th or 95th percentile, or weights greater than 120% of median weight for height. Using reference standards from growth charts can be a problem in that children vary greatly in the timing and coordination of weight and height growth spurts. Childhood obesity is a particular problem because it is extremely difficult to treat and tends to persist into adulthood. The combination of parents, who may unwittingly establish a pattern of overfeeding, and inactivity contributes to the problem of obesity. Working with children on appropriate food habits and exercise is essential. Encouraging a child to adopt a pattern of eating that allows growth into his or her weight has met with more success than attempting to bring about an actual weight loss. Sound programs for treatment or prevention should be individualized, nutritionally sound, psychologically sound, supportive of social needs, diversified, and based on the premise that there is a wide range of acceptable body sizes and shapes.[6]

Dental caries

Dental caries affect 98% of all American children.[27] Diet and nutrition have an important role in preventing or causing the development of dental caries. Cariogenicity of a child's diet is related more to frequency of intake of sticky suger-containing foods that cling to teeth than to the total amount of sugar in the diet. Preventive actions include restricting sugary foods to mealtimes, brushing teeth immediately after eating sugary foods, and decreasing the practice of allowing infants and children to go to sleep with a bottle containing juice, milk, or other sugar-containing fluid.

Atherosclerosis

In the CSFII of 1985, young children (1 to 5 years) had an average dietary intake of 35% of total calories from fat, 14% of total calories from saturated fats, and 233 mg cholesterol per day. For children 6 to 19 years of age, average dietary intakes are 36% of calories from total fat, 14% of calories from saturated fats, and 249 mg and 205 mg cholesterol per day for females and males, respectively. Recent studies suggest that atherosclerosis begins in early childhood and that cholesterol levels in children are predictors of levels in adults, but whether there should be universal screening for children's cholesterol levels has been debated. The National Cholesterol Education Program (NCEP) Expert Panel on Cholesterol in Children and Adolescents recommends two strategies to reduce elevated cholesterol levels: a population approach and an individualized approach.[36] The individualized approach is directed toward identifying and treating individual children and adolescents with high cholesterol levels and who have a familial history of premature heart disease or parental hypercholesterolemia. The population approach for dietary intervention for children 2 years and older has the following nutrient recommendations: nutrition adequacy should be achieved by a variety of foods; energy (calories) should be adequate to support growth and development and to reach or maintain desirable body weight; consumption of saturated fatty acids should be less than 10% of total calories; consumption of total fat should be an average of no more than 30% of total calories from all fat; and consumption of dietary cholesterol should be less than 300 mg/day.[20,31,36]

Feeding Patterns

In reviewing the food habits of any child, it is important to keep in mind nutritional requirements, culture, socioeconomic status, and family dynamics as they influence the individual. By age 18 months to 2 years, many toddlers are quite adept at feeding themselves. Individual dietary preferences appear, and the child should be allowed to choose food he or she likes. Toddlers often prefer small, frequent feedings of finger foods and often reject or simply pick at a prepared meal. This behavior should not alarm the parent or be perceived as a challenge to parental authority.

Parents who are distraught over the eating patterns of 2- and 3-year-old children often can be reassured that psychogenic anorexia and atypical (by adult standards) eating behavior are normal during this period of experimentation.

Parents should be aware that the period of maximum growth has been completed by the end of the first year. Between 1 and 5 years growth slows and is reflected by a proportional decline in nutrient intake on a weight-adjusted basis.

By age 5 years, children can effectively use knives and forks. There are increased opportunities for socializing through school experiences with exposure to new foods and new practices. Asking children to assist in preparing or serving a new food often will permit them to overcome reluctance to experiment with new foods. Table 7-16 describes food intake according to food groupings and number of servings at different stages of the life cycle.

Guidelines for Patient Management

The expected health outcomes for a normal child include the following:
- Child maintains weight for height between 5th and 95th percentile on NCHS growth chart.
- Child maintains height for age between 5th and 95th percentile on HCHS growth chart.

Table 7-16. Food guide for healthy adults to meet the special nutrients needs associated with stages of the life cycle

Age group	Fruits and vegetables				Breads, cereals, grains			Milk products (Nonfat or low-fat)	Protein food		Fats and oils†
	Vitamin A	Vitamin C	Other	Total	Whole grain	Other	Total		Vegetable protein (As a substitute for 1 serving of animal protein)	Total animal and vegetable (Low-fat/lean)	
Toddler											
1-2 years	1	1	3-7	5-9	4 or more	3-7	7-11	2 (whole milk only)	3 or more/week	3-4 oz	2 tsp
2-3 years	1	1	3-7	5-9	4 or more	3-7	7-11	2	3 or more/week	3-4 oz	6 tsp
Children											
4-6 years	1	1	3-7	5-9	4 or more	3-7	7-11	2	3 or more/week	3-4 oz	8 tsp
7-10 years	1	1	3-7	5-9	4 or more	3-7	7-11	2	3 or more/week	5-7 oz	8 tsp
Teens and young adults, female											
11-18 years	1	1	3-7	5-9	4 or more	3-7	7-11	3	3 or more/week	5-7 oz	8 tsp
19-24 years	1	1	3-7	5-9	4 or more	3-7	7-11	3	3 or more/week	5-7 oz	6 tsp
Teens and young adults, male											
11-14 years	1	1	5-7	7-9	4 or more	3-7	7-11	3	3 or more/week	7 oz	8 tsp
15-18 years	1	1	5-7	7-9	5 or more	4-6	9-11	3	3 or more/week	7 oz	10 tsp
19-24 years	1	1	5-7	7-9	5 or more	4-6	9-11	3	3 or more/week	7 oz	8 tsp

Adapted from Kizer KW: *The California daily food guide: dietary guidance for Californians*, Sacramento, 1990, California Department of Health Services.
* Physically active individuals and children going through growth spurts may require larger amounts of food. Extra foods are not included in the California Guide and may add significant amounts of fat, sugar, sodium, and calories. A regular pattern of meals and snacks distributed throughout the day is recommended.
† Select nonfat or low-fat food choices. When higher-fat food choices are selected, limit or reduce the fats and oils used in preparation or at the table. At least half of the fat should be from unsaturated sources.

- Child does not deviate more than 25 percentile points from his or her established growth pattern (height or weight) on NCHS growth chart.
- Child's hemoglobin and/or hematocrit determinations are within acceptable levels.
- Child consumes types and amounts of food in frequencies appropriate for age and weight for height.

Nutrition Screening and Assessment

Anthropometric Assessment

The following anthropometric measurements should be completed for a preschool child:

Weight
Stature (standing height)
Head circumference
Chest circumference
Triceps skinfold

From school age through adolescence, the following measurements should be taken:

Weight
Stature (standing height)
Triceps skinfold

Weight. Children who can stand without assistance are weighed standing on the scale and wearing only lightweight undergarments. The scale should be in an area that ensures privacy. The child stands over the center of the platform of the scale with heels together. The reading is made when the child is standing still. Weight of a child should be recorded to the nearest 100 g (0.1 kg or ¼ lb). Consistency of technique and choice of weight units is important to avoid unnecessary sources of errors.

Stature. Children between 2 and 3 years of age can be measured in the recumbent or standing position, depending on their ability to cooperate during the procedure. It is essential to note whether length or stature (standing height) was measured because length is greater than stature by up to 2 cm (nearly 1 in). Thus integration of measurements will be difficult if it is not known whether length or stature was measured or if length was measured on one occasion and stature on another.

Children older than 3 years of age should be measured standing. Measurements of stature require a measuring stick or a nonstretchable tape attached to a vertical, flat surface, such as a wall. A guide for a right-angle headboard also is needed. Movable measuring rods attached to platform scales are too unsteady to ensure accurate measurement.[22] The child should wear only underclothes, so that the stance can be seen clearly, and stand with bare heels close together, legs straight, arms at the sides, and shoulders relaxed. Two people may be needed to measure the stature of an uncooperative child, but usually only one is required. The child's knees should be straight with heels on the floor and with head, shoulder blades, buttocks, and heels touching the wall.

The child should be asked to stand tall, take a deep breath, and look straight ahead so the line of vision is perpendicular to the body. Then the headboard is lowered against the guide onto the crown of the head. The measurer's eyes should be level with the headboard to avoid errors. With headboard in place, the measurement is read and recorded to the nearest 0.1 cm (⅛ in). NCHS growth charts should be used to monitor the child's growth (see Figs. 7-4 and 7-5).

Head circumference. Head circumference should be measured routinely in infants and children until they are 36 months of age.

Triceps skinfold thickness. Triceps skinfold thickness is a measurement of a double length of skin and subcutaneous fat on the back of the upper arm.

Biochemical Assessment

Because anemia is a problem in this age group, the initial screening should include hemoglobin and hematocrit determinations. Acceptable levels are:

Age (Both Sexes)	Hemoglobin	Hematocrit
12-23 months	>11 g	>33%
2-4 years	11.2 g	34%
5-7 years	11.4 g	34.5%
8-11 years	11.6 g	35%

Total serum cholesterol levels are completed using 170 mg/dl and 110 mg/dl LDL cholesterol as a cutoff point for children age 2 through 17 years with familial risk factors.[36] Blood lead levels should be completed on children age 6 to 72 months, using the cutoff point of 10.0 μg/dl.[4] Guidelines for nutritional assessment and intervention in infants and children are described in Table 7-7.

Dietary Assessment

Techniques of dietary assessment are discussed in detail in Chapter 15.

Clinical Assessment

Screening children for hypertension has become routine in many clinics. For children age 3 through 17 years, the following cutoff points for blood pressure are used.[23]

Degree of Risk	Cutoff	
Normal	Systolic and diastolic blood pressure <90th percentile for age and sex	
High normal	Systolic and/or diastolic blood pressure 90th-95th percentile for age and sex	
	3-5 years	107 mm Hg/69 mm Hg
	6-9 years	113 mm Hg/72 mm Hg
	10-12 years	119 mm Hg/77 mm Hg
High	Systolic and/or diastolic blood pressure >95th percentile for age and sex	
	3-5 years	116 mm Hg/76 mm Hg
	6-9 years	122 mm Hg/78 mm Hg
	10-12 years	126 mm Hg/82 mm Hg

Nutrition Intervention, Counseling, and Education

Head Start is a model day-care program that was initiated as an 8-week summer program by the Office of Economic Opportunity in 1965. It is now a full-year program administered by the Administration of Children, Youth and Families, Department of Health and Human Services. The goal is to provide low-income preschool children with a comprehensive program based on their special educational, psychological, emotional, health, and nutrition needs. Nutrition education is provided to the children and their parents with the meal service as an educational tool.

Nutrition education, depending on each state, is emphasized in school curriculum both in elementary and secondary schools. A major vehicle for nutrition education is the School Breakfast and School Lunch Programs administered by U.S. Department of Agriculture and state departments of education. In 1977 Congress passed Public Law 95-166 as part of the National School Lunch Act and Child Nutrition Amendments, which authorized the Nutrition Education Training Program (NET). NET funds support projects to teach children about the relationship of food and health, train food service personnel, instruct teachers to teach nutrition in their classrooms, and develop and use innovative classroom materials and curricula. The use of the Dietary Guidelines for Americans is being emphasized in both the classroom and meal service settings. This effort should be encouraged for all schoolchildren.

The American Heart Association has the School-site Program for students in grades prekindergarten through 12 to develop heart-healthy habits. The Heart Treasure Chest is for day-care centers, kindergarten, and schools for 3 to 5-year-olds; it focuses on the importance of a healthy heart and how to develop positive diet and exercise habits. The Getting to Know Your Heart program is designed for grades kindergarten through 6 to educate students about controllable factors (smoking, nutrition, and exercise) that contribute to heart disease and stroke.

The American Cancer Society's Changing the Course program is a health education curriculum for elementary through secondary grades. It is designed to educate children about the relationship between nutrition and health and to encourage them to adopt lifelong eating patterns that are health-promoting and at the same time may also lower their risk of developing certain cancers and other chronic conditions. In addition to the curriculum, there is an implementation guide for school food service providers to make gradual changes in school meals and food choices.

The pediatrician's office and the health clinic are available to children and their parents for nutrition and medical services.

Referral

Several food assistance programs are available to children, including WIC, School Breakfast, School

Lunch, Summer Feeding, Special Milk, and Child Care Food programs. In addition, food stamps and commodity foods are available to their families. Table 7-13 briefly describes these programs. The box on p. 36, in Chapter 2, describes the food programs in detail.

Assuring Quality of Health and Nutrition Care for Children

Quality assurance standards have been set for the normal child (Table 7-17). These standards provide a basis for evaluating the quality of care for community nutrition programs that serve infants and children.[19]

ADOLESCENTS

Adolescence, the transition from childhood to adulthood, is accompanied by a series of physical, physiological, biochemical, hormonal, and psychological changes. A time of wide variability in norms of growth, it lasts nearly a decade with no specific beginning or end. Progress in the individual is characterized by orderly sequence, but there is marked variation between sexes and between individuals in timing, intensity of change, and deviation in the process.

This progressional period is usually described in two phases: pubescence and adolescence. *Pubescence*, which includes the adolescent growth spurt (average age is 9 to 13 for females and 12 to 16 for males), begins with the first increase in hormonal secretion and appearance of secondary sex characteristics (increase in breast size in females and external genitalia in males and appearance of pubic hair) and ends when sexual reproduction becomes possible. *Adolescence* (average age is 10 to 17 years for females and 12 to 21 years for males) is the period beginning with the appearance of sexual maturity and terminating with the cessation of growth in stature.

Adolescence is thought of as a nutritionally vulnerable period for two reasons. First, the dramatic increase in physical growth and development during the transition from childhood to adulthood creates great demands. Although there is a gradual movement from pubescence to adolescence, there are few identifiable points of demarcation. During pubescence, which lasts an average of 2 to 3 years, there is a peak velocity of increase in stature and weight preceding menarche in girls and spermatogenesis in boys.

In normal healthy girls, on the average, the growth spurt begins at 9.6 years; peak height velocity at 11.8 years; stage 2 breast development at 11.2 years; and menarche at 12.4 years. Normal variations around the mean are noted, as for any biological phenomenon, but menarche before 9 years and after 16 years of age is considered outside the normal range. A relatively large component of weight gain is body fat.

Males begin their pubescent growth spurt approximately 2 years later than females. The onset of male adolescence is accompanied by production of gonadotropin, which stimulates enlargement of the testes in the 9- to 12-year age range. Skeletal growth continues at an accelerated rate, reaching a peak of approximately 10.3 cm (4 in) at age 14.1 years. Associated changes in muscle mass, voice, and physical skills are noted. Linear growth almost ceases at approximately age 18 years, although some individuals continue to grow taller well into their twenties.[26] Weight gain is more of an increase in muscle mass.

Hormonal Influences

Although the sex hormones exert a major controlling influence, many other hormones participate in adolescent development. Growth hormone, somatotropin, a polypeptide produced by the pituitary, is highly species-specific and is necessary for growth, but its role in adolescent growth has yet to be fully described. Growth hormone stimulates protein anabolism at the cellular level. The thyroid hormones, triiodothyronine (T_3) and thyroxine (T_4), influence overall body growth and skeletal maturation. The metabolic effects of these thyroid hormones include increases in oxygen consumption, heat production, nitrogen retention, protein synthesis, glucose absorption, glycolysis, and gluconeogensis.

Insulin has an indirect effect on growth by increasing the uptake and metabolism of glucose, glycogenesis, and synthesis of fatty acids. It also stimulates the transport of amino acids into the cells

Table 7-17. Model criteria for quality assurance in ambulatory care of normal child*

Criteria — Identify outcome (O) and process (P)	Critical time	Exceptions†	References
1. Child maintains weight for height between 5th and 95th percentile on NCHS growth charts (O)	1 year to puberty	Less than 2500 g birth weight until 18 months	Fomon SJ: *Nutritional disorders of children,* DHEW Pub (HSA) 77-5104, Rockville, Md, 1977, US Government Printing Office *Growth charts with reference percentile for girls and boys 2 to 18 years,* DHEW, Atlanta, 1976, Centers for Disease Control
2. Child maintains height for age between 5th and 95th percentile on NCHS growth charts (O)			
3. Child does not deviate more than 25 percentile points from his or her established growth pattern (height or weight) on NCHS growth chart (O)	1 year to puberty		Fomon SJ: *Nutritional disorders of children,* DHEW Pub (HSA) 77-5104, Rockville, Md, 1977, US Government Printing Office
4. Child's hemoglobin and/or hematocrit determinations are within acceptable levels as outline below (O)			Pilch SM, Senti FR, editor: *Assessment of iron nutrition status of the U.S. population based on data collected in the Second National Health and Nutrition Examination Survey, 1976-1980,* Bethesda, Md, 1984, Federation of American Societies for Experimental Biology, Life Science Research Office
Hemoglobin Hematocrit 11.0 g 33% 11.2 g 34% 11.4 g 34.5% 11.6 g 35%	1-1.9 years 2-4.9 years 5-7.9 years 8-11.9 years	Higher altitudes	Yip R, Johnson C, Dallman PR: Age-related changes in laboratory values used in diagnosis of anemia and iron deficiency anemia, *Am J Clin Nutr* 39:427, 1984 CDC criteria for anemia in children and child-bearing-aged women, *MMRW* 38:400, 1989.
5. Child consumes types and amounts of foods in frequencies appropriate for age and weight for height as specified in agency protocol (O)	1 year to puberty	None	Pipes PL: Nutrition in infancy and childhood, ed 4, St Louis, 1989, The CV Mosby Co.

Updated from Kaufman M, editor: *Guide to quality assurance in ambulatory nutrition care,* Chicago, 1983, American Dietetic Association.
*One year up to puberty; weight for height from 5th up to and including the 95th percentile for age and sex; no medical complications (physical handicaps, mental retardation, or other syndromes).
†Lost to follow-up applies to all criteria.

and catalyzes the incorporation of amino acids into protein.

Estrogen influences the development and maintenance of secondary sex characteristics and reproductive functions. They result in significant morphological, physiological, and behavior changes by regulating the secretion of follicle-stimulating hormone (FSH) and luteinizing hormone (LH) by the pituitary, thereby increasing uterine weight and inducing vaginal cornifications.

Progesterone, secreted by the corpora lutea of the ovarian cortex, causes changes in the uterine endometrium and is responsible for the cyclic changes in the vagina and also acts in the maturation of breast function.

The physiological sequence of development that occurs during the growth spurt results in a high demand for calories and nutrients to support optimum growth.

Nutrient Requirements

Peak nutrient requirements occur during the years of maximum growth. For practicality, the RDAs during the adolescent period are divided by chronological rather than maturational or biological age groups: 7 to 10 years (prepubescent), 11 to 14 years (junior high or middle school), 15 to 18 years (high school), and 19 to 24 years (college), with separation by sex after 11 years of age.[10] The RDAs for males and females ages 11 to 14 years and 15 to 18 years are shown in Table 7-18.

There are few direct experimental data on which to base nutrient requirements for adolescents, specifically for vitamins and minerals. Except for energy, values such as the RDA are extrapolated from adult or child studies. Nutrient needs are greatest during the pubescent growth spurt and gradually decrease as the individual achieves physical maturity. The adolescent growth spurt contributes

Table 7-18. Recommended dietary allowances for adolescents

	Males		Females		Pregnant females	
	11-14 years	15-18 years	11-14 years	15-18 years	11-14 years	15-18 years
Weight (kg)	45	66	46	55	46	55
Energy (kcal)	2500	3000	2200	2200	2500	2500
Protein (g)	45	59	46	44	60	60
Vitamin A (μg RE)	1000	1000	800	800	800	800
Vitamin D (μg)	10	10	10	10	10	10
Vitamin E (mg TE)	10	10	8	8	10	10
Vitamin C (mg)	50	60	50	60	70	70
Folate (μg)	150	200	150	180	400	400
Niacin (mg)	17	20	15	15	17	17
Riboflavin (mg)	1.5	1.8	1.3	1.3	1.6	1.6
Thiamin (mg)	1.3	1.5	1.1	1.1	1.5	1.5
Vitamin B_6 (mg)	1.7	2.0	1.4	1.5	2.2	2.2
Vitamin B_{12} (μg)	2.0	2.0	2.0	2.0	2.2	2.2
Calcium (mg)	1200	1200	1200	1200	1200	1200
Phosphorus (mg)	1200	1200	1200	1200	1200	1200
Iodine (μg)	150	150	150	150	175	175
Iron (mg)	12	12	15	15	30	30
Magnesium (mg)	270	400	280	300	320	320
Zinc (mg)	15	15	12	12	15	15

From Food and Nutrition Board, National Research Council, National Academy of Sciences: *Recommended dietary allowances*, ed 10, Washington, DC, 1989, National Academy Press.

about 50% to adult body weight and 15% to final adult height. The peak energy value for females is at 11 to 24 years (2200 kcal), but for males it is much later and of greater magnitude, 3000 kcal at 15 to 18 years. The male thus has a higher allowance for energy within which to meet the requirements for other essential nutrients. The female, whose energy needs are less, must select foods of high nutrient density to meet all of her nutrient needs without exceeding the energy allowance.

Energy

The requirements for energy vary widely from one individual to another, not only because of different timing and magnitude of somatic growth, but also because of variations in physical activity.

Age or weight alone is not a useful predictor of energy needs. Combinations of kilocalories, kilograms, and age and kilocalories, kilograms, and centimeters are more useful tools. The single measure that best expresses energy requirements is height in adolescence because it usually correlates well with physiological development.

Protein, Carbohydrates, and Lipids

The protein allowances, like those for energy and other nutrients, follow the growth pattern. During adolescence the highest protein allowance for males begins at 15 years (59 g) and persists through adulthood; for females the protein allowance peaks at 11 to 14 years (46 g). Most adolescents consume protein in excess of these amounts. Limitation of either protein or energy during the accelerated phase of growth has been repeatedly demonstrated to inhibit growth.

No allowances have been established for carbohydrates or lipids. Carbohydrates are of particular importance to the adolescent who participates in athletic competition.

Vitamins and Minerals

The paucity of information concerning vitamin and mineral requirements of adolescents is emphasized by several authors. Few data are based on measurements of adolescents, and recommended levels are extrapolations from adult or child studies with a built-in safety factor. With the increase in energy demands, rate of tissue synthesis, and skeletal growth associated with adolescence, it can be expected that vitamin needs are elevated.

To meet the increased energy demands, higher-than-normal adult levels of thiamin (B_1), riboflavin (B_2), and niacin (B_3) are necessary. Folate and vitamin B_{12}, both required for tissue growth, have increased requirements. In addition, skeletal growth necessitates adequate vitamin D intake. Vitamins, A, C, and E are all essential to keep this new tissue in working order.

Calcium. Calicum needs are greater during adolescence than in either childhood or adulthood. During the growth spurt about 45% of the adult skeletal mass is formed. Consequently, the RDA standard for calcium increases from 800 mg for children 7 to 10 years old to 1200 mg for both males and females at 11 to 18 years of age. The need to consume good sources of calcium such as dairy foods is important for bone health during adolescence and beyond.

Iron. Adolescents need iron to maintain hemoglobin as well as their iron mass during growth periods. The recommended intake level of 12 mg/day for males 11 to 18 years, an additional 2 mg/day more than children, is to cover the pubertal growth spurt that occurs between 10 and 17 years. In females the recommended intake level of 15 mg/day, starting at age 11 years, an additional 5 mg/day more than children, is to cover the pubertal growth spurt and menstruation, which begins age 10 or soon after and continues through the menstrual years.

The need for iron increasess during the adolescent growth spurt, particularly for males, because of the expansion of blood volume and muscle mass. Females require less iron for growth but must replace iron lost in menstrual flow. Iron needs are related closely to lean body mass, with males requiring 42 mg/kg of weight gain and females needing 31 mg/kg of weight gain. When growth is rapid, males require more iron than menstruating females, but once growth slows down, the female's iron needs surpass those of the male.

Although iron is most easily absorbed from meat, absorption from plant sources, such as beans and green vegetables, can be tripled by eating these foods with foods high in ascorbic acid. The major sources of iron are in fortified cereals and flour products. To meet the RDA of 12 to 15 mg, adolescents must consciously select iron-containing foods of high iron availability.

Zinc is necessary for growth and sexual maturation. The recommended allowance for men is 15 mg/day and women 12 mg/day. It has been shown that many adolescents consume far less than they need, especially girls, who often consume less than half the RDA. Zinc deficiencies can result in growth retardation.

Psychological and Environmental Influences and Health Consequences

The nutritional health of American youths is better than in past decades. Overt nutrient deficiency diseases are not a public health problem except for iron deficiency. Instead of nutrient deficiency, there are now problems of dietary imbalance and excess.[32] Certain dietary habits among adolescents may continue into adulthood, and along with other factors increase the risk for chronic diseases (e.g., osteoporosis, heart disease, and some types of cancer). Inadequate nutrition during adolescence may retard or stunt linear growth, lower resistance to infections and disease, impair learning ability and performance, adversely affect the ability to function at peak physical capacity, and diminish quality of life and life span for those with chronic illness.[28]

Many factors infringe on and modify the adolescent's diet. Most teenagers are preoccupied with physical appearance, body shape and size, and peer acceptance. A strong desire to be lean and to have a particular body image can result in inappropriate weight reduction, dietary aberrations, and selective widely distributed nutrient deficiencies. Chronic dieters are at high risk for inadequate diets. In adolescent females such behavior may lead to the eating disorders, anorexia nervosa and bulimia nervosa.

Obesity

Males at age 10.5 years normally have 5.3 kg of fat, which is 16% of their body weight. This increases to 9 kg of fat, or 12.9% of body weight, by age 18 years. Females at age 10.5 years have 8.14 kg of body fat, and by age 18.5 years have 14.24 kg of fat, or 25% of their body weight.[12] The correlation of cardiovascular risk factors and distribution of body fat is strong in upper segment obesity (waist-to-hip ratio) in adults with glucose intolerance, hyperlipidemia, and hyperinsulinemia. There is evidence of a genetic predisposition to juvenile obesity. Obesity also appears to cluster in families so that intervention plans need to center around the family to include teaching appropriate lifestyles, physical activity, and concern with body image rather than a restrictive dietary program.[28]

Atherosclerosis

Major risk factors have been identified in adults: age, sex, family history and genetic factors, hyperlipidemia, cigarette smoking, hypertension, and diabetes, several of which have their origins and behavioral development during adolescence. Altering cigarette smoking behavior, controlling blood pressure in hypertensive individuals, preventing obesity through physical activity and weight control, and promoting lowering serum cholesterol require more emphasis with adolescents.

Anorexia Nervosa

Anorexia nervosa is an eating disorder with serious underlying developmental and psychological disturbances. It is a syndrome of self-induced starvation characterized by voluntary refusal to eat due to fear of becoming fat, as well as by extreme weight loss, amenorrhea, and body image disturbances. Surveys establish the prevalence at about one case in 100 adolescent girls. Treatment and management of anorexia nervosa depend on the stage and severity of the problem. Interventions include nutritional, medical, and psychological support. There is a strong resistance to treatment, with a high incidence of relapse or partial recovery.

Bulimia Nervosa

Bulimia nervosa is a disorder distinct from anorexia nervosa. This syndrome is characterized by recurrent episodes of gorging or binge eating with self-induced vomiting, abuse of laxatives and diuretics, and vigorous exercise, but also a maintenance of normal weight and body shape. Today many teens are using vomiting (hyperemesis) as a form of weight control. The behavior may be reinforced on athletic squads or when groups of young people such as college students live together.

Substance Abuse

Substance abuse in adolescents is a public health problem of major significance. Tobacco, alcohol, and illicit drugs are the substances most used and abused by adolescents. In a 1988 national survey of high school seniors, 63.9% reported alcohol use in the previous 30 days and 4.2% reported daily consumption; 2.7% reported daily marijuana use, and 0.2% reported daily cocaine use.[18] Chronic users are more vulnerable to nutrition problems because of either inadequate intake or in the case of alcohol, maldigestion and malabsorption. Alcohol use is as high among females as among males. Of particular concern is the pregnant adolescent who consumes alcohol and may have a marginal diet, because of her risk of producing a child with fetal alcohol syndrome. Young people differ from adults in that they tend to drink less regularly but consume larger amounts at a time—binge drinking.

Tobacco

Cigarette smoking continues to be prevalent among teens despite the evidence of negative health effects. Besides cigarettes, there is an increased use of smokeless tobacco by children and adolescents. Complications of regular use of this substance include periodontal disease, oral cancer, hypertension, and dependence.

Sports and Athletics

Optimal nutrition is a basic requisite for training and maintaining good physical performance. Diets of athletes must supply optimal amounts of energy, protein, water, fat, carbohydrates, vitamins, and minerals. Energy is needed for growth as well as for the extra energy expended with activity. Adequate hydration is a principal concern for adolescents; fluid should be replace before, during, and after exercise. A problem associated with inappropriate weight loss in females is amenorrhea, thought to be caused by the change in the ratio of lean body mass to body fat. At particular risk are female athletes, particularly swimmers, runners, and dancers who train intensely, with loss of body fat and concomitant gain in lean body mass.

By contrast, adolescents who exercise infrequently run a high risk of becoming obese. Lack of exercise, coupled with boredom that results in increased food intake, puts the adolescent in double jeopardy for excessive accumulation of body fat.

Fast foods, fad diets, skipped meals, snacking, and high-carbohydrate foods are facts of life in our society. Condemnation of such dietary practices does little to win the adolescent's confidence. Many fast foods are adequate sources of energy and selected nutrients. However, continued intake of a single class of foods eliminates variety and balance, whereas skipping meals habitually can result in a low intake of selected nutrients or uncontrolled eating binges. Both practices are unhealthy.

When nutritional guidance is needed, it should be provided without preconceived or culturally induced biases about the importance or quality of a particular food. A rational approach is to determine the nutritional contribution of the particular food to the adolescent's overall daily needs. Figure 7-6 describes the interrelationships of factors influencing adolescent food consumption patterns. A prudent diet in moderation with appropriate snacks provides a diet that meets the nutrient requirements of adolescents.

Guidelines for Patient Management

The outcomes expected in working with adolescents include the following:

- Weight and height does not differ by more than 25 percentile points from his or her established growth patterns as plotted on NCHS growth chart.
- Adolescents consume appropriate types and amounts of food.
- Hematocrit and hemoglobin meet acceptable standards as follows:

Age (years)	Hemoglobin	Hematocrit
Both sexes		
8-11	11.6 g	35%

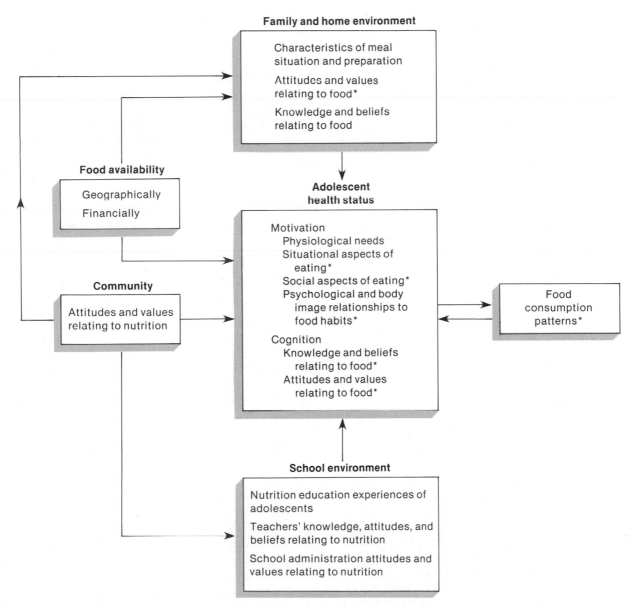

Figure 7-6. Interrelationships of factors influencing adolescent food consumption pattern. *Factors investigated in the survey described and conducted in Edmonton.
Redrawn from Lund LA, Burk MC: *A multidisciplinary analysis of children's food consumption behavior,* University of Minnesota's Agriculture Experimental Station Technical Bulletin 265, Minneapolis, 1965, University of Minnesota Press.

Age (years)	Hemoglobin	Hematocrit
Male		
12-14	12.3 g	37%
15-17	12.6 g	38%
≥18	13.6 g	41%
Female		
12-14	11.9 g	35.5%
15+	12 g	36%

Nutrition Screening and Assessment

Anthropometric Assessment

Height, weight, and skinfold thickness measurements should be completed as described for children.

Biochemical Assessment

Because iron deficiency is prevalent among adolescents, hemoglobin and hematocrit determinations should be completed. In addition, assessments of serum cholesterol levels should be completed for those individuals with familial risk for cardiovascular disease.

Clinical Assessment

Screening adolescents for hypertension should be routine in clinics. For individuals 13 through 18 years the following cutoff points for blood pressure are used:[23]

Degree of risk	Cutoff
Normal	Systolic and diastolic blood pressure <90th percentile for age and sex
High normal	Systolic and/or diastolic blood pressure 90th-95th percentile for age and sex
	10-12 years 119 mm Hg/77 mm Hg
	13-15 years 126 mm Hg/78 mm Hg
	16-18 years 134 mm Hg/83 mm Hg
High	Systolic and/or diastolic blood pressure >90th percentile for age and sex
	10-12 years 126 mm Hg/82 mm Hg
	13-15 years 136 mm Hg/86 mm Hg
	16-18 years 142 mm Hg/92 mm Hg

Information collected should include drug and alcohol consumption, including tobacco. Table 7-19 describes the guidelines for nutritional intervention for adolescents.

Nutrition Intervention, Counseling, and Education

Health Care Settings

The biological, psychosocial, developmental, and nutritional issues for adolescence are complex, interrelated, and unique. Adolescent-oriented nutrition services in health care settings are beginning to be developed. There are adolescent centers that have all of their staff trained in adolescent issues. Other clinical areas, such as weight reduction clinics, eating disorder clinics, lipid research centers, prenatal care clinics, hospital inpatient units including juvenile justice facilities, and rehabilitative units dealing with drug and alcohol addictions, require adolescent nutrition counseling expertise. Adolescent care in prenatal clinics is even more important, given the evidence that adequate nutrition during pregnancy reduces the prematurity rate and the subsequent number of low-birthweight infants.[28]

School-Based

Schools can have the greatest impact on assisting young people in becoming healthy adults and having healthier and successful lives. A comprehensive school health program that includes nutrition education can establish an understanding of the relationship between personal health and behavior. Nutrition education must be part of the curriculum of any comprehensive school health program. Within a school, the school cafeteria is the learning laboratory for nutrition education. Messages from the classroom should be consistent with the foods offered in the cafeteria.

The American Cancer Society's Changing the Course program, a health education curriculum, is also written for intermediate and secondary grades. Besides the curriculum, there is an implementation guide for school food service providers to make gradual changes in school meals and food choices.

The American Heart Association Schoolsite Program includes the Heart Decision program, which is for the middle school, grades 7 through 9, to teach students the relationship between lifestyle and health, and that the risk of cardiovascular disease in adulthood may be significantly lowered by

Table 7-19. Model criteria for quality assurance in ambulatory care of normal adolescent*

Criteria — Identify outcome (O) and process (P)	Critical time	Exceptions†	References
1. Adolescent's weight/height does not differ by more than 25 percentile points as plotted on NCHS growth charts (O)	Throughout puberty and adolescence		Barnes HV: *Physical growth and development during puberty* (appendix 1), DHEW Pub 79-5234, *Adolescent Health Care: A Guide for BCHS Supported Programs and Projects,* US Government Printing Office
2. Adolescent's hemoglobin and/or hematocrit determinations meet acceptable standards as follows (O)	8-11.9 years	Higher altitudes: nonnutrition	Pilch SM, Senti FR, editor: *Assessment of iron nutrition status of the U.S. population based on data collected in the Second National Health and Nutrition Examination Survey, 1976-1980,* Bethesda, Md, 1984, Federation of American Societies for Experimental Biology, Life Science Research Office
Hemoglobin Hematocrit			Yip R, Johnson C, Dallman PR: Age-related changes in laboratory values used in diagnosis of anemia and iron deficiency anemia, *Am J Clin Nutr* 39:427, 1984.
11.6 g 35%			CDC criteria for anemia in children and childbearing-aged women, *MMRW* 38:400, 1989.
Females			Food and Nutrition Board: *Recommended dietary allowances,* ed 10, Washington, DC, 1989, National Academy Press
11.8 g 35.5%	12-14.9 years		
12.0 g 36%	15-17.9 years		
12.0 g 36%	≥18 years		
Males			
12.3 g 37%	12-14.9 years		
12.6 g 38%	15-17.9 years		
13.6 g 41%	≥18 years		
3. Adolescent consumes appropriate types and amounts of foods as specified in agency protocol (O)	Throughout puberty and adolescence		

Updated from Kaufman M, editor: *Guide to quality assurance in ambulatory nutrition care,* Chicago, 1983, The American Dietetic Association.

*Puberty and adolescence: no medical complications (chronic diseases, physical handicaps, mental retardation, or other syndromes); not underweight or overweight; nonpregnant.

†Lost to follow-up applies to all criteria.

adopting healthy habits at a young age. The Heart Challenges program is a curriculum for high school, grades 10 through 12, which focuses on three major risk factors for heart disease: nutrition, exercise, and smoking.

Referral

Pregnant adolescents may be referred to prenatal care, maternal and infant care programs, and food assistance programs such as WIC, food stamps, and school lunch, which are described in Table 7-17. In addition, physical fitness programs and bona fide weight reduction programs are also available in the community.

Assuring Quality of Health and Nutrition Care for Adolescents

Quality assurance standards have been set for the normal adolescent (see Table 7-19). They provide a basis for evaluating the quality of care.[19]

SPECIAL HEALTH CARE NEEDS

Crippled Children's Services, established by Title V of the Social Security Act of 1935, was recently renamed State Programs for Children with Special Health Care Needs. This name change reflects the extension of these programs from their original focus on children with orthopedic handicaps to children with physical disabilities, sensory impairments, developmental disabilities, and chronic illnesses. Public Law 99-457, the Education of the Handicapped Act Amendments of 1986, establishes strong incentives for states to expand public education to all handicapped children between 3 and 5 years of age and provide discretionary programs for handicapped children from birth through 2 years of age. The concept of community-based, family-centered coordinated care and early intervention services are central to the legislation. Nutritionists and dietitians are identified in the law as qualified personnel who provide developmental services.

The estimated number of children with special health care needs is between 10% to 20% of pediatric population, depending on the definition and degree of disability. Individuals include those at risk of physical or developmental disabilities or who are affected by chronic medical conditions caused by or associated with genetic or metabolic disorders, physical birth defects, prematurity, trauma or infections (including human immunodeficiency virus [HIV] infection), or perinatal exposure to drugs and subsequent serious emotional or behavioral disorders or mental retardation.[11] The increase in prevalence rates over the years is attributed to better detection and diagnosis, increased survival of high-risk infants through neonatal intensive care, and increased infection and exposure to drugs. Table 7-20 summarizes the prevalence of chronic conditions and their associated nutrition problems.

Altered Nutrient Requirements

Energy

The special needs child has the same nutrient requirements for optimal growth, development, and health as an unaffected child with the multiple risk factors related to the condition(s) superimposed. These nutritional risk factors are shown schematically in Figure 7-7. Energy needs may be increased or decreased, depending on the child's disorder. The conditions requiring increased energy needs are pulmonary dysfunctions and bronchopulmonary dysplasia. Conditions that result in inactivity or lack of ambulation require decreased energy needs. Spina bifida or cerebral palsy conditions can have either increased or decreased energy requirements.

Individual Nutrients

Metabolic disorders have different nutrient requirements. Children with genetic or chromosomal disorders have altered nutrient needs due to the altered genetic material.

Drug-Nutrient Interaction

Children with special health care needs often require chronic medication. Long-term use of anticonvulsants affects metabolism of calcium and vitamin D. The effects of these medications on nutritional status need to be studied.

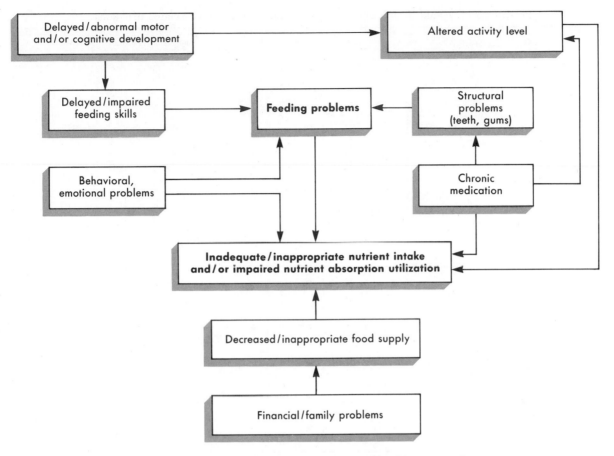

Figure 7-7. Nutritional risk factors in children with special health care needs. Redrawn from Baer MT, Farnan S, Mauer AM: *Children with special health care needs.* In Sharbaugh CO, editor: *Call to action: better nutrition for mothers, children, and families,* Washington, DC, 1991, National Center for Education in Maternal and Child Health.

Feeding Problems

Feeding problems are common with multiple etiologies. The problem can be a structural defect or muscular dysfunction that affects the child's ability to suck, swallow, chew, or self-feed. Developmentally delayed children may not progress normally in reaching the milestones leading to independence in feeding, regardless of whether physical and medical problems have been resolved.[2]

Nutritional Assessment

Anthropometric Assessment

Length or height and weight. Growth is the most important indicator of tthe individual's nutritional status. Population-specific growth charts are available for certain syndromes; linear growth and rate of weight gain can be evaluated for conditions with a clear deviation from the norm, such as Down's and Turner's syndromes. It is advisable

Table 7-20. Prevalence of certain chronic conditions with associated nutrition-related problems

Disorder	Prevalence estimates per 1,000 (and range)	Altered nutrient needs	Altered energy needs/intake	Problems with oral cavity	Nutrient deficiencies	Constipation/diarrhea	Poor appetite	Delayed feeding skills	Malabsorption	Nutrient-drug interactions	Maladaptive behaviors	Lack of knowledge	Difficulty understanding diet	Does not limit intake	Inappropriate feeding practices
			Child-related									Caregiver-related			
Asthma	38 (20-53		●		●		●			●					
Moderate to severe	10 (8-15)														
Visual impairment	30 (20-35)							●		●					
Impaired visual acuity	20														
Blind	0.6 (0.5-1)														
Mental retardation	25 (20-30)		●	●	●			●		●					●
Hearing impairment deafness	16														
	0.1 (0.6-1.5)														
Congenital heart disease	7 (2-7)	●	●		●		●		●	●		●			
Severe congenital disease	0.5														
Seizure disorder	3.5 (2.6-4.6)	●								●		●			
Cerebral palsy	2.5 (1.4-5.1)		●	●	●	●	●	●		●		●		●	●
Arthritis	2.2 (1-3)	●	●									●			
Paralysis	2.1 (2-2.3)		●			●		●			●	●		●	
Diabetes mellitus	1.8 (1.2-2.0)											●	●	●	
Cleft lip/palate	1.5 (1.3-2.0)		●	●				●				●			●
Down's syndrome	1.1		●	●	●			●			●	●		●	●
Sickle cell disease	<1.0	●			●										
Neural tube defect	<1.0		●			●				●				●	
Autism	<1.0						●			●	●				●
Cystic fibrosis	<1.0	●	●		●	●	●		●	●		●	●	●	●
Hemophilia	<1.0														
Acute lymphocytic leukemia	<1.0	●	●		●	●	●			●					
Phenylketonuria	<1.0	●			●							●	●	●	
Chronic renal failure	<1.0	●	●		●	●	●			●		●	●		
Bronchopulmonary dysplasia		●	●		●				●	●					
AIDS		●	●	●	●	●	●	●	●	●		●			
Gastrointestinal disorders		●			●	●	●		●						

Example of nutrition problems and factors contributing to high nutritional risk

Baer MT, Farnan S, Mauer AM: *Children with special health care needs*. In Sharbaugh CO, editor: *Call to action: better nutrition for mothers, children, and families*, Washington, DC, 1991, National Center for Education in Maternal and Child Health. Adapted from: Dwyer JT, Freedland J: *Nutrition services*. In Wallace HM, Ryan G Jr, Oglesby A, editors: *Maternal and child health practices*, ed 3, Oakland, 1988, Third Party Publishing Co.

to use Z-scores from the median on the NCHS charts for individuals below the 5th percentile.

Skinfold. Assessment of tricep and subscapular skinfolds can provide information relative to the child's fat reserves in addition to measurement of arm circumference for muscle mass.

Biochemical Assessment

Individuals on medications for long periods of time are vulnerable to drug-nutrient interactions. Routine biochemical determinations should be conducted to prevent potentially serious nutrient deficiencies.

Diet and Feeding Assessment

Nutrient analysis of food records is vital to identify the adequacy of an individual's diet. Feeding evaluation for a special health care needs child is essential. A comprehensive picture would include assessment of oral structure and function, neuromotor abilities, developmental level, and mother-child interaction, along with observation of the feeding situation.[2]

Nutrition Intervention, Counseling, and Education

The nutrition concerns of this special population vary from critical (metabolic disorder controllable by diet only) to those being similar to other children. An interdisciplinary team assessment approach is critical for nutrition care planning. Components of the plan should integrate a family service plan with respect to the priorities of the child's disorder. Depending on the child's developmental evauations, parents may require intensive nutrition counseling. Children with chronic conditions may have frequent hospitalizations, during which nutrition care plans may be interrupted for long periods. Close coordination between community-based staff, hospital personnel, and the family is needed to assure that the long-term nutrition goals or new recommendations are understood and implemented.[2]

Referral

Community referrals should be as close to home as possible while at the same time ensuring high-quality care. Formation of good networks can maximize the resources and establish linkages to include Title V programs, WIC and other food assistance programs, other local clinics and developmental centers, and other services in the community. Nutrition services for children with special health care needs are in an evolutionary state. New opportunities are available for improving nutrition services through comprehensive health care because of the new legislation, changing population, home health care, high-technology treatment, multiagency involvement, and the focus on family-centered and community-based delivery of services.

SUMMARY

A healthy child grows at a genetically predetermined rate that may be compromised or accelerated by undernutrition, imbalanced nutrient intake, or overnutrition. Physical growth is one of the major criteria used to assess the nutritional status of infants and children.

Nutrition assessment, counseling, and education provide the framework for high-quality nutrition care. These components of nutrition services should be considered integral parts of health programs that provide both food and nutrition services to infants, children, and adolescents and to those individuals with special health care needs.

REFERENCES

1. Andrews EM, Clancy KL, Katz MG: Infant feeding practices of families belonging to prepaid group practice health plan, *Pediatrics* 65:678, 1980.
2. Baer MT, Farnan S, Mauer AM: *Children with special health care needs.* In Sharbaugh CO, editor: *Call to action: better nutrition for mothers, children, and families,* Washington, DC, 1991, National Center for Education in Maternal and Child Health.
3. Brown JE: Nutrition services for pregnant women, infants, children, and adolescents, *Clin Nutr* 3:104, 1984.
4. Centers for Disease Control, Division of Nutrition: Pediatric nutrition surveillance system, Atlanta, 1990, unpublished data.
5. Committee on Nutrition, American Academy of Pediatrics: Measurement of skinfold thickness in childhood, *Pediatrics* 42:538, 1968.
6. Dwyer J, Arent J: *Child nutrition.* In Sharbaugh CO, editor: *Call to action: better nutrition for mothers, children, and families,* Washington, DC, 1991, National Center for Education in Maternal and Child Health.
7. Endres BE, Rockwell RE: *Food, nutrition, and young child,* ed 2, St Louis, 1985, CV Mosby Co.
8. Fomon SJ: *Infant nutrition,* ed 2, Philadelphia, 1974, WB Saunders Co.
8a. Fomon SJ: *Nutritional disorders of children,* DHEW Pub (HSA) 77-5104, Rockville, Md, 1977, US Government Printing Office.

9. Fomon SJ: *Nutritional disorders of children: prevention, screening and follow-up*, DHHS Pub (HSA) 76-5612, Rockville, Md, 1976, US Government Printing Office.

10. Food and Nutrition Board: *Recommended dietary allowances*, ed 10, Washington, DC, 1989, National Academy Press.

11. Garza C, Cowell C: *Infant nutrition*. In Sharbaugh CO, editor: *Call to action: better nutrition for mothers, children, and families*, Washington, DC, 1991, National Center for Education in Maternal and Child Health.

12. Haschke F: *Body composition during adolescence*. In WJ Klish, Kretchmer N, editors: *Body composition measurements in infants and children: report of the ninety-eighth Ross conference on pediatric research*, Columbus, Ohio, 1989, Ross Laboratories.

13. Human Nutrition Information Services: *Nationwide food consumption survey 1977-1979*, preliminary report 11, US Department of Agriculture, Washington, DC, 1982, US Government Printing Office.

14. Human Nutrition Information Services: *Nationwide food consumption survey continuing survey of food intakes by individuals*, report 85-1, US Department of Agriculture, Washington, DC, 1985, US Government Printing Office.

15. Institute of Medicine: *Nutrition during lactation*, Washington, DC, 1991, National Academy Press.

16. Jelliffe DB, Jelliffe PEF: *Early infant nutrition*. In Winick M, editor: *Nutrition: pre- and post-natal development*, New York, 1979, Plenum.

17. Johnson CL and others: *Basic data on anthropometric measurements, regular measurements of hip and knee joints for selected age groups (1-74 years of age), U.S., 1972-1975*, National Health Examination Study, NHANES 1, Washington, DC, 1981. US Government Printing Office.

18. Johnson L, Bachman J, O'Malley P: *Drug use, drinking and smoking: national survey results from high school, college, and young adult population 1975-1988*, Rockville, Md, 1989, US Department of Health and Human Services.

19. Kaufman M, editor: *Quality assurance in ambulatory nutrition care*, Chicago, 1983, American Dietetic Association.

20. Lavee RM: Commentary. Should children, parents and pediatricians worry about cholesterol? *Pediatrics* 89:509, 1992.

21. Lonnerdal B, Forsum E, Hambraes L: A longitudinal study of protein, nitrogen and lactose contents of human milk from Swedish well nourished mothers, *Am J Clin Nutr* 29:1127, 1976.

22. Moore WM, Roche AF: *Pediatric anthropometrics*, Columbus, Ohio, 1982, Ross Laboratories.

23. National Heart, Lung, and Blood Institute: Report of the second task force on blood pressure control in children, *Pediatrics* 79:1, 1987.

24. Owen GM: Measurements, recording and assessment of skinfold thickness in childhood and adolescence: report of a small meeting, *Am J Clin Nutr* 35:629, 1982.

25. Owen GM, Paige DM: *Infancy*. In Paige DM, editor: *Manual of clinical nutrition*, Pleasantville, NJ, 1983, Nutrition Publications.

26. Paige DM, Owen GM: *Childhood and adolescence*. In Paige DM, editor: *Manual of clinical nutrition*, Pleasantville, NJ, 1983, Nutrition Publications.

27. Palmer CA: *Diet and nutrition: crucial factors in the dental health of children*. In Bourne GH, editor: *World review on nutrition and diet*, 8:131, 1989.

28. Story M, Heald F, Dwyer J: *Adolescent nutrition: trends and critical issues for the 1990s*. In Sharbaugh CO, editor: *Call to action: better nutrition for mothers, children, and families*, Washington, DC, 1991, National Center for Education in Maternal and Child Health.

29. Tanner JM: Growth and maturation in adolescence, Nutr Rev 39:43, 1981.

30. US Department of Health and Human Services: *Natural health and nutrition examination survey* (NHANES I) Washington, DC, 1975, US Government Printing Office.

31. US Department of Health and Human Services: Expert panel on blood cholesterol levels in children and adolescents, *Pediatrics* 89:495, 1992.

32. US Department of Health and Human Services, Public Health Service: *The surgeon general's report on nutrition and health*, DHHS Pub (PHS) 88-50210, Washington, DC, 1988, US Government Printing Office.

33. US Department of Health and Human Services, Public Health Service: *Child health USA '90*, Washington, DC, 1990, US Government Printing Office.

34. US Departtment of Health and Human Services, Public Health Service: *Healthy people 2000: national health promotion and disease prevention objectives*, DHHS Pub (PHS) 91-50212, Washington, DC, 1991, US Government Printing Office.

35. US Department of Health and Human Services, Public Health Service, Centers for Disease Control: *Preventing lead poisoning in young children*, Atlanta, 1991, US Government Printing Office.

36. US Department of Health and Human Services, Public Health Service, National Institutes of Health: *National cholesterol education program, report of the expert panel on blood cholesterol in children and adolescents*, Pub (NIH) 91-2732, Washington, DC, 1991, US Government Printing Office.

FOCUS ON THE ADOLESCENT: HEALTH RESOURCES—PROFESSIONAL MATERIALS

The Health of America's Youth. A data book highlighting statistics on adolescents including population statistics, health status, and health services utilization (1990).

The Forgotten Child in Health Care, Children in the Juvenile Justice System. Select papers from a two-part conference held in June 1988 and August 1989, sponsored by the Department of Maternal and Child Health, School of Hygiene and Public Health, The John Hopkins University (1990).

Proceedings from the 1989 State Adolescent Health Coordinators' Conference. The conference was sponsored by the University of Minnesota Adolescent Health Program held in Denver, Colorado, August 8-10, 1989.

Pregnancy and Childbearing Among Homeless Adolescents: Report of a Workshop. This document is a synopsis of the meeting convened in October 1989 by the National Institute of Mental Health and the Bureau of Maternal and Child Health and Resources Development, US Public Health Service. The meeting brought together selected national experts on homeless youth as well as representatives from several programs around the country and staff from a number of federal agencies. The purpose of the meeting was to share effective treatment models and to develop a set of recommendations to assist federal agencies in policy making, program development, and information dissemination (1989).

Child and Adolescent Health Profile: Resource Directory. The Child and Adolescent Health Project was undertaken both to develop a comprehensive picture of the health status and needs of New York's population under age 19 and to provide a replicable model for other states to use in obtaining and presenting similar information about their own population (1988).

Promoting the Health of Adolescents, Proceedings from the 1990 State Adolescent Health Coordinators' Conference (1991).

Adolescent Health: Abstracts of Active Projects FY 1991. Publication provides information regarding the adolescent component of programs supported by the Federal Maternal and Child Health Bureau (1991).

Adolescent Health: Catalog of Products. This publication is a catalog of products (journal articles, videotapes, curricula materials, patient education materials, etc.) which have been produced by SPRANS projects which focus on adolescent health, and includes a comprehensive collection of materials dealing with a wide range of topics (1990).

Adolescent Fathers Directory of Services. This directory lists one hundred and fourteen programs targeted toward young men. The Association of Maternal and Child Health Programs' Committee on the Health of School Age Children and Adolescents surveyed MCH program directors, directors of adolescent programs and adolescent training programs, and school bases clinics to determine current services, funding sources, staffing, and outreach information to determine what services are available to the target population.

The Health of America's Youth: Current Trends in Health Status and Utilization of Health Services. This chartbook brings together a number of existing data sets on adolescent health status by utilizing census data and existing national surveys that identify risk behaviors in adolescents and youth (1991).

AIDS and Adolescents: Exploring the Challenge. Journal of Adolescent Health Care, May 1989, Volume 10: Number 3 (Supplement).

Adolescent Substance Abuse: Risk Factors and Prevention Strategies. Maternal and Child Health Technical Information Bulletin. (1991).

MCH Program Interchange: *Focus on Adolescent Sexuality* (June 1990) and *Focus on Adolescent Substance Abuse* (August 1991).

For information regarding copies of these publications contact:
National Maternal and Child Health Clearinghouse
(NMCHC)
38th and R Streets, NW
Washington, DC 20057
(202) 625-8410

Source: *ASTPHND Fall Newsletter* Supplement 1991.

APPENDIX 7-1

Neuromuscular and psychosocial development in infants

Neuromuscular	Psychosocial	Implications for Feeding
Birth to 1 month		
Sucking and swallowing reflex present at birth	Early emotional and psychological and social attachment of mother and infant may determine future aspects of infant's personality	Oral reflex is a definite adaptive food-seeking reflex for survival
Stimulus in mouth leads to rhythmical sucking and swallowing pattern		On satiety, infant withdraws head from breast or bottle and falls asleep
Tongue protrusion predominates	Mother's feeding practices determine exposure of tactile stimulation, which is essential to infant's physical and emotional growth	If infant's needs are satisfied through food and love, trust develops between child and mother

Continued.

Neuromuscular and psychosocial development in infants—cont'd

Neuromuscular	Psychosocial	Implications for Feeding
Birth to 1 month—cont'd		
		Feeding is the main means for infant to establish human relationship with mother
Month 2		
Corners of mouth are well approximated but not very active in sucking; an open gap separates the lateral portions of the lips	Infant recognizes mother's face	Infant is an individual who shapes his own behavior and feeding schedule
Opens mouth widely to grasp nipple once it has touched lips	Infant learns to equate mother with food	Infant learns to equate mother with food
Hands often open	Strong emotional bond develops between mother and infant and can be viewed as beginning of social interaction of infant	Infant eats about five times per day and sleeps through the night
Tonic grasp disappearing		
Month 3		
Lip movement begins to refine; lower lip pulls in; may smack lips	More tactile stimulation exists with breastfed infant	Infant recognizes bottle or breast as source of food
Tongue protrusion still present but may swallow with less protrusion	Basic trust factor (if established) is manifested in infant responses to mother	Milk runs out of the sides of the mouth when nipple is withdrawn
Infant can hold onto an object without focusing on it	Infant ceases to cry with hunger when mother approaches	Infant still does not readily accept the cup
By end of third mouth, control of head and eyes is achieved	Infant stares into mother's face on feeding; shows response to human voice	
Month 4		
Smacking and pouting of lips	Infant in self-control	Important to watch infant for readiness of introduction of solid foods, since their introduction may influence lifelong dietary behavior
True negative pressure suck begins	Breastfeeding is significant in emotional development of infant	Schedule should be developed for the individual infant on demand to prevent overfeeding; self-demand feeding satisfies hunger in a natural way
Grosser back and forth movement of tongue and mandibular action beneath nipple disappears	Infant vocalizes through musical cooing; smiles and increases body activity	
Maintains grasp when object placed in hand	Can distinguish familiar people and knows mother's voice	Breastfeeding creates a more intense sense of intimacy and closeness because of skin contact
Rooting reflex gone		Feeding considered a psychocommunication and sociocultural exchange between mother and baby
Bite reflex disappearing		
Lifts head and chest when placed on stomach		
Month 5		
Beginning of hand-eye coordination is seen	Infant anticipates feeding	Feed only as long as infant desires
Head is steady now when infant is in a sitting position	Infant turns head aside to surroundings when satisfied	Beginning to sit when propped up
	Seeks out social stimulation and smiles to get attention	Feed infant when he is hungry
		Infant will open mouth for spoon and close mouth over it

Neuromuscular and psychosocial development in infants—cont'd

Neuromuscular	Psychosocial	Implications for Feeding
Month 5—cont'd Lower lip becomes more active; lips purse at the corners and nipples are held more firmly Strong sucking has developed Parts lips in process of shifting foods and in swallowing Tendency to eject food from mouth because of dominance of tongue projection Bite reflex disappears Munching stage evolves Normal swallowing occurs Gag reflex strong until chewing of solids Pats and holds bottle or breast	Development of hunger rhythm occurs Strengthening of trust is through feeding	Food is secured through sucking from the spoon Spoon feeding is difficult because of tongue projection as spoon is removed Considerable spilling milk running from the mouth
Month 6 Lower lip moves into internal position Lips purse together at corners Draws in lower lip when spoon is removed Pouts lips in process of shifting food in the mouth and during the swallow Normal bite begins Sucking is volitional Tongue is held poised in gutteral position Mouth poses to receive the spoon Hand and arm movements refine, and finger-feeding is seen Takes objects to mouth Helps with the spoon Can sit with support	Hungry infant who is fed learns to trust parents, and the foundation for a healthy personality is facilitated Interaction with others during feeding influences infant's acceptance and response to food Infant will show a preference for the individual who gives him the most care By the end of 6 months, crucial attachment rather than responsiveness occurs	Holding and cuddling the baby during bottle-feeding encourages warm communication between parent and infant Developmentally infant is ready for solid foods; any attempt to feed solid foods before this time can be viewed as a form of force-feeding Stages of addition of solid food to infant's diet should be individualized to infant Food should never be forced on infant Use a small spoon that easily fits into infant's mouth
Month 7 Keeps mouth tightly closed Chewing begins with action of tongue moving food around in the mouth Normal gag reflex present Starts eating solids without choking Teeth erupt Good lateral movement of tongue	Infant is more active socially; expresses wishes for contact but may also refuse it Attachment to mothering person is shown by infant's recognition of and pleasure in being with her Develops self-awareness and awareness of surroundings; is developing own personality	Soft, chewable foods may be introduced Introduce solids at a time when infant is in a more sociable and experimental mood; do not force new food if infant cries or fusses at the time it is introduced; wait until infant is in a better mood

Continued.

Neuromuscular and psychosocial development in infants—cont'd

Neuromuscular	Psychosocial	Implications for Feeding
Month 7—cont'd Reaches with one hand instead of two Transfers objects from hand to hand Holds bottle alone		
Month 8 Sits freely without support and has good head and body control Licks spoon with lips Bites a nipple, spoon, or rim of cup Chokes easily when drinking from a cup Inferior scissor grasp developed Reaches for spoon or cup with hand and head Expresses satiety by playing, razzing of the lips, or moving his arms actively	Infant becomes vocal and initiaties social contact and mimics adult behavior Mother's attitude is important in developing self-demand feeding schedule	Feeding time is one of social interaction for infant Feeding begins to occur in a regular pattern Infant should be allowed to use hands in feeding Infant shows eagerness or cries when food is prepared Infant may fuss or push food away when he does not like it
Month 9 Drinks from bottle independently When drinking from cup, fluids spill from corners of mouth Infant can bite off correct amount of food Table foods are easily chewed Teeth: eruption of lower and upper lateral incisors Pincer movement of thumb and forefinger developed Has developed coordination of hands	Demonstrates separation anxiety when separated from mother Necessity of fixing a schedule may cause tension and conflict	Set a feeding pattern, maintaining a variety of foods so all nutrients will be included in diet
Month 10 Tongue is drawn back within mouth and may be depressed in anticipation of feeding Tongue projection may occur again around 1 year when child explores with tongue to lick food morsels off lower lip	Infant mimics adult model in behavior and vocalizes for attention Expresses needs and feelings During feeding, infant demands a plaything to keep hands busy On final satiety, infant turns head to one side and keeps lips pursed	Infant may be offered fruit juices by the cup Offer bite-sized pieces of food for infant to pick up in self-feeding

Neuromuscular and psychosocial development in infants—cont'd

Neuromuscular	Psychosocial	Implications for Feeding
Month 10—cont'd		
Can handle bottle alone: shown by grasping bottle and bringing it to mouth		
Pincer grasp is becoming apparent with infant grasping small objects of food with thumb and index finger		
Pokes with index finger at nipple or at food in dish		
Finger-feeds small pieces		
Month 11		
Infant begins to walk, holds to stand, and cruises	Infant shows an understanding of adult words and gestures such as "Give it to me" and "Hand it over"	May introduce more table foods
Feeding behavior matures		Provide small bite-sized pieces of food for the infant to eat by finger-feeding
Drinks fairly continuously, four to five swallows at a time	During feeding, hands rest on side or tray top and by the end of the meal, infant is ready to play	Encourage self-feeding with help
Drinks fluids from a cup that is held for him; may begin to hold cup		
Begins self-spoon feeding with help		
Finger-feeding; much of mealtime is messy		
More interested in feel of food than finger-feeding; may put food back into dish		
Chewing is more refined		
Month 12		
Pattern of feeding solid foods has changed from sucking to rotary chewing	Infant becomes quieter on feeding and shows a growing interest in self-feeding	Finger-feeds most of meal
Upper lip draws in		Begins self-feeding with utensils
Lower lip sweeps over food on upper lip		
Deliberate spitting occurs		
Tongue projection may occur again as tongue becomes freer and child explores with it		
Tongue is drawn back within mouth and may even be depressed in anticipation of feeding		
Increased neuromotor coordination occurs		
Rotary chewing is present in solid food eating		

8 Nutrition in the Adult Years

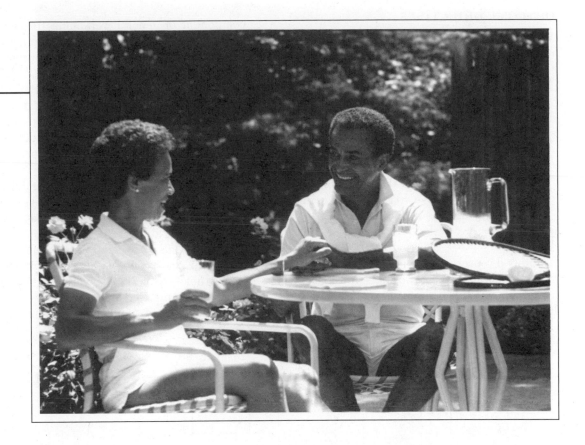

GENERAL CONCEPT

Maintenance of health, prevention of acute disease, and chronic disease risk reduction are primary goals for adults. Health promotion objectives must be understood, accepted, and adopted as early in life as possible because many chronic diseases begin early in childhood, if not sooner. The consequences of many nutrition-related diseases can be avoided, or at least delayed, if healthful lifestyle practices are adopted early and followed over the long term.

OUTCOME OBJECTIVES

When you finish this chapter, you should be able to:

- Cite examples of *Healthy People 2000* objectives for the United States as they relate to the adult population.
- Review the energy and nutrient needs of adults.
- Know the risk factors for major nutrition-related chronic diseases of adults.
- Apply client management strategies for chronic disease risk reduction in the adult population.
- Develop an innovative strategy for nutrition intervention programs in the community.

THE ADULT YEARS

Adulthood represents the longest period of the life cycle, spanning ages 21 to 60. It interfaces with adolescence and the senior years. Nutrition is an important aspect of healthful behavior and a major component of general well-being throughout the adult years. Whereas genetics determine our propensity for developing a number of chronic diseases (e.g., obesity, hypercholesterolemia, hypertension), the occurrence and extent of these diseases are determined by lifestyle choices. Early adulthood is often accompanied by vigor and vitality; however, the processes of aging and disease are already in progress. Many physiological functions decrease with age.

During adulthood, careers are established and families are started. Today's adults are faced with caring for their aging parents as well as their growing children. No longer is the traditional family of two parents and 2.4 children the American norm (Fig. 8-1). The "typical" American mother does not stay at home while father works; 52% of married women are employed outside the home. The number of family households has decreased while the

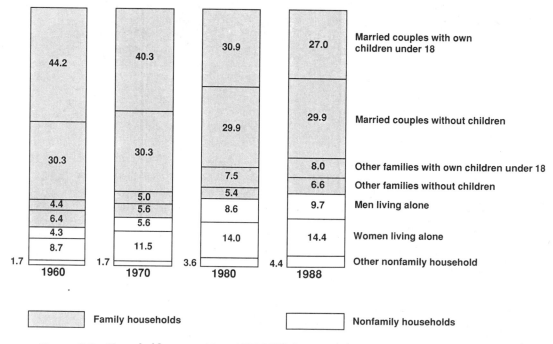

Figure 8-1. Household composition: 1960-1988 (in percent).
Reprinted with permission. U.S. Department of Commerce, Bureau of the Census; *Changes in American family life*, Current Population Reports, Special Studies, Series P-23, No 163, 1989, The Department.

number of nonfamily households has increased. The number of men and women living alone has also increased.

The heterogeneous group comprising adulthood were classically subgrouped as follows:

Young, single or married adults or couples without children

Young adults (single or married) with young children (the young family)

Maturing families with all school-aged children

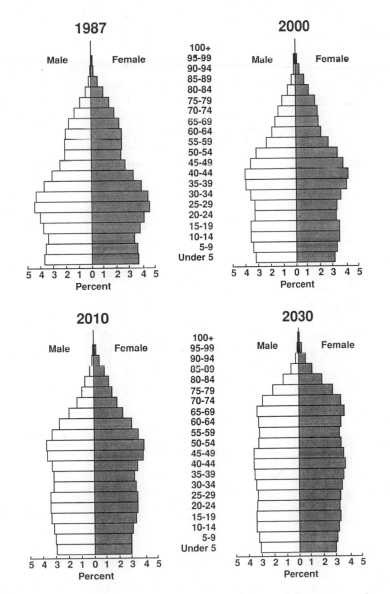

Figure 8-2. Estimates and projections of the age distribution of the U.S. population, by sex: 1987, 2000, 2010, 2030.

Reprinted with permission from Taeuber C, editor: *Statistical handbook on women in America,* published by The Oryx Press, 4041 N. Central at Indian School Rd., Phoenix, AZ 85012.

Middle-aged to "upper" middle-aged, single adults or couples without children at home

Currently, other adult groups not traditionally cited are growing in number and gaining importance. They include:

Single or living alone throughout life

Childless couples throughout life

Older (middle-aged) couples and individuals (married or single) starting a family (not shown in Fig. 8-1)

Most adults will be a part of several subgroups in this phase of the life cycle. The nutritional needs and concerns of each subgroup may differ. Thus it is important to recognize that the needs and concerns for any one individual change during the 40 years spanning adulthood.

The following major demographic shifts have markedly altered American food choices. Foods must not only be nutritionally adequate and tasty but also convenient to prepare, meet ethnic tastes, and be safe. For many, food costs are also a significant consideration. Integrating all these concerns into an healthful, active lifestyle is a primary goal of adulthood.

Demographic Characteristics

Gender and Age

More than half of the U.S. population is female. The median age of the population has increased for both males and females. Baby boomers, those born between 1946 and 1964, represent the bulge in the age distributions for 1987, 2000, and 2010 (Fig. 8-2) and account for the projected dramatic increase in our elderly population. After the year 2030, the number of individuals over 85 years (especially women) is projected to increase significantly. Overall, life expectancy in 1988 was 75 years old (Fig. 8-3). For white males, life expectancy was 72.3

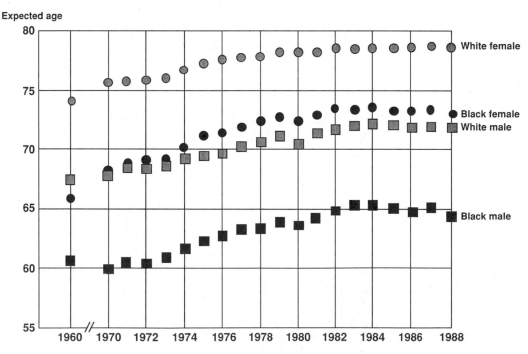

Figure 8-3. Life expectancy at birth, according to race and sex, United States, 1960 and 1970-1988.
Source: National Center for Health Statistics, National Vital Statistics System. In *Health United States*, DHS no. 91-1232, Hyattsville, Md, 1991, United States Department of Health and Human Services, National Center for Health Statistics.

years, whereas for white females it was 78.9. For black males, life expectancy was 65 years, and for black females it was 73.5 years.

Minority Population

Between 1980 and 1988, the white population in the United States increased 6%. During the same period, the Asian population increased 70% because of increases in immigration. The American Indian population increased 19% because of a high birth rate. The Hispanic population increased 34% while the black population, the largest minority in the United States, increased 13% between 1980-88 (Fig. 8-4). These figures are based on census data, which may underestimate minority populations.

Poverty

There are significant economic differences among population groups in our society. Approximately 10% of the U.S. white population had incomes below the poverty level in 1988. In contrast, about one third of the minority population lives in poverty; 32% of blacks, 27% of Hispanics, and 28% of American Indians had incomes below the poverty level in 1988. However, only 13% of Asians fell into this category.

Women who are the single heads of a family and elderly women are more likely to be poor than the population as a whole. The poverty rate of black female-headed families is higher than that of other families.

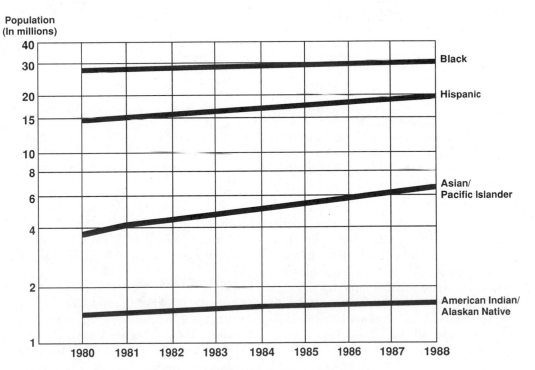

Figure 8-4. Minority populations in the United States, 1980-1988.
Source: U.S. Bureau of the Census, Current Population Surveys, 1990. In *Health United States*, DHS no. 91-1232, Hyattsville, Md, 1991, United States Department of Health and Human Services, National Center for Health Statistics.

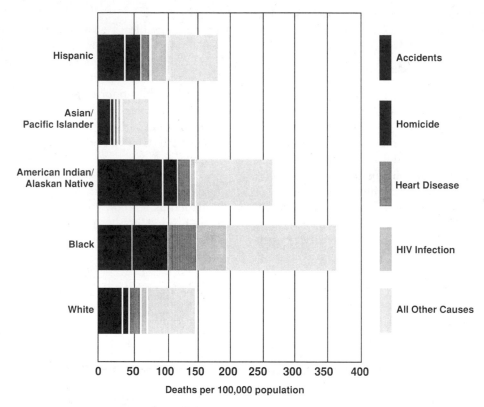

Figure 8-5. Death rates for selected causes for persons 25-44 years of age, according to race/ethnicity: United States, 1988.
Source: National Center for Health Statistics, National Vital Statistics System, and U.S. Bureau of the Census, Current Population Surveys. In *Health United States,* DHS no. 91-1232, Hyattsville, Md, 1991, United States Department of Health and Human Services, National Center for Health Statistics.

Death Rates

The death rate for black adults (25-44 years old) is 2.5 times higher than for white adults (Fig. 8-5). The death rate for Asians is low, about half the death rate for whites. The leading cause of death for all groups was unintentional injuries, although diseases of the heart, a modifiable cause of death, represented a significant cause of mortality for middle-aged adults, especially for blacks, American Indians, and Alaskan Natives.

Health Status

Between 1985 to 1988, 25% to 33% of blacks, American Indians, and Hispanics were in fair or poor health compared to Asian American and white adults between the ages of 45 and 64 years. Even with 12 or more years of education, blacks and American Indians were twice as likely to be in fair or poor health than whites and Asian Americans.

Cigarette Smoking

Cigarette smoking is considered to be the single most avoidable cause of death in the United States. About 400,000 lives are lost yearly from lung cancer, cardiovascular disease and chronic, obstructive pulmonary disease.

Smoking rates are high among black (39%), American Indian (37%) and Puerto Rican (37%) males as compared to Asian (25%) men. White men had smoking rates that were intermediate (30%).

Smoking rates are lower for females than males. They are, nonetheless, higher for American Indian (31%), black (29%), and white (28%) women than they are for Asian women (12%).

Health Coverage

Between 1980 and 1986, the proportion of persons who were uninsured increased from 12% to 15%. Health care coverage is available to essentially all persons older than 65 years of age. Less than 60% of the black population had private health care coverage between 1980 and 1983. Other vulnerable groups are Puerto Ricans and Mexican Americans: approximately 35% of the Mexican-American population younger than 65 years of age had no health care coverage during 1983 to 1986, compared with 16% of the white and Asian-American population.

Physiological Changes

During adulthood, there are many physiological changes (Fig. 8-6). Physiological systems function maximally in adolescence and early adulthood.

Throughout adulthood there is a loss in vitality and functionality of these systems. By age 70, these changes are significant. Initially, these changes are imperceptible, and over the years the changes become noticeable. The rate of decline of the physiological systems varies. Among individuals, genetics and lifestyle practices (e.g., diet, exercise, alcohol, and tobacco use) affect the aging process.

Some changes in physiological functions that occur with aging impact on nutrition:

1. Muscle mass decreases and body fat increases with age, even when body weight does not change, although more typically, there is an increase in body weight as well as body fat with age. The decrease in muscle mass relates to the decrease in basal metabolic rate (BMR) that occurs throughout adulthood. A small but measurable decline is apparent by age 30 and continues at a rate of 2% per decade. Regular exercise slows the loss of muscle mass associated with aging.

2. Accretion of cortical (peripheral bone) skel-

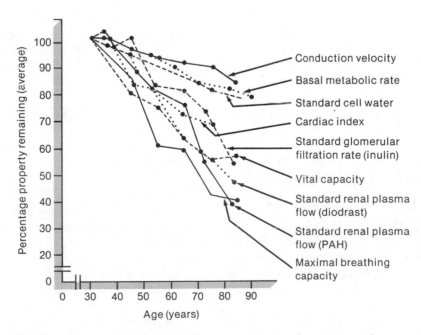

Figure 8-6. Age changes in physiological functions, expressed at percent of mean value at age 30.
Redrawn from Shock NW: *J Am Diet Assoc* 56:491, 1970.

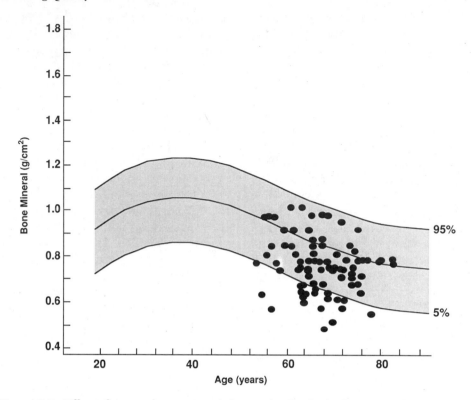

Figure 8-7. Effect of age on bone mineral density (mid-radius) of women. The center line represents age regression, whereas the upper and lower lines represent 90% confidence limits. Reprinted with permission from Riggs BL and others: Different changes in bone mineral density of the appendicular and axial skeleton with aging, *J Clin Invest* 67:328, 1980, by permission of the American Society for Aging.

etal mass continues to age 30 and decreases thereafter (Fig. 8-7). The rate of decrease is greatest between the ages of 40 and 60. Vertebral skeletal mass decreases in women throughout adulthood, including early adulthood (Fig. 8-8).

Intellectual Functioning

Although morphological and biochemical changes occur during the transition through adulthood to the elderly years, new research has shown that intellectual functioning can be maintained well into old age. In many individuals, there is a decline in cognitive ability during aging; however, it has been reported that attitudinal flexibility, an active lifestyle, and the absence of family discord can help to maintain intellectual functioning.[29] Therefore, a

lifestyle that includes involvement in a broad spectrum of intellectual and problem-solving activities appears to be important to maintain intellectual acuity in old age.

Characteristics of the Adult Years

During the adult years, there are many lifestyle changes. These behavior changes are characteristic of different generations that comprise the adult group:

Physical activity generally decreases with age, although more Americans are participating in a program of regular exercise.

Vitamin and mineral supplement use occurs in about one third of the adult population. Multivitamin and vitamin C supplements are used most frequently, and calcium and iron sup-

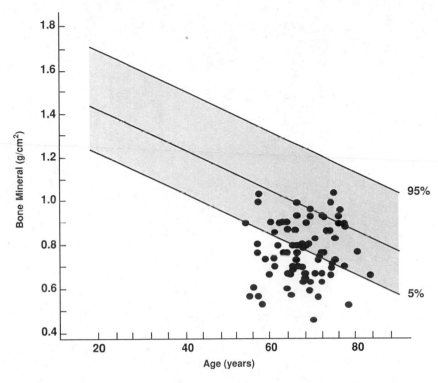

Figure 8-8. Effect of age on bone mineral density (lumbar vertebrae) of women. The center line represents age regression, whereas the upper and lower lines represent 90% confidence limits.

Reprinted with permission from Riggs BL and others: Different changes in bone mineral density of the appendicular and axial skeleton with aging, *J Clin Invest* 67:328, 1980, by permission of the American Society for Aging.

plements also are popular. Women and whites are more likely to use supplements. Use increases with level of education.

Nutritional Issues

Since the 1970s, nutritional concerns have shifted from nutrient deficiencies to nutrient excesses and the special nutritional issues of specific adult groups. Chronic disease risk reduction has become a major emphasis of public health nutrition.[7,33] Although this is an important aspect of contemporary nutrition practice, equally important and even more relevant for some individuals are other relatively common nutritional needs that also should be addressed in community nutrition practice. Dealing with these special issues may frequently

take precedent over intervention for chronic disease risk reduction.

Nutrient and Energy Requirements

The Recommended Dietary Allowances (RDAs) for adult males and females at ages 19 to 24, 25 to 50, and older than 50 are presented in Table 8-1.

The use of the RDAs is described as follows by the Food and Nutrition Board of the National Academy of Sciences:

> They are typically used for planning and procuring food supplies for population subgroups, for interpreting food consumption records of individuals and populations, for establishing standards for food assistance programs, for evaluating the adequacy of food supplied in meeting national nutritional needs, for

Table 8-1. Recommended dietary allowances for the adult years (revised 1989)

Category*	Age (years)	Protein (g)	Fat-soluble vitamins				Water-soluble vitamins							Minerals						
			Vita-min A (μg RE)†	Vita-min D (μg)‡	Vita-min E (mg α-TE)§	Vita-min K (μg)	Vita-min C (mg)	Thia-min (mg)	Ribo-flavin (mg)	Niacin (mg NE)‖	Vita-min B6 (mg)	Fo-late (μg)	Vita-min B12 (μg)	Cal-cium (mg)	Phos-phorus (mg)	Mag-nesium (mg)	Iron (mg)	Zinc (mg)	Iodine (μg)	Sele-nium (μg)
Males	19-24	58	1,000	10	10	70	60	1.5	1.7	19	2.0	200	2.0	1,200	1,200	350	10	15	150	70
	25-50	63	1,000	5	10	80	60	1.5	1.7	19	2.0	200	2.0	800	800	350	10	15	150	70
	51+	63	1,000	5	10	80	60	1.2	1.4	15	2.0	200	2.0	800	800	350	10	15	150	70
Females	19-24	46	800	10	8	60	60	1.1	1.3	15	1.6	180	2.0	1,200	1,200	280	15	12	150	55
	25-50	50	800	5	8	65	60	1.1	1.3	15	1.6	180	2.0	800	800	280	15	12	150	55
	51+	50	800	5	8	65	60	1.0	1.2	13	1.6	180	2.0	800	800	280	10	12	150	55

The allowances, expressed as average daily intakes over time, are intended to provide for individual variations among most normal persons as they live in the United States under usual environmental stresses. Diets should be based on a variety of common foods in order to provide other nutrients for which human requirements have been less well defined.

*Weights and heights of reference adults are actual medians for the U.S. population of the designated age, as reported by NHANES II. The use of these figures does not imply that the height-to-weight ratios are ideal.

†Retinol equivalents. 1 retinol equivalent = 1 μg retinol or 6 μg β-carotene.

‡As cholecalciferol. 10 μg cholecalciferol = 400 IU of vitamin D.

§α-Tocopherol equivalents. 1 mg d-α tocopherol = α-TE.

‖1 NE (niacin equivalent) is equal to 1 mg of niacin or 60 mg of dietary tryptophan.

Table 8-2. Factors for estimating daily energy allowances at various levels of physical activity for men and women (ages 19-50)

Level of activity	Energy expenditure* (kcal/kg per day)
Very light	
Men	31
Women	30
Light	
Men	38
Women	35
Moderate	
Men	41
Women	37
Heavy	
Men	50
Women	44
Exceptional	
Men	58
Women	51

*REE (Resting Energy Expenditure) was computed from formulas in Table 8-1 and is the average of values for median weights of persons ages 19 to 24 and 25 to 74 years: males, 24.0 kcal/kg; females, 23.2.

designing nutrition education programs, and for developing new products in industry.[9]

They are most appropriately applied to groups, but an estimate of an individual's probable risk of nutrient deficiency can be made with sufficient dietary intake information taken over a period of time.

Energy needs vary considerably among adults. Energy expenditure is principally a function of gender, body mass, and level of physical activity. A simple method for estimating energy allowance is presented in Table 8-2.

Nutrient Intakes

In a nationwide food consumption survey, the mean intakes of vitamins A, C, B_{12}, thiamin, and riboflavin met or exceeded the 1989 RDAs for adults. The intake of vitamins B_6 and E were slightly below the RDA (but more than two thirds of the RDA). In general, the intakes of vitamins were within the recommended level. Iron intake for women 12 to 50 years of age was approximately two thirds of the recommended daily intake (15 mg). Zinc and magnesium intakes for both men and women were approximately 75% of the RDA. Copper intakes of men and women were below the lower range recommended.

In addition to iron, calcium is another problem nutrient for women. Women consumed approximately 600 mg of calcium per day—200 mg/day less than recommended.

Nutrient and Food Consumption Trends

Nutrient intake changes since the 1960s are reflective of generational differences[25]:

- A change in the nutritional practices of Americans in recent years is consistent with contemporary dietary recommendations for chronic disease risk reduction. The percentage of calories from fat have decreased from 42% to about 36% to 37% in 1984.
- Saturated fatty acid intake decreased from 18% to 20% of calories to about 14% of calories.
- Polyunsaturated fatty acid intake increased from 2% to 4% of calories to about 7.5% of calories.
- Dietary cholesterol intake decreased from about 600 mg/day to less than 400 mg/day.

Food Intake Changes

Changes in the consumption of certain foods throughout the life cycle reflect generational differences.

Milk and milk products. Consumption of these foods decreases in both males and females after 18 years of age. Women typically consume less milk than men. Women in the 35- to 50-year age group have the lowest milk consumption of any group in the life cycle.

Cereals and grains. Intake is lowest for women who are aged 19 to 50. Interestingly, cereal and grain consumption increases in both men and women after age 50.

Meat, poultry, and fish. Consumption is higher in men than women. The intake of meat, poultry, and fish decreases in both men and women after age 65.

Fruits and vegetables. Consumption increases considerably after age 50.

Alcohol Consumption and Nutrition

Per capita alcohol consumption is equal to 160 calories/day.

Women's Special Nutritional Issues

Energy Intake during the Menstrual Cycle

Some researchers have shown that women tend to consume fewer calories (about 200) per day for approximately 2 weeks before ovulation than after ovulation.[12] This difference may be due to the slight increase in energy requirements that have been reported during the premenses and menses phases of the menstrual cycle.

Premenstrual Syndrome (PMS)

PMS is defined as a cluster of physical, emotional, and psychological symptoms that some women experience 7 to 10 days before menstruation. The cause of PMS is unknown but may be related to the hormonal milieu prior to menstruation. There is no evidence to suggest that PMS is caused by a nutrient deficiency. There is some evidence, however, to suggest that a nutritional supplement may reduce the severity of PMS symptoms in some women,[17] but this is as yet a controversial issue that requires further investigation. Some women benefit from weight loss, a nutritionally adequate diet, regular exercise, avoidance of alcohol and tobacco, and reduced caffeine intake.

Effects of Oral Contraceptive Agents (OCAs) on Nutritional Status

The OCA preparations used today have approximately one tenth the level of estrogen and progesterone originally used. Therefore, their side effects are less or nonexistent compared with earlier reports. Because OCAs reduce menstrual blood loss, fewer nutrients are lost in menstrual blood. Most notably, iron is conserved. Although OCAs affect the metabolism of other nutrients (Table 8-3), well-nourished women do not require nutrient supplements.

Nutrient Requirements of Cigarette Smokers

Cigarette smokers have a higher vitamin C requirement than nonsmokers because cigarette smoking increases the metabolism of vitamin C. In addition, cigarette smokers absorb 10% less vitamin C. The RDA for vitamin C is 100 mg/day for persons who smoke 20 or more cigarettes per day.

Dietary Supplements

Despite statements issued by professional medical and nutrition societies promoting the concept that healthy people can obtain all necessary nutrients by eating a variety of foods, many adult Americans use dietary supplements. Reasons given for supplement use include uncertainty about nutrient adequacy of foods, a desire to attain perceived improved physical status, and as self-treatment for illness. Professionals are concerned about the nonprescriptive use of supplements. Overdoses of single nutrients, such as vitamins A and D, can be harmful. Large doses of some nutrients may interact with other nutrients and interfere with their absorption, metabolism, excretion, and hence their requirements. Additionally, supplementation may mask diagnosis of some chronic diseases.

In 1989, the National Center for Health Statistics issued the results of a survey conducted in 1986 documenting vitamin and mineral supplement usage in the United States.[20] During 1986, more than one third of the U.S. adult population consumed nonprescription supplements, with women consuming them more frequently (Fig. 8-9). Usage differed between races and education levels. About two fifths of white adults, one fifth of black adults, and less than one third of Hispanic adults used supplements (Fig. 8-9). Supplement usage was higher as income and educational level increased. People living in western states consumed more supplements than in other regions of the country.

Single-vitamin and vitamin-mineral combination products were the two most common types used by women. Men most frequently used single vitamins and multivitamins. Women and men under 45 years of age were more likely to take broad-spectrum vitamins (those containing A, B vitamins, C, D, and E and at least one mineral such as cal-

Table 8-3. Effects of oral contraceptives on nutrients

Nutrient	Effect on blood concentrations and metabolism
Energy-yielding nutrients	
Carbohydrate	Elevated fasting glucose
	Elevated insulin
Lipid	Elevated triglycerides
	Elevated low-density lipoprotein (LDL) cholesterol
	Lowered high-density lipoprotein (HDL) cholesterol
Protein	Elevated coagulating proteins
	Lowered albumin
Vitamins	
Folate	Lowered (in some studies)
Riboflavin	Lowered (in some studies)
	Impaired enzyme activity (in some studies)
Vitamin A	Elevated retinol (lowered liver stores)
	Elevated retinol-binding proteins
	Lowered carotene
Vitamin B_6	Lowered
Vitamin B_{12}	Lowered in serum; normal in red blood cells
Vitamin C	Lowered in leukocytes, thrombocytes, and platelets
Vitamin E	No effect
Vitamin K	Elevated clotting factors (and lowered response to anticoagulants)
Minerals	
Copper	Elevated
Iron	Elevated
Zinc	Lowered
Water	Retained temporarily

Data from Dimperio D: *Effect of oral contraceptives on nutrient status*, presentation at the Conference on Nutrition for Pregnancy, Lactation, and Infancy on 13 February 1987, in Gainesville, Fla; and Tyrer LB: Nutrition and the pill, *J Reprod Med* 29:547, 1984.

cium, phosphorus, iodine, iron, magnesium, copperr, zinc, or manganese). Women over 45 were more likely to use specialized products; men over 45 used these products equally.

Both men and women consumed vitamin C more than any other supplement. Calcium and iron were the minerals most frequently consumed by women. Iron was the single mineral most frequently consumed by men. Some of these supplement users were consuming certain vitamins far in excess of the RDA. For 10% of adult male and female users, vitamins E, C, thiamin, riboflavin, B_6, and B_{12} were consumed in quantities greater than 15 times the RDA. All of the minerals were consumed at less than 200% of the RDA or the Estimated Safe and Adequate Daily Dietary In-

takes levels. Side effects have been noted for excessive intake of certain nutrients, including water-soluble vitamins such as vitamins C and B_6.

Drug-Nutrient Interactions

Although some dietitians and nutritionists consider drug-nutrient interaction a problem associated with the elderly, younger adults frequently use both prescription and over-the-counter medications for a variety of problems. Thus nutrition educators need to be aware of the potential effects of drug-nutrient interactions in the adult population.

Drugs and nutrients can interact in three primary ways: a drug and nutrient can react together to form a new product; a drug or nutrient can affect the gastrointestinal tract and ultimate absorption

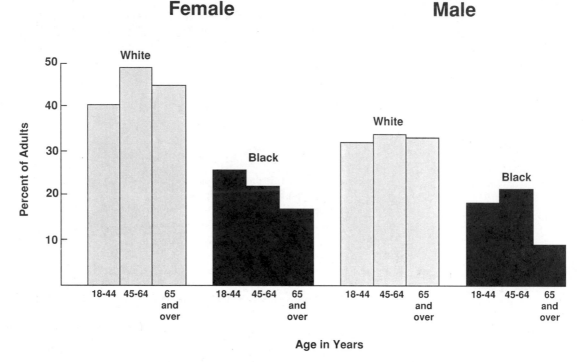

Figure 8-9. Percentage of adults in the United States using vitamin and mineral products by age, race, and sex in 1986.
Reprinted with permission from Moss AT and others: *Use of vitamin and mineral supplements in the United States: Current users, types of products and nutrients,* Advanced data from vital health statistics No 174, Hyattsville, Md, 1989, National Center for Health Statistics.

of either; and a drug can impair the use of nutrients. The occurrence of an interaction is dependent on the drug, the food consumed, and the pattern of food consumption. Risk of interaction can be reduced by adjusting the dosage of drug, the timing of drug intake, and the timing of food intake.[28]

The following are some common drug-nutrient interactions.[28] Long-term use of aspirin can promote chronic gastrointestinal blood loss. Diuretics can promote loss of body potassium. Antacids containing aluminum hydroxide can reduce phosphorus absorption. Dietary calcium can reduce the absorption of the antibiotic tetracycline. Carbonated drinks can cause some drugs to dissolve in the stomach rather than in the intestines, where they are more easily absorbed into the blood. A combination of alcohol and depressants (tranquilizers, barbitu-

rates, or painkillers) can slow performance skills, judgment, and alertness to dangerously low levels.

Usually physicians and pharmacists assume the role of providing advice on drug-nutrient interactions. However, nutrition educators can suggest the following: read labels on prescription and over-the-counter drugs; question the physician or pharmacist about how a drug may react with foods and beverages; and tell a physician about any unusual symptoms. Such simple messages can help increase awareness of potential problems and prevent adverse reactions.

Nutrition Services for Adults
Domestic Food Assistance Programs
The most commonly used food program for non-pregnant American adults is the Food Stamp Pro-

Table 8-4. Cost of food at home per week for food plans, June 1991, U.S. average

Age group	Thrifty plan	Low-cost plan	Moderate-cost plan	Liberal plan
Family of two				
20-50 yr	$49.80	$ 62.90	$ 77.70	$ 96.60
51+ yr	47.30	60.70	74.80	89.20
Family of four (couple 20-50 and children)				
1-2 yr & 3-4 yr	72.50	90.40	110.70	135.90
6-8 yr & 9-11 yr	83.10	106.30	132.90	160.10

gram.[18] Food stamps help low-income households purchase a nutritionally adequate diet. Monthly benefits are based on household size and income and on the cost of the Thrifty Food Plan (Table 8-4). This plan represents the least costly of four representative food plans developed by USDA's Human Nutrition Information Services. The plan assumes that food for all meals and snacks is purchased at the store and prepared at home. Estimates of amounts of food for each plan are computed from food consumption survey data. Average participation in the Food Stamp Program was 20.2 million households in 1990, costing an estimated $3.5 billion in benefits.

The Temporary Emergency Food Assistance Program is another federally funded program available to nonpregnant adults. Through this program, food is directly distributed by designated food banks to low-income families. The amount of food distributed varies with the availability of government surplus food supplies.

Many privately funded food assistance programs exist in local communities throughout the United States. Funding agencies include churchs, local government, private industry, and nonprofit groups.

Nutrition Education Services

A variety of governmental agencies (both federally and locally funded), as well as nonprofit groups and private industry, offer nutrition education services to the U.S. adult population. The USDA's Cooperative Extension Service provides education through a variety of programs including the Expanded Food and Nutrition Education Program (EFNEP). EFNEP, established in 1968, serves low-income households with children under the age of 18 in both rural and urban areas.[26] Using paraprofessional staffing from within the community, the program provides participating families with basic information on food and nutrition and assists them in learning how to incorporate this information into menu planning and improved family diets. Common areas of inquiry for county extension agents include general nutrition topics as well as food safety and food preservation issues. Programs delivered by extension agents include application of dietary guidelines, weight management strategies, child and infant nutrition, and food safety.

NUTRITION-RELATED HEALTH PROBLEMS

Dietary factors are associated with five of the ten leading causes of death in the United States: coronary heart disease, some types of cancer, stroke, non–insulin dependent diabetes mellitus (NIDDM) and atherosclerosis.[24] In addition, other chronic diseases such as osteoporosis and allergies are associated with a nutrition component. Advances in medical technology throughout the twentieth century have increased survival rates of adults stricken with chronic diseases in their young and middle adult years and thus increased their life span. Childhood mortality and deaths from infectious diseases have increased. In the area of nutrition-related illness, focus has shifted from pre-

Table 8-5. *Healthy People 2000* objectives

Objectives	Prevalence
Health status	
Reduce coronary heart disease deaths to no more than 100/100,000 people.	Age-adjusted: 135/100,000 (1987)
Reverse the rise in cancer deaths to achieve a rate of no more than 130 per 100,000.	Age-adjusted: 133/100,000 (1987)
Reduce overweight to a prevalence of $\geq 20\%$ among people ≥ 20 years.	26% for people 20-74 (1976-80); for men, 24%; for women, 27%
Risk reduction	
Reduce dietary fat intake to an average $\leq 30\%$ of calories and average saturated fat intake to $< 10\%$ of calories among people 2 years of age and older.	For people 20-74 (1976-80): 36% of calories from total fat; 13% from saturated fat; 36% and 13% for women 19-50 (1985)
Increase complex carbohydrate and fiber-containing foods to ≥ 5 daily servings for vegetables (including legumes) and fruits, and to ≥ 6 daily servings for grain products.	2½ servings of vegetables and fruits; 3 servings grains for women 19-50 (1985)
Increase to at least 50% the proportion of overweight people ≥ 12 years who have adopted sound dietary practices combined with regular physical activity to attain appropriate body weight.	30% overweight women; 25% overweight men aged 20 and older (1985)
Increase to at least 30% the proportion of people ≥ 6 years who engage regularly, preferably daily, in light to moderate physical activity for at least 30 minutes per day.	22% over 18 were active for at least 30 minutes ≥ 5 times weekly; 12% ≥ 7 times weekly (1985)
Increase calcium intake so at least 50% of people aged 5 and older consume ≥ 2 servings daily of foods rich in calcium.	15% women & 23% men aged 25-50 consumed ≥ 2 servings (1985-86)
Decrease salt and sodium intake so at least 65% of home meal preparers prepare foods without adding salt, at least 80% of people avoid using salt at the table, and at least 40% of adults regularly purchase foods modified or lower in sodium.	54% in women aged 19-50 who served as main food preparer did not use salt in preparation (1985); 68% also did not use salt at the table; 20% of all people ≥ 18 years of age regularly purchased foods with reduced salt and sodium (1988)
Increase to at least 85% the proportion of people ≥ 18 years of age who use food labels to make nutritious food selections.	74% used labels in 1988
Increase to at least 50% the proportion of worksites with > 50 employees that offer employees nutrition education/weight management programs.	17% offered nutrition education activities and 15% offered weight management activities in 1985.

Adapted from *Healthy people 2000: national health promotion and disease prevention,* Washington, DC, 1991, Department of Health and Human Services, Public Health Service.

vention of acute dietary deficiency diseases to health promotion. Through personal choices, adults have many opportunities to change established practices and adopt lifestyles that can significantly shape their long-term health prospects.

The U.S. Department of Health and Human Services document *Healthy People 2000*[11] identifies objectives for nutrition-related issues specific to adults. The objectives for both health status and risk reduction, along with baseline prevalence, are listed in Table 8-5.

Obesity and Weight Management

Caloric intake and energy expenditure are the two major modifiable components of body weight. Over the past 25 years, dietitians and nutritionists have focused efforts on modifying caloric intake. More recently, attention also has been given to the health benefits of increased physical activity. Awareness of energy consumed and energy used is critical to the prevention and treatment of obesity.

A large portion of the U.S. adult population is overweight (Table 8-6). The prevalence of obesity has not declined over the last two decades despite intense attention to the problem.[5] The rate varies depending on racial origin, cultural and socioeconomic conditions, and physical status. Indeed, obesity is multifactorial, reflecting both genetic and environmental influences. Although heredity plays a critical role, some persons who are predisposed to obesity may not become obese. Propensity to obesity does not assure expression of obesity. Environmental factors significantly influence the onset of obesity.

Obesity is an independent risk factor for development of NIDDM, gallbladder disease, hypertension, cardiovascular diseases, and some cancers.[7] Distribution of fat appears to play an important role in relation to increased risk of death, stroke, heart disease, and NIDDM. Centrally located fat (based on waist to hip ratio) appears to be more of a health risk than peripherally located fat (Fig. 8-10).

Despite consensus within the scientific community that obesity represents a major public health problem, there is a lack of consensus over

Table 8-6. Overweight prevalence by population group

Overweight prevalence	1976-80 Baseline*
Low-income women aged 20 and older	37%
Black women aged 20 and older	44
Hispanic women aged 20 and older	
Mexican-American women	39†
Cuban women	34†
Puerto Rican women	37†
American Indians/Alaska Natives	29-75‡
People with disabilities	36§
Women with high blood pressure	50
Men with high blood pressure	39

Data from *Healthy people 2000: national health promotion and disease prevention,* Washington, DC, 1991, Department of Health and Human Services, Public Health Service.
*Baseline for people aged 20-74.
†Baseline for Hispanics aged 20-74.
‡1984-88 estimates for different tribes.
§1985 baseline for people aged 20-74 who report limitation in activity due to chronic conditions.

the definition of obesity. A variety of standards have been used: weight for height tables based on people applying for life insurance, body mass index (BMI = weight in kilograms divided by height in meters, squared), percent of body fat, waist to hip ratio, and weight for body frame size based on a representative sample, to name a few.

The third edition (1990) of *Nutrition and Your Health: Dietary Guidelines for Americans*[33] advises maintenance of healthy weight and presents a chart relating body weight to height and age (Table 8-7). Healthy weight is defined as meeting three criteria: a weight within the suggested range for height and age, a fat distribution pattern that is not associated with a high risk of morbidity and mortality, and absence of any medical condition for which weight loss is indicated.

Incidence of major weight gain is twice as high in women and highest in persons aged 25 to 34 years.[34] Initially overweight women gain the most weight. In those persons not initially overweight, the incidence of becoming overweight in a 10-year period is the same for men and women and highest in those aged 35 to 44 years. Although new research

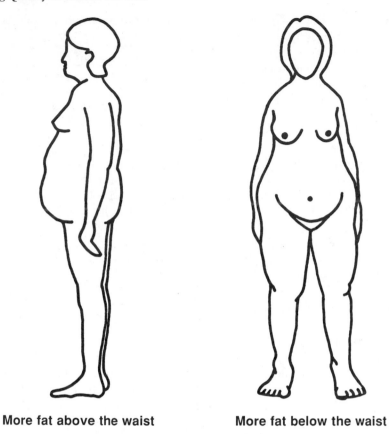

More fat above the waist   **More fat below the waist**

Figure 8-10. Distribution of body fat.

suggests that people can be slightly heavier as they age without risk to health,[2] it is clear that attention must be focused on prevention of obesity. Prevention is important during the entire life span, but focus during early adulthood on healthful lifestyle habits is critical to avoid weight gain in midadulthood.

Lack of physical activity increases the risk of becoming overweight.[32] Television viewing, along with lack of weekly exercise, has been independently associated with increased prevalence of obesity in adult men and women. As television viewing time increases, exercise tends to decrease and snacking increases. It can be debated that either obesity leads to decreased exercise or vice versa.

Whichever the initial cause, the relationship of decreased activity and increased weight remains.

In minority populations, obesity represents a major public health problem.[1,21] However, the impact of obesity is dependent on the population group. Compared with whites, many minority populations have higher rates of obesity but lower rates of coronary heart disease, except for blacks, who have higher rates of both.

Recognition of the health consequences associated with obesity, combined with social acceptance of "thin is beautiful," has led a significant number of Americans to spend $2 billion annually in attempts to lose weight. Individual approaches include use of over-the-counter liquid diet drinks and

Table 8-7. Suggested weights for adults

Height*	Weight in lb†	
	19 to 34 years	35 years and over
5'0"	97-128‡	108-138
5'1"	101-132	111-143
5'2"	104-137	115-148
5'3"	107-141	119-152
5'4"	111-146	122-157
5'5"	114-150	126-162
5'6"	118-155	130-167
5'7"	121-160	134-172
5'8"	125-164	138-178
5'9"	129-169	142-183
5'10"	132-174	146-188
5'11"	136-179	151-194
6'0"	140-184	155-199
6'1"	144-189	159-205
6'2"	148-195	164-210
6'3"	152-200	168-216
6'4"	156-205	173-222
6'5"	160-211	177-228
6'6"	164-216	182-234

Derived from National Research Council: *Diet and health: implications for reducing chronic disease risk*, Washington, DC, 1989, National Academy Press.
*Without shoes.
†Without clothes.
‡The higher weights in the ranges generally apply to men, who tend to have more muscle and bone; the lower weights more often apply to women, who have less muscle and bone.

foods, physician-administered liquid diet programs, pharmacological aids, and physical devices, as well as adherence to specific diet regimens found in numerous books. Group programs abound. Some require purchase of special foods or supplements; others only offer social support. Many follow established guidelines for a safe weight loss program (see the box at right).

Unfortunately, well over 90% of people who have lost weight regain at least the amount lost, and sometimes more. Many of these people go through several rounds of dietary restrictions leading to weight loss, followed by a regaining of weight, then further weight loss, and regaining, and so on. This pattern is referred to as weight cycling or yoyo dieting. Recent evidence suggests such fluctuations in body weight may negatively affect health, independent of obesity, and may tend to increase body weight over time.[16]

Many authorities express concern over the overwhelming failure of reliance on food restriction and behavior management techniques as the sole means of maintaining healthy weight in most overweight individuals.[10] Some have suggested evaluation of the standard practice of placing every overweight individual into a weight loss program. Others have suggested incorporating relapse prevention techniques, such as those used in substance abuse programs, along with increasing physical activity into current weight management philosophy. Much research remains to be done in the area of prevention and treatment of obesity.

Physical Activity

Many obese adults tend to eat fewer calories to lose weight, but few resort to increasing physical activity to achieve the same end. This disturbing fact reflects the sedentary lifestyle of U.S. adults, the

WEIGHT LOSS PROGRAMS

Characteristics of a sensible weight loss program
- Weight loss of ½ to 1 lb/week
- Stresses *new* habits:
  Increase physical activity
  Low-fat, affordable, practical eating habits (calories adjusted to meet individual needs)
  Change food and eating habits
- Positive mental image
- Lifetime commitment and monitoring

Characteristics of questionable weight loss programs
- Author not a nutrition authority
- Forbidden food lists
- Use supplemental food or pill
- Use secret scientific formula
- Anecdotal reports
- Fewer than 1000 calories
- No medical supervision
- No maintenance plan

relatively high emphasis placed on diet as a means of weight reduction, and the lack of recognition of the impact of physical activity on health status.

Regular physical activity can help prevent and manage coronary heart diseases, hypertension, NIDDM, osteoporosis, obesity, and mental health problems such as depression and anxiety.[15] It is also associated with decreased rates of colon cancer and stroke. Physically active people, on the average, tend to outlive more sedentary people.

Regular physical activity is defined in *Healthy People 2000* as "exercise which involves large muscle groups in dynamic movement for periods of 20 minutes or longer, 3 or more days a week, and which is performed at an intensity of 60 percent or greater of an individual's cardiorespiratory capacity."[11] Even light to moderate activity (requiring sustained, rhythmic muscular movements) below levels recommended for cardiovascular fitness can have significant health benefits. However, less than half the adult American population exercises more than three times weekly for 20 minutes, regardless of intensity.

It is unclear what types and amounts of physical activity are required for health benefits.[4] Increased energy expenditure enhances weight reduction and may favorably affect blood pressure, platelet aggregation, and glucose tolerance. Aerobic exercise enhances cardiovascular function. Exercises to increase muscular strength and flexibility may protect against disabilities and injuries. Individuals can select from a variety of activities (Table 8-8) to develop a personalized physical activity plans suited to their own preferences and adapted to meet their own health needs.

Coronary Heart Disease

Coronary heart disease (CHD) is the leading cause of death in the United States. There are approximately 1 million deaths annually from heart and blood vessel diseases, nearly as many as all other causes of death combined. One fourth of all Americans have some form of cardiovascular disease. The major modifiable risk factors for CHD are hypercholesterolemia (elevated total and low-density lipoprotein [LDL] cholesterol levels), hypertension,

and cigarette smoking. Excessive body weight and long-term physical inactivity are other controllable risk factors. The major nonmodifiable risk factors are family history of premature CHD, male gender, and increasing age. Other risk factors are a low high-density lipoprotein (HDL) cholesterol concentration (less than 35 mg/dl), and non–insulin dependent diabetes mellitus.

The National Cholesterol Education Program (NCEP)[22] defines a desirable blood cholesterol level as less than 200 mg/dl, a borderline blood cholesterol level as 200 to 239 mg/dl, and high blood cholesterol as more than 240 mg/dl. LDL cholesterol is the atherogenic (or unfavorable) lipoprotein fraction and is classified as follows: a desirable LDL cholesterol level is less than 130 mg/dl, a borderline LDL cholesterol is 130 to 159 mg/dl, and a

Table 8-8. Steps to increase calorie expenditure

Activity	Calories expended per hour*	
	Man†	Woman†
Sitting quietly	100	80
Standing quietly	120	95
Light activity:	300	240
Cleaning house		
Office work		
Playing baseball		
Playing golf		
Moderate activity:	460	370
Walking briskly (3.5 mph)		
Gardening		
Cycling (5.5 mph)		
Dancing		
Playing basketball		
Strenuous activity:	730	580
Jogging (9 min/mile)		
Playing football		
Swimming		
Very strenuous activity:	920	740
Running (7 min/mile)		
Racquetball		
Skiing		

Derived from McArdle et al, *Exercise physiology, energy, nutrition, and human performance*. Philadelphia, 1986, Lea & Febiger.
*May vary depending on environmental conditions.
†Healthy man, 175 lb; healthy woman 140 lb.

high LDL cholesterol is more than 160 mg/dl. The average cholesterol level for the adult U.S. population is 210 to 215 mg/dl. More than half of adult Americans have a blood cholesterol level of more than 200 mg/dl. The goal of the NCEP is to reduce the average blood cholesterol level to less than 200 mg/dl by the year 2000.

Diet is the primary treatment for an elevated blood cholesterol level. The NCEP has recommended that essentially all Americans (over 2 years of age) reduce consumption of saturated fatty acids, total fat, and cholesterol and achieve and maintain an ideal body weight. The Step-One has been recommended for all Americans[23]:

- Less than 10% of total calories should come from saturated fatty acids
- An average of 30% or less of total calories should come from all fat
- Dietary energy levels to reach or maintain a desirable body weight
- Consumption of less than 300 mg of cholesterol per day

Adoption of the Step-One diet can result in a 10% to 15% reduction in blood cholesterol levels, which in turn is expected to lead to a 20% or greater reduction in CHD. For individuals with an elevated plasma total (and LDL cholesterol) level, diet therapy is recommended at least 6 months before drug therapy is initiated. A Step-Two diet (less than 7% of calories from saturated fatty acids and less than 200 mg of cholesterol per day) is recommended for individuals who need to be treated more aggressively to lower their plasma cholesterol level.

A goal of *Healthy People 2000* is that 75% of adults have had their blood cholesterol checked within the preceding 5 years. In 1988, 59% of people 18 years and older have had their blood cholesterol checked at least once.

Hypertension

Hypertension generally is defined as systolic blood pressure more than 140 mm Hg, diastolic blood pressure more than 90 mm Hg, or a condition requiring antihypertensive medication. Approximately 30% of adults have hypertension. Almost two thirds of these individuals are aware of their condition, although only about 24% have achieved hypertensive control. A causal relationship has been demonstrated between hypertension and the development of CHD.

Familial, genetic, and environmental factors are thought to play a role in the development of hypertension. The genetic predisposition for developing hypertension appears to remain latent until activated by environmental factors. The higher incidence of hypertension in blacks than in whites is suggestive of a strong hereditary influence.

Several dietary factors are thought to affect blood pressure.[30] Obesity and habitual high alcohol intake are related to elevated blood pressure. Central deposition of fat (android obesity), more so than peripherally deposited fat (gynoid obesity), is associated with hypertension. Some individuals are responsive to a habitual high-salt diet. A high-potassium diet seems to be protective against the development of hypertension. Some evidence suggests an inverse relationship between blood pressure and calcium intake, as well as level of physical activity.

Blood pressure control is a major objective of the Department of Health and Human Services. The goal for the year 2000 is to have blood pressure control in 50% of the hypertensive population (up from 24% in 1982 to 1984) and to have at least 90% of individuals with hypertension taking action to control their elevated blood pressure.

Diabetes Mellitus

Diabetes is defined as a metabolic disorder characterized by elevated blood glucose levels and impaired carbohydrate utilization caused by an insulin deficiency. Six to 10 million Americans have diabetes, of which only 5% to 10% have insulin-dependent diabetes mellitus (IDDM) and more than 90% have non-insulin-dependent diabetes mellitus (NIDDM). There appears to be a strong genetic component in the development of IDDM. NIDDM is associated with unknown genetic factors, aging, and insulin resistance associated with obesity (especially android versus gynoid obesity).

Relative body weight is the only factor that consistently has been related to the prevalence of NIDDM. A higher calorie and fat intake are positively related to the incidence of NIDDM, perhaps because of the positive relationship reported between percentage of body fat and percentage of calories from fat.

A calorie-restricted diet to lose weight and maintain weight loss is the primary treatment of NIDDM. Because the leading cause of death among individuals with NIDDM is CHD, a fat- and cholesterol-modified diet also is recommended. In addition to a Step-One diet for control of weight, blood cholesterol, and blood glucose, a diet high in soluble fiber is recommended because it has been shown to lower blood cholesterol and glucose levels.

Healthy People 2000 goals for diabetes include reducing deaths and severe complications from diabetes as well as the incidence of diabetes to 2.5:1000 people (from 2.9:1000 people). The risk reduction objectives for diabetes include reducing the prevalence of overweight and increasing the proportion (by 30%) of people who exercise regularly. Another objective is to have 75% of persons with diabetes receive formal patient education.

Cancer

Although it is not possible to quantify precisely the contribution of specific dietary components to individual cancers, the National Research Council (NRC)[24] concluded that approximately one third of all cancer mortalities in the United States may be related to diet. Indeed, exact mechanisms have yet to be established for either the carcinogenic or anticarcinogenic effects of specific dietary factors. However, there is strong evidence from both epidemiological and animal studies to suggest that specific food components affect specific sites in the development of neoplasms.

Cancers of the gastrointestinal tract have been positively associated with alcohol (esophageal and colorectal), salt-preserved foods (stomach cancer), and dietary fats (colorectal and prostate cancers). Consumption of fresh fruits and vegetables has an inverse association with stomach cancer. High intakes of vegetables have a strong inverse association with colorectal cancer.

Comparison of data from different countries suggests a positive association between breast and prostate cancers and high fat intakes.[3] High alcohol intake has also been associated with breast cancer. Consumption of foods contaminated with mycotoxin (i.e., aflatoxin) has been positively associated with development of liver cancer. Additional food components implicated in the initiation of cancer include heterocyclic amines, and N-nitroso compounds.[27] Broiling, frying, and barbecuing protein-rich, high-fat, low-carbohydrate foods, such as meats, at high temperatures so that the meat burns, can cause formation of heterocyclic amines. N-nitroso compounds are formed by the interaction of amines and nitrosating agents such as nitrite or nitrous oxides. This happens in cured meats and salt-dried smoked fish.

Cancers of the lungs and bladder are most clearly associated with exposure to tobacco and certain industrial chemicals. However, plant foods, especially fruits and green and yellow vegetables appear to have a protective effect against lung cancer. β-carotene and other carotenoids, vitamin C, fiber, and selenium are specific dietary components identified as possible protective agents.

Finally, obesity appears to be associated with an increased risk of the development of cancer of the endometrium and gallbladder. Some have suggested that obesity is also involved with development of breast cancer.

Epidemiological techniques such as case control and cohort studies associating specific dietary factors to human carcinogenesis have been either inconclusive or conflicting.[8] This may be from methodological problems: measuring dietary fat intake (especially from past years) is imprecise and often unreliable, smaller differences in dietary habits exist between people living within a country when compared to people living in other countries, and the genetic component is difficult to assess in population studies. These problems result in a dilution of strong relationships and make detecting weak relationships difficult. Perhaps long-term intervention studies in susceptible populations will provide the answers that population studies have yet to give us.

However, after extensive literature review, the

NRC proposed the following general dietary recommendations to lower cancer risk:

Increase fruit, vegetable, and grain consumption

Limit intake of alcohol, salt-preserved and cured foods, and fats

Maintain healthy body weight

Osteoporosis

Osteoporosis is a multifactorial and complex disorder of the skeletal system characterized by bone loss and increasing skeletal fragility. The skeletal system consists of two types of bones: cortical bones comprise the rigid appendicular skeleton, whereas trabecular bone is spongy, providing strength and elasticity to vertebral skeleton. Osteoporosis is usually not apparent until minimal trauma causes a fracture, most typically in the hips, wrists, or vertebrae. Although associated primarily with postmenopausal white women, osteoporosis is a common condition affecting about 24 million Americans. It is the major cause of approximately 1.3 million bone fractures yearly in the United States alone.

It is estimated that 50% of women over 45 years of age have osteoporosis. Gradual decrease in estrogen secretion following menopause is directly correlated to reduction in bone mass. Reduced estrogen levels result in reduction of intestinal calcium absorption, as well as in an increase in calcium bone resorption. However, ethnic and genetic differences, decreasing physical activity, cigarette smoking, alcohol intake, adiposity as measured by body mass index, reproductive history, and low bone calcium reserves may play selective roles.

Peak bone mass is achieved 5 to 10 years after longitudinal bone growth has ceased. Once peak bone mass is reached, it remains stable until age 40 to 45. Thereafter, bone is lost at a yearly rate of about 0.2% to 0.5%, except in women just before and for about 10 years after the onset of menopause, when the rate increases. There appears to be a strong genetic relationship between mothers and daughters affecting both the level of peak bone mass and the amount of postmenopausal bone loss. In a recent study, women demonstrated a continuous significant loss of cortical bone despite the level of dietary intake of calcium. There was no difference in the amount of bone loss whether women consumed less than 800 mg of calcium daily or greater than 1350 mg daily. Low dietary calcium intake during preadolescent and pubertal years may result in lower peak bone mass.

In the United States, the prevalence of osteoporosis is lower among blacks than whites. White women are two to three times more likely to suffer a hip fracture than black women and men of both races. This difference appears to be from higher bone density, skeletal calcium content, total body potassium, and muscle mass in blacks.

Calcium supplementation is inferior to estrogen replacement therapy in the treatment or prevention of osteoporosis. Estrogen slows cortical bone loss and completely prevents trabecular bone loss. Recent evidence suggests that the use of sodium fluoride is not an acceptable treatment. More reasonable strategies to reduce the risk of developing osteoporosis are suggested in *Healthy People 2000*: "increase to at least 90 percent the proportion of perimenopausal women who have been counseled about the benefits and risks of estrogen replacement therapy for prevention of osteoporosis" and "increase calcium intake so at least 50 percent of people aged 25 and older consume two or more servings [of food rich in calcium] daily."[11]

Alcohol Abuse

The use of alcohol has declined in the last 10 years as evidenced by lowered alcoholic beverage sales and tax data.[14] The consumption of hard liquor declined 21% between 1978 and 1986. Wine and beer sales have remained stable. This decline may be the result of growing social intolerance regarding the effects of alcohol abuse. However, alcohol abuse is still a major problem in the United States, with more than 18.5 million Americans considered alcohol abusers. It is estimated that 9% of adults over 21 years old consume more than two drinks daily. The economic costs of alcohol abuse are estimated to be more than $70 billion each year, primarily from decreased productivity.

Excessive alcohol consumption increases the risk for heart disease, high blood pressure, neurological diseases, and many other disorders. Alcohol is the major contributor to development of liver cirrhosis, the ninth leading cause of death in the United States. Alcohol is involved in more than 50% of all motor vehicle accidents and fatal intentional injuries (homicides and suicides). Disproportionately more blacks (70%) and Native Americans suffer from alcohol abuse.

The nutritional consequences of alcohol consumption are related to the amount of alcohol consumed. Light drinkers simply add extra calories, whereas moderate to heavy drinkers displace as much as half their energy with alcohol. Yet alcohol abusers are no more obese than the rest of the population.[6] In recent years the nutritional status of the drinking population has improved. This has enabled scientists to demonstrate the toxic effects of alcohol on the liver independent of malnutrition.

Alcohol abuse can lead to primary malnutrition, in which alcohol replaces consumption of other foodstuffs. Alcohol abuse also can lead to secondary malnutrition by decreasing nutrient digestion, absorption, or utilization or by increasing nutrient demands. As consumption of alcohol increases, the percentage of energy from protein, fat, and carbohydrates decreases. Dietary nutrient quality also declines with significant decreases in vitamins A and C, thiamin, calcium, iron, and fiber. Nitrogen excretion increases, resulting in a higher protein requirement for alcohol abusers.

Although some studies suggest beneficial effects of moderate alcohol intake in lowering coronary heart disease risk, these studies have not demonstrated a causal relationship. It is generally recommended that alcohol not be consumed because of the risk of addiction. If consumed, alcohol intake should be limited to the equivalent of less than 1 oz of pure alcohol per day. This is the amount in two cans of beer, two small glasses of wine, or two average cocktails.

NUTRITIONAL ASSESSMENT

Nutritional assessment is an important part of providing nutrition services and is discussed in Chapter 15. Dietary intake data, anthropometric measurements, biochemical analyses, clinical evaluation, and psychosocial-economic status assessment are approaches commonly used to provide an adequate appraisal of an individual's nutritional status. Guidelines for assessing nutritional status along with intervention strategies for the adult appear in Table 8-9. Client involvement and awareness at each step of the assessment process are essential.

Dietary Assessment

Data from major nutrition surveys—the Ten-State Nutrition Survey, the National Health and Nutrition Examination Surveys (NHANES), USDA Food Consumption Studies, as well as data from studies by individual investigators—are used to assess the nutritional status of adults in the United States (see Chapter 15).

It is difficult to compare or categorize findings of studies of nutritional status of adults reported in the literature over time because the RDAs have been revised ten times since their inception in 1941. Differences in dietary methodology have also resulted in some inconsistencies in reported intake among similar population groups. Common intake data are collected using the 24-hour recall, food records, or diet histories. Recent reports suggest most people tend to underreport their normal intake, thus causing scientists to question the validity of dietary intake data.[19]

In addition, some investigators use 100% of the RDA as their standard of adequate intake, whereas others use various levels of the RDA as standards. A further complication exists because food composition tables have changed as food production techniques have changed, and analyses have been more sophisticated. Values used 10 years ago for the same food product may be quite different from current ones, making comparisons difficult.

Anthropometric Variables

Weight, height, and body site measurements are easily obtained and are useful if edema is not present. Calculation of body mass index (weight in kilograms divided by height in meters, squared) and waist-hip ratios provide the educator with additional tools for determining counseling strategies.

Table 8-9. Nutrition assessment and intervention guidelines in community nutrition for adults

Nutritional assessment component	Methods	Risk and problem indicated	Intervention guidelines	Referral sources
Anthropometric Height Weight Skinfold thickness Arm circumference	Use standardized equipment for measuring—balanced scales, steel or nonstretch measuring tapes and calipers Use standardized height and weight tables to determine weight status (as shown in 1990 Dietary Guidelines) Use BMI to determine weight status Use waist-hip ratio to determine site of fat deposition For skinfold thickness, use measurements according to Durnin-Womersley procedure for triceps, biceps, subscapular, and suprailiac skinfolds to determine body fat	Moderate to underweight (BMI: < 16 for men; < 15 for women Moderate overweight (BMI: for men: 25-30; for women: 24-29) Severe overweight (BMI: for men: > 30; for women: > 29) Waist-hip ratios: for men: > 1.0; for women: > 0.8	Adjust recommended weight to higher than average for overweight and lower than average for overweight/obese If weight loss of more than 10 lb in a year or below the lowest weight for height standard, determine reason for recent weight loss Adjust nutrient density of diet to compensate for increased or decreased energy requirement Adjust activity level as an adjunct to decreased energy intake to assist weight reduction to reduce BMI and waist-hip ratio	Reputable weight management program Registered dietitian and public health nutritionist Reputable physical fitness program and recreational facilities Worksite health promotion program
Biochemical Hemoglobin Hematocrit Serum cholesterol and other lipids Blood glucose	Use standardized laboratory equipment and laboratory quality control procedures Compare biochemical values to (1) Centers for Disease Control standards for hemoglobin and hematocrit adjusted for age, sex, and altitude; (2) National Cholesterol Education Program Guidelines, (3) National Diabetes Data Group, National Institutes of Health	Anemia Elevated cholesterol (> 200 mg/dl) Elevated low-density lipoprotein cholesterol—LDL-C (> 130 mg/dl) Low HDL-C (< 35 mg/dl)	Diet modifications to increase number of foods that are high in iron sources Diet modifications to decrease total fat (< 30% of calories), saturated fat (< 10% of calories), and cholesterol (< 300 mg/day) energy intake is appropriate to achieve and maintain healthy body weight Adjust personal diet modifications using diabetes exchange list	Public, private, and voluntary agencies State/local health departments State/local heart associations State/local diabetes associations Community hospitals Registered dietitian and public health nutritionist

BMI, Body mass index.

Continued.

Table 8-9. Nutrition assessment and intervention guidelines in community nutrition for adults—cont'd

Nutritional assessment component	Methods	Risk and problem indicated	Intervention guidelines	Referral sources
Clinical Medical history Blood pressure Chronic disease risk factor questionnaire family history, diabetes, and stress Physical fitness Smoking Dental Socioeconomic status	Use clinical assessment and physical examination data to determine if one or more signs indicate nutrition-related diseases Use questionnaire to determine risk factors for cardiovascular disease Use a sphygmomanometer and blood pressure procedures established by the Joint National Committee on Detection, Evaluation and Treatment of High Blood Pressure Use treadmill test for physical fitness Use lung function test for smoking and other respiratory problems Examine oral cavity, condition of teeth and gums, and oral hygiene	Hypertension (blood pressure > 140/90 mm Hg) Risk of heart attack, stroke, and certain cancers (lung, esophagus, bladder) increases with number and severity of risk factors such as overweight, fat intake, hypertension, elevated cholesterol, smoking, inactivity, and stress	Encourage adherence to drug and diet modifications Develop personalized intervention plan on desirable life-style modifications that include diet and exercise	Stop-smoking clinics Food Stamp Program Cooperative extension services Emergency food programs
Dietary evaluation: 3-4 day food record, 24-hour recall, including one weekend day; food frequency	Determine quantity and quality of diet with special consideration given to alcohol, total fat, saturated fat, cholesterol, sodium, sugars, and fiber intakes	Alcoholism Drug abuse Marginal intakes of essential nutrients, which could lead to nutritional deficiencies Excessive intakes of food/nutrients, which could lead to future nutritional problems	Investigate causal factors in substance abuse and suggest coping mechanism Adjust diet modifications in relation to other indicators that contribute to dietary amelioration	Alcoholics Anonymous Public, private, or voluntary behavioral health agencies/programs Consulting registered dietitians or public health nutritionists
Psychosocial Life-style Cooking, shopping, eating Family structure Income Ethnicity Literacy level	Determine environmental factors affecting food procurement, choices, and preparation	Lack of facilities for food purchase and preparation Lack of financial and other resources	Adjust recommendations to overcome limitations	Public, private, or voluntary agencies

Clinical Assessment

Medical history, complete physical examination, blood pressure measurements, chronic disease risk questionnaires, family history, stress factors, physical fitness, smoking history, alcohol consumption information, and dental evaluation are reviewed with the client. Skin, hair, teeth, gums, lips, tongue, and eyes are examined. Because of rapid cell turnover of epithelial and mucosal tissue, hair, skin, and mouth are susceptible to nutritional deficiencies.

Biochemical Assessment

Examination of a metabolite in blood or urine represents a sensitive measurement of nutritional status. Sometimes tissues such as hair, fingernails, and even bone and liver are examined. Immunological measurements are useful in assessing malnutrition. Plasma total cholesterol measurement is recommended for virtually all adults, followed by a lipoprotein analysis when plasma total cholesterol is greater than 240 mg/dl.

Psychosocial-Economic Assessment

Information about lifestyle, attitudes about food, nutrition and health, home life, food procurement and preparation facilities, economic situation, literacy level, and ethnicity should be collected. This information is important in establishing an effective counseling relationship with the client.

Comparison of individual assessments with standardized measurements are made. Following assessment, the dietitian or nutritionist is ready to counsel the adult client about normal nutrition, based on Dietary Guidelines, making all appropriate dietary modifications. The educator needs to remain aware of the economic, social, emotional, and environmental factors affecting each client in order to tailor counseling to individual needs.

ASSURING QUALITY OF HEALTH CARE

Specific guidelines for patient management have emerged that incorporate specific expected health outcomes in a health promotion–disease prevention model. These guidelines are recommendations for evaluating the quality of care that provide quality assurance standards.

- Client maintains acceptable weight and height based on Dietary Guideline standards.
- Client maintains acceptable Body Mass Index.
- Client maintains acceptable waist-hip ratio.
- Client does not deviate more than 25% from usual weight.
- Client maintains blood pressure of less than 140/90 mm Hg.
- Client maintains plasma cholesterol levels less than 200 mg/dl.
- Client does not smoke.
- Client consumes no more than one drink daily (female) or two drinks daily (male). (One drink equals 12 oz regular beer, 5 oz wine; 1½ oz distilled 80 proof spirits.)
- Client consumes adequate amount of nutrients, fiber, and water with caloric intake to maintain acceptable weight.
- Client maintains hemoglobin level between 12 to 15 g.
- Client reviews appropriate types and amounts of food as defined by Dietary Guidelines.
- Client participates in regular physical exercise for periods of 20 minutes or longer, 3 or more days a week, performed at an intensity of 60% or greater of individual's cardiorespiratory capacity.

NUTRITIONAL INTERVENTION FOR CHRONIC DISEASE RISK REDUCTION

Community and public health dietitians and nutritionists have exciting new job opportunities and challenges. As discussed previously, many nutrition goals have been identified to reduce the risk associated with the major chronic diseases. There is a growing need for nutrition intervention programs targeted to specific groups representing different ages, ethnicity, gender, and literacy and income levels. Public demand for these programs is increasing as more individuals become health conscious. Many adults are committed to improving the quality of their own lives as well as that of their families. By implementing effective and successful intervention programs, dietitions and nutritionists can have an impact on the health of individuals, groups, and even whole communities.

How are individuals and groups given important

nutrition messages? Communitywide nutrition intervention programs are relatively new. Many community nutritionists have not received formal training in design, implementation, and evaluation of these programs. Although this new responsibility may seem overwhelming at first, two things can be done to simplify the process. Working with individuals, groups, teams, and other organizations to form partnerships will be beneficial in planning and delivering programs. In addition, careful plan-

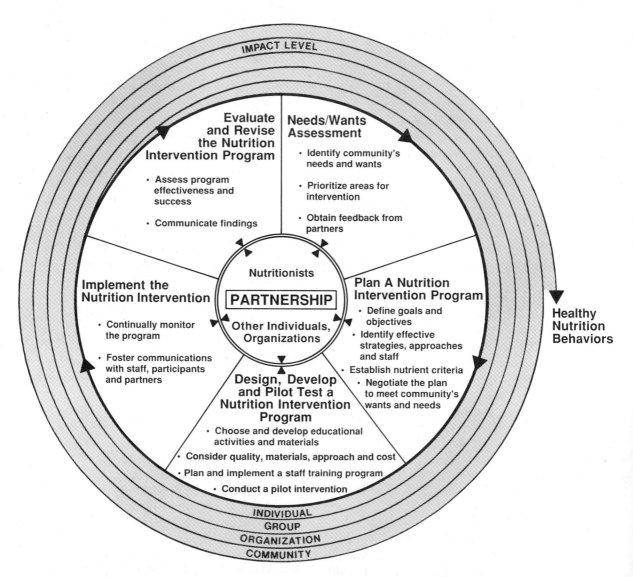

Figure 8-11. A diagrammatic representation of the nutrition intervention planning and delivery process.

ning at every step will assure achievable program goals.

The Process

A new publication, *Nutrition Intervention in Chronic Disease: A Guide to Effective Programs*[13] provides detailed instructions for planning, implementing, and evaluating nutrition intervention programs aimed at chronic disease risk reduction in a community setting. The author, Darlene Lansing, M.P.H., R.D., draws on her extensive experience as well as that of many of her colleagues. The following section is a brief introduction to the nutrition intervention program planning, implementation, and evaluation process (Fig. 8-11).

GUIDELINES FOR DELIVERING NUTRITION INTERVENTION PROGRAMS

Step 1. Establish Successful Nutrition Intervention Partnerships

Partnerships are new entities created when two or more organizations (or individuals) exchange information, work together, share resources, or solve problems. Partners find mutual goals, share tasks, make joint decisions, and act cooperatively. Partnerships organize the community to support health promotion and chronic disease prevention activities by sharing their expertise and resources.

Partnerships should be involved in all aspects of the nutrition intervention program process. A more comprehensive needs assessment is possible and a larger-scale intervention program can be realized when teams with mutual goals are built. Possible partners for nutrition intervention programs in the community include the categories given below.

Individuals

Other health professionals and dietitians and nutritionists, leading community figures (businesspersons, government officials, clergy), and well-known persons such as athletes, coaches, and entertainers.

Groups and Organizations

Schools, colleges, churches, businesses, shopping malls, county extension agencies, professional health-related and other organizations (American Heart Association, American Cancer Society, American Diabetes Association, Lions Club, Kiwanis), children's groups (Boy and Girl Scouts, 4-H clubs, fraternities and sororities), and PTAs.

Other

Local television, radio, newspapers.

Step 2: Nutrition Assessment: Identify Community's Needs and Wants

There are three important areas of inquiry. First, a community profile, including demographic data, health statistics, and social networks (schools, churches, civic organizations), should be developed. Second, the health and nutrition needs of target community groups should be identified. Collecting these data might be as simple as telephoning a state or community health office. Alternatively, this information may have to be collected via networking with colleagues, discussions with other professionals, listening to local radio and television programs, and reading local newspapers. Finally, talk with community leaders to identify perceived needs of community members (e.g., With what do they want help?).

Following this needs assessment, specific goals can be prioritized. After deciding on a focus, it is important to get feedback from other colleagues, health professionals, and members of the community.

Step 3: Plan the Community Nutrition Intervention

Considerable time and effort is needed to organize the nutrition intervention program. Partners should identify strategies to achieve the major intervention goal(s). Additional partners should be recruited, both to evaluate the nutrition intervention program and to help make it successful.

Step 4: Negotiate a Plan to Meet the Community's Wants and Needs

Partners then need to negotiate objectives and specific activities. The budget, timeline, and a contingency plan are defined. It is essential that a registered dietitian or nutritionist establish these nutrient criteria. These criteria are *not* negotiable. Nutrient criteria are standards by which food products are judged, for example, less than "*x*%" in saturated fatty acids, cholesterol, or fat. If a "Lite Fare" at restaurants is established, it will be essential to decide which entrées and other foods will be placed in this special category. Likewise, if you are identifying lean cuts of meat, it is essential first to define *lean* in terms of the nutrients targeted for intervention. In addition to negotiation of objectives, program evaluation strategies should be identified to assess program effectiveness. Examples of evaluation strategies include interviews with participants, telephone follow-up surveys, logs of intervention activities (observations, comments of participants, etc.), pretest and posttest knowledge evaluations or risk factor assessments, dietary health, or anthropometric data.

Step 5: Design, Develop, and Pilot Test a Nutrition Intervention Program

A successful program that is completed on time, at the projected cost, with quality maintained, is guided by a specific action plan. The development of effective educational module(s) should include decisions about content and format of participant activities.

A training program for persons implementing the program is essential to ensure quality. These persons should be trained, evaluated, and given feedback.

Before a major intervention program is implemented, a pilot study is recommended. It is often worth the time and investment to assure program quality. Ideas, strategies, goals, and materials should be evaluated by individuals outside the partnership. Potential problems are frequently identified and subsequently prevented.

The community should be informed of intervention activities, particularly via media coverage. Partners may report activities in different ways, including supermarket videos, fliers, strategic placement of pictures and materials, newsletters, and community meetings.

Step 6: Implement and Evaluate the Nutrition Intervention Program

The key to keeping the program on track is effective communication among the staff. Staff responsibilities must be clearly delineated. Frequent meetings to discuss project progress, staff activities, problems, and budget will achieve intervention goals.

It is important to monitor all staff and target groups activities closely, especially during the early stages. This often is accomplished through the use of written logs, diaries, and reports, as well as frequent meetings.

Step 7: Revise the Intervention Program, If Needed

A formal program evaluation is essential for planning a more effective nutrition intervention program at a later date. All data, both quantitative and qualitative, are analyzed. In addition, oral and written staff evaluations and suggestions should be collected. Participant feedback also should be summarized.

Finally, staff should be recognized for their efforts. All other program participants and networking partners should be informed of the results of the intervention. Professional peers as well as members of the community also should be informed. This activity will be beneficial in establishing new and continued nutrition intervention partnerships.

The Impact

Nutrition intervention programs can be delivered to individuals, groups of all sizes, organizations, communities, and even whole populations. The process of developing and delivering nutrition intervention programs on a small- or large-scale basis is similar in each case and is guided by the steps defined in Chapters 13 to 18 and in Figure 8-11. The magnitude of the nutrition intervention depends on the goals of the organization and available resources. It is important to appreciate advantages and limitations associated with each intervention approach:

Intervention Approach	Advantages	Limitations
Individual	Highly individualized and personalized; can be intensive with extensive follow-up; educational materials cost can be very low; chances for successful behavior modification are good	Reaches a limited number of people; small impact on community health; cost per person is high; important health or nutrition issues may not be addressed
Group	Group interactions may facilitate desired behavior change; important nutrition message(s) can be targeted to groups' individuals with similar needs or characteristics; can reach a relatively large number of individuals	Different learning styles and goals of group members may limit program effectiveness
Organization	Organization support can facilitate behavior change; major nutrition problems and issues can be addressed; can have an impact on the health of an organization's members or employees; cost per individual can be relatively low	Intervention is not individualized; organization support may be too strong and certain related policies (e.g., negative incentives for certain behaviors) may hurt employee or member morale

All approaches have been shown to be effective and have led to desired behavior changes that have reduced the risk of many chronic diseases. Dietitians and nutritionists must be flexible in the approaches they use, consider the advantages and disadvantages of all intervention approaches, and be prepared to use any approach that is justified for a given situation. Gaining experience with the smaller-scale approaches first will be beneficial in planning and delivering larger-scale nutrition intervention programs that will have a greater health impact by virtue of reaching a larger audience.

Program Examples

Many different nutrition intervention programs can be planned and delivered to individuals, groups, organizations, and communities. The following represent ideas that have proved to be effective for other nutritionists.

Nutrition Intervention Approaches for the Individual

Individualized counseling
Chronic disease risk assessment
Personalized nutrition program
Personalized fitness program (e.g., one-on-one instructor)
Supermarket tour
Food preparation instruction (cooking instruction, recipe modification)
Restaurant tour

Nutrition Intervention Approaches for Groups

Group classes (weight management, blood cholesterol lowering, exercise, cooking, etc.)
Print materials, refrigerator guides, shopping guide
Blood cholesterol screening with follow-up intervention planned
Contests (weight loss, recipe, fitness, etc.)
Family activities
Activities in health care provider offices (videos, print materials)
Healthful nutrition potluck dinners
Low-fat gourmet clubs
Supermarket and restaurant tours

Nutrition Intervention Approaches for Organizations

Chronic disease risk assessment (via questionnaires, taking measurements such as blood cholesterol and blood pressure)

Classes during breaks, lunch hour, and after work

Video programs shown in the cafeteria

Nutrition information provided for cafeteria, snack bar, and vending food items; provision of healthier alternatives in cafeteria, snack bar and vending machines.

Health celebrations (serve healthful foods at social occasions)

Contests

Nutrition column in in-house publications

Posters, fliers

Nutrition Intervention Approaches for Communities

Mass media approaches: messages on television and radio and in the newspaper

Supermarket and meat market programs that educate consumers about healthful food choices

Incentives, coupons

Brochures

Videos

Point-of-purchase nutrition information

Cooperative extension activities

Virtually all of these strategies can be effective. The challenge now is to decide which to try first. Choice of program will be guided by many factors such as organizational and personal philosophy, the population you are working with, time, and resources of the nutrition intervention partnership. Following are examples of strategies that have proven effective for others.

INNOVATIVE STRATEGIES

COMMUNITY: THE FOUR HEART RESTAURANT PROGRAM

Pawtucket Heart Health Program
Mary Lynne Hixson, M.A., R.D., Intervention Coordinator

One of the earliest nutrition interventions of the Pawtucket Heart Health Program (PHHP), a 10-year cardiovascular disease prevention study, was the Four Heart Restaurant Program. A Better Eating Around Pawtucket (BEAP) Committee, comprised of community volunteers and leaders, facilitated the initial implementation of the program in 1983. This committee recognized this unique opportunity for nutrition education to reach large numbers of people, including those not easily reached through traditional education programs.

The impetus for restaurants to get involved with PHHP as a community partner in promoting heart health to the people of Pawtucket was primarily to increase their community visibility through association with a recognized, credible health program. With the growing public awareness of cholesterol in the late 1980s, offering heart-healthy menu selections became a marketing edge to attract and retain health-conscious patrons.

The cornerstone of the Four Heart program was a heart logo printed next to the menu items that met the Four Heart Restaurant criteria for less fat, sodium, and cholesterol. In addition, a menu explanation statement was required to identify the program sponsor (PHHP) and to explain the nutritional features of the labeled foods.

A formal written agreement between the restaurant and PHHP described the responsibilities of each partner and the terms of the agreement. The written agreement minimized misunderstandings, encouraged compliance, and facilitated program success.

Staff training was an integral component of the Four Heart Program. Informed, involved, and ethusiastic staff were essential to program success. To facilitate staff training, *Menu Labeling for Heart Health* was developed in 1989. This training package allows a manager or designated trainer to train staff on the menu labeling program.

Variations on the menu labeling concept were developed in collaboration with selected restaurants looking to create a nutrition marketing edge. A Four Heart Breakfast Menu was developed in response to a competitor's introduction of Egg Beaters to its breakfast menu. Another three-restaurant chain developed a three-color Heart Healthy Menu that exclusively included heart-healthy menu items along with the calories, fat, and content of each.

Collaborations between dietitians and nutritionists and restaurateurs can be mutually beneficial. However, the approach and expectations must be realistic. Although restaurants have not been a traditional outlet for nutritional information, the increasing awareness of health and food choices has created a marketing niche for nutrition education through restaurants.

COMMUNITY: EDUCATING CONSUMERS IN THE SUPERMARKET
Jo Ann S. Carson, R.D./L.D., EatRite Supermarket Tours

Supermarket tours are an increasingly popular means of impacting the diets of healthy adults. In Dallas at Tom Thumb supermarkets and Simon David stores, consumers concerned about excessive calories, fat, and sodium learn to select the healthiest foods right from the shelves.

Carson, a registered dietitian and director of the Clinical Dietetics Program at the University of Texas Southwestern Medical Center at Dallas, teaches EatRite Tour participants to keep the nutritional value of products in perspective. They arrange cheeses in order from those highest in fat to those lowest in fat. They rate cereals based on the amount of fiber and fat per serving. At the meat counter, EatRite shoppers learn that ground sirloin contains less fat than typical ground turkey, and that ground breast of chicken or turkey is even leaner. Participants like the hands-on opportunity and the chance to get answers about products right there on the shelf.

Support from the supermarket is critical to successful tours. A formal request to the supermarket or supermarket chain will likely be approved when the benefit of bringing new customers and increasing consumers' expenditures is clearly evident. The tours in Dallas were originated by Leni Reed, RD, in 1984. Dietitians and other professionals now purchase Reed's Supermarket Savvy R kits for use in developing their own tours across the country. Whether organized as an adjunct to a hospital or fitness center's nutrition program or as part of a dietitian's private practice, supermarket nutrition tours can be a valuable tool in helping the public make healthier food choices.

COMMUNITY: SPORTS NUTRITION
Genda Potter, M.S., R.D.
Sports and Cardiovascular Nutritionist

Among athletes, there is a growing interest in nutrition. Unfortunately, dietitians and nutritionists have not been a major source of information for athletes, and the sources on which they rely are not always accurate. Consequently, athletes are exposed to an abundance of misinformation, and reports of nutrition knowledge among athletes indicate many misconceptions about food and its effect on performance.

Motivated by these circumstances, Potter developed a 30-minute slide program with an audiotape covering four major topics about which athletes have misconceptions: The Athlete's Basic Diet, Pregame Meals, Fluids, and Ergogenic Aids. The unique program is designed to be used either in a group setting or as a self-instruction program. It is divided into four self-contained modules that can be shown separately or together as a complete program. In addition, study questions with answers for each module, a pretest, and a posttest are also included.

COMMUNITY OUTREACH: INTERNATIONAL FOOD INFORMATION COUNCIL
Sheila Owens, B.S., Communications Coordinator; Clare Regan, M.S., R.D., Nutritionist

The International Food Information Council (IFIC) is a nonprofit organization recognized by health professionals nationwide as a credible resource for sound scientific information on food safety and nutrition.

Through established and ongoing partnerships with organizations including the American Dietetic Association, the Food and Drug Administration, and the American Academy of Family Physicians, IFIC has launched numerous nutrition education programs to help health professionals stay informed about current food and nutrition information.

IFIC's scientific white papers and consumer brochures on food topics are provided to health professionals regularly. *Food Insight,* IFIC's award-winning bimonthly newsletter, reaches more than 20,000 key professionals and media in the health and nutrition fields.

IFIC participates in professional meetings nationwide by sponsoring educational exhibits and giving presentations on food information. In conjunction with the American Dietetic Association Foundation, IFIC also sponsors educational workshops and seminars on food and nutrition.

Often referred to as the critical link among health professionals, scientists, food manufacturers, government officials and the media, IFIC serves to build a better understanding of nutrition and food ingredient issues worldwide.

WORKSITE WELLNESS: LIFEKEY PROGRAM
Electronic Data Systems Corporation
Patricia A. Volz-Clarke, M.S., R.D., Manager
Supervisor, LifeKey Health and Fitness Division

Lifekey, the wellness division with EDS, was formed in 1984. Committed to providing programs that aid employees in understanding total wellness and in achieving balance and personal development in all areas of life, services are offered in four areas: Family Services, Fitness and Recreation, Personal Health, and Personal Effectiveness. This total approach to wellness is a drastic change in direction for corporate fitness programs.

Family Services
Every family environment is different and, as such, the Lifekey Family Services programs are extremely diverse in an attempt to provide something for everyone. Educational opportunities that enhance awareness and knowledge of parenting issues assist in identifying and acquiring new skills. Topics such as pregnancy, self-esteem, communication with teenagers, child care selection, and traits of a health family are addressed.

Fitness and Recreation
Lifekey operates fitness centers at four locations exclusively for employee use. These centers provide state-of-the-art equipment, on-side professional assistance, educational materials, and a variety of activity classes. Employees can undergo a fitness assessment that evaluates their present fitness levels; a Lifekey professional reviews the results and helps the employees establish personal goals.

Walk for Health is Lifekey's extremely popular national 4-month program designed to promote walking as a practical lifetime activity. Lifekey also offers a wide variety of recreational activities. Employees can play on company-sponsored volleyball, basketball, and softball teams.

Personal Health
Personal health has been the major emphasis of corporate wellness programs since their origins. Traditionally these programs have been medically based, with rigid standards of right, wrong, good, and bad behavior. Lifekey's personal health programs are designed to provide the necessary information for individuals to make their own health choices and feel good about them.

Choices for Life is a program independent of body weight and scales that encourages participants to abandon short-term diets and adopt a long-term attitude toward weight management by choosing and making small, achievable lifestyle changes. The HeartChek program provides employees with infor-

mation about their total cholesterol, blood pressure, and body mass index. These measurements are followed by a presentation that encourages participants to look at their results and set up an individual plan of action.

Personal Effectiveness
Lifekey's personal effectiveness classes and programs are designed with personal awareness and self-responsibility in mind.

In stress management, the classes include Relax and Refresh, which discusses various relaxation techniques, and Time for Myself, which highlights strategies for finding and using personal time.

Lifekey Discovery is an experientially based work-group-tailored program designed to foster self-worth, encourage individual responsibility, and strengthen performance. Topics include problem solving, trust, group cohesiveness, conflict resolution, and healthy risk taking.

The direction that EDS's health and fitness division has taken is by no means unique in corporate wellness. The field is changing from traditional medically based intervention and education programs to more holistic "people-based" programs. A successful wellness intervention program does not necessarily mean that it is an illness prevention program.

STATE: CALIFORNIA'S 5 A DAY—FOR BETTER HEALTH CAMPAIGN
Susan B. Foerster, M.P.H., R.D., and Dileep Bal, M.D., M.P.H., California Department of Health Services; and Lorelei DiSogra, Ed.D., R.D., and Brian Krieg, M.M.M., California Public Health Foundation

The California Department of Health Services' 5 A Day—for Better Health Campaign promotes the importance of eating at least five servings of fruits and vegetables every day. Major funding for this project came from the National Cancer Institute (NCI). The grant was awarded in 1986.

The intervention channels selected to reach the public were mass media, retail grocers, and state government. A produce industry steering committee was formed, and a campaign format chosen. Stragetic planning with the industry was conducted over a 6-month period. Implementation plans were developed, along with a mission statement and evaluation protocols. The campaign began in 1988 and continued for 3 years. In 1989 and 1991, statewide telephone dietary surveys of 1000 randomly selected adults were conducted.

Fifteen grocery chains with more than 1750 stores are now participating in the campaign. Media coverage has been extensive. The California Departments of Health Services, Education, and Aging are all promoting the eating of five servings of fruits and vegetables in their activities as part of the state's new dietary policy.

This state program gave impetus to a nation-wide "Five A Day" Program to reach children. Under the leadership of Dole Food Company's Director of Nutrition, Dr. Lorelei DiSogra, a children's nutrition education program has been launched in response to critics of food advertisements targeted to children. An American Academy of Pediatric (AAP) public service announcement (PSA), funded by Dole Food Company, encourages children ages 5 to 10 to eat five or more servings of fruits and vegetables a day as part of a balanced diet. This PSA exemplifies the linkages of systems—the AAP, the produce industry, and a food company as a result of Rep. Ron Wyden's (D-OR) critique of Saturday morning advertising for children.

HOSPITAL-BASED CORPORATE HEALTH PROMOTION: FITWEIGH NUTRITION

Jean Storlie, M.S., R.D., President, JS Associates, formerly, ProActive Health of ArcVentures, Inc., Rush-Presbyterian–St. Luke's Medical Center

In 1986 Rush-Presbyterian–St. Luke's Medical Center (RPSLMC) formed ProActive Health through its for-profit subsidiary, ArcVentures, Inc., to package, market, and distribute the hospital's employee wellness programs to local business and industry. Jean Storlie, RD with a master's degree in adult fitness and cardiac rehabilitation, was hired to spearhead this new business venture.

The first program to be developed was FitWeigh Nutrition, a weight loss and nutrition education program based on 8 years of Storlie's research and program development work in eating habits and weight control. In 1980 Storlie developed a program model based on nutrition, exercise, and behavior modification.*

FitWeigh Nutrition became the prototype for a series of other life-style modification courses, including FitStress Stress Management Course and FitQuit Smoking Cessation Program. All programs use an application of goal-setting theory developed by Shield.

In this approach, the behavior change process is broken down into a series of ten steps or goals (Fig. 8-12). Each week, one step is introduced, background

*Originally developed as a master's thesis (Storlie J: *Development and evaluation of NUTREXERCISE: a weight control program*, Master's thesis, La Crosse, Wisc, 1982, University of Wisconsin–La Crosse).

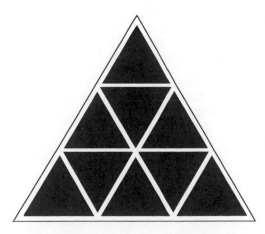

▲ I will eat at least three meals daily.

▲ I will decrease my food portion sizes.

▲ I will reduce the amount of empty calorie foods I eat.

▲ I will exercise at least___ times per week.

▲ When faced with conflict, I will analyze a situation and plan a solution.

▲ I will reduce the amount of fat I eat.

▲ I will make low-calorie food selections when given a choice.

▲ When special events occur, I will be flexible and adapt my plan to the best of my ability.

▲ I will not let my emotions dictate my eating.

▲ Next Step: I have accomplished all nine steps and will be a role model for others.

Figure 8-12. Ten steps in the behavior change process. Reprinted with permission from ArcVentures, Inc.

information is presented, and participants discuss how to integrate the goal into their life. Participants personalize goals and monitor achievement in a pocket-size goal-setting booklet that is reviewed by the instructor. The first 10 to 15 minutes of the following class is devoted to a goal-setting discussion in which participants share their successes and problems. At the completion of this discussion, participants nominate and vote on the "most inspirational" class member for the week, and the winner takes home a rotating award.

From 1987 to 1990, the program was delivered by ProActive Health staff to 393 employees from nine different companies in Chicago, including Ford Motor Company, Motorola, the Chicago Mercantile Exchange, and Proctor & Gamble. In response to a request from Ford Motor Company, a blue-color version of FitWeigh Nutrition was also created.

In 1989 ProActive Health responded to demands in the professional market to launch a licensing program by making FitWeigh Nutrition and the other life-style courses available for marketing and delivery by professionals in their settings. During the next 2 years, 20 organizations signed licensing contracts, and 92 of their instructors were trained to deliver FitWeigh Nutrition. They, in turn, delivered the program to 2319 participants. In 1991 ArcVentures sold the marketing and distribution rights to Health Fitness Corporation, a national corporate fitness company based in Minneapolis.

SUMMARY

Adulthood, the longest period in the life cycle, spans the time between adolescence and the senior years. Nutrition becomes a major component of general well-being throughout the adult years. The occurrence and extent of chronic diseases, such as obesity, coronary artery disease, diabetes, cancer and osteoporosis, are determined by lifestyle choices made during these years. Early adulthood is often accompanied by vigor and vitality; however, the processes of aging and disease are already in progress. Physical and psychological changes affect nutritional status; conversely, nutritional status affects physical and psychological well-being. Nutrition intervention during the adult years aims at reducing the risk and extent of chronic disease.

REFERENCES

1. Bouchard C, Knowler WC: Obesity and cardiovascular disease in minority populations, *Am J Clin Nutr* 53:1507S, 1991.
2. Calloway CW: New weight guidelines for Americans, *Am J Clin Nutr* 54:171, 1991.
3. Carroll KK: Dietary fats and cancer, *Am J Clin Nutr* 53:1064S, 1991.
4. Casperson CJ: Physical activity epidemiology: concepts, methods and applications to exercise science, *Exerc Sport Sci Rev* 7:423, 1989.
5. Centers for Disease Control: *MMWR* 1991.
6. DeCastro JM Jr, Orozco S: Moderate alcohol intake and spontaneous eating patterns of humans: evidence of unregulated supplementation, *Am J Clin Nutr* 52:246, 1990.
7. Dietary Guidelines Advisory Committee: *Report of the Dietary Guidelines Advisory Committee on the dietary guidelines for Americans*, Hyattsville, Md, 1990, US Department of Agriculture, Human Nutrition Information Service.
8. Doll R: An overview of the epidemiological evidence linking diet and cancer, *Proc Nutr Soc* 49:119, 1990.
9. Food and Nutrition Board, National Academy of Science: *Recommended dietary allowances*, ed 10, Washington, DC, 1989, National Academy Press.
10. Goodrick GK, Foreyt JP: Why treatments for obesity don't last, *J Am Diet Assoc* 91:1243, 1991.
11. *Healthy people 2000: national health promotion and disease prevention*, Washington, DC, 1991, Department of Health and Human Services, Public Health Service.
12. Jarasuk U, Beaton GH: Menstrual cycle pattern: in energy and macronutrient intake, *Am J Clin Nutri* 53:442, 1991.
13. Lansing D: *Nutrition intervention in chronic disease*, Public Health Service publication no 535-281, Atlanta, 1991, Centers for Disease Control.
14. Leiber CS: Alcohol and nutrition: an overview, *Alcohol Health Res World* 13:197, 1989.
15. Leon AS: *Effects of physical activity and fitness on health*. In National Center for Health Statistics: *Assessing physical fitness and physical activity in population-based surveys*, DHHS publication No (PHS) 89-1253, Hyattsville, Md, 1989, Department of Health and Human Services.
16. Lissener LD and others: Variability of body weight and health outcomes in the Framingham population, *N Engl J Med* 324:1839, 1991.
17. London RS, Bradley L, Chiamori NY: Effect of a nutritional supplement on premenstral symptomatology in women with premenstrual syndrome: a double-blind longitudinal study, *J Am Coll Nutr* 10:494, 1991.
18. Matsumoto A: Recent trends in domestic food programs, *Food Rev* 14:31, 1991.
19. Mertz W and others: What are people really eating? the relation between energy intake derived from estimated diet records and intake determined to maintain body weight, *Am J Clin Nutr* 54:291, 1991.

20. Moss AJ and others: *Use of vitamin and mineral supplements in the United States: current users, types of products and nutrients*, advance data from vital health statistics No 174, Hyattsville, Md, 1989, National Center for Health Statistics.

21. *Obesity and cardiovascular disease in minority populations*, *Am J Clin Nutr* 53:1507S, 1991.

22. National Cholesterol Education Program: Report on detection, evaluation and treatment of high blood cholesterol in adults, *Arch Intern Med* 148:36, 1988.

23. National Cholesterol Education Program: *Report of expert panel on population strategies for blood cholesterol reduction*, NIH publication No 90-3046, Washington, DC, 1990, NHLBI.

24. National Research Council: *Diet and health: implications for reducing chronic disease risk*, Washington DC, 1989, National Academy Press.

25. Putnam JJ, Allshouse JE: *Food consumption, prices and expenditures, 1968-89*, USDA statistical bulletin No 825, Washington, DC, 1991, Department of Agriculture.

26. Randall MJ, Brink MS, Joy AB: EFNEP: an investment in America's future, *J Nutr Educ* 21:276, 1989.

27. Ricker AS, Preussman R: Chemical food contaminants in the initiation of cancer, *Proc Nutr Soc* 49:133, 1990.

28. Roe DA: *Handbook on drug and nutrient interactions: a problem oriented guide*, ed 4, Chicago, 1989, American Dietetic Association.

29. Schaie W: Midlife influences upon intellectual functioning in old age, *Int J Behav Dev* 7:463, 1984.

30. Slater E and others: Metabolic and Nutritional Factors in Hypertension, *Hypertension* Supplement I, 18(3):I21-I25, 1991.

31. *Statistical handbook on women in America*, Phoenix, 1991, Oryx Press.

32. Tucker LA, Bagwell M: Television viewing and obesity in adult females, *Am J Public Health* 81:908, 1991.

33. US Department of Agriculture, US Department of Health and Human Services: *Nutrition and your health: dietary guidelines for Americans*, ed 3, Washington, DC, 1990, US Government Printing Office.

34. Williamson DF and others: The 10-year incidence of overweight and major weight gain in U.S. adults, *Arch Intern Med* 150:665, 1990.

CHAPTER

9 The Elderly

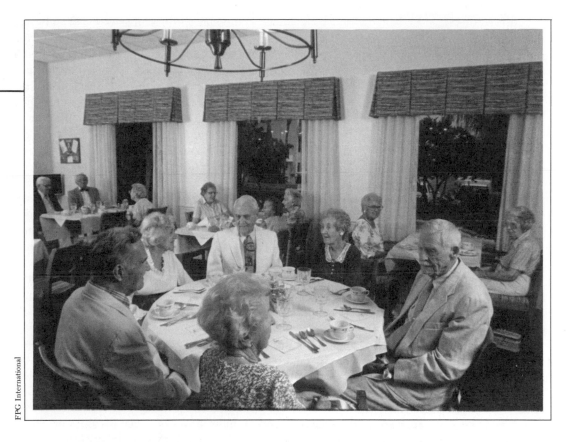

FPG International

GENERAL CONCEPTS

This chapter describes some of the special nutrition-related problems of aging individuals and what is known of their nutritional needs. Distinctions are made between aging itself and the effects of disease and other disabilities that may be associated with age but that are not age dependent. Guidelines for managing some common nutrition-related problems are provided. Because physical activity levels and exercise are so important in determining energy needs and preventing or treating obesity, recommendations on this topic are also provided. Services that should be provided at the local level and some innovative models for delivering such services are highlighted.

The chapter focuses on the second 50 years of life, with special attention to the upper decades, recognizing the limitations of any chronological definition of age. The rationale for choosing such a definition is that many preventive and curative nutritional measures that have a positive influence on later health are best begun early in maturity. This is coincident with the sixth decade of life, during which the changes in sex hormones associated with the menopause in women and the climacteric in men usually occur.

OUTCOME OBJECTIVES

When you finish this chapter you should be able to:

- Describe the goals for the year 2000 for older adults, some sources of data that document progress in reaching them, and reasons why they are important.
- Describe the major nutrition-related problems of older Americans and how they may affect functional status and quality of life.
- Enumerate major characteristics of older people that are useful for screening out those at increased risk of malnutrition and poor general health.
- Detail some of the additional nutritional and other assessment measures that are necessary to confirm or eliminate nutritional factors increasing risks.
- Review effective intervention measures that may be useful for preventing, controlling, or ameliorating nutrition problems in older Americans.
- Recognize the need for prioritizing and focusing interventions to maximize improvement in function and quality of life, as well as in morbidity and mortality.
- Implement appropriate nutritional screening, assessment, and intervention measures in aging Americans.
- Become familiar with some innovative programs that are aimed at realizing goals for promoting health and preventing disease in aging Americans.

WHO ARE AGING ADULTS?

Who are aging Americans? In a sense, all Americans fall into this category because from the moment of conception, the aging process begins in each one of us. Traditionally, terms such as *aging Americans, older adults,* and *the elderly* were reserved for those who had reached the legal retirement age.

Supported in part by Contract 53K06 5-10 to Tufts University for the US Department of Agriculture Human Nutrition Research Center on Aging at Tufts University.

Over the past decades, not only have legal requirements changed but also it is apparent that from the physiological standpoint age-based cutoffs have little meaning. Chronological age is a poor indicator of physiological age because age-related changes occur at different rates in different people and, within individuals, at different rates within cells and organ systems. At any given chronological age after 60, Americans today are healthier than their parents or grandparents were. Therefore, age-related definitions for singling out individuals who were especially vulnerable from the nutritional standpoint are now often not meaningful under 80 or 85 years of age. To get a better view of risks, we must probe more deeply into individual characteristics, particularly those that indicate differential rates of aging, disease, and disability in various individuals in the sixth, seventh, and later decades of life.

Individuals older than 50 years of age, and particularly after age 65, have special physiological, psychological, and social needs as well as vulnerabilities. They deserve special consideration in crafting community, public health, and health care measures in nutrition. History shows that during times of war or social disruption, older individuals are especially vulnerable. For example, during the famine in northwestern Holland at the end of World War II, weight losses, signs and symptoms of protein calorie malnutrition, and anemia were especially high among civilians older than 60 years of age.[26]

Some of the causes for increased vulnerability of older people are pathological because of a variety of environmental insults, including chronic and degenerative diseases and disabilities, and other insults that some people experience. Other causes are truly age-related physiological changes in cells, organs, and organ systems. The rates of these changes vary in different people.

As an example, consider the many possible changes that occur in the gut with aging. Frequently, loss of teeth and alterations in taste and smell occur. Changes are apparent in gastrointestinal function. Weakening of the gastroesophageal sphincter may increase the potential for reflux esophagitis. Gut motility may decrease, slowing transit time and increasing risks of constipation. Production of acid and intrinsic factor in the stomach decreases, with potential effects on the absorption of nutrients. Pancreatic secretions also decline in some respects, potentially altering digestion of large loads of macronutrients. Similar changes have been described in other organ systems with aging.

In addition to these age-associated physiological changes, of even greater importance in terms of human health are the physiological alterations due to inborn or acquired diseases. Many of the most common diseases among the elderly, such as cardiovascular disease, are modifiable, even though risks for them may be partly genetic. Others, such as lung cancer, can be largely prevented by alterations in personal behaviors such as smoking. The increased vulnerability of older people involves not only physiological but also social and environmental factors. Among older Americans past and present, physiological stressors differ from those in younger people. Nevertheless, many diet-related diseases associated with imbalance and excess as well as with deficiency are present in all of the American population, including the elderly.

GOALS FOR THE YEAR 2000

Our country's latest seminal document on health promotion and disease prevention goals for the year 2000 presents worthy health goals for aging Americans.[60] The overall goal is to prevent older Americans from being disabled and to help those with disabilities to prevent further declines and preserve function. More specifically, it is hoped to increase the span of healthy life, that is, life that permits independent function, not just a longer life. At age 65 today, Americans have on the average about 16.4 years of life remaining. About 12 of these years are likely to be a period of healthy life during which the individual is able to carry out basic activities associated with daily living. Increasing the span of healthy life involves decreasing the number of days of restricted activity older people suffer. This is to be accomplished by addressing a variety of the preventable or treatable conditions

of old age, many of which have nutritional implications.

Two other specific objectives for older Americans are to reduce health disparities and to achieve better access to preventive services. Although we have made considerable progress as a nation in decreasing the disparities between socioeconomic groups in expectation of life at birth, the differences by race and social class are still considerable at age 65 years. Therefore, greater efforts aimed at altering environments, health and social services, and personal habits that affect health, particularly among groups that are lagging behind in their health status, deserve attention.

Several of the Year 2000 goals for maintaining vitality and independence in older people are particularly relevant with respect to nutrition. Reducing the incidence of adverse drug reactions lessens the likelihood that medications will cause undernutrition and malnutrition. Similarly, the objective focused on reducing suicide deaths by early interventions among older people reduces depression, a common cause of poor nutrition, especially in men. Prevention of influenza and pneumonia by use of vaccines decreases the likelihood that these diseases will lead to secondary malnutrition. More attention to hydration will help to prevent heat-related deaths, which are all too common among elderly individuals today.

The Year 2000 nutrition goals chiefly address health status and risk reduction. The nutrition goals applying to older Americans that involve health status objectives are to reduce coronary heart disease deaths to 100 and cancer deaths to no more than 130 per 100,000. In addition to screening for breast, uterine, prostate, colon, and oral cancers, dietary measures may be helpful for some cancers. Decreasing smoking, even in the elderly, can have a positive effect on heart disease, chronic obstructive pulmonary disease, and perhaps on lung cancer. Overweight should be reduced to no more than 20% among adults up to age 74; at present it is at about 76% for all adults. Obesity is even higher in certain subgroups, such as black and Hispanic females, low-income women, and individuals who have high blood pressure. Much of the type II diabetes mellitus in older people responds well to weight loss.

Risk-reduction objectives involving nutrition include lowering fat to 30% of calories and saturated fat to no more than 10% of calories. Also, complex carbohydrate and fiber–containing foods should increase to five or more servings of fruits and vegetables and to six or more servings of grain products. Individuals should also consume at least two servings of calcium-rich foods daily. Although osteopenia is often far advanced by old age, keeping calcium intakes up can slow the loss of bone to some extent. It remains to be seen if such measures can lower the prevalence of falls and fractures, which operate to inhibit independent living for many older Americans. Salt and sodium intakes are to be decreased so that at least 65% of home meal preparers do not add salt, at least 80% of individuals avoid using salt at the table, and at least 40% of adults regularly purchase foods modified or lower in sodium. It is suggested that at least 85% of all Americans, including older adults, should use food labels to make nutritious selections. Also the proportion of overweight individuals who adopt sound dietary practices combined with regular physical activity should rise to at least 50%.

The physical activity and fitness health status objectives for older adults also include the overweight and the coronary artery disease goals. For risk reduction goals, it is hoped that at least 30% of adults will engage in regular (preferably daily) light to moderate physical activity for at least a half hour a day. Light to moderate activity includes rapid walking, swimming, cycling, dancing, gardening, and yardwork. In addition, it is hoped that at least 20% of older adults will engage in vigorous physical activities for at least 20 minutes three times a week. Vigorous physical activities include activities that increase heart rate to about 60% of its maximum. Another goal is to decrease to no more than 22% the people 65 and older who engage in no leisure activity; today it is 43%. It is recommended that at least 35% of the older population regularly perform physical activities enhancing and maintaining muscular strength, muscular endur-

ance, and flexibility. This is particularly important for maintaining functional status. Among the useful activities in this regard are home maintenance, yardwork, and gardening. Finally, it is important that at least 40% of all individuals 65 and older participate in community physical activity programs each year.

NUTRITION-RELATED PROBLEMS

The nutrition-related problems associated with aging play a significant role in limiting the span of healthy lives and are among the causes of health disparities among Americans. Personal health habits, access to preventive and curative health services, and aging itself are partly responsible for them. Nutrition-related effects are influenced by the physiological changes that occur in different organs and systems as individuals age, but they also result from environmental, social, and economic factors.

The major factors that increase risk of poor nutritional status in older adults are described next. The indicators that can be used to further corroborate the presence of malnutrition are summarized later in this chapter.

Inappropriate Food Intake

Amounts of food and fluid intakes and also the types of food eaten may be inappropriate in older people. These shortfalls arise because of either personal choices or environmental factors. For example, one recent survey of 55- to 74-year-olds found that the vast majority failed to consume the minimum number of servings of fruits and vegetables daily[46]; such patterns of intake increase risks of deficiencies for certain vitamins and minerals as well as dietary fiber. Other older individuals have inappropriate or inadequate intakes because of self-imposed or medically prescribed dietary modifications. Finally, alcohol abuse may be involved.

Screening for Inappropriate Food Intake

Some simple screening items that may help to identify those who are at risk in this area include the following:

1. Does not have enough food each day
2. Several days each month without any food
3. Poor appetite
4. Daily intakes are less than recommended number of servings, or alcohol use is excessive
5. Individual has special dietary practices, is on a special diet either physician- or self-prescribed, or complains about problems with meeting special dietary needs; individual has multiple diet prescriptions or has unusual dietary practices
6. Goes 6 or 8 hours or longer during the day without food or liquids
7. Eats one meal a day or less
8. Eats the same foods every day

Poverty

Annual incomes under about $6,000 per person per year are currently considered to constitute poverty in older people. Many means-tested services for older people use a threshold of approximately 125% of poverty. By such definitions, in recent years about 17% of men and 42% of women older than 65 years of age reported incomes that would make them eligible for economic assistance to help subsidize food, housing, medical, and other expenses.[57]

Individuals who are poor and who do not receive supportive services have an increased risk of undernutrition. An unknown number of them may actually be suffering from protein calorie malnutrition (PCM) or other dietary deficiency diseases. Some of the elderly poor who suffer from PCM become ill because they are malnourished and take in too little food. Others become malnourished because they are ill.

Screening for Poverty Status

Some ways to screen to see if poverty may be present include:
1. Income is less than $6000 per year; less than $35 per week spent on food
2. Person is unable to buy needed food or prefers not to spend money on food

3. Individual refuses to participate in income assistance programs in spite of evident need

Social Isolation

Social isolation also increases the likelihood of poor nutritional status in older Americans. Eating and appetite are strongly influenced by social factors. Social isolation may occur because of lack of social support systems in the community, loss of spouse or friends, distance from family or other concerned individuals, or psychological factors such as depression that cause the individual not to seek help or to reject help if it is offered.

Living locations may be isolated. When cooking, food storage, and transportation facilities are lacking in living arrangements, the person is also at risk. When the individual has physical or psychological disabilities, risks of social isolation may be further heightened. Presently, only about a fifth of the elderly use community services. Increased social interaction can sometimes have positive impacts on food intake as well as general health and well-being.[53]

Screening for Social Isolation

Some screening items that may reveal social isolation are:
1. Lives alone, exhibits concern about home security, rejects help
2. Housebound
3. Lost a spouse or other loved one in the past year
4. Contact with family or friends less than once a week
5. Usually eats alone

Dependence and Disability

Ability to perform self-care activities, especially those involving behaviors critical to food getting, food preparation, and eating, can be crudely assessed using functional status indicators, such as the Activities of Daily Living and the Instrumental Activities of Daily Living.[35] These rather crude and insensitive measures do pick up major difficulties in eating, walking, and other activities that are important in living independently, such as food purchasing and handling money. When they are limited, this may be a warning sign of impending risk to nutritional status.

Disabling conditions, especially those that limit manual dexterity or make it necessary to use assistive devices to eat, increase risk of malnutrition. Almost 20% of Americans living at home who are 65 years and older have difficulties in walking, 2% have trouble eating unassisted, 10% have trouble shopping, 8% in preparing meals, 8% in doing light housework, 20% in doing heavy housework, 5% in using the telephone, and 5% in managing money—all important tasks for assuring good food intakes.[41]

Extreme inactivity, which eventually can give rise to disuse atrophy, immobility owing to extreme frailty, and diseases such as arthritis of the hips, knees, and hands, may cause dependency on others for getting food or eating. The need for assistive devices such as walkers, wheelchairs, and modified dishes or utensils for preparing or consuming food is associated with increased nutritional risk because they mean that preparing and consuming food are more difficult.[61]

Inability to read or write in any language and especially in English makes it difficult to communicate needs and can further increase dependency on others, as well as isolating the older person socially in many settings.

Screening for Nutrition-Related Functional Problems

A change from independence to dependence on two of the Activities of Daily Living, which assess self-care abilities (e.g., bathing, dressing, toileting, transfer from bed to chair, continence, feeding), or in one of the nutritionally relevant skills in the Instrumental Activities of Daily Living (e.g., ability to shop for groceries or prepare one's own meals) are indicators of poor nutritional status.

Screening for functional status problems that includes questions on need for assistance with bathing, dressing, continence, toileting, eating, walking, transportation, and food preparation begins to get at these issues. Of particular importance is a report that the individual has trouble self-feeding,

cooking, getting to the grocery store, or shopping for food.

Acute and Chronic Diseases or Conditions

Diseases of both an acute and chronic nature, including multiple illnesses and disabilities, are prevalent among older Americans, particularly those in their late 70s and 80s.[4] Diseases cause impairments at the cellular and organ level, which in turn may be followed by disability and losses in everyday personal functions such as eating that are required for independent living. Eventually they may also lead to limitations and handicaps that affect behavior, social relationships, and the ways older people are regarded in the larger society.

The most common conditions with nutritional implications in people over 65 years of age are arthritis, hypertension, heart disease, orthopedic impairments, chronic sinusitis, diabetes mellitus, cataracts, deafness or hearing loss, hemorrhoids, blindness, arteriosclerosis, and constipation. The presence of events such as recent hospitalization, surgery, trauma, or infection or need for special routes or assistance in feeding all suggest increased nutritional risk. When acute or chronic disease is present, particularly if it is extensive, it is also a warning sign of possible malnutrition.

Evidence from national nutritional monitoring of the general population indicates that protein calorie malnutrition (PCM) and other dietary deficiency diseases due solely to lack of food are somewhat rare in the United States today. However, sampling frail, sick, poor older Americans is difficult. These are the very groups most likely to have inadequate diets and insecure food access.[3] Monitoring systems are not yet in place that are sufficiently sensitive to provide good evidence on the presence or absence of PCM in older populations. Thus PCM may occur when money for food, food access, or food availability is limited and other unavoidable expenses are high. Also, if the individual fails to eat because of some other reason, such as lack of orderly eating habits, inability to obtain or prepare food, lack of acceptable food, psychological factors, and lack of social support, risk is also elevated.

Protein calorie malnutrition commonly coexists with chronic illness, and poor older people may have this added risk for its presence. A preceding or accompanying disease may precipitate PCM by increasing energy needs or altering absorption or metabolism of protein and other nutrients.

Smaller-scale surveys suggest relatively high prevalence rates of PCM among dependent, homebound, elderly persons and among subgroups such as the demented or chronically ill with multiple other illnesses who are living at home, in nursing homes, and in acute care hospitals. Although there is disagreement on appropriate standards to use, PCM prevalence rates in nursing homes, other long-term care facilities, and even acute care hospitals are higher.

Abnormalities of body weight, such as recent involuntary gain or loss of weight, as well as the presence of obesity or underweight, predict both increased risk of illness and death. Older people who are extremely overweight or underweight have higher death rates; underweight is particularly highly associated with mortality in the very old.[55] Risks of decubitus ulcers and systemic infections are also elevated among those who are underweight.[49] The causes of involuntary and unexplained weight loss in the elderly vary. Among them are depression, undiagnosed cancers, reactions to medication, and hyperthyroidism.[56] Often several causes are involved.

Obesity is very prevalent in older Americans, regardless of what standards are used to measure it. Using a body mass index (BMI) of about 27, which is the 85th percentile for younger adults, more than a third of all older men and women are obese. Counting only those people who are very severely overweight, with a BMI of 30 (which corresponds to the 95th percentile of younger adults), more than 10% of all men and perhaps 15% of all women are at risk.[11] Dietary factors associated with five of the ten leading causes of death in our country that are worsened by obesity include coronary artery disease, some types of cancer, stroke, non-insulin-dependent diabetes mellitus, and atherosclerosis.

Alcohol abuse may also increase nutritional risk.

Body water is lower in older people, metabolism is often slowed, and they more often take medications that enhance the effects of alcohol, factors that increase the risks of alcohol abuse and problem drinking at all levels of drinking. In addition, energy from alcohol is virtually devoid of other nutrients, making it difficult for older people to increase the quality of their diets if alcohol constitutes a major source of calories.[2] The prevalence of alcohol abuse is difficult to determine in the elderly and probably is underestimated. Among 65- to 74-year-olds, about 43% of the population drink; of those older than 75 years of age, about 30% drink.[59] Many older abusers live isolated or alone. Their drinking is less likely to cause run-ins with legal authorities, family and friends may conceal their abuse, and their lifestyles are such that job-related discovery is rare. Early identification of alcohol abuse, especially in those who have just begun their problem drinking, is important.

Cognitive or emotional impairments also affect the nutritional status of many elderly people. After 80 years of age, approximately 20% of all people suffer from some type of dementia, and these rates rise steadily over age 65.[34] Low body mass is quite common in demented elderly people, including outpatients, even after taking account of the other illnesses they may be suffering.[6] In nursing homes the prevalence is even higher. Depressive disorders are also common in nursing homes as well as in the general population, and they may alter appetite and weight. The reasons that weight loss is more common among such individuals in institutions include inability to shop for, prepare, and eat food because of the cognitive impairment, possible impairments in taste and smell due to drugs or to the underlying illness, depression and lack of appetite, the presence of other illnesses that go unrecognized, and, in some agitated patients, increased energy needs.[25]

Tooth loss, mouth pain, and other oral health problems are common in the elderly.[30] Dental disabilities include total lack of teeth; poorly fitting dentures; periodontal disease; decayed, missing, and filled teeth; dry mouth; facial pain; and difficulties with chewing. The prevalence of oral cancer rises with age, particularly among heavy alcohol abusers and smokers. When these disorders are present, eating may be extremely difficult. By age 50, many Americans have lost their teeth. Those who still have them often have one or more missing teeth, 42% have untreated caries at the roots of the teeth (root caries), 5% have untreated crown caries, 40% have gingivitis, and 17% have periodontitis.[44] After age 85, the majority of individuals are totally edentulous, and many, perhaps the majority, have denture-related problems. Caries, particularly root caries, also increase with age. Oral health affects chewing, swallowing, and the type of diet that can be eaten. At the very least, oral health problems detract from the joy of eating and the taste of food, and they may also cause pain, alterations in diet, and thus heightened malnutrition.

Sensory impairments such as blindness make getting food and eating more difficult, particularly if the individual has not adapted to loss of sight. Deafness may also increase risks of poor nutritional status because it may contribute to social isolation and make use of devices such as the telephone more difficult.

Screening Items for Disease

Several simple questions can help to identify those who are likely to have diseases with nutritional implications:

- Hospitalization or surgery in past 6 months
- Problems with memory loss, making it difficult to shop, cook, or eat
- Sadness and depression, with little interest in shopping, cooking, and eating
- Chronic diseases, especially those involving dietary modifications
- Tooth loss or mouth pain: missing, loose, or rotten teeth, dentures that do not fit, mouth sores that do not heal, bleeding or sore gums, more than a year since the last dental visit
- Involuntary loss or gain in weight: losses or gains of more than 10 pounds in 6 months, reported weight 20% over or under best or desirable weight

Many other diseases and conditions are caused in part by diet and also have nutritional implications. They include osteomalacia, which is often due to low vitamin D intakes or disordered vitamin D metabolism; folic acid deficiency, and vitamin B_{12} deficiency. Common causes of poor nutritional status are alcoholism, cognitive impairment, and chronic renal insufficiency. When individuals who are ill with any cause complain of anorexia, early fullness after eating, nausea, difficulty in swallowing, changes in bowel habits, and fatigue, possible nutrition-related causes may be involved.

Signs of malnutrition are vague enough that they are rarely diagnostic. They include angular stomatitis of the mouth, pressure ulcers or other poorly healing wounds, evident loss of subcutaneous fat and muscle mass during clinical examination, and fluid retention. Pressure sores are also signs of increased nutritional risk because their presence is associated with poor nutritional status.[8] They all may indicate malnutrition and should be noted.

The most useful major biochemical indicator of poor nutritional status is serum albumin level below 3.5 g/dl. Other laboratory tests that may be helpful for confirming the presence of malnutrition include reduced serum albumin or other serum proteins with shorter half-lives, such as prealbumin and transferrin; low red blood cell folic acid; iron deficiency anemia; increased blood urea nitrogen (BUN); and low serum ascorbic acid.

Unfortunately, food intake, anthropometric measurements, findings from physical diagnosis, other signs and symptoms, and laboratory tests are rather nonspecific, and none of them alone suffices for declaring that a person is malnourished. However, taken together with dietary and other evidence, they may be diagnostic.

Chronic Medication Use

Among the elderly living in the community, almost a quarter take at least five medications, and the majority of all older adults are taking more than one medication.[37] Nearly half of all nursing home residents take more than five medications. Both physician- and self-prescribed medications can increase risks of poor nutritional status, owing to the effects of drugs on absorption, metabolism, and drug-nutrient interactions.

Nutritional quackery and overuse of vitamin,

mineral, and other nutrient supplements are thought to be common among older Americans.[39] Some preparations such as very large doses of vitamin D can cause toxicities. Use of others is fraught with hazard because it is often associated with delays in seeking medical help for health problems.

Screening for Inappropriate Medications

Some screening questions that can tap possible problems related to drugs and other medications that may be affecting appetite are:

1. Use of three or more prescribed medicines daily
2. Use of over-the-counter or vitamin or mineral tablets daily, especially if more than three of these are used
3. Excessive preoccupation with and use of unproven nutritional or other remedies

NUTRITIONAL NEEDS

The Recommended Dietary Allowances (RDAs) are standards commonly agreed upon for assessing and planning to meet nutrient needs at various ages.[23] For most nutrients, the present RDAs do not provide separate recommendations by age beyond 51 years. This is not because such recommendations are not desirable or necessary but rather because there are few data on which to base them.

Decreased calorie recommendations are the most striking changes in nutrient needs for older adults in the RDA. For the population as a whole, recommendations decrease by 6% from ages 51 to 75 years and by another 6% after 74 years of age, the lowered recommendations being due to declines in lean body mass and in physical activity among older adults. However, it is not clear that these decreases are an inevitable part of growing older. Currently there is a great deal of interest in the hypothesis that it is possible to preserve lean body mass into old age by lifelong vigorous physical activity.

If older people stay physically active, in addition to gains in fitness and limberness, their energy needs and the amount of foods they can eat while maintaining energy balance stay high, making it easier to meet nutrient needs. Sustained or increased physical activity and exercise might prevent declines in lean body mass and hence in resting metabolism (which is due chiefly to lean body mass), as well as increasing discretionary and nondiscretionary physical activity and energy outputs needed to move the body about. Another current hypothesis is that growth hormone therapy can increase lean body mass, even in the very old. The major problem with this therapy is that it is extremely expensive and the side effects are not yet clear.

Water requirements are often forgotten in discussions of nutrient needs but are particularly important among the aged. Thirst mechanisms are weak, body water is low, ability to concentrate the urine decreases, and many of the elderly are on diuretics that cause obligatory losses of water. Thus older people must learn to drink even when they are not thirsty to avoid dehydration.

Mineral needs of aging individuals are presently being actively investigated. The major difference in mineral RDAs for older as compared with younger adults is that needs for iron decrease in females owing to cessation of menses and hence slower iron losses after the menopause. Calcium recommendations are currently similar to those suggested for younger adults, but there is evidence that in women some but not all of the calcium loss that occurs with aging, especially on very low calcium intakes, can be stopped by providing somewhat larger amounts of calcium than the current RDA and, even more importantly, by estrogen replacement therapy, particularly in women who begin with low bone density.[51] Recommendations vary from about 1000 to 2000 mg of calcium to achieve these effects. A recent consensus development conference on the subject emphasized that high calcium intakes are important, but that they are not substitutes for estrogen therapy in blunting losses after menopause.[12]

Dietary protein recommendations are also similar to those for younger adults. Good health can be maintained among older people who have no debilitating disease on protein intakes of less than 1 g/kg desirable body weight or less. The RDA for men and women over 51 years of age is currently 0.8 g/kg or an average of about 63 g for reference males and 50 g per day for reference females.[23] Of course, if the older individual is ill, additional protein may be needed for rehabilitation. Whether very low protein intakes offer any advantage in slowing progression of early chronic renal disease is a topic of much current investigation.

Recommendations for aging adults differ very little from those earlier in adulthood for most of the vitamins. One exception is vitamin D. It may need to be provided to elderly shut-ins who live in inclement climates. Other elderly persons whose well-founded zeal for preventing skin cancer includes use of very effective sunblocks when they go outdoors also need supplementary D in RDA amounts. Vitamin D deficiency may contribute to osteomalacia and also to osteoporosis through its effects on increasing bone loss and discouraging bone apposition.

Elderly people's intakes of vitamins are not markedly different from that of younger persons but are more variable. Vitamin intakes may be dangerously low among the very old and frail who suffer from many diseases and use many medications. Among the vitamins that may be particularly low are vitamins A, C, B_6, and riboflavin. Rates of atrophic gastritis also rise with age; both it and pernicious anemia may cause vitamin B_{12} deficiency. For such patients a vitamin-mineral supplement at RDA levels is a sensible precaution.

Needs for essential fatty acids (linoleic acid and α-linolenic acid) are small and thought not to change with age. Consumption of the essential fatty acids is high among adults and appears to be more than adequate among the elderly. For example, linoleic acid consumption is between 4% and 10% of calories, whereas only about 1% to 2% of calories are thought to be needed. α-Linolenic acid, an omega-3 fatty acid, is thought to be about 0.5% of usual energy intakes.

At present the RDAs do not make recommendations for intakes of certain other substances, such as dietary cholesterol, dietary fiber, or amount and type of fat. However, another committee of the Food and Nutrition Board of the Institute of Medicine, National Academy of Sciences, has made recommendations on intake levels. A recent authoritative report on diet and health addresses intakes for healthy older people of constituents for which the RDAs do not provide guidance.[11] Another recent report, *The Second Fifty Years: Promoting Health and Preventing Disabilities*, makes recommendations for all healthy adults, including the elderly.[5] This recent population-based panel report of the National Cholesterol Education Program, like the National Academy of Sciences report, suggests that intakes of fat be approximately 30% of total calories, with not more than 10% from saturates, polyunsaturates, or monounsaturates[43] for older Americans. The pros and cons of this recommendation are discussed elsewhere.

GUIDELINES FOR MANAGEMENT

Screening

Often too little is done to prevent unnecessary nutrition-related problems in the elderly because they are not recognized until after they already have caused significant disruption to normal function. The Preventive Health Services Task Force report of the U.S. Public Health Service[61] has made many useful recommendations for instituting prevention measures for older adults in primary health care settings. It suggests yearly health examinations that include dietary intake, physical activity, and functional status reports by the patient. Physical examinations should include, among other things, height, weight, blood pressure, need for hearing and assistive devices, and an oral health examination. Laboratory and diagnostic tests recommended include total serum cholesterol, dipstick urinalysis, and periodic tests of thyroid function and fecal occult blood. Physicians must remain alert for symptoms of depression, abnormal bereavement, changes in cognitive function, medications that increase risk of falls, tooth decay and deteriorated dental health, and signs of physical abuse and neglect. If primary physicians are more active in carrying out these recommendations, many problems may be cured that are now overlooked. They can also help by indicating to their patients that nutrition is a high priority for maintaining good health.

Not everyone who needs nutritional help or

other types of health care sees a physician, and many problems may arise between visits. Therefore, vigilance in other settings and between visits to the physician is also needed. A new approach to identifying nutritional and health problems involves nutrition screening and referral in primary care and community settings. The motivation for this program, the Nutrition Screening Initiative, is that it is more efficient and effective to find and treat preventable nutritional and other health problems than to wait until they become acute. It proposes a broad-based approach to nutrition screening that starts in the community and then proceeds, if necessary, into the health services system.[45] (See also Appendix 15-2.)

The process begins with stimulating greater nutrition awareness among older people in a variety of nonmedical settings. It gives particular attention to those who may be at risk or who may need nutritional or health services. The kinds of issues that are important in increasing risk to nutritional and general health can be easily remembered by the word *determine* (*d*isease, *e*ating poorly, *t*ooth loss or mouth pain, *e*conomic hardship, *r*educed social contact, *m*ultiple medications or drugs, *in*voluntary weight loss or gain, *n*eed for assistance with self-care, and *e*lder of very advanced age, that is, 80 years or older).

The next step is to collect information on these and other issues from individuals by using a screening form on which characteristics are easily determined by questioning the individual. The types of information that can be collected vary, but at a minimum some of the characteristics that tap factors related to these problems should be obtained. In some circumstances it might be appropriate for the elderly person to complete a checklist covering these points himself; in other situations a social service or health care worker might ask the questions of clients.

The details about characteristics that are useful to consider in screening older people were discussed earlier in this chapter. Tools for screening that include all of these items are now available from the Nutrition Screening Initiative.[45]

Some of the needs identified by this type of screening do not require health care. Rather, they involve preventive interventions such as home-delivered meals, assistance with shopping or cooking, congregate meals programs, or nutrition education. Others require further referral. For example, physicians need to be contacted if there are increases or decreases in weight, if body weights are outside recommended limits to begin with, or if the person has other health complaints or questions. A registered dietitian should be consulted for problems in the food area.

Unfortunately, no screening instrument is available that reflects only dietary deficits or correctable nutritional problems. Rather, the types of questions asked reflect both health status and disease severity as well. Therefore, nutrition screening tools actually screen for many aspects of both nutritional and general health, and they pick out for further assessment individuals who have deficits in both. This shortcoming does not mean that such screens are not useful or that screening should not be done. To the extent that they highlight problems that can be prevented or ameliorated better when they are identified early, especially among individuals who otherwise would not be recognized as suffering from a disease that can be treated, they perform an important function. When they identify disease rather than nutritional problems, some of them can also be dealt with even if they cannot be prevented. These screening tools are simple enough to apply in community settings in which older Americans live as well as in health care settings. Thus they stand a chance of recognizing individuals who may be at nutritional risk and channeling them into the health or other services that may be able to correct deficits.

Assessment

The major difference between screening and assessment is that assessment is done in a health care setting in which laboratory and clinical examination is possible. Confidentiality can be better assured, and patients or those who are intimately familiar with their health and nutritional status can be questioned directly, rather than having to rely on records. Also the length of time required increases.

INDICATORS OF POOR NUTRITIONAL STATUS: DIET

Individuals whose characteristics on preliminary screening are such that nutritional problems appear to be present need referral to a physician or other qualified health care professional for additional assessment. Significant and sustained reduction of dietary intakes below RDAs indicates that food intake is insufficient in one or more respects.[11] For screening purposes, insufficient intake is usually present if an individual consumes less than the recommended minimum from one or more of the five food groups (i.e., two servings of milk or milk products, two servings of meat or meat alternates, two servings of fruits, three servings of vegetables, and six servings of breads and cereals). These crude measures of intake may need to be followed up. Further information, obtained by asking the patient to keep a dietary record, observation of the patient eating (especially if disability is present), feeding assessment, or keeping intakes and output information, may be helpful. Also of concern are imbalances in food intakes. In older individuals, *Dietary Guidelines for Americans*[58] is a good general guide, but it needs to be individualized to some extent in the elderly because diseases or conditions may be present that also require diet therapy. Nevertheless, failure to consume fat, saturated fat, cholesterol, sugar, and salt in moderation deserves further assessment. More than 1 oz of alcohol a day in women or 2 oz in men also should be a cause for concern. The nutrition interview should also probe risks of poor nutrition due to the living environment. Absence of a stove or refrigerator, inadequate heating or cooling, nonuse of food programs if income is very limited, and concerns about home security and safety may indicate that food is difficult to obtain or prepare. When no specific nutritional problem is present but the individual is poor or functionally dependent, referral to community social service and food programs may still be in order. The problems the individual has with food getting and availability, the social circumstances of eating, appetite, and in meeting special dietary needs, as well as types of unusual dietary practices, need documentation.

Fluid intakes and signs of fluid balance–related problems, such as dehydration and constipation, need to be assessed. Water is a nutrient that is often forgotten but extremely important in older adults, whose thirst is not always a good indicator that they are appropriately hydrated. Histories of decreased fluid intake, fever, vomiting, diarrhea, diabetes, chronic renal disease, and use of diuretics often place individuals at nutritional risk of dehydration. If an individual exhibits decreased skin turgor and dry mouth and mucous membranes that are not easily explained by other factors, dehydration may be present. A good preventive target is at least 1 to 2 quarts of fluid per day.

Constipation, the passage of small, dry stools after straining and difficulty, is often due to lack of water or low fiber intake in the elderly.[7] The use of laxatives and the presence of constipation are often not mentioned unless they are probed for directly. Increased fluid and fiber intakes, more physical activity, and regular meals and bowel habits are all helpful. These measures often can eliminate the need for laxatives.

INDICATORS OF POOR NUTRITIONAL STATUS OF OTHER TYPES

The nutrition-related aspects of assessment involve, in addition to diet, a more definitive functional assessment; a fuller history and physical; actual measurements of height, weight, skinfolds, and body fat distribution; laboratory tests; and a complete review of medications. Many of these functions may be performed by the dietitian, nutritionist, or another health professional. Regardless of who performs them, they need to be taken into account in order to devise a sound nutrition plan.

It is helpful during further assessment of the patient to observe performance of the activities of daily living or at the very least to obtain additional information from spouse, friends, or others who know how the individual is functioning. It is best to assess physical disability and dependence by clinical observation as well as by questioning. Dietitians and nutritionists can be particularly helpful by making and recording observations in food and eating domains and by communicating these recommendations to other members of the health care team. The Activities of Daily Living (ADL) and Instrumental Activities of Daily Living (IADL) assessment questionnaires are functional status indicators that can be administered by dietitians, nutritionists, or other health professionals.[35] Ability to perform self-care activities, especially those involving behaviors critical to getting food, food preparation, and eating, can be roughly assessed with them. Although these measures are rather insensitive, they do pick up major difficulties in eating, walking, and other activities that are important in living independently, such as purchasing food and handling money. When these functions are limited, this may be a warning sign of impending risk to nutritional status. A change from independence to dependence on two of the Activities of Daily Living, which assess self-care abilities (e.g., bathing, dressing, toileting, transfer from bed to chair, continence, feeding) or in one of the nutritionally relevant skills in the Instrumental Activities of Daily Living (e.g., ability to shop for groceries or prepare one's own meals) are indicators that poor nutritional status may be present.

More definitive and less subjective information on mental and cognitive status can be obtained in health care settings than in community settings. One way of doing this is by use of short questionnaires. Physicians, dietitians and nutritionists, and other health professionals who are trained to administer these questionnaires can do so successfully; they have already been validated with allied health professionals as administrators.

If the Folstein Mini Mental Status questionnaire score is under 26,[22] this suggests that the individual's capability for memory, language, abstract thinking, arithmetic, reading, writing, and orientation to time, place, and person may be limited, thus increasing nutritional risk. Occasionally the dementia or memory changes may be due to nutritional problems, such as dehydration or vitamin B_{12} deficiency caused by pernicious anemia, but more usually, although the consequences of decreasing nutritional status are still significant, the causes are not nutritional.

Depression questionnaires tap another risk factor for poor nutritional status. Depression also contributes to poor nutritional status because it is often associated with anorexia, inability or disinclination to seek help, and confusion. Among the depression scales that are particularly useful, a score under 15 on the Beck Depression Scale or a score greater than 5 on the Geriatric Depression Scale (GDS) may also indicate problems.[35] They can be administered by dietitians and nutritionists after appropriate training.

Anthropometric measurements, rather than reports, are mandatory for sound nutritional assessment. All patients who are seen in health care settings should be weighed and measured on a regular basis. Scales should be calibrated frequently, and weights should be taken in a standardized fashion. Anthropometric measurements should be taken, rather than relying on reports, because elderly people often remember measurements from an earlier time. Measurements should be done on a well-standardized scale. It is best to use a knee height measurement if deformity or kyphosis prevents accurate measurement.

Significant weight loss over time is an indicator of poor nutritional status. Loss of more than 10 pounds or loss of more than 5% of previous body weight in a month, 7.5% in three months, or 10% or more in 6 months is significant.[42] When weight for height is less than 80% of desirable weights for height, underweight indicative of poor nutritional status is present.[28] Losses of weight are also suggested by reductions below the 10th percentile compared to usual body weights. Weight for height can be assessed by using knee height if deformity or kyphosis prevents accurate measurement.[10] Midarm muscle circumferences below 10% of desirable levels and triceps skinfold thicknesses below 10% of standards are suggestive of muscle wasting.

Obesity is considered significant if the body mass index is over 27 or weight is over 120% of desirable. Although the standards for obesity are still evolving, even the more liberal limits in the *Dietary Guidelines for Americans* only suggest gains of 10-15 pounds from normal weights in young adulthood.[58] Excessive gains in weight are also suggested by increases above the 95th percentile in triceps skinfolds.[27] Significant gains in weight are indicators of possible nutritional problems. Obesity is also suggested by triceps or subscapular fatfold thicknesses over the 95th percentile; triceps skinfold measurements and measurements of midarm muscle circumference should be taken in a standardized fashion; if not taken correctly, they are highly unreliable and not diagnostic.

Body fat distributions indicating abdominal adiposity increase risk for many chronic degenerative diseases that are associated with obesity. Waist to hip ratios over 1.0 in males or 0.8 in females indicate increased risk in these regards and suggest that weight reduction may be needed.

The medical history and physical examination during nutritional assessment follows up the clues that were provided by earlier screening. Many diseases and conditions are caused in part by diet and also have nutritional implications. A few deficiency diseases also are especially prevalent in older persons. They include osteomalacia, which is often due to low vitamin D intakes or disordered vitamin D metabolism; folic acid deficiency (especially frequent in elderly alcoholics), and vitamin B_{12} deficiency, associated with pernicious anemia. Iron deficiency anemia is relatively rare, although anemias of chronic disease or due to occult and unrecognized blood loss are common. Thus anemias should always be further assessed in older people. Certain diseases are especially common as causes of poor nutritional status among older people. They include unrecognized infections, alcoholism, cognitive impairment, chronic renal insufficiency, and other chronic degenerative diseases stemming from a variety of causes. Discovering these diseases often requires extensive and involved medical workups. Emphasis in nutritional assessment is on how to make changes in diet or eating that will maximize functioning and quality of life.

Patients' complaints about their health must be carefully assessed by a physician who is knowledgeable in geriatric medicine. The signs and symptoms of problems often are different in older than in younger people. When individuals who are ill complain of anorexia; fatigue; early fullness after eating; nausea; problems with their mouths, teeth, or gums; difficulty in chewing or swallowing; or changes in bowel habits, possible nutrition-related causes may be involved. A history of bone pain and fracture suggests that mobility and getting food may be difficult, increasing nutritional risks.

Clinical examination for signs of malnutrition may be helpful in assessment. Skin changes, including the presence of skin ulcers, may also suggest increased nutritional risk. Signs such as angular stomatitis of the mouth, pressure ulcers or other poorly healing wounds, evident loss of subcutaneous fat and muscle mass during clinical examination, and fluid retention may indicate malnutrition and should be noted.

The most useful major indicator of poor nutritional status involving biochemical tests is a serum albumin level below 3.5 g/dl. Serum cholesterol levels under 160 mg/dl are often present in undernutrition but also when other pathology is present. Serum cholesterol levels over 240 mg/dl are potential warning signs of hyperlipidemia and should trigger additional assessment of lipoprotein levels and ratios. Other laboratory tests may be helpful for confirming the presence of specific types of malnutrition. They include reduced values for other serum proteins with shorter half-lives than serum albumin, such as prealbumin and transferrin, low red blood cell folic acid, iron deficiency anemia, increased blood urea nitrogen (BUN), and low serum ascorbic acid. However, these tests are not usually appropriate or available on a routine basis. Unfortunately, these signs and symptoms, anthropometric measurements, and laboratory tests are rather nonspecific. None of them alone suffices for declaring that a person is malnourished. Taken together with dietary and other evidence, however, they may be diagnostic.

INTERVENTIONS

The ability to function independently into old, old age depends in part on factors we can control ourselves, such as lifetime nutritional habits, including maintenance of healthy weights, prudence in current dietary intakes, and avoidance of substance abuse, among other factors. Nutrition is not a panacea, however. Aging well depends on access to adequate and comprehensive gerontological care.

Other important factors include genetics; personal characteristics such as intelligence, motivation, curiosity, and religious or philosophical convictions; social characteristics such as maintaining an active social life, responsibility for others, family integrity, and intimacy; financial independence; and age-adaptable living arrangements in the physical environment.[52]

Older people respond differently, but mostly enthusiastically, to various kinds of screening programs in the community.[29] They are particularly interested in diagnosis-related information and in obtaining further advice.

The U.S. Preventive Health Services Task Force's recommendations[63] for the content of routine visits by primary physicians include counseling of a general nature on diet and exercise, substance use, injury prevention, and other primary prevention measures. Particular attention is suggested to ensuring moderation in intakes of fat, especially saturated fat, dietary cholesterol, and sodium. By substituting complex carbohydrate foods like breads, cereals, pastas, rice, and potatoes for fattier foods, fat can be decreased without causing undesirable weight loss. At the same time, counseling must ensure that energy balance is maintained and that intakes of calcium are satisfactory. Alcohol and other drug use needs to be examined and suggestions made for reducing use or changing medications if intakes are inappropriate or excessive. In addition, patients may need referrals to community programs, such as the congregate and home-delivered meals programs funded under Title III of the Older Americans Act or similar programs. Other community support programs that are also sometimes available can provide assistance with shopping or meal preparation, social interaction, and support to combat isolation (which may prevent the isolation and lack of social relationships that discourage some older people from eating). Other programs help with transportation needs to help older people obtain food. When they are not available, health professionals have an obligation to work to make them so. Senior gardening programs have proven to be very successful in many places.[32]

Nutrition education to help older Americans sharpen their skills in making healthier nutrition choices is needed as well, but it must be reality based and tailored to older people. Often general recommendations for younger people are inappropriate, given health and other limitations, or culturally inappropriate. Recently, special programs for black elderly people, for native Americans, and for other special groups have been developed. The USDA's cooperative extension programs have successfully developed programs for altering diet and physical activities in more healthful directions from the standpoint of cardiovascular health.[33] Congregate meal programs are excellent sites for nutrition education of older people.

Preventive and health promotion actions are essential, but they alone are not enough. Screening and assessment of nutritional status are useful only when they are coupled with interventions to address nutritional problems that are identified. Older Americans also have a right to a range of nutritional interventions all across the entire continuum of health care and social services, including clinical care for the control or amelioration of diseases and conditions. Thus counseling of patients and preparation of meals to assure adequate intakes of protective nutrients, to avoid imbalances and excesses, and to control chronic degenerative diseases with dietary implications are mandatory.

Many therapeutic interventions involving nutrition are available. Many dietary modifications can improve the health and function of older people. The secret in implementation is to prioritize among the older person's various needs, concentrating on nutrition and other interventions that stand the best chance of success and of improving function. Space does not permit a description of the entire spectrum of nutritional interventions that are vital signs of good health care. They have been described at length elsewhere.[16] Among the helpful interventions for major malnutrition-related causes of disability are obesity treatment, treatment of chronic degenerative diseases requiring nutritional support (such as hypertension, hyperlipidemia, diabetes mellitus, renal disease, cancer, chronic obstructive pulmonary disease, and gastrointestinal conditions). Deficiency diseases, which are often complicated by other problems, include protein calorie malnutrition, anorexia and undernutrition due to inappropriate medications, dehydration, and constipation. Inadequate physical activity and exercise need to be dealt with. Alcohol abuse, constipation, and other problems such as burns, arthritis, and osteoporosis also may require nutritional measures for amelioration. Referral for dental care is needed when poor dentition or other oral health problems impede food consumption. Counseling and treatment of active alcoholics or problem drinkers are also necessary; because they are often debilitated, nutrition counseling may also be in order.

A small but significant number of older Americans reside in institutions such as long-term care facilities. An even smaller number are hospitalized. These individuals are especially challenging from the nutritional standpoint because their health and functional status are much poorer than those of older people living in the community. They are afflicted with all of the many illnesses described here.

Intakes of energy and other nutrients are sometimes low among residents of nursing homes and acute care facilities, even though sufficient food is provided. Among the causes of low intakes are the presence of disease itself, untreated dehydration, very poor oral health, very low physical activity, unsuitable meal environments, too many meals too close together, poor understanding by staff on how to feed older people (particularly those who need feeder assistance), lack of ready availability of snacks and supplements, and many other factors. Some of these factors are amenable to change; others are not. Special diets should be prescribed and provided for institutionalized elderly people who need them for various chronic conditions. Special feeding routes involving enteral and parenteral nutrition for individuals who are unable to eat by mouth are also called for at times. At the same time, dietitians and nutritionists are key in ensuring that foodborne disease outbreaks are avoided. Because the elderly are at particularly high risk for serious morbidity from foodborne disease, nursing homes should practice careful food handling, preparation, and storage. In addition education needs to be provided to food handlers, and active infection control programs to handle outbreaks must be in place. The most common foodborne diseases in nursing homes are *Salmonella* infection, most commonly due to egg-related contamination, and staphylococcal food poisoning.[38] Nutrition professionals have an important role to play in altering food preparation, food service, and eating environments, as well as providing therapeutic dietary prescriptions to maximize food intake in nursing homes.

EXAMPLES OF COMMON PROBLEMS

Older Americans have the highest prevalence of elevated serum cholesterols of any age group in the nation. Because rises in serum cholesterol with age do not occur in all countries, it does not seem that cholesterol metabolism changes with aging so that the entire rise in serum cholesterol is inevitable. There is some limited evidence that the activity of the low-density lipoprotein (LDL) cholesterol receptor in the liver declines with age so that LDL removal is less and that this accounts for some of the age-associated serum cholesterol rise, but as yet this speculation has not been proven in humans. Some rare individuals also have genetic predispositions that permit them to maintain low serum cholesterol levels even when their diets are high in saturated fat and cholesterol, and they may have reached old age for this very reason.[31]

In the population as a whole, increased LDL cholesterol remains an independent factor increasing risk even into extreme old age, although it is somewhat less potent than it is in younger individuals. Elevated high-density lipoprotein cholesterol provides some protection against heart disease in older as well as younger people. Obesity and excessive intakes of dietary fat, particularly saturated fat, and of dietary cholesterol are risk factors for coronary artery heart disease even in older adults. However, the atherosclerotic process probably takes decades rather than years to develop to the point where health is clinically impaired. The utility of diet-related preventive measures undertaken late in life, although possibly of benefit, is still unclear.

Some recent commentators have argued that for older people it is too late to achieve significant risk reduction for atherosclerosis by instituting dietary measures, and other expensive medical measures are now being used to deal with coronary artery disease in older people. For example, many older people have coronary artery bypass surgery or angioplasty to replace atherosclerotic vessels. It makes sense to delay the buildup of atherosclerotic plaque and to try to keep grafted arteries free of plaque as long as possible, by dietary and other means. Also, older people often live in families and eat meals that are prepared for people of younger ages who clearly stand to benefit from heart-healthy eating patterns. Risks of cancers of the colon, prostate, and breast, which may be associated with the type or amount of fat, also persist into old age, providing another possible rationale for stressing moderation in dietary fat intakes. Among older people who are extremely sedentary, high-fat, calorie-dense diets may increase risks of excessive calorie intakes and hence risks of obesity and associated diseases, such as non-insulin-dependent diabetes, high blood pressure, and gallstones.

There is little evidence that moderate decreases in dietary fat intakes from current levels are dangerous to older people if diets remain adequate in energy and other nutrients. Years ago when polyunsaturated fats were often substituted for saturated fats without lowering total fat intakes, it was claimed that excessive amounts of omega-3-polyunsaturated fatty acids caused cancer. However, more recent evidence does not support this.[15] Finally, although there is substantial evidence that very low serum cholesterol levels (below 150-160 mg/dl) are associated with increased morbidity and mortality, this is not a cause-and-effect relationship; rather, very low serum cholesterols often indicate the presence of other disease. Therefore, there are good reasons for lowering serum cholesterol levels, even among many of the elderly.

The National Cholesterol Education Program's Population Based Panel Report provided dietary advice for older adults similar to that for the young.[43] Namely, it suggested limiting total fat to 30% of calories, with no more than 10% of calories from saturates or polyunsaturates, and the remainder from monounsaturates. These and the *Dietary Guidelines for Americans*[58] represent reasonable goals toward which older Americans can strive. However, the knowledge base is still incomplete, and these recommendations must be interpreted in the light of the person's entire health profile. Fat modification is a particularly difficult issue on which to make general statements because older individuals may suffer from many complex disorders, each of which has dietary implications and each of which may require dietary alterations. They also are frequently afflicted with other health problems that need urgent attention. It is not possible to ameliorate every aspect of diet or health at once. Appropriate prevention and therapy focus on the problem that is most likely to affect quality of life, function, and morbidity. Thus priority setting needs to be done between informed patients and health care providers, given each individual's particular health characteristics. Active medical management of high serum cholesterol levels is usually restricted to the limited group of older individuals who are most likely to benefit from long-term therapy.[14] Both older men and postmenopausal women who are healthy and have active lifestyles and a good prognosis for an extended lifetime are good candidates for preventive and therapeutic efforts. In contrast, very old, frail, debilitated patients who are suffering from dementia, arthritis, osteoporosis, malignancy, or already very severe coronary disease need to be considered on an individual basis.

Dietary modification downward in amount of fat and cholesterol is the first step in treatment. Although it remains to be determined if changes in the omega-6 fatty acids:omega-3 fatty acids ratio interferes with immunological processes and aggravate inflammatory disorders, the best advice at present is that the nature of dietary fatty acids consumed by the elderly as well as by other groups should consist of less saturated and more unsaturated (both monounsaturated and polyunsaturated) fat. A goal is 30% of total calories, with no more than 10% from saturates and 10% from polyunsaturates. Increased amounts of food sources (not supplements) of the omega-3 fatty acids may be helpful, but supplements of fish oil may have undesirable and unknown effects and also add calories.

There is little reason for older Americans to eat more fat and cholesterol than they now eat, and a good case can be made for many to reduce current consumption levels of fat and saturated fat. However, recent studies of eating habits over the past decade suggest that overall intakes of dietary fat are not higher than in the rest of the population to begin with among the elderly and that they have not changed much.[48] This state of affairs may be due in part to lack of sound nutrition education, such as confusion about the difference between cholesterol in foods and cholesterol in blood, the relative strength of various dietary influences on serum cholesterol levels, and the extent of food choice changes that are necessary and how to go about making them without making undue sacrifices in the realm of taste.

It is important that fat intake not be reduced without substituting calories from other sources because the energy intakes of many elderly people are already often quite low. Sudden, drastic, unsupervised changes in fat intakes without appropriate caloric substitutions may precipitate weight loss. If anorexia is a problem, overzealous restriction of fat and substitution of a diet higher in bulk from complex carbohydrates and fiber might cause undesirable weight loss. For these reasons, prudence is warranted. Gradual changes help to avoid such complications. If energy intakes are very low, a vitamin-mineral supplement at RDA levels may be in order. The recent emphasis in advertising and some health promotion campaigns on foods to avoid rather than on foods to eat may have led some elders to make unwise, unbalanced, and inadequate food choices that they think are "healthy." Like others, the elderly must recognize that all foods, in moderation, can be included in a heart-healthy diet. In any event, individualized age- and condition-specific guidance is needed, especially for patients on medications and those who have other health problems.

Modifications in soluble dietary fiber, which also has a small lipid-lowering effect, are also helpful because many of the elderly have diets that are very low in fiber. Fruits, vegetables, and whole-grain products provide dietary fiber, vitamins, and minerals.

The extent to which dietary changes can or should be made varies from person to person. If the individual is a smoker or a poorly controlled diabetic, action on these risk factors may take precedence. If serum cholesterol levels are very high, drug therapy may be utilized as well.

The current edition of the *Recommended Dietary Allowances*[23] treats all adults over age 51 as one group for specific nutrient recommendations other than energy because of the lack of data on nutrient requirements in older people. Prudence is warranted in approaching dietary changes in the elderly in view of the gaps in our knowledge and the many illnesses and conditions that many older people suffer. The most appropriate and beneficial dietary changes an older person can make depend on individual health priorities, risks, and desires, as jointly arrived at by physician and patient and communicated to the dietitian or nutritionist. *Dietary Guidelines for Americans*[58] is a suitable framework on which to build individualized recommendations.

Obesity and weight control measures need to be individualized for elderly people who need to lose weight. There is still a good deal of dispute about the most appropriate weight goals for older Americans. These issues are discussed at length elsewhere.[18] There is little evidence that older individuals who are already at healthy weights gain more weight as they get older. Involuntary losses of weight may indicate disease or other adverse life events that need remediation and should not be automatically regarded as good in themselves. In most instances, all other things being equal to at least age 80, weight goals similar to those for younger adults are appropriate. However, these standards are based on mortality data from younger individuals, whereas the obesity-related problems most immediately relevant to the elderly person's situation are the morbidities and consequent decrements in quality of life that might be averted if obesity were lessened or prevented. If the older individual is not obese and not suffering from obesity-associated symptoms, there is nothing to be gained from restricting calories simply to reduce weight to some theoretical ideal level because among the elderly very low body weights also carry risk. If they are overly fat, as many older people are, even losses of 5 to 10 pounds may alter glucose tolerance, blood pressure, pain in weight-bearing joints, and other health indicators in more favorable directions. Therefore, even relatively modest weight losses may be helpful in improving quality of life and function. Among those who are confined to their homes or to an institution because of infirmities, a worthwhile goal may be simply to stave off future weight gains, which may worsen weight-associated conditions and make care more difficult. After age 80, because of losses of bone, water, and lean body mass, generalization about appropriate weight goals is difficult, and indications for weight reduction must be evaluated on an individual basis. Weight reduction is best achieved by physical activity as well as dietary measures when it is needed. It is now recognized that low energy outputs in older people are neither inevitable nor desirable. When possible, more physically active lives should be encouraged in people of all ages, including the elderly. Among the elderly obese, energy intakes are usually very low, particularly in very old individuals, because lean body mass and thus resting energy expenditure as well as physical activity are low. Vigorous physical activity may not be possible owing to other infirmities. Under such circumstances, only modest energy deficits and very gradual weight loss are in order to avoid unduly rigorous deprivation in dietary intakes and unnecessary depletion of lean body mass.[17]

Malnutrition occurs more frequently in ambulatory elderly patients who are poor, socially isolated, and above age 70, have multiple chronic diseases, and have had relatively recent changes in mental status than in others in the same age group.[41] Although undernutrition due solely to lack of food is rare, it does occur, owing both to poverty and to abuse and neglect. For these reasons it is important to screen the elderly not only for weight status and disease-related factors[36] but also for so-

cial and functional status[19] and to utilize food programs, nutritional counseling, and other social and medical interventions, as appropriate.

PHYSICAL ACTIVITY, EXERCISE, AND OBESITY RECOMMENDATIONS

More than half of all Americans over 65 years of age and at least a third of those aged 45 to 64 are currently less active than the levels experts consider appropriate, based on the 1990 objectives for the nation for promoting health and preventing disease.[9] Regular exercise and physically active lifestyles are associated with improved function and lessened symptoms of some of the chronic degenerative diseases and may also decrease mortality.[54] Also, immobility is associated with increased risk of institutionalization. Thus improvements in functional capacity through appropriate choices of physical activity and exercise are important in addition to dietary measures in improving quality of life among the elderly.

Obviously choosing appropriate forms of physical activity for older adults requires special care because they vary even more than younger persons in exercise tolerance and health status. Guides are now available for doing this.[20] Briefly, older adults should be urged to engage in light to moderate physical activity for at least 30 minutes a day. They should all engage in some leisure activity. Moreover, more accommodations need to be made for them so that they have increased access to hiking trails, parks, and other community recreational facilities. For those whose health status is impaired, individualized exercise and physical activity programs are needed.

SERVICES AT THE LOCAL LEVEL

The goals of nutrition programs for the elderly in the community are to promote independent living, to help support the frail elderly, and to provide networking and advocacy with and for them.

The continuum of community nutrition support begins with the well elderly who are relatively independent. The continuum also should, but does not always, include support of those who are frail and semidependent and need help to continue to live at home through maintaining community links to those who are institutionalized.[47] Nutrition education and counseling programs are gradually becoming more widely available.

For the well elderly who are able to care for themselves at home, services include the various food programs of the U.S. Department of Agriculture, such as food stamps and commodity supplemental foods and the Congregate Meals Program sponsored by the Administration on Aging of the U.S. Department of Health and Human Services. Services to combat food emergencies due to homelessness, inadequate or uncertain food supplies, and illness are also available in some municipalities. Community-sponsored programs have encouraged restaurants to provide low-priced meals that permit elders to dine out in the afternoon and early evening at reduced cost. Older Americans are often very interested in nutrition, and well-crafted community nutrition education programs at senior citizen centers and elsewhere attract rapt audiences if the topics are really those that the elderly want and need. These programs include supermarket tours and cooking demonstrations with special attention to good choices for those who have health problems that require special dietary management, discussions of nutrition topics that are currently being discussed in the mass media, and explanations of policy changes and means of obtaining access to food assistance programs or other services for elders.[52] Congregate meals for the elderly provided by Title III C of the Older Americans Act and meetings at senior citizen centers sponsored by churches and other groups are sites that are frequently ripe for such programs. Excellent guides are now available for menu planning and incorporating innovative educational programs into such settings.[50] The American Association of Retired Persons has produced several slide-tape programs, complete with notes, with useful materials for such presentations.

For older Americans living at home who need more support to continue semi-independent living, food shopping, transportation, and assistance services are often sponsored by the area agencies on aging, churches, community businesses, or voluntary groups. Homemaker and chore services provide reliable individuals who can assist the elderly living at home with meal planning, shopping, and other necessary tasks to maintain independence. Those who are frail—that is, impaired in their abilities to perform the activities of daily living without considerable help or afflicted with diseases and conditions that make usual ambulatory care inappropriate—need additional supportive services, including accessible outpatient nutrition counseling integrated with comprehensive primary care for the geriatric patient with a special focus on maintaining independent function. Counseling and nutrition support through home health services and community visiting nurse associations help these individuals deal with their special problems. Home-delivered meal programs, home health aides, and other homemaker services help to overcome potential problems in getting, preparing, and eating food. Nutrition, cooking, and food-related education may help those who assist in the care of the frail elderly. If the individual is unable to eat without assistance, dietitians and nutritionists specializing in rehabilitation medicine and occupational therapists are available in many community hospitals for consultation on the use of assistive devices and appropriate methods for feeding the individual if necessary. Some communities have sheltered housing that permits the older person to live independently, while providing some nursing and other assistance services on site. In other communities day-care services that provide sheltered settings, supervision, and one or more meals a day are available for elderly persons with particular impairments. Such services are helpful in assisting caretakers with older persons who are demented and unable to stay at home all day. Respite care services provide temporary support of elderly persons living at home when their usual caretakers are unable to carry out their usual functions owing to special circumstances or to emotional stress and fatigue. Hospice services that assist in supporting palliative nutritional care at home or in a sheltered group care facility in the community for those who are terminally ill are also becoming available.

Finally, community nutrition programs must continue to provide services to older Americans who are institutionalized and who return home after stays in institutions. Retirement homes, board and care facilities providing some personal care for older people, and nursing homes providing both intermediate and skilled care must all provide for the food and nutritional needs of their residents. Usually some monitoring and surveillance of standards for these services is provided by state licensing boards and by the conditions required for participation in Medicare and Medicaid programs. However, the realities of time and money available to accrediting agencies make it impossible to assure that the standards of nutritional care and food services are always met. The involvement of community nutrition services in providing advocacy, education, and technical assistance to those who operate these programs can do much to ensure that high-quality services are provided. Nutrition education of patients has a somewhat different focus than it does among the free-living and healthier elderly because most of institutionalized patients' food is provided by the facility and their health status is usually compromised. Therefore, education of staff at all levels is also essential. Also vital is involvement of community nutritionists in assisting with transitions from one level of care to another so that special dietary needs are adequately dealt with as the individual moves from one setting to another. Such transitions include discharges from acute care hospitals to long-term care facilities, homes, and hospices. Advocacy and networking to improve food and nutrition programs and services for older Americans in all settings must continue.

Nutrition and other services for older Americans today vary enormously at the local level. Several resources are available for guiding the organization in use of local resources.[21] Several organizations at the local level in most communities provide services to older Americans:

- County health departments
- Visiting nurse associations
- Cooperative extension offices
- Local chapters of voluntary groups, such as the Gray Panthers, American Association of Retired Persons, Older Women's League, Red Cross, and church-based social services
- Congregate or home-delivered meal sites
- Departments of nutrition, geriatrics, or dietetics in local hospitals

SERVICES AT THE STATE AND NATIONAL LEVEL

The Administration on Aging is the part of the federal government that has the specific mission of looking after federally sponsored services for older Americans. The National Center for Health Promotion and Aging at the federal level coordinates state and local health-related efforts and serves as a clearinghouse for them. The National Institutes of Aging at the National Institutes of Health is devoted to fundamental and applied research on all aspects of aging.

Although there are few well-organized and wide-scale truly national efforts, a few particularly valuable services are likely to be present nationwide. They include:

- State commissions and units on aging and state public health departments
- Area Agencies on Aging, located in each region of the country in the U.S. Department of Health and Human Services Regional Office
- State or local American Dietetic Association chapters

NEW DIRECTIONS

The model of public health or community nutrition that is based solely on providing primary prevention services to the elderly is outdated. It is particularly inappropriate for dealing with and ameliorating health problems faced by the growing numbers of very old, impaired, and disabled people who are trying to live more or less independently in the community.[24] The nutritional problems they face involve control and amelioration of disease-related disabilities, not simply primary prevention. Public health and community nutrition efforts, which have traditionally focused on primary preventive services, are inadequate for dealing with these problems, as are strategies designed primarily for young or middle-aged individuals whose health and life circumstances are very different from those of the elderly. One hopeful development is the dawning recognition that public health nutrition can and should also involve diet therapy and ameliorative measures. During the next few decades, both preventive and curative health services involving nutrition must be extended beyond physician offices and clinics and into all the settings in which the elderly live if we are to maximize their ability to live and function independently for as long as possible. A large number of specific health problems with nutritional implications are now often left to visiting nurse services or home care companies, but those generalists who provide such nutritional care at present often lack specific training in clinical nutrition, dietetics, geriatrics, and gerontology.

Better cross-training of generalist health professionals in the delivery of nutrition services, extension of the scope of dietetic and nutrition services into new settings (such as home care and an active instead of simply a consultative role in visiting nurse associations), and better integration of health care services with community social services will be required to deal with the needs of ill older people living in the community.

INNOVATIVE MODELS

Some hopeful innovative developments for lessening the nutrition problems of older Americans are in place and are described in this section. Others are suggested in recent documents.[1]

The American Association of Retired Persons has developed a series of useful programs in such topics as eating a good diet, making living and food preparation arrangements suitable and safe, and sources for obtaining devices for help with eating. It also has an active program for helping older people recognize and avoid quackery and fraud, including nutrition-related quackery.

The elder hostel program combines travel and attendance at short-course classes in special sessions at various colleges in this country and abroad. At some, nutrition is among the course offerings.

"Retirement courses" that focus on the foodways of older adults and assistance with special nutrition-related questions and problems are increasing in popularity.[13] Many older people change their food purchasing, preparation, and consumption habits in the years after they retire, and they are often ready for advice about nutrition at that time.

The Nutrition Screening Initiative is a 5-year project devoted to promoting routine nutrition screening and better nutrition care in America's health care system, particularly among the elderly. It is a joint effort of the American Academy of Family Physicians, the American Dietetic Association, and the National Council on Aging. Among its efforts was a consensus conference that reached agreement among a group of medical, social service, and nutrition experts on standards to use in screening and assessment of older people. It is also actively involved in extending screening into primary health care and other community settings.

Hospital discharge planners are beginning to be more sophisticated about taking into account patients' needs for nutritional services after discharge. In some hospitals, dietitians and nutritionists function on the social service staff as discharge planners. They help to link older persons to the entire range of services in the community.

Several home care services now include a full-time dietitian or nutritionist who functions as a consultant, referral source, and quality control expert in addition to providing limited amounts of direct nutritional care to patients who need special enteral and parenteral support. In addition, the dietitian or nutritionist is active in professional education. Another hospital-based program is a nutrition support clinic for older and younger patients requiring special routes for the provision of nutrition. Still a third service provides complete home medical care services to the very old and frail, including visits by the physician to the patient's home.

Apartment houses and other congregate living arrangements for older people now sometimes include staffing by nurse clinical specialists on site, with 24-hour on-call services to deal with the health problems of individuals living in the unit. A few such services also include periodic visits by a dietitian or nutritionist.

One department store chain has developed a

"department" that is actually a health promotion club for older Americans. Membership fees are low. In addition to having a place to meet, a variety of social and educational programs are provided, including programs on nutrition education.

In many parts of the country walking clubs for older people are now popular. In some places, local parks and recreation departments have cooperated and plotted out an appropriate measured walking course. Mall walking is another activity that is gaining in popularity. Many malls have established hours, before the stores open, when the facility is totally available to walkers. For those older people who are on their own and fear for their security, mall walking is a pleasant and safe activity. In some communities, fitness classes for older people are available with various types and levels offered for those at different fitness levels or for those with special problems. People find it more fun to work with others who are close to their own levels with respect to fitness and skill. Wellness programs in which nutrition education and exercise are combined are also popular. These programs are further enhanced by the fun and social activities that follow the exercise and discussion sessions.

More good ideas for innovative programs at the local level can be obtained from the National Resource Center on Health Promotion and Aging, which is part of the AARP, at 601 E Street, NW, Washington, D.C. 20049.

SUMMARY

The goal of all preventive and curative efforts among aging adults is to extend the years of healthy life and function as long as possible. It is best accomplished by earlier identification of nutrition- and health-related problems and of social and economic problems that may threaten independence. Realizing the goal requires greater integration of public, private, and voluntary services aimed at improving the nutritional status of older people than is yet present. Also, more efforts must be devoted to the task. Therefore, older Americans themselves must be intimately involved in these efforts.

The blueprint for making progress has been provided by the *Year 2000 Goals for Promoting Health and Preventing Disease,*[60] which was recently released by the U.S. Department of Health and Human Services. It recognizes that changing the American diets, including the diets of older Americans, will require efforts not only in the health services but also in our educational systems, the mass media, the food industry, and government programs.

In conclusion, professionals and others who deal with older Americans need a view of nutrition that focuses on living, quality of life, and function rather than solely on the clinical aspects of treatment. More attention should be given to achieving greater integration of preventive and curative health services and to assuring that the social, emotional, and economic supports all of us need as we grow older are provided. Doing this is a worthy agenda for the twenty-first century.

REFERENCES

1. Abdellah FG, Moore SR, editors: *Surgeon General's workshop: health promotion and aging,* Washington, DC, 1989, US Department of Health and Human Services.
2. Adams WL and others: Alcohol intake in the healthy elderly: changes with age in a cross sectional and longitudinal study, *J Am Geriatr Soc* 38:211, 1990.
3. Anderson SA and others: *Core indicators of nutritional state for vulnerable and difficult to sample populations,* Bethesda, Md, 1990, Life Sciences Research Office, Federation of American Societies for Experimental Biology.
4. Barry PP, Ibarra M: Multidimensional assessment of the elderly, *Hosp Pract* [Off], p 117, April 15, 1990.
5. Berg RL, and Cassells SS, editors: *The Second Fifty Years: Promoting Health and Preventing Disabilities,* Institute of Medicine, 1990, National Academy Press, Washington, DC.
6. Berlinger WG, Potter JF: Low body mass index in demented outpatients, *Am Geriatr Soc* 39:973, 1991.
7. Block G, Lanza E: Dietary fiber sources in the United States by demographic group, *J Natl Cancer Inst* 79:83, 1987.
8. Braneis GH and others: The epidemiology and natural history of pressure ulcers in elderly nursing home residents, *JAMA* 264:2905, 1990.
9. Caspersen CI, Christenson GM, Pollard RA: Status of the 1990 physical fitness and exercise objectives: evidence from the National Health Interview Survey 1985, *Public Health Rep* 101:587, 1986.
10. Chumlea WC, Roche AF, Mukherjee D: Nutritional assessment of the elderly through anthropometry, Columbus, Ohio, 1984, Ross Laboratories.
11. Committee on Diet and Health: *Recommendations to reduce chronic disease risk,* Washington, DC, 1989, Institute of Medicine, National Academy Press.

12. Consensus Development Conference. Conference report: consensus development conference: prophylaxis and treatment of osteoporosis, *Am J Med* 90:107, 1991.

13. Davies L: Retirement courses: should they include nutrition? *J R Soc Health* 110:20, 1990.

14. Denke MA, Grundy SM: Hypercholesterolemia in elderly persons: resolving the treatment dilemma, *Ann Intern Med* 112:780, 1990.

15. Dolecek TA, Grandits G: *Dietary polyunsaturated fatty acids and mortality in the Multiple Risk Factor Intervention Trial (MRFIT)*. In Simopoulos AP and others, editors: *Health effects of omega 3 polyunsaturated fatty acids in seafoods, World Rev Nutr Diet*, Basel, Karger 66:205, 1991.

16. Dwyer JT: *Screening older Americans' nutritional health: current practices and future possibilities*. Washington, DC, 1991. Nutrition Screening Initiative.

17. Dwyer JT: Treatment of obesity: conventional programs and fad diets. In Bjortorp P, Brodoff BN, editors: *Obesity*, Philadelphia, 1992, JB Lippincott.

18. Dwyer JT: *Medical evaluation and assessment of obesity*. In Blackburan G, Kanders B, editors: *Obesity* (in press).

19. Elam JT and others: Comparison of subjective ratings of function with observed functional ability of frail older persons, *Am J Public Health* 81:1127, 1991.

20. Evans W, Rosenberg I: *Biomarkers*, New York, 1991, William Morrow.

21. Fallcreek S, Mettler M, editors: *A healthy old age: a source book for health promotion with older adults*, New York, 1984, Haworth Press.

22. Folstein MF, Folstein SE, McHugh PR: Minimental state: a practical method for grading the cognitive state of patients for the clinician, *J Psychiatr Res* 12:189, 1975.

23. Food and Nutrition Board, Subcommittee on the Tenth Edition of the RDA: *Recommended dietary allowances*, Washington, DC, 1989, National Academy Press.

24. Ford AB, and others: Impaired and disabled elderly in the community, *Am J Public Health* 81:1207, 1992.

25. Franklin CA, Karkeck J: Weight loss and senile dementia in an institutionalized elderly population, *J Am Diet Assoc* 89:790, 1989.

26. French CE, Stare FJ: Nutritional surveys in Western Holland, J Nutr 33:649, 1947.

27. Frisancho AR: New norms of upper limb fat and muscle areas for assessment of nutritional status, *Am J Clin Nutr* 34:2540, 1981.

28. Frisancho AR: New standards of weight and body composition in frames, size and height for assessment of nutritional status of adults and the elderly, *Am J Clin Nutr* 40:814, 1984.

29. Gans KM and others: A cholesterol screening and education program: differences between older and younger adults, *J Nutr Educ* 22:275, 1990.

30. Gift HC: Issues of aging and oral health promotion, *Gerodontics* 4:194, 1988.

31. Gotto AM: Cholesterol intake and serum cholesterol level, *N Engl J Med* 324:912, 1991.

32. Hackman RM, Wagner EL: The senior gardening and nutrition project: development and transport of a dietary behavior change and health promotion program, *J Nutr Educ* 22:262, 1990.

33. Hermann JR and others: Effect of a cooperative extension nutrition and exercise program for older adults on nutrition knowledge, dietary intake, anthropometric measurements, and serum lipids, *J Nutr Ed* 22:271, 1990.

34. Institute of Medicine: *Depression*. In Berg RL, Cassells JS, editors: *The second fifty years: promoting health and preventing disability*, Washington, DC, 1990, National Academy Press.

35. Katz S, Stroud MW: Functional assessment in geriatrics: a review of progress and directions, *J Am Geriatr Soc* 37:267, 1989.

36. Kubena KS and others: Anthropometry and health in the elderly, *J Am Diet Assoc* 91:1402, 1991.

37. Lamy PP, Michocki RJ: Medication management, *Clin Geriatr Med* 4:623, 1988.

38. Levine WC and others: Food borne disease outbreaks in nursing homes 1975-87, *JAMA* 255:2105, 1991.

39. Levy AS, Schucker RE: Patterns of nutrient intake among dietary supplement users: attitudinal and behavioral correlates, *J Am Diet Assoc* 87:754, 1987.

40. Life Sciences Research Office: *Nutrition monitoring in the United States: an update report on nutrition monitoring prepared for the US Department of Agriculture and the US Department of Health and Human Services*, Washington, DC, 1989, US Government Printing Office.

41. Manson A, Shea S: Malnutrition in elderly ambulatory medical patients, *Am J Public Health* 81:1195, 1991.

42. National Center for Health Statistics: *Current estimates from the National Health Information Survey United States, 1985 Vital and Health Statistics series 10, no 160, 1986*. In Fulton JP, Katz S: *Aging and rehabilitation: advances in state of the art* by Brody SJ, Riff GE, editors, New York, 1986, Springer.

43. National Cholesterol Education Program Population Based Panel Report, National Cholesterol Education Program, National Heart, Lung and Blood Institute, Washington, DC, 1990, Department of Health and Human Services.

44. National Institute of Dental Research: *Oral health of United States adults: national findings*, US Department of Health and Human Services (NIH) Pub 87-2868 Washington, DC, 1987, US Government Printing Office.

45. Nutrition Screening Initiative: *Report of nutrition screening a: toward a common view*, Washington, DC, 1991, Nutrition Screening Initiative.

46. Patterson BH and others: Fruit and vegetables in the American diet: data from the NHANES II survey, *Am J Public Health* 80:1442, 1990.

47. Phillips HT, Gaylord SH, editors: *Aging and public health*, New York, 1985, Springer.

48. Popkin BM, Haines PS, Patterson R: Dietary changes among older Americans, *Am J Clin Nutr* 55:823-839, 1992.

49. Potter JF, Schafer DF, Bohi RL: In hospital mortality as a function of body mass index: an age dependent variable, *J Gerontol* 43:M59, 1988.

50. Rhodes SS, editor, and Gerontological Nutritionists: *Effective menu planning for the elderly nutrition program*, Chicago, 1991, American Dietetic Association.

51. Riggs L, Melton LJ: Involutional osteoporosis, *N Engl J Med* 314:1676, 1986.

52. Roe D: *The elderly in our society*. In Roe D, editor: *Geriatric nutrition*, ed 3, Englewood Cliffs, NJ, 1992, Prentice Hall.

53. Ryan KC, Bower ME: Relationship of socioeconomic status and living arrangements to nutritional intake of the older person, *J Am Diet Assoc* 89:1805, 1989.

54. Shephard RJ: The scientific basis of exercise prescribing for the very old, *J Am Geriatr Soc* 38:62, 1990.

55. Tayback M, Kumayika S, Chee E: Body weight as a risk factor in the elderly, *Arch Intern Med* 150:1065, 1990.

56. Thompson MP, Morris LK: Unexplained weight loss in the ambulatory elderly, *J Am Gerontol Soc* 39:497, 1991.

57. US Bureau of the Census: *Projections for the population of the United States by age, sex, and race, 1989 to 2080*, Current Population Report Series P 25, No 1018, Washington, DC, 1989, US Bureau of the Census.

58. US Department of Agriculture, US Department of Health and Human Services: *Dietary guidelines for Americans*, ed 3, Washington, DC, 1990, US Government Printing Office.

59. U.S. Department of Health and Human Services, National Institute on Alcohol Abuse and Alcoholism: *Toward a national plan to combat alcohol abuse and alcoholism: A report to the United States Congress*, Washington, DC, 1981, US Government Printing Office.

60. U.S. Department of Health and Human Services, Public Health Service: *Healthy people 2000: national health promotion and disease prevention objectives*, DHHS Pub (PHS) 91-50213, Washington, DC, 1991, US Government Printing Office.

61. U.S. Preventive Health Services Task Force: *Clinical guide to preventive services*, DHHS, Washington, DC, 1990, U.S. Government Printing Office.

62. Williams ME: Identifying the older person likely to require long term care services, *J Am Geriatr Soc* 35:761, 1987.

63. Woolf SH and others: The periodic health examination of older adults: the recommendations of the US preventive services task force part II screening test, *J Am Geriatr Soc* 38:933, 1990.

PART

3

Developing Effective Community Nutrition Strategies

10 Managing Change with Nutrition Education

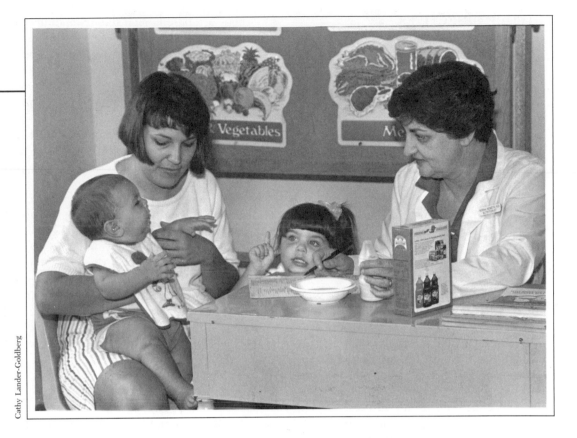

GENERAL CONCEPT

Successful nutrition education in the community involves learning to manage change in people's eating behaviors and the forces that shape it. This chapter describes a multilevel approach for understanding how people make food choices and change eating patterns and introduces six theoretical frameworks that elaborate on this approach. Next, nutrition education applications of models for behavior change, including individual-level nutrition counseling, group programs, and community- or population-based approaches to improving nutrition, are presented.

OUTCOME OBJECTIVES

When you finish this chapter, you should be able to:

- Identify two or more ways in which an understanding of human behavior is important for delivering effective nutrition services.
- Describe the characteristics of the changing environment of eating behavior that create a dynamic context for nutrition education.
- Explain the value of a multilevel approach for understanding how people make food choices, and specify the key concepts of six models for understanding and influencing dietary behavior.
- Describe the key elements of applications of nutrition education to promote healthy eating patterns at each of three levels.

WHY UNDERSTANDING BEHAVIOR IS IMPORTANT

Promoting healthy eating behavior is the central goal of nutrition education. For nutrition education to be effective, the educator must understand health behavior related to nutrition and transform that knowledge into useful strategies to enhance health. This understanding then needs to be combined with technical knowledge about nutrition and dietary recommendations. It also needs to be put into practice in the community, because healthy dietary patterns can be truly effective only if they are sustained over the long term. This means that attention must be directed not only at understanding individual food consumption but also toward the forces affecting behaviors of the many different people involved in the production, sale, supply, purchase, and preparation of food.

Understanding eating behavior establishes the foundation for why we think certain strategies will be successful. It makes possible a conceptual, analytical way of thinking about what we do. It allows us to generalize our experience and that of others, allowing us to recognize different types of dietary change, different kinds of individuals and communities, and various constraints on delivering nutrition education. Recommendations for changing eating habits are more likely to have an impact if they are based on an understanding of factors that affect food choices.[26]

As is the case for many lifestyle behaviors that influence health and disease, people do not always think about food choices as health actions on a daily basis. Yet behavior change for better nutrition often requires changes in well-established daily habits. With eating behavior in particular, it is important to remember that most diet-related health problems develop gradually and do not present immediate or dramatic symptoms. Recommendations for dietary change are usually restrictive; that is, they involve giving something up, and they may be incompatible with personal and family eating habits. In addition, there may be barriers such as food costs, access, and the skill, time, and effort necessary for food preparation that constrain compliance with both health-promoting and therapeutic diets.[6] When they are based on an understanding of the determinants of food choices, nutrition education strategies have a much greater chance of producing positive change.

FOOD CHOICE IN A CHANGING ENVIRONMENT

We live in a rapidly changing environment. Major social changes over the past few decades have transformed the way we live, work, play, and eat. There are more women in the work force, changes in family structure, rapidly emerging computer technologies, an information explosion, and increases in the speed of communication.

The food supply in the United States has also changed dramatically. It has changed in the face of new production and preparation techniques, the societal changes just mentioned, and consumer interest in healthier products. Some changes, such as the production of leaner beef and pork products, make healthier foods more accessible. More processed food products are being produced and marketed with a health focus. Reduced-calorie, low- and reduced-sodium, high-fiber, and cholesterol-free products now abound on grocery shelves.[8]

New product developments are a way of life in the competitive food industry. Each year thousands of new products appear on the shelves of supermarkets. Yet many of the new products would not make very nutritious contributions to the diet. The challenge of making informed choices is growing as time pressure to select and prepare food while maintaining busy schedules leaves less time for consumers to learn about what is available.

The changing environment presents new and continual challenges for nutrition education. We need to find new ways to reach people that fit into their lives. We cannot rely on memorization of information but need to equip people with skills and tools to navigate the ever-changing scenery. Our advice cannot be rigid, but must be adaptable for a variety of lifestyles and eating environments. New trends in the way people eat and the roles of food in their lives challenge nutrition educators to remain current and anticipate changes that lie ahead.

A MULTILEVEL APPROACH IS NECESSARY

Nutrition education in the community includes not only instructional activities but also organizational efforts, policy directives, environmental activities, and community-level programs. The development, maintenance, and change of eating patterns are determined not only by individual factors but also by many social, cultural, and environmental influences. Physiological and psychological factors, acquired food preferences, and knowledge about foods are significant individual determinants of food intake. Interpersonal or social factors are also important: family ties and other close relationships often affect food purchase, preparation, and consumption. Socioeconomic status, economic change, and social support have an important impact on eating patterns that may even be reflected in the prevalence of nutrition-related diseases. Culture, geography, and food availability may increase or limit the range of food choices.

A multilevel, ecological perspective is necessary to a broad understanding of nutrition behavior and the opportunities for nutrition education. Behavior both affects and is affected by multiple levels of determinants.[10,15] McLeroy and associates[15] have identified five distinct sets of factors comprising an ecological perspective on health promotion:

1. *Intrapersonal factors*—characteristics of the individual, such as knowledge, attitudes, behavior, and skills

2. *Interpersonal processes and primary groups*—formal and informal social network and social support systems, including family, work group, and friendship networks

3. *Institutional factors*—social institutions with organizational characteristics and formal (and informal) rules and regulations for operation

4. *Community factors*—relationships among organizations, institutions, and informal networks within defined boundaries

5. *Public policy*—local, state, and national laws and policies

This chapter focuses on three distinct levels of understanding and changing dietary behavior: the intrapersonal, or individual, level; the interpersonal level; and the organizational-community level (see Chapter 12). These levels often overlap and should be considered as working in combinations. Each successively "higher" or "larger" level incorporates concepts from the "lower" or "smaller" level; thus groups are made up of individuals, and communities are composed of individuals and groups. Comprehensive community nutrition education efforts draw on understanding and strategies from each level at various times.

MODELS FOR UNDERSTANDING AND INFLUENCING DIETARY BEHAVIOR

Using a multilevel perspective, this section presents six theoretical models that are particularly useful for understanding the determinants of dietary behavior and the processes of changing eating patterns to improve health. The models each include two theories at the intrapersonal, interpersonal, and organizational-community levels.[7]

The first four models—consumer information processing (CIP), stages of change, social cognitive therapy (SCT), and relapse prevention—all fall within the broad category of cognitive-behavioral models. Cognitions are personal thought processes used as frames of reference, including knowledge, beliefs, expectations, attitudes, and perceptions. In cognitive-behavioral models, behavior is viewed as linked with, and even reciprocally related to, cognitions. In a general sense, these models view behavior as mediated through people's knowledge of what to do, what they think about it, and how these merge within their personal worlds.

The last two models—community organization and diffusion of innovations—concern how we can more effectively spread the adoption of healthier eating habits within and among organizations and communities. They are important to community nutrition because a populationwide impact depends on widespread practice of healthy behaviors and not just an accumulation of individual changes.

For each of the six models, a brief statement of the rationale for applying it to nutrition behavior and education is first presented: how does it help us understand eating behavior, so that it can inform more effective nutrition education strategies? It is followed by a description of the central elements of the theory that are applicable to nutrition education. The next section of this chapter illustrates practical adaptations of these models for nutrition education in the community. Throughout, the focus is on how to use and benefit from the use of the models in designing and delivering nutrition education services.

Consumer Information Processing

Rationale

Knowledge is necessary, but it is not sufficient to enable people to follow guidelines for healthy eating.[6,26] Knowledge of disease processes in nutrition-related conditions has not consistently been found to be associated with healthy eating. However, instrumental or how-to knowledge about how to choose nutritious foods *is* necessary for people to be able to follow guidelines for healthy eating. Although basic nutrition knowledge is at an all-time high, many people lack an understanding of how to apply specific nutrition advice to the foods they eat every day.[8] Misconceptions and misinterpretations of nutritional guidance reduce the chances that people will make wise food choices.

The nutrition information environment can be complex and confusing. Because nutrition education contains a great deal of information and because people need to apply it in everyday situations, nutrition educators must rely heavily on printed materials. Even the best oral communication to patients or consumers can result in misunderstanding and memory failure over time. However, many nutrition education materials are written at too sophisticated a level in terms of their wording and concepts. It is clearly important to understand how people use information and to pay careful attention to the way information is presented if nutrition education is to be effective.

Description

Consumer information processing (CIP) theory grew out of the study of consumer behavior in the late 1970s. It has its roots in the domain of cognitive psychology, mainly in the areas of human problem solving and information processing.[24] A central premise of CIP is that individuals can process only a limited amount of information at one time.[2]

CIP is not a single unified theory but rather a conceptual framework that draws on theories of cognition, decision making, and behavior change. From a CIP perspective, consumer decision making is a multistage process of information acquisition and evaluation (search), decision making, use, and learning. As set forth by Bettman, the CIP framework assumes a continuous and reciprocal interaction among elements.[2,24] The central processes in Bettman's model are information acquisition and evaluation; people tend to seek only enough information to make a satisfactory choice, not necessarily the best choice. In addition, people develop heuristics or rules of thumb to help them make choices within their limited information-processing capacity.[2]

There are several implications of consumer information processing theory for nutrition education. One relates to the minimum necessary conditions for consumers to make use of nutrition information: it must be available, it must be considered useful, it must not be confusing, and it must be processable within the effort and comprehension level of the individual. It should also be placed so it is easily accessible at the time of decision making.[24] Thus effective nutrition information should be tailored to the comprehension level of the audience, matched to their past experience and lifestyles, be readily visible, and be portable or available at or near the point of food selection. Information that indicates that specific food items are healthier food choices, presented at the point of choice, has the greatest chance of being easy to use with limited effort.

Concepts from consumer information processing can improve our ability to provide useful nutrition information for making healthy food choices. The elements of CIP can be used during program development, for example, in needs assessment and pretesting of communications. By using CIP concepts, it is possible to match the most effective type, format, and quantity of information with a specific target population.

Stages of Change
Rationale
Changes in eating patterns involve multiple steps and adaptations over time. People may or may not be "ready" to try to change at a given time. For example, even when people are informed that they are at risk for serious health problems that can be controlled through dietary change, some do not successfully modify their eating patterns. This may be true of a person with multiple risk factors or for whom dietary risk is asymptomatic (such as a high blood cholesterol level). It may be that, because of competing demands and the need to set priorities, nutrition does not get much attention even when it is clearly warranted.

A great deal of research in the area of smoking cessation and substance abuse has indicated that people vary in their "readiness" to change.[20] Emerging research on adoption of low-fat eating patterns in healthy populations suggests that this idea also applies to nutrition behavior.

Irrespective of medical need or medically diagnosed risk, people may be at various stages of receptivity for learning and using nutrition advice. By applying this idea to the process of dietary change, interventions can be designed to reach, motivate, and teach people who are more or less ready to make significant attempts to improve their eating behavior.

Description
The stages of change model is part of a broader transtheoretical model of the behavior change process developed by Prochaska and DiClemente.[20] The central assumption of the model is that behavior change is a dynamic process involving several distinct stages. At any point in time, people may be at various stages along a continuum of change readiness: precontemplation (unaware, not interested in change), contemplation (thinking about changing), determination or preparation (becoming determined to change), action (actively modifying habits or environment), maintenance (maintaining the new, healthier habits), or relapse (returning to the old behavior).[20]

People are believed to recycle and repeat rather than to move through the stages in a straight line, and they can enter or exit at any point. Moreover, the stages appear to be similar whether people seek professional help or attempt change on their own.[20]

The stages of change model has direct application to nutrition education. Program strategies must be available to match people's stage in the change process, or they will not be reached at all. For example, if someone with high cholesterol who is consuming a high-fat diet has not begun to think about changing, there is no point in providing detailed nutrition information and food preparation tips. It would be more effective to try to increase that person's awareness and personal health concern before introducing action strategies.

The stages of change model has important implications not only for planning nutrition education strategies but also for the way success is defined in nutrition education and counseling: it suggests that movement through the stages is a mark of effectiveness, not just the traditional end points of behavior change or maintenance. This way, a wider range of intermediary steps can be viewed as successful, or at least positive, outcomes that eventually may lead to improved eating behavior.

Social Cognitive Theory
Rationale
As discussed earlier, it is widely recognized that food choices are determined by a complex set of

factors within individuals, in their primary social groups, and in the environment. Their personal knowledge and beliefs, the beliefs of important others, and the accessibility of foods all influence what they eat.[14,26] The relative importance of healthfulness and other qualities of food (taste, cost, convenience, etc.) are weighed in the context of the environment and social influences. The importance of family support and social support from others involved in the process are important to initiating and maintaining dietary changes.

Given the importance of both personal factors and social and environmental influences on the development of eating habits and the process of dietary change, social cognitive theory (SCT) suggests fruitful directions for designing and implementing nutrition education programs.

Description

SCT postulates dynamic relationships among personal factors, the social and physical environment, and observable behavior.[1] These dynamic relationships are conceptualized in the central construct of reciprocal determinism, which means that a person can both be an agent for and a respondent to change.

In SCT, change is considered to be mediated by cognitive factors rather than in a strict "behaviorist" stimulus-response manner.[1] SCT is the cognitive version of social learning theory and comes from a long tradition of learning theory that has, over the years, placed increasing emphasis on cognitive processes as important forces along with behavioral responses to external reinforcements (e.g., reward and punishment).[19] SCT incorporates the basic concepts of behavior modification in conjunction with cognitive, interpersonal, and environmental influences on behavior.

Social cognitive theory includes many concepts, only a few of which are highlighted here. They include environment, observational learning, reinforcement, self-control, and self-efficacy. Environment is defined as all factors physically external to a person that can influence behavior. These factors might include, for example, access to healthy food choices or social support for losing weight. Observational learning takes place when someone watches another person's behavior and the outcomes (reinforcements) of that behavior. It suggests the use of credible role models, perhaps a friend or relative who has successfully improved his or her eating pattern and experienced positive feelings as a result.

Reinforcement is the response to a person's behavior, which can be positive reinforcement ("reward") or negative reinforcement (no external reward). Reinforcement can also be internal to a person, such as a feeling of pride or accomplishment. Self-control of behavior involves a person observing his or her own behavior, setting personal goals, evaluating achievement of goals, and rewarding himself or herself. Behavioral self-regulation (or "behavior modification") techniques, such as setting specific goals, gradual change, and self-monitoring, are activities based on self-control that are common features of weight management and nutrition counseling programs.[6]

The concept of self-efficacy from SCT appears to be quite useful as a basis for fostering dietary behavior change. Self-efficacy is defined as an individual's estimate of his or her chances of success at mastering a given type of behavior; it is synonymous with self-confidence about performing a specific type of behavior.[1] Behavioral and cognitive strategies such as setting small goals, monitoring, and self-reward can be used to increase self-efficacy and improve the motivation to try new healthy foods or to maintain recommended dietary changes.

Several SCT concepts are applicable to community nutrition education. In group programs, activities like cooking demonstrations and group problem-solving sessions can provide opportunities to learn, practice, and observe healthy eating patterns and to receive social support for new habits. In self-help or self-managed interventions, individuals might work through the process of setting realistic goals, monitoring their achievement, and progressively making strides toward healthier eating.

Relapse Prevention

Rationale

The health impact of nutritious eating can be achieved only if desirable habits are maintained over a period of time. Yet it is widely recognized that many people who begin programs of behavior change eventually return to their previous habits. Many people return to their previous habits, or relapse, fairly soon after they initiate changes. The phenomenon of relapse is widely recognized for addictive behaviors such as drug abuse, problem drinking, smoking, and eating disorders.[13,21] Although it is more difficult to define nonaddictive dietary change (e.g., lowering dietary fat), relapse can be considered as one end of a continuum in which change fails to be maintained after time.

Relapse prevention theory can provide the underpinnings for useful strategies in nutrition education in that it focuses on an important point in the behavior change process that is often given too little attention. It fits well with the stages of change model (in which the last stage is maintenance or relapse) and is consistent with the orientation of social cognitive theory.

Description

Relapse prevention theory encompasses a wide range of strategies for preventing relapse in long-term behavior change.[13] It is based on the idea that addictive behaviors are habit patterns that have been overlearned. These patterns can be changed through self-management or self-control procedures, particularly through developing ways to change expectations of oneself in new environments. For example, if a person eats a high-calorie dessert while trying to maintain a recently achieved weight loss, he or she might feel guilty, label himself or herself as weak, and go on to eat even more fattening food. The goal of relapse prevention would be to break the negative chain of thinking that seemed to make that course of behavior inevitable.

Relapse prevention encourages individuals to develop problem-solving skills to help strengthen their commitment and ability to continue new be-

haviors. Examples of techniques for dietary self-management using relapse prevention training include developing skills to deal with stressful or challenging situations (for example, learning to say no while being a gracious guest), fostering new cognitions (attitudes, attributions) about one's ability to control behaviors, and developing a daily lifestyle that includes health-promoting behaviors such as exercise and stress management techniques.[13]

Community Organization

Rationale

To promote desirable dietary behaviors in the population, we need focus on the public as a whole and not only on subgroups who are at high risk. Healthy diets during pregnancy, adequate childhood nutrition, adoption of low-fat eating patterns, and weight control (or prevention of overweight) are populationwide goals not limited to people who exhibit risk factors.

The concept of working with populations, and not just individuals, is central to the field of community nutrition. Thus it is essential that we make an effort to understand and learn to work with people through the social structures that are the context for their eating behavior. When communities provide an environment to support healthy nutrition and engage in collective action to encourage healthy lifestyles, the potential for change is multiplied.

Description

Community organization is the process by which community groups are helped to identify common problems or goals, mobilize resources, and in other ways develop and implement strategies for reaching goals.[16] A community can be defined by geographical, political, or organizational boundaries or by shared interests and concerns. Central concepts in community organization include empowerment, development of community competence, participation, and community-based issue selection.[16] Community organization is not a single theory per se; rather, it is derived from an amalgamation of theories of social change, including social support and systems perspectives.

Community organization is usually characterized by several different models of practice, the most widely known being Rothman's typology of three models[23]: locality development (or community development), social planning, and social action. Locality development emphasizes process, especially development of consensus and cooperation, capacity building through leadership development, and building a group identity. Social planning is task oriented and focuses on problem solving—usually with assistance from an outside expert. Social action focuses on increasing a community's problem-solving ability *and* achieving concrete changes, often for a group that is considered disadvantaged. The three models may overlap, but most community organization endeavors can be placed in one of these categories.[23]

Community nutrition education can invoke each of the three models in appropriate circumstances. The Minnesota Heart Health Program, a communitywide cardiovascular risk reduction program, used a blend of locality development and social planning to enhance the sense of local ownership for improved heart health through improved diet, exercise, hypertension control, and smoking cessation.[3] The delivery of nutrition education for older adults through senior center meal programs would be an example of the social planning model. A social action approach to community organization for improved nutrition might involve the parents lobbying the school administration for healthier meals and expanded nutrition education curricula at schools.

Different models of community organization require various levels of involvement and direction by dietitians and nutritionists. A social planning strategy might be planned and delivered primarily by professionals. With a locality or community development program, a professional can act as a behind-the-scenes organizer, provide training, and offer technical assistance. Social action requires the professional to take a back seat and be available to provide assistance and encouragement only when the community wants it.

Diffusion of Innovations

Rationale

The past two decades have brought increasing understanding of and consensus on the relationship of nutrition and health and on the most important dietary practices for maintaining health and preventing disease (for example, the Dietary Guidelines, *Healthy People 2000*, the *Surgeon General's Report on Nutrition and Health*, and the National Academy of Sciences' *Diet and Health* report) (see Chapter 1). The recommendations that have emerged are not "new" ideas. Still, the wider endorsement of what constitutes a healthy eating pattern has given the goal of societal or population-wide adoption of healthy diets important new momentum.

Nutrition education aims to first understand and then accelerate the wider adoption of healthy nutrition and its integration into social organizations and society at large. In order for public health nutrition goals to truly take root, informal and formal social groups and organizational structures must be receptive to and supportive of changes in individuals and the environment. Toward that end, the concepts of diffusion of innovations focus attention on communication and interpersonal influence processes and their effects.

Description

Diffusion is defined as the process through which an innovation is communicated through channels over time among members of a social system.[22] An innovation is an idea, practice, service, or object that is considered new by an individual or social group. Efforts of nutrition educators to communicate about what healthy eating patterns are and how they can be incorporated into everyday life establish those patterns as innovations.

According to diffusion theory, certain characteristics of innovations increase the chances that they will be widely adopted. Successful innovations are compatible with existing value systems and lifestyles; they are flexible and seen as more advantageous than previous practices; they are reversible (allow for making choices repeatedly over time), low risk, and are perceived to have greater benefits than their costs.[22] Thus nutrition educators can promote healthy eating if they maximize and emphasize these features.

Several stages of functionally differentiated behavior are involved in the adoption process, whether applied to an individual, a group, or an organization. They are awareness, interest, evaluation, trial, and finally adoption.[22] Personal experience and the experience of those in social networks are also important to the continued use of an innovation.

The communication of innovations influences the rate and extent of adoption. A key generalization of diffusion theory is that different information sources have greater importance at various stages of adoption. Media sources (such as broadcast media and print materials) are most effective in promoting awareness and interest. Interpersonal sources of communication, especially from respected individuals and peers, become more important during the later stages of evaluation, trial, and adoption.[22] Further, respected people in one's social arena, or opinion leaders, provide an important link between media and interpersonal influence.

Some diffusion systems are passive, and in those systems individuals must seek out information on an innovation for themselves. So-called active systems seek out potential users of innovations and attempt to influence their use. Health promotion and nutrition education tend to be active diffusion systems.

Diffusion processes are similar to the processes of behavior change proposed by Bandura[1] in social cognitive theory, with the main difference being that diffusion theory emphasizes the broader nature of social change, with social learning models stressing intrapersonal and interpersonal processes. Several principles of diffusion, which are also consistent with SCT, can improve the effectiveness of behavior change efforts: selecting an optimal setting for introducing innovations, creating the preconditions for change, implementing a demonstrably effective intervention early on, and disseminating the innovation through successful examples.[1] Taken together, these concepts under-score the importance of identifying opportunities to enhance diffusion of nutrition education in an organization or community over a period of time.

APPLICATIONS OF MODELS TO NUTRITION EDUCATION STRATEGIES

This section presents the application of the six theoretical models to nutrition education in the community. Each application, like the art of delivering nutrition services in the community, does not strictly follow the lines of a single model. However, each application emphasizes one of the levels: individual, group, or community or population. These applications illustrate the translation of conceptual frameworks into practical strategies in real-world settings.

Individual Level Applications
Nutrition Counseling
Nutrition counseling aims to help individuals develop and implement eating plans for improving health or controlling risk factors and disease processes. Nutrition counseling may be appropriate in promoting healthy eating during pregnancy, child feeding, weight loss, cholesterol management, diabetes management, and a variety of other situations. Whether health maintenance or a therapeutic diet is the goal, a one-to-one relationship between the client (or patient) and a nutrition counselor is the heart of the behavior change process.

A "traditional" model of nutrition counseling involves a one-to-one relationship and repeated sessions over a period of time. This model is not feasible for many clients, so it is essential to consider alternative models for nutrition counseling. Two models are presented here: brief dietary counseling and comprehensive individual counseling. It is important to develop alternative strategies if your client load is heavy, time is limited, or you are short of staff (all common scenarios in community nutrition).

Both the brief dietary counseling and comprehensive individual counseling approaches are based on a cyclical sequence of assessment, treatment, and evaluation and monitoring.[25] The main difference is that the brief dietary counseling is designed to focus on the client's readiness for change and follow through accordingly. It is unique in not assuming that all patients are equally motivated, ready, or interested in attempting dietary changes.

The four components of brief dietary counseling are assessment of risks, assessment of readiness to change behavior, motivation or action planning, and follow-up. Assessment of risks involves reviewing the client's health profile and any available information about risk indicators, coexisting risk factors, family history, and eating patterns. This provides a starting point and informs the counselor about the urgency of change and the possibility of multiple behavior change issues for the client (e.g., the need to stop smoking as well as reduce dietary fat). A brief discussion of the risks (or health needs) with the client, or verification that he or she understands the health problems, establishes initial contact.

Assessment of readiness to change behavior is the next step. After explaining the benefits of a modified diet to the client, the counselor asks if the client is interested in attempting change at this time. (In other words, is he or she at the contemplation or determination stage?) The question can be as simple as "Are you interested in developing a low-fat eating pattern at this time to lower your cholesterol?" If the answer is "yes" or "maybe;" the counselor moves to an assessment of past dietary change experience, barriers counseling, and action planning. If the patient says "no," the counselor moves quickly to the motivation phase and follows up at a later date.

Motivating the precontemplator involves two basic elements: personalizing the benefits of change and increasing the awareness and opportunities for thinking about changing. It is best to emphasize the benefits of dietary change rather than the risks of not changing. To increase awareness, available sources of information can be suggested, and everyday opportunities for trying small changes can be pointed out (such as substituting frozen yogurt for ice cream). Clients should be encouraged to think about when (not whether) they will be ready to try some dietary changes. Follow-

up can be a phone call or raising the matter of change at the next clinic visit.

If the client is definitely or possibly interested in changing his or her eating pattern, motivation involves assessment of past dietary change experience and barriers counseling. First the counselor should ask about previous efforts to make dietary changes. The nature of the changes, whether outside help was sought, and the success or problems with change provide important information for the next step, barriers counseling, which is a discussion of the most important obstacles or barriers that the patient thinks will stand in the way of adopting a new eating pattern. It is useful in anticipating and dealing with problem situations. The counselor can be prepared with suggestions and ways to overcome the most common barriers (see the box on p. 265). This is also a good time for problem solving in which the client can develop his or her own solutions. Barriers counseling involves helping a client develop ways to manage the environment.

Action planning is the phase in which the counselor makes suggestions for beginning the dietary change process in earnest. The counselor should recommend suitable intervention modalities for the client, such as written educational materials, comprehensive counseling, or group education. The goal and referral should be written down—not only on the client's record but also on a card or page that the client can take home.

It is helpful to advise the client that you will follow up on your discussion with either a phone call or a later visit. The follow-up should be routine and include reinforcement and encouragement as well as problem solving to deal with unanticipated difficulties.

Comprehensive nutrition counseling is desirable when there are fewer constraints on time and when the client or patient is committed to addressing the process of dietary change in some depth. "Comprehensive" counseling can be anything from a single "full-length" encounter of 30 to 45 minutes to regular and repeated individual sessions for 6 months or more. The goals of comprehensive nutrition counseling are to work with the client to set goals, solve problems, and take action to make di-

BARRIERS COUNSELING

1. *I like the foods I eat now; I would have to give up my favorite foods.*
2. *I don't know how to fit low-fat foods into the way I eat.*
   - Even though adopting a low-fat eating pattern means making changes in how you eat, you don't have to *give up* the foods you like. You might have to cut down on the foods you like or plan for those choices, however.
   - Small, gradual changes are the key.
   - Often you can eat the same *type* of foods by only having to change the way the food is prepared or the portion size.
3. *I don't know which foods I can eat on a low-fat diet; there are too many things to remember.*
   - It seems complicated at first, but once you learn some basic ideas and begin to pay attention to what you eat, choosing foods will get easier.
   - Some of the guides, books, manuals you can read or classes you can attend will include convenient wallet-size reminder cards; the tipsheet from our office should be helpful also.
   - Learning to read labels can go a long way in helping you choose low-fat foods.
4. *I'm too rushed; it's too much work to buy or fix low-fat foods.*
5. *I eat out a lot.*
   - It's easy to learn ways to cook low-fat foods without too much work; once you pick out some low-fat foods that are your favorites, you will find it even easier.
   - Often you can partially prepare foods in advance and save time in the long run.
   - Some of the foods need *less* preparation; for example, fresh fruit and foods that do not need heavy sauces or frying.
   - Once you learn some basic ideas and tips, you will find it easy to choose low-fat foods when eating out.
6. *Someone else buys and prepares my food.*
   - In that case, you will want to have that person work with you as you try to develop a low-fat eating plan.
7. *I enjoy having a drink with my friends.*
8. *I drink when I feel anxious.*
   - If you usually have more than two drinks (or the equivalent) at one occasion, try drinking nonalcoholic beverages (juice, mineral water, soda) instead of alcohol some of the time.
   - If "binge" drinking, even periodic, is present, consider referral for counseling.

---

etary changes that improve health or reduce risk. The process is ideally one in which responsibility is shared and the client is an active participant; eventually the client adopts and maintains new behavior patterns so that treatment is no longer needed.[11,25]

The core of comprehensive counseling is the counseling relationship—a "therapeutic alliance" between the client and counselor based on liking, respect, and trust that is conducive to positive client change. Several qualities of the counselor are important: expertness, credibility, empathy, warmth, self-disclosure, and a compatible match with the client.[11]

A wide variety of counseling methods are available to help people change. Most are based on some combination of social cognitive theory and the related behavior modification or behavioral self-regulation models described earlier. Figure 10-1 depicts the cyclical counseling process and its context for the nutrition counselor. Within this general process, theory-based strategies address both individual behavior and interpersonal processes. Analysis of behavior during client evaluation usually involves eating-pattern assessment, often in the form of a food diary, to aid the understanding of eating patterns and relevant situational triggers. Goal setting occurs next as part of treatment, and often small achievable goals are set at first. Behavioral contracting is a frequently used formal method of setting goals and making a commitment for change. Rewards can be planned as reinforcements for reaching goals. Most clients find that long-term change is best achieved through gradual, stepwise goal attainment rather than by attempting to make major changes all at once.

Maintenance of behavior change is also an important area of attention in comprehensive nutri-

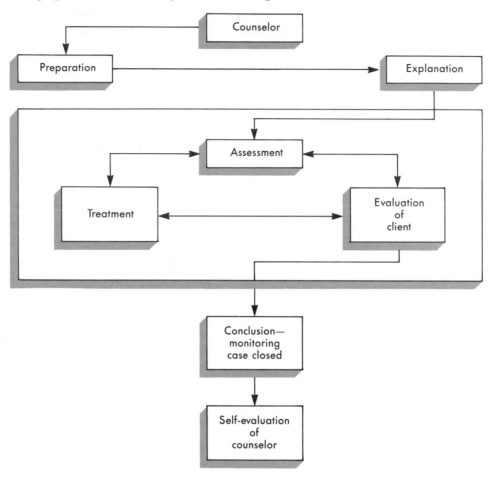

Figure 10-1. Model for nutrition counseling.
Reprinted from Snetselaar LG: *Nutrition counseling skills: assessment, treatment, and evaluation*, ed 2, with permission of Aspen Publishers, Inc., 1989.

tion counseling. When substantial progress toward implementing a behavior change plan has been made, techniques of relapse prevention should be considered. Self-management strategies such as self-talk, problem solving, and behavioral rehearsal can all be useful. Periodic reinforcement from a counselor—by telephone or in person—can also enhance behavioral change maintenance. Referral to group programs or support groups may also be worthwhile at this point.

Clearly, both individual- and interpersonal-level models of understanding and changing behavior

can and should be employed successfully during these processes.

Nutrition Education Materials

Nutrition education often involves communicating concepts that need to be applied to a vast array of food choices in everyday situations. Therefore, printed nutrition education materials are important components of the educational process, both when used alone and as adjuncts to nutrition counseling. Because they are the tools that clients or patients will have to rely on outside of face-to-face educational situations, their development and selection warrant special attention.

It is essential that educational materials be accessible and understandable to the individuals for whom they are intended. However, in nutrition education, concern about technical accuracy of the content has often taken priority over readability and ease of comprehension. Educational materials may be written at too sophisticated a level in terms of wording and concepts. Few of the widely available nutrition education materials (i.e., those distributed by the government and major health organizations) are suitable for people without high levels of literacy.

Strategies based on the concepts of consumer information processing (CIP) are useful in tailoring printed nutrition materials to the audience. Information acquisition, processing, and evaluation should be low-effort tasks for the users of these materials. Thus nutrition educators should be familiar with the range of reading levels and cultural backgrounds of their clients and communities, and evaluate printed nutrition education materials accordingly. There are simple formulas to evaluate readability (i.e., reading grade level) of printed materials. When new materials are developed, they should be pretested on people similar to the clients who will later receive them. In face-to-face nutrition education contacts, the provider can go through, mark, and explain some of the more difficult words or concepts so that the client will not be confused when using the materials.

In general, it is best not to overload learners with too much information, which will only make it harder for them to identify and absorb the key points. At the same time, it is important to be prepared to provide additional guidance to those who may want more information. If people request more information or want to seek it out (e.g., in books that can be recommended as credible sources), they are more likely to be motivated to make use of it.

Interpersonal Level Applications
Small Groups

Small group nutrition education programs can be used to supplement or be substituted for individual nutrition counseling. They often use strategies similar to those described for one-to-one counseling but with the added element of a group setting. Group education is commonly offered for people trying to lose weight, and it is increasingly being used for cholesterol management education. In small groups that have been studied, nutrition education based on social cognitive theory and concepts of self-directed change has been found to be more effective than traditional didactic methods.[26] Such groups address not only the nutrition information needed to follow a healthy eating plan but also techniques of self-monitoring, goal setting, and achieving gradual changes that are reinforced along the way.[6]

Social Support

Social support can involve interacting with positive role models and problem solving through discussion with people who have shared problems or nutrition needs. Social support can be incorporated into small group programs or fostered in other ways. Buddy systems can create focused support systems, or family members can be invited to attend group programs. People attending nutrition education programs can also learn skills for involving families in dietary change outside the program setting.

One strategy for mobilizing social support for nutrition education is the worksite weight loss competition program. Weight loss competitions combine group support and self-management. Typically, workers sign up to participate as part of a team, which develops a unique identity and identifies ways to encourage success among its members. A classroom program may also be included. Group members strive to increase one another's self-efficacy, and rewards are used as reinforcements for various amounts of weight loss or for reaching goals more successfully than other groups. Competitions have been especially popular among men and can reach many employees at a fairly low cost.[9]

Peer Education

Peer education can be effective for enhancing observational learning (a concept from SCT) through role models and is particularly useful with youth and cultural minority groups. School-based programs have made extensive use of peer leaders to establish and improve a variety of health behaviors. Successful peer-led cardiovascular nutrition education programs for tenth-grade students in California used nutrition information, skills training for behavior change, and relapse prevention training to avoid a return to previous habits. Training and practice in how to resist peer pressure stressed increasing self-confidence and problem-solving skills, strategies that are based on social cognitive theory and relapse prevention.[26]

Interpersonal methods of nutrition education have many advantages. Key assets include the ability to reach people more efficiently than individual counseling, providing opportunities for engaging social support, and motivating participants through rewards that are relevant to group members.

Community- and Population-Level Applications

Community- or population-based strategies make it possible for nutrition education to reach wide audiences and achieve greater impact. These efforts, often called *environmental* strategies, reach populations through influencing the availability of healthy food, access to information for making food choices, and the accessibility and appeal of nutrition education experiences.[8] As indicated earlier, they incorporate individual and interpersonal level approaches but go a step further—institutions and communities are partners with community nutrition personnel in developing and delivering them.

Effective population-based nutrition interventions require that nutrition and health professionals collaborate with organizations that serve as hosts or loci for programs. These organizations and organizational components are gatekeepers for enhancing nutrition in populations. They include social units such as workplaces, schools, and hospitals and food outlets such as cafeterias, supermarkets, and restaurants. These organizations are complex structures with various levels of management.[4]

Population-based interventions often involved longer and more complex start-up periods than individual or small group programs. Feedback and evidence of success come more slowly. However,

the potential result is much greater when these interventions are implemented effectively. In order to deliver these services, dietitians and nutritionists need to master not only the skills of individual and interpersonal education but also methods based on community organization and diffusion theories.

Two applications of community-level models are presented here: point-of-purchase supermarket programs, and an initiative to increase the availability of healthy foods in a school food service. Examples of other community level models are presented in Chapter 8, where the Pawtucket Cholesterol Screening Campaign[12] and the Minnesota Heart Healthy Program Eating Patterns Campaign[8,17] are discussed in detail.

Point-of-Choice Nutrition Information

This program is a community approach to communication of nutrition information to guide food selections in food establishments such as supermarkets, cafeterias, and restaurants. The premise behind these efforts is that information at the point of decision making will increase awareness or serve as a reminder to promote selection of healthier foods. The informational component of point-of-choice (or point-of-purchase, P-O-P) interventions is related to consumer information processing; the effort needed to seek and use information is greatly decreased. P-O-P interventions also draw on diffusion theory: information is presented to maximize the apparent benefits and relative advantages of healthier food choices (the *innovation*).

In evaluation studies of P-O-P nutrition information programs, varying degrees of success have been found. The largest program evaluations were in grocery stores, and the most effective strategies include brand-specific information. Much remains to be learned about how to create successful point-of-choice programs. It appears that simple, specific comparing information that is highly visible is most likely to have an impact.[8]

Increasing the Availability of Healthy Foods

Making more nutritious food available to people in community settings removes one of the greatest barriers to healthy eating. Increasingly, institutions and their food services, as well as commercial food outlets, are showing an interest in providing healthier food choices. This can be accomplished through changes in food preparation or by introducing new menu offerings. *Healthy People 2000*, the national health promotion objectives, includes objectives that call for school and worksite food service managers to follow and promote the U.S. Dietary Guidelines.

School-based efforts to increase the variety of healthy food choices can directly influence the foods consumed by students, staff, and teachers and also reinforce classroom nutrition education curricula. The Go for Health project, a diet and exercise program for elementary school children in Texas, used a planning group of food service managers and project staff to design changes in menu planning, food purchase, recipe selection, and food preparation practices to offer reduced fat and sodium meals.[18] In two New England boarding schools, changes in food purchase and preparation decreased sodium use and changed the fat composition of foods served, resulting in lower intakes of sodium and saturated fat, along with increased healthy offerings that students felt were acceptable and palatable food choices.[5] In both these examples, close collaboration with school food service staff was a core component of the interventions. Concepts of community organization, diffusion of innovations, and social cognitive theory all contributed to the successful implementation of these environmental programs.

Community- and population-level nutrition intervention strategies often gain momentum and resources when they are part of larger, comprehensive health promotion programs. When this is the case, nutrition staff are challenged to collaborate successfully and at the same time to establish their leadership of the nutrition component.

SUMMARY

The central goal of nutrition education is to promote healthy eating behavior. Successful nutrition education in the community involves managing change in people's eating behavior and the forces that shape it. A central thrust of community nutrition is aiming to both understand and influence not only individuals but also groups, organizations, and populations.

This chapter presented a multilevel approach for understanding how people make food choices and demonstrated how this can be translated into strategies for facilitating change in eating patterns. The ecological perspective includes several levels: intrapersonal factors, such as knowledge, attitudes, behavior, and skills; interpersonal processes and primary groups, including social networks, support systems, and families, friends, and co-workers; institutional and community factors, or features of social organizations and institutions and their interrelationships; and public policy at all levels of government.

Of the many models for understanding behavior, six theoretical frameworks have been described that are most useful for understanding factors affecting eating patterns and the processes of improving them. The models at the individual level are consumer information processing (CIP) and stages of change. CIP addresses how people seek, evaluate, and use information to make choices and how nutrition educators can increase the usability and impact of information they provide. The stages of change model has as its central premise the idea that people may be at various levels of readiness to change and that increasing awareness and motivation may be most important at one point in time, if someone is not ready to take action.

Social cognitive theory (SCT) and relapse prevention are related models incorporating individual and interpersonal concepts. Social cognitive theory (the cognitive version of social learning theory) postulates reciprocal relationships between individuals, their environments, and behavior. It incorporates concepts of behavior modification such as goal setting, self-monitoring, and reinforcement and emphasizes the role of self-efficacy for successfully achieving behavior change. Relapse prevention theory focuses on similar concepts, with special application to the maintenance of change.

Community organization and diffusion of innovations are important foundations for achieving populationwide impact. Community organization concerns ways to activate communities and foster their sense of ownership of health-enhancing efforts. Diffusion of innovations addresses ways to optimize communication and adoption of new ideas and programs in populations.

Examples of how these models for change have been applied in nutrition education included, at the individual level, brief dietary counseling, comprehensive nutrition counseling, and effective nutrition education materials; at the interpersonal level, group education, social support activation, and peer education; and at the population level, cholesterol screening campaigns, an eating pattern campaign in a heart disease prevention program, point-of-choice information, and changes in cafeteria food offerings.

Dietitians and nutritionists have a leadership role in designing, implementing, and evaluating nutrition education. Using your behavior change skills and collaborating with other professionals and community members, you can help to improve health through better nutrition.

REFERENCES

1. Bandura A: *Social foundations of thought and action: a social cognitive theory*, Englewood Cliffs, NJ, 1986, Prentice Hall.
2. Bettman JR: *An information processing theory of consumer choice*, Reading, Mass, 1979, Addison-Wesley.
3. Carlaw R and others: Organization for a community cardiovascular health program: experiences from the Minnesota Heart Health Program, *Health Educ Q* 11:243, 1984.
4. DiSogra L, Glanz K, Rogers T: Working with community organizations for nutrition intervention, *Health Educ Res* 5:459, 1990.
5. Ellison RC and others: The environmental component: changing school food service to promote cardiovascular health, *Health Educ Q* 16:285, 1989.
6. Glanz K: Nutrition education for risk factor reduction and patient education: a review, *Prev Med* 14:721, 1985.
7. Glanz K, Lewis FM, Rimer BK, editors: *Health behavior and health education: theory, research, and practice*, San Francisco, 1990, Jossey-Bass.
8. Glanz K, Mullis RM: Environmental interventions to promote healthy eating: a review of models, programs and evidence, *Health Educ Q* 15:395, 1988.
9. Glanz K, Seewald-Klein T: Nutrition at the worksite: an overview, *J Nutr Educ* 18(suppl):1, 1986.
10. Green LW, Kreuter MW: *Health promotion planning: an educational and environmental approach*, ed 2, Mountain View, Cal, 1991, Mayfield.
11. Kanfer FH, Goldstein AP, editors: *Helping people change: a textbook of methods*, ed 3, New York, 1986, Pergamon Press.
12. Lefebvre RC and others: Community intervention to lower blood cholesterol: the "Know Your Cholesterol" campaign in Pawtucket, Rhode Island, *Health Educ Q* 13:117, 1986.
13. Marlatt GA, Gordon JR: *Relapse prevention*, New York, 1985, Guilford Press.
14. McCann BS and others: Promoting adherence to low-fat, low-cholesterol diets: review and recommendations, *J Am Diet Assoc* 90:1408, 1990.
15. McLeroy KR and others: An ecological perspective on health promotion programs, *Health Educ Q* 15:351, 1988.
16. Minkler M: *Improving health through community organization*. In Glanz K, Lewis FM, Rimer BK, editors: *Health behavior and health education: theory, research, and practice*, San Francisco, 1990, Jossey-Bass.
17. Mittlemark M and others: Community-wide prevention of cardiovascular disease: education strategies of the Minnesota Heart Health Program, *Prev Med* 15:1, 1986.
18. Parcel GS and others: School promotion of healthful diet and exercise behavior: an integration of organizational change and social learning theory interventions, *J Sch Health* 57:150, 1987.
19. Perry CL, Baranowski T, Parcel GS: *How individuals, environments, and health behavior interact: social learning theory*. In Glanz K, Lewis FM, Rimer BK, editors: *Health behavior and health education: theory, research, and practice*, San Francisco, 1990, Jossey-Bass.
20. Prochaska JO, DiClemente CC: Transtheoretical therapy: toward a more integrative model of change, *Psychother Theory Res Pract* 19:276, 1982.
21. Rimer BK: *Perspectives on intrapersonal theories in health education and health behavior*. In Glanz K, Lewis FM, Rimer BK, editors: *Health behavior and health education: theory, research, and practice*, San Francisco, 1990, Jossey-Bass.
22. Rogers EM: *Diffusion of innovations*, ed 3, New York, 1983, Free Press.
23. Rothman J, Tropman JE: *Models of community organization and macro practice: their mixing and phasing*. In Cox FM and others, editors: *Strategies of community organization*, ed 4, Itasca, Ill, 1987, Peacock.
24. Rudd J, Glanz K: *How individuals use information for health action: consumer information processing*. In Glanz K, Lewis FM, Rimer BK, editors: *Health behavior and health education: theory, research, and practice*, San Francisco, 1990, Jossey-Bass.
25. Snetselaar LG: *Nutrition counseling skills: assessment, treatment, and evaluation*, ed 2, Rockville, Md, 1989, Aspen.
26. Thomas PR, editor: *Improving America's diet and health: from recommendations to action*, Washington, DC, 1991, National Academy Press.

Working with Industry: Alliances, Coalitions, and Partnerships for Dietitians and Nutritionists

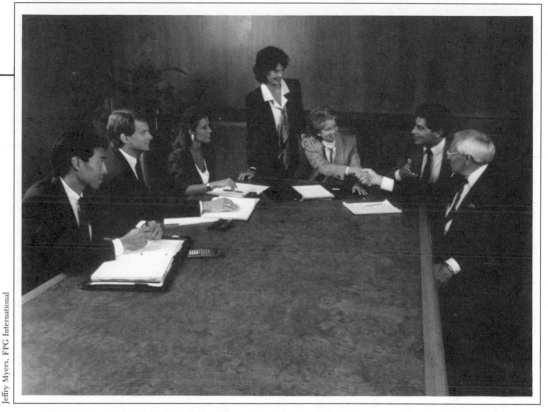

GENERAL CONCEPT

The world is undergoing massive changes that extend to two areas of major concern to dietitians and nutritionists—health care and business. One of the immediate consequences is that the health care field has become too complex for dietitians and nutritionists to "go it alone." As a result, major adjustments will have to be made in the way their services are structured and delivered.

The key to the future is likely to be in cooperative ventures—partnerships, alliances, coalitions—joining forces with others who have access to customers and potential customers.

These partnerships with the private sector enable the good nutrition message to be broadcast more widely and permit dietitians and nutritionists to communicate through the mass media, multiplying the effect and scope of the message. In addition, industry provides resources and perspectives perhaps otherwise unavailable.

Those who develop and excel in the area of private sector partnerships will move in the vanguard of health care and will continue making important contributions to the health and well-being of American society.

OUTCOME OBJECTIVES

When you finish this chapter, you should be able to:

- Describe the importance of closer cooperation between dietetics and the private sector.
- Explain how dietitians and nutritionists can benefit from industry partnerships.
- Understand the four key steps in building partnerships.
- Understand how to apply marketing skills in working with the private sector.

CHANGES IN HEALTH CARE AND INDUSTRY

Every period in the history of civilization has been marked by change. Arguably, however, the contemporary world is undergoing change that is broader and deeper than at any other time in history. Technology, politics, societal mores, economics, communications, and transportation—no area of life is exempt from change. At the present rate of change, without any acceleration, in just 20 years the world will be virtually unrecognizable.

The winds of change also are buffeting two areas of major concern to dietitians and nutritionists—health care and business—and the results will necessitate major adjustments in the way dietetic services are structured and delivered.

The present-day health care environment is a highly charged one. New delivery systems, advanced technology and treatment, changing demographics, the wellness movement, the graying of America, and escalating costs are creating a climate fraught with challenges and opportunities.

One of the immediate consequences of the changes is that the health care field has become too complex for dietitians and nutritionists to "go it alone." That is true in the larger arena as well. Despite occasional exceptions, the day of the rugged individualist, the solitary hero or heroine struggling alone against great odds, seems relegated to the pages of history.

Today, those who want to excel are increasingly looking to work together in partnerships, alliances, coalitions, and networks. There are many desig-

nations for working together, and there are some nuances of difference between the terms, but the bottom line is that whatever the language, the underlying message is, as the fabulist Aesop put it, "Union gives strength."

In the business world, corporations that have been competitors, such as IBM and Apple, have linked resources to develop compatible computer systems. Similarly, Time Inc. and Warner Communications merged to form a giant conglomerate spanning magazines, motion pictures, cable and broadcast television, book publishing, and other areas.

Japanese and American automobile companies, once perceived as locked in a death struggle, now often cooperate in joint ventures. Rosabeth Moss Kanter, former editor of the *Harvard Business Review*, writes of "more than eight thousand person-visits by U.S.-based Ford employees to Japan—and so much traffic between Detroit and Tokyo in general that many U.S.-Tokyo flights now originate in Detroit rather than Chicago."[1] She also reports on other rival businesses working together, for example, "The Center for Advanced Television Studies, formed by ABC, CBS, NBC, PBS, RCA, and five other companies to improve the quality of television transmission."[1]

The key to the future for dietitians is likely to be in such cooperative ventures—partnerships, alliances, coalitions.

Former American Dietetic Association (ADA) president Anita L. Owen, MA, RD, told a workshop on building partnerships at the University of Minnesota Heart Health Program, "The past few years has produced a flurry of books peering into the twenty-first century. All describe trends that offer the potential for more economic prosperity, social progress, and scientific advancement than the world has ever known. One of the themes that is pervasive throughout all of the crystal balling is the need to develop partnerships or broad-based coalitions to survive."[8] She cited an Association Management prediction that "successful coalitions will be those that bring together new and varying interests and broad-based support. . . . If a large and diverse coalition can be put together, one that represents consumer and professional groups, and industry, Congress and the public will pay attention. The issues must prove to be good for everyone or it just will not fly."[8]

The ADA has recognized the need for these relationships beyond the boundaries of the dietetic profession and has more than 90 different partnerships in place, many through its recently inaugurated National Center for Nutrition and Dietetics in Chicago. They cover the full spectrum of "age-oriented" groups and associations ranging from the National Council on Aging to the American Academy of Pediatrics. The ADA's campaigns also include all organizations involved in prevention and health maintenance such as the American College of Sports Medicine and the American Heart Association. Recently, ADA joined with professional groups concerned about the aging to provide input to the federal government on reform regulations for nursing homes.

The association promotes networking and also fosters staff alliance activities, encouraging individual dietitians to assume leadership roles in their areas of expertise.

To capitalize on the activities of the ADA and its practice groups, individual dietitians in all areas of specialty have to develop a keen understanding of partnership building and learn how to utilize it in their own activities. Individual dietitians and nutritionists must understand—as the association has—that to thrive, perhaps to merely survive, in the immediate and long-term future they must recognize the importance of joining forces with others who have access to customers and potential customers. They must shed the "go it alone" mentality, identify potential allies—those with a commonality of interests—and build coalitions and partnerships. See the box at right for a listing of areas where dietitians and nutritionists can develop alliances.

Although dietitians and nutritionists generally recognize the value of collaborative efforts with fellow health care professionals and are increasingly comfortable in these partnerships, it is fair to say that they have not been as aggressive in pursuing similar relationships in the business world.

EXAMPLES OF AREAS IN WHICH DIETITIANS AND NUTRITIONISTS CAN DEVELOP ALLIANCES

- Hospitals: Nurses enjoy prestige and influence and often have the ear of administrators. Dietitians and nutritionists can ally themselves with nurses to convince administrators of the importance of nutrition services.
- Community: In their communities, individual dietitians and nutritionists can work with those key organizations and individuals with an interest in health and nutrition.
- Industry: The private sector is perhaps the single most critical area for dietitians and nutritionists who wish to function in the vanguard of health care in the future. They must develop comarketing ventures with companies and businesses that have complementary skills. Kanter writes: "Many joint ventures form because one partner is eager to learn something from the other—get a piece of technology, learn how to manage a process, gain technological expertise. . . . A second opportunistic use of joint ventures is to gain fast access to new markets."[1]
- Politics: Working in the political arena is challenging but can produce enormous dividends. A key is identifying players—including elected officials—who share common health and nutrition views and working toward mutual goals. Often in the political arena, dietitians and nutritionists will be working with other health care practitioners who in different settings may be competitors. Therefore, it is crucial that these joint ventures show dietitians and nutritionists in the best light: as total professionals who understand science and communicate it effectively. At the organizational level, ADA is active in Washington, DC, where it maintains an office of government affairs. Individual dietitians and nutritionists can work at all levels—federal, state, and local—to promote the cause of good nutrition.

PERSPECTIVES ON PRIVATE BUSINESSES

Many business leaders and executives recognize the benefits of such partnerships from their private sector standpoint. American business, like much of the rest of society, is undergoing sweeping and deep changes. Corporations that once were perceived as focusing exclusively on the bottom line, profits and losses, cash flow, and stock dividends are now in increasing numbers becoming more public-spirited, even in turbulent economic times. They are widely marketing and publicizing their new altruistic programs in order to differentiate their corporations and their products.

Corporate America has always had its share of philanthropists, but the modern, visionary business leader has realized that corporations do not operate in a vacuum, that everything in society—the environment, education, health, safety, the standard of living, the quality of life—is a legitimate concern of the business world.

They understand that the economic health of the country and the strength of society are built upon the status of the many millions of individual Americans. Increasingly, companies have begun to assume the role of "good corporate citizen." That kind of volunteerism in business is what President George Bush refers to when he speaks of a "thousand points of light."

Corporate giants like IBM and American Express are among the companies that are plugged into the world around them. American Express is a pioneer in "cause-related" marketing, which links contributions to local cultural institutions and events to credit card expenditures by customers. IBM, a perennial leader in corporate giving, supports health-related charities, assists local hospitals in controlling health care costs, and donates equipment and money to elementary schools. In addition, it provides research grants to colleges and universities in areas that directly relate to IBM's operations—engineering, business, and management.

Some corporations focus their efforts on improving America's institutions. Popular industry ventures include the "adopt-a-school" programs, endowing scholarships for outstanding high school students, and awarding grants to not-for-profit organizations to encourage volunteerism. Many of these efforts originate in a corporation's charitable foundation or corporate giving department, but marketing executives also are interested in partnerships. They want credible sources to help communicate the concept of their products.

Some companies, particularly those that do business within the health care profession, focus much of their marketing on building relationships with health care professionals and creating programs for them. Dietitians and nutritionists have two kinds of opportunity in working with companies: joint ventures in marketing activities and corporate sponsorship or grants, that is, working together for common goals as compared to outright financial support in the form of grants.

It is important, however, to retain perspective, to remember that, no matter how public-spirited, no private concern or individual is in business to lose money. Survival dictates that all but nonprofit organizations must operate in the black, and even the nonprofit operation must function on a pay-as-you-go basis. Consequently, American corporations still must keep their primary focus on the bottom line.

The key for dietitians and nutritionists is to make the opportunity a win-win situation for both, a partnership in which the corporation gets concept communication and dietitians and nutritionists get visibility. Obviously, dietitians and nutritionists know their own goals; it is important that they understand the needs and objectives of the proposed partner as well.

Dietitians and nutritionists who develop and excel in this area will move in the vanguard of this emerging alliance between health care and business and continue making important contributions to the health and well-being of American society.

THE BENEFITS TO DIETITIANS AND NUTRITIONISTS OF INDUSTRY PARTNERSHIPS

American health care is undergoing a veritable revolution, one driven in part by skyrocketing health care costs. In 1986, $458 billion was spent on health care in the United States. This represents nearly 11% of the gross national product (GNP)—the total value of goods and services produced in any given year. It surpasses what we spend on housing and soon will top food expenses. By the year 2000, the annual health care bill is expected to top 15% of the GNP.

In the past, much of the burden was assumed

by the federal government; now it is falling on the private sector. At the beginning of the 1980s, corporations were spending about $60 billion a year for employee health care. In the early years of this decade, it is estimated that the total will soar to between $350 and $400 billion annually.

Citing *Healthy People: The Surgeon General's Report on Health Promotion and Disease Prevention*, Owen suggests that what has actually emerged in our society in the past decade is a redefinition of health—from the mere absence of disease to the existence of a positive state of health in the whole person.[8]

> It represents an emerging consensus among scientists and the health community that the nation's health care strategy must be dramatically recast from treatment-oriented approaches to emphasizing the prevention of disease. The health care environment has changed—the consumer, not the provider, is now in control. . . . Dietitians should monitor this movement carefully, retool our skills if necessary to meet the needs of today's changing consumers. In terms of partnerships, this approach will require working with a whole new cast of characters.[8]

The new health care environment, with its advanced technology, focus on costs, and emphasis on new public attitudes, makes it necessary for dietitians and nutritionists to change the way they offer and provide their services. One of the keys is through alliances and partnerships with business and industry.

How Dietitians and Nutritionists Benefit

How can dietitians and nutritionists benefit from industry partnerships? In the framework of the current upheaval in the health care field, on the surface this is a question that is easy to answer. Most practicing dietitians and nutritionists would have specific responses; most likely there would be a great deal of similarity in their answers.

At their most basic, these partnerships strengthen the impact of the good-nutrition message, and enable it to be broadcast more widely. They permit dietitians and nutritionists to communicate through the mass media, thus multiplying the effect and scope of the message. In addition,

industry provides resources and perspectives perhaps otherwise unavailable to dietitians and nutritionists.

With these shifts in health care, dietitians and nutritionists need support from outside the profession, support that can complement their own education, experience, and expertise. The business end of the partnership should provide the vision, perspective, and business strategies that can move key health and nutrition issues to the forefront and position dietitians and nutritionists for a major role in present and future health care.

Positioning

Positioning is a key to the future for dietitians and nutritionists. According to marketing experts Ries and Trout, who helped popularize the concept, positioning is "an organized system for finding a window in the mind. It is based on the concept that communication can only take place at the right time and under the right circumstances." They describe it as "a new approach to communications . . . the first body of thought that comes to grips with the difficult problem of getting heard in our overcommunicated society."[9]

In the context of health care, that description can be altered and broadened to include ensuring that dietitians and nutritionists are in the right spot at the right time, poised and prepared to capitalize on opportunities. It is precisely the resources, prestige, and power of major corporations that can help dietitians and nutritionists get heard.

Networks

Networking is a relatively new term for a practice that probably has been going on for centuries. As the world grows more complex and health care more sophisticated, it is one of the single most important elements in communicating with the public, with fellow health care professionals, and with the private sector. That is true as well in many other aspects of professional life.

Just what is networking? According to Naisbett, "Networks are people talking to each other, sharing ideas, information, and resources. . . . The important part is not the network, the finished product, but the process of getting there—the communication that creates the linkages between people and clusters of people."[7]

In more concrete terms, networks can have a myriad of functions: creating new markets and meeting the needs of customers, increasing job opportunities and career advancement, providing up-to-date information, enhancing one's power base, helping to cope with problems, and establishing national and international connections in the public and private sectors.

As in all relationships, some networks are better—more effective—than others. High-quality networking results from building mutually supportive relationships that are marked by both giving and receiving.

It is self-evident that corporations will have built networks quite different than those in the health care profession. It is likely that private-sector networks extend throughout the business and financial worlds, into the highest reaches of government, the media, and foundations, both domestically and internationally. Those business networks represent a unique opportunity for dietitians and nutritionists to extend their contacts and bring the message of good nutrition and good health to publics not ordinarily reached through health care contacts.

Resources

The private sector has cash and people resources generally unavailable to health care professionals and, in most cases, their associations.

Mass audience advertising is a proven, effective, and measurable way to reach the general public, yet it is financially far out of the reach of most health-related campaigns. At last count, a full-page color ad in *Time* was selling for $120,130; a similar placement in *TV Guide* is $112,900. Television is even more expensive: a 30-second prime-time network spot on a program like "Wonder Years" is $303,660, plus the cost of production. Even a $1 million budget can be exhausted quickly.

When health care joins forces with the private sector it can utilize the resources of private industry, and tie a health care message to an existing campaign, the result is a bigger bang for the buck.

Similarly, tapping into the expertise and experience of private sector personnel in marketing, quality control, financial matters, and research complements the strengths of individual health care practitioners and of the profession. The resulting joint effort is powerful and effective.

For example, the health care profession and Nabisco's Fleischmann products are involved in a joint venture. Published by the Center for Healthcare Communications, *Nutrition Update* is designed for dietitians and nutritionists and features handout materials for distribution to patients. The publication is supported by a grant from Fleischmann's Margarine, Fleischmann's Light and Extra Light, and Egg Beaters. Its advisory committee is comprised of registered dietitians and nutritionists and physicians. As an example, the Winter 1991 issue focused on worksite cholesterol education efforts. The magazine included information on strategies, guidelines, and tactical plans for implementing such a program and pullout information, including steps to lower cholesterol.

Reach

Closely linked to resources is the ability of private sector entities to reach mass audiences and enable dietitians and nutritionists to address large numbers of customers and potential customers. In addition to the financial support necessary, corporations generally have well-established channels for distributing their sales messages.

An exciting campaign, Healthy Start—Food to Grow On, was launched in 1991 by the Food Marketing Institute, the American Academy of Pediatrics, and the American Dietetic Association. A nationwide nutrition effort, Healthy Start brings together 41,000 pediatricians, 62,000 registered dietitians, and 1600 food retailers and wholesalers. This powerful alliance designed its campaign to "encourage families with young children ages 2 to 6 to make better food choices." Through the reach of the Food Marketing Institute, informational kits were distributed to 1600 of its supermarket members. Materials also are available in grocery stores, in pediatricians' offices, and through registered dietitians and nutritionists.

At the core of the campaign are four informational brochures on basic nutrition:

- *Right from the Start: ABC's of Good Nutrition for Young Children*
- *What's to Eat? Healthy Foods for Hungry Children*
- *Feeding Kids Right Isn't Always Easy: Tips for Preventing Food Hassles*
- *Growing Up Healthy: Fat, Cholesterol and More*

Supermarkets also can distribute a quarterly *Healthy Start* newsletter and a parent-child activity booklet for children ages 5 and 6. Each retail outlet also is provided with promotional suggestions, ideas for events, and a list of professional nutrition resources.

Visibility

Through its networks, resources, and extended reach, the private sector is able to help health care professionals heighten their visibility.

Although dietitians and nutritionists are respected among their fellow health care professionals for the excellence of their education, training, and performance, they traditionally are not highly visible to the public at large.

One of the ways this situation is being rectified is a clear illustration of how visibility can be increased through cooperation with the private sector. Seven years ago, the American Dietetic Association developed its Ambassador Program with the active support of Ross Laboratories. The Ambassador Program was designed to train registered dietitians in media relations, and its mission is to create a positive environment that makes it easier for every dietitian to do her or his job.

At last count, 83 trained spokespersons were prepared to speak knowledgeably to the media on nutrition topics and to comment on breaking news stories. In addition, more than 20 national ambassadors and at least one trained spokesperson in each state are ready to step before the cameras or comment to reporters.

The ambassadors function as marketing agents for every dietitian and nutritionist and for the profession as a whole. The program has been so successful that it has become a prototype for other professional organizations, which are following ADA's lead and establishing similar projects.

Prestige

Prestige is a less tangible benefit of working with private industry, but it is no less real than the other advantages previously cited. When a corporate giant like IBM, American Express, or Xerox lends its name and resources to a program, the recipient benefits in terms of prestige. The fact that a major corporation with no direct benefit to itself supports a project like the ADA Ambassador Program gives that venture added clout. Similarly, highly respected and visible industry leaders lend their personal prestige when they become involved in a cause.

According to Judy Dodd, president of the American Dietetic Association:

> The participation of a major corporation in a health care project can mean the difference between success and outright triumph. When respected corporate leaders put their prestige behind a venture, it is a signal to the rest of the business world that this is something special, something worthwhile. It creates interest and can generate additional support in the business community and in government. In the same way, it tells the public that people in power are willing to back this effort with money and other resources, so it must be important. It makes people in all walks of life pay attention.

A prime example of a partnership between business and health care that is built around networking and benefits all parties is the Nutrition Screening Initiative (NSI) launched in the spring of 1991. NSI is a coalition of powerful and prestigious associations and individuals in medicine, health care, and aging. It is being led by the 68,000-member American Academy of Family Physicians, the 62,000-member American Dietetic Association, and the influential National Council on Aging, with the support of Ross Laboratories.

This 5-year campaign to promote routine nutritional screening and better nutrition treatment in the U.S. health care system also involves a blue ribbon advisory committee of 35 key health and medical organizations and professionals.

By bringing Ross and its resources into the mix, NSI is able to use the company's networks to bring its message to key legislators in the federal government. It also can more effectively focus on its prime target audience, a demographic segment Ross is knowledgeable about through its product marketing and sales efforts.

The end result will be an improvement in the way health care is delivered, particularly to senior citizens.

It is apparent that dietitians and nutritionists can benefit in a variety of ways from partnership relationships with public-minded, health-oriented private businesses and corporations. What, in turn, is private industry looking for in relationships with dietitians and nutritionists? How can they help meet the objectives and needs of private industry?

WHAT INDUSTRY LOOKS FOR FROM DIETITIANS AND NUTRITIONISTS

At first glance, it might appear that with its networks, resources, and other assets the private sector is bringing more to the relationship than the dietitian or nutritionist. Close examination reveals, however, that dietitians and nutritionists have much to offer industry in terms of quality and in impact.

The captains of industry want to know more about dietetics and nutrition because that is an area of interest for their customers. To fill that need, they are hiring more dietitians and nutritionists to work on staff, often in new or unconventional positions. There are already a substantial number of such specialists in business and communications. For the same reason, companies are receptive to partnerships and alliances with dietitians.

A recent study examined the attributes for employability in industry.[2] These same qualities are equally relevant for dietitians and nutritionists seeking partnerships. Current and prospective employers were questioned, as were 300 members of the Dietitians in Business and Communications Practice Group. The majority of both groups found the most influential attribute to be "communications skills." Clinical experience also was considered important.

The respondents did not agree as completely on other qualities. Employers and prospective employers ranked an MBA as the second most important; dietitians and nutritionists ranked it in fifteenth place. Conversely, dietitians and nutritionists placed registration status—the RD—as fourth on their list; business people ranked it as the least important of all qualities.[2]

The study also reported that employers look to dietitians and nutritionists to increase health care sales, enhance the credibility of the organization, and help them understand customer needs and expectations. It also underscored the fact that dietitians and nutritionists have much to offer as partners to private industry. The benefits dietitians are able to bestow can be assigned to three basic categories: credibility, networking, and the ability to target a message.

Credibility

Health care professionals generally and dietitians and nutritionists specifically have an extremely positive public image. Credibility and rapport with patients are common attributes. They have a reputation for being altruistic and dedicated to serving the health and well-being of society. Who enjoys more respect than the physician, the nurse, and the dietitian and nutritionist? Patients and the public in general do not usually perceive of these professionals as selling anything other than good health.

A recent example of a joint venture in which the private sector partner, in this case a publisher, derives benefit from the prestige of health care involves a magazine, *Healthy Kids*. Described as "the magazine for parents from the American Academy of Pediatrics," *Healthy Kids* is issued quarterly by Cahners Publishing Company. It is available through approximately two thirds of U.S. pediatricians, who distribute the publication—bearing their own imprint—in waiting rooms and offices throughout the country. It is effective because it is tied to the American Academy of Pediatrics.

Networking

Just as private industry has its own business-oriented networks, health care professionals have long been establishing relationships in their own field.

Dietitians and nutritionists in particular have a very tight, highly effective organizational network. Through ADA's district, state, and affiliate associations and its house of delegates, word travels fast among 62,000 members. Dietitians and nutritionists learn quickly about a company with an excellent reputation for nutrition and health.

Moreover, dietitians and nutritionists have strong networks through the entire health care field, not just nationally, but internationally as well. The professional network built on the credibility of dietitians and nutritionists is a most effective way for a corporation to accomplish its strategic objectives.

Targeting

One of the major advantages the private sector derives from working with the dietetic profession is the ability to market its goods, services, and concepts to targeted audiences. Whether it is 62,000 dietitians and nutritionists, an estimated 2 million nurses, 68,000 family physicians and general practitioners who each average 5876 patient visits per year, or 31,000 pediatricians who on an average see more than 6000 children and parents annually, the influence of these professionals is enormous.

More than half of ADA's members belong to a practice group (see Chapter 18). A cooperative message can be communicated to the market segments served by a given practice group in a timely and cost-effective manner. For example, a company interested in reaching a target audience concerned with diabetes would be able to deliver its message through the ADA's Diabetes Practice Group. Similarly, communications with the elderly, young mothers, or any of a number of other special groups can easily be targeted through a partnership with the ADA.

Although dietitians and nutritionists cannot match the private sector's financial resources and power to mount multimedia advertising campaigns, they can draw on their experience, expertise, and networks to identify and market to specific groups in and outside the profession.

HOW DIETITIANS AND NUTRITIONISTS AND INDUSTRY WORK BEST TOGETHER

One of the prime prerequisites for a mutually beneficial relationship is for the partners to retain autonomy. Failure to do so can seriously damage the credibility of all participants. This priority is emphasized by Mullis and Shannon, who suggest that when both parties are autonomous "the relationship is open and positive, and the contribution each has to offer is viewed as essential to the success of the program."[6]

In everything they do, especially in their dealings with the public, the private sector, their fellow practitioners, and other members of the health care team, dietitians and nutritionists must enhance their reputation by always demonstrating the highest standards in performance and in values. No matter what the financial pressures—income or the employer's bottom line—dietitians and nutritionists must never lose sight of their professional goal: to foster good health through good nutrition.

As dietitians and nutritionists increasingly function as marketers—for their services and for their profession—the credibility that marks the health care field becomes still more important to them as individuals. Credibility is something that is obtained the old-fashioned way, by earning it. Once earned, it is an asset to protect. Without credibility, even the best product or service will struggle for acceptance.

One of the most striking examples is Tylenol, which has become a textbook case of successful crisis management. Its manufacturer, Johnson & Johnson, was able to overcome a product tampering panic, rebuild the credibility of Tylenol, and restore the product as a market leader. Meyers, the former chairman of American Motors and an expert in crisis management, writes, "Whenever the public at large is involved, the most important thing is to protect your credibility. With it, you can recover; without it, you are in for lasting damage."[5]

The best course is to be protective of credibility in the first place and, whenever possible, anticipate and avoid events that could damage it. Dietitians and nutritionists need to maintain and enhance that credibility by emphasizing a strong science background. The credibility of physicians is built, in part, by the confidence the public has in their training and expertise.

FOUR KEY STEPS IN BUILDING PARTNERSHIPS

Once the reasons for forming partnerships and the principles that must be observed in the process are understood, it is appropriate to address how to proceed. The four key steps are:

- Situational analysis
- Writing proposals
- Presentation of the proposal
- Delivering what has been promised

Situational Analysis

The general who launches a campaign before analyzing the enemy, the terrain, and the conditions is courting military disaster. The dietitian or nutritionist who approaches a partnership without research and situational analysis is risking failure or, worse, a loss of respect and credibility.

Situational analysis is becoming informed and knowledgeable before approaching the target company or organization. It involves conducting a gap analysis, which, simply put, is finding a need and filling it. In building partnerships, gap analysis means determining what is special about the proposed relationship and demonstrating that it will fill a unique role. It requires that dietitians and nutritionists draw on their knowledge of the potential partner, their own services, and marketplace conditions and then demonstrate the benefits of working together. Those benefits may be enhanced prestige, reaching new audiences, or cost savings.

The necessary knowledge can be acquired through library research, reading annual reports, and talking to experts in the field, including security analysts, former employees, friends, and friends of friends. The goal is to acquire as much knowledge as possible and to understand the prospective partner's products, goals, personnel, and corporate ethos and philosophy. In some quarters this process is described as "knowing the customer."

Whatever the appellation, the end result is the ability to demonstrate compellingly the benefits of the partnership to the corporation and to prove that the alliance is a win-win situation. Mullis and Shannon suggest:

> To be successful collaborators, dietitians and food marketers must be willing to listen and recognize one another's needs. All of them need to be flexible and willing to seek ways to accommodate one another's positions and values. . . . Dietitians who function successfully in collaborative programs must have credibility in the community and be able to establish strong, empathetic community relationships. Other competencies important to successful collaborations are organizational skills, the ability to persuade or create intention to change, and the ability to communicate how to make the change . . . they must be able to thrive within the dynamic atmosphere of community activism. . . . Those [food marketers] most likely to be interested in involvement will have a commitment to human welfare.[6]

Writing Proposals

An effective proposal has focus; it covers one or two major points compellingly and concisely. The best proposal is built around the satisfaction of a company's need or the solution to a problem.

It is called *customer focus*, which is built on knowing the customer, in this case the company that is being pitched. To develop this focus on the customer, dietitians and nutritionists must differentiate between what they think the customer needs or wants and what is actually needed or wanted. No one can attain that information by guessing. It is imperative that dietitians and nutritionists base their proposals on facts, not assumptions.

Mackay, chairman and chief executive officer of a multimillion-dollar envelope company and a best-selling author, writes:

> Knowing your customer means knowing what your customer really wants. Maybe it is your product, but maybe there's something else, too: recognition, re-

spect, reliability, concern, service, a feeling of self-importance, friendship, help—things all of us care more about as human beings than we care about mail or envelopes.[4]

Knowing the customer, determining specific needs, and identifying who wants a product and who wants friendship, help, or respect involve research, as does learning the business goals and good works objectives of a corporation. That research can be as complex as an extensive survey, or it can be as basic as the old-fashioned methods of careful conversation and attentive listening.

Proposals should also be keyed to opportunities. One person's problem is another's opportunity. A corporate chief executive officer may be experiencing difficulty in reaching a particular market segment, for example, mothers of newborn babies. Dietitians and nutritionists, through the appropriate ADA practice group, have a pipeline to those very people. The corporation has a problem; dietitians and nutritionists have an opportunity.

Over the last 5 years, the federal government has issued a number of initiatives to guide the public on preventive health measures. Recently the Surgeon General released *Healthy People 2000*, developed by the U.S. Department of Health and Human Services. The initiative focuses on health problems and goals such as decreasing the incidence of obesity and increasing breastfeeding. Obesity and the disinclination of some women to breastfeed are problems; solving them are opportunities for dietitians and nutritionists. There are 21 such opportunities in *Healthy People 2000* (see Chapter 1), and it is a virtual game plan for dietitians and nutritionists in the coming years.

Changing federal regulations on food labeling have created confusion. That, too, is an opportunity for dietitians and nutritionists and those companies that want to promote consumer education. There is a tendency among many consumers to look at food as risk-avoidance behavior instead of as a pleasurable experience. That is a problem, but it also is a challenging opportunity. Can dietitians and nutritionists find ways to present nutrition advice positively and appealingly? Who can be their partners in the effort?

Identifying opportunities is not equal to capitalizing on them. Opportunities are not permanent. By their very nature they are transient and call for timely action. Some people describe such circumstances as the "window of opportunity." When the window is open, dietitians and nutritionists must be ready with their services and their programs. They cannot wait until circumstances are perfect. Those who do are never ready for action.

The Nutrition Screening Initiative, which is an example of networking in action, also illustrates the principle of the window of opportunity. The NSI campaign, which aims at making nutrition assessment as integral a part of health care as a blood pressure or pulse reading, is an idea whose time has definitely come. It is the culmination of years of "growing" a market and of promoting the need for nutrition screening to expand that market.

Presentation of the Proposal

To be effective in presenting a partnership proposal, it is wise to develop a strategy. That strategy should include who (the person to whom the presentation will be made), what (the content of the proposal), where (at the corporate headquarters, at a neutral site), and how (written, oral, or both; in person or by mail, telephone, or fax).

Proposals are not always presented to the top executive of a company. Often a middle manager or someone in the ranks can open the proper door. Recognizing who actually makes things happen in any organization is part of knowing the customer. Business lore is filled with tales of secretaries who were the real power behind the throne.

Developing allies within an organization and then working with those people can help get the job done. Understanding the political climate, practicing communication and presentation skills, utilizing audio and visual aids as appropriate, and, most of all, supporting the presentation with evidence, hard facts, and proof can enhance the chances of success.

Kanter suggests that two kinds of information are required for effective partnership participation: technical knowledge and knowledge of partnership activities and political intelligence.[1]

Deliver What Has Been Promised

Few things in life are as frustrating—or disappointing—as dealing with someone who does not deliver on a promise. It is easy and perhaps tempting to tell potential customers precisely what they want to hear and to make the promise it takes to close the deal today.

However, there are two reasons to make sure that the promise can be backed. The first is that integrity is involved. Once compromised, integrity cannot easily be recaptured or rebuilt. The second is that an unfulfilled promise is, at the least, counterproductive. The goal is usually a continuing relationship. Relationships cannot be built on the foundation of hollow promises.

It also is important to monitor results, make changes and adjustments as necessary, and exercise quality control. Experience is a great teacher for willing students. It also is important to share results and experiences to build trust and bring partners into the loop so their experience and expertise can be applied to making the venture a success.

Those with experience in marketing may recognize these four steps. They are, in fact, marketing principles that have been used with success for years by professionals in all fields.

Mackay has an excellent explanation of marketing that can be applied by dietitians and nutritionists to pursuing partnerships and generally in positioning themselves in the changing health care environment: "Marketing is not the art of selling. It's not the simple business of convincing someone to buy. It is the art of creating conditions by which the buyer convinces himself."[4]

PERSONAL QUALITIES FOR SUCCESS

Developing and polishing personal qualities and skills can enhance the prospects for success in partnerships, as well as in most other areas of professional and private life.

Of these, the single most important may be communication skills. It is no accident or coincidence that the respondents in the Kirk, Shanklin, and Gorman study ranked communication skills at the top of their list of influential attributes.[2]

Expressing oneself clearly and forcefully is essential in both speaking and writing. The best ideas in the world wither and die in their formative stages if they are not transmitted to others, presented in understandable form, and shared with customers or target audiences.

Very few people are born communicators. Generally the great communicators have worked at it and continue to do so. They study the channels of communication, learn techniques, practice speaking and writing, critique their own performances, and know that communication consists of both transmission and feedback.

Consequently, they also listen. They hear and heed what the other person has to say. They give the speaker full attention, and they think about what they are hearing. That, too, is part of knowing the customer.

Dietitians and nutritionists who want to play a major role in forging partnerships with the private sector also would do well to focus on leadership and management skills. The profession needs both, and they are complementary but different.

John P. Kotter, professor of organizational behavior at the Harvard Business School, writes that management involves functions like "planning and budgeting, organizing and staffing, problem solving," while leadership deals with "establishing direction, aligning people, motivating and inspiring," and developing a vision. "The real challenge," he continues, "is to combine strong leadership and strong management and use each to balance the other."[3]

It is apparent how each—the leader and the manager—fits into partnership building and what roles they will play. Individuals can develop ability as a leader or as a manager. There are many courses and books; there are role models to follow. Much of the essence of self-development can be distilled into self-confidence or self-esteem, vision, focus, political or organizational savvy, and willingness to take risks.

SUMMARY

There are many yardsticks for a successful partnership. Perhaps the most basic is pragmatic: Does it work? Does it make sense? Are the partners compatible? Does it satisfy the objectives and needs of both partners?

Kanter lists the "Six I's of Successful Partnerships." With only slight variation, they are valid for dietitians and nutritionists and partnerships:

- "The relationship is *I*mportant, and therefore it gets adequate resources, management attention and sponsorship; there is no point in going to the trouble of a partnership unless it has a strategic significance.
- "There is an agreement for longer-term *I*nvestment, which tends to help equalize benefits over time." For dietitians and nutritionists, that investment could be translated instead into a long-term commitment.
- "The partners are *I*nterdependent, which helps keep power balanced."
- "The organizations are *I*ntegrated so that the appropriate points of contact and communication are managed."
- "Each is *I*nformed about the plans and directions of the other."
- "Finally, the partnership is *I*nstitutionalized— bolstered by a framework of supporting mechanisms, from legal requirements to social ties to shared values, all of which in fact make trust possible."[1]

As the environment of health care continues to change and as technology continues its revolution, there will be innumerable problems and opportunities for all dietitians and nutritionists, no matter what their specialty. There will be enormous new areas for cooperation with corporate America. The challenge through the next decade and into the next century is to identify and capitalize on those opportunities by marketing services, products, and concepts that solve problems. As Kanter observes:

Today the strategic challenge of doing more with less leads corporations to look outward as well as inward for solutions to the competitiveness dilemma, improving their ability to compete without adding internal capacity. Lean, agile, post-entrepreneurial companies can stretch in three ways. They can pool resources with others, ally to exploit an opportunity, or link systems in a partnership. . . . Strategic alliances and partnerships are a potent way to do more with less.[1]

Dietitians and nutritionists who know their customers and understand needs and wants and how to fill them are the best positioned to convert problems into opportunities to work in those strategic alliances and partnerships.

When discussing the relationship between health care professionals and corporate America, some people are inclined to focus exclusively on the business aspects of a situation, and sometimes the broader vista is overlooked. For dietitians and nutritionists who deal with nutrition and health matters, maintaining perspective is essential, even when they are engaging in basically business activities. By focusing on the message of dietetics and nutrition and by maintaining focus on a vision, they are, above all, promoting better understanding of nutrition and better eating practices.

From a pragmatic point of view, dietitians and nutritionists should bear in mind that industry values people with leadership and managerial abilities and marketing skills. It respects talented marketers, leaders, and managers. As the private sector and health care continue to move closer together, those dietitians who have developed and excelled as marketers, leaders, and managers will be able to move in the vanguard of these emerging partnerships and alliances.

That, in turn, will enable dietitians and nutritionists to continue making important contributions to the improvement of the health and well-being of American society—for the present and for future generations.

REFERENCES

1. Kanter RM: *When giants learn to dance*, New York, 1990, Simon and Schuster.
2. Kirk D, Shanklin CW, Gorman MA: Attributes and qualifications that employers seek when hiring dietitians in business and industry, *J Am Diet Assoc* 89:494, 1989.
3. Kotter JP: *A force for change: how leadership differs from management*, New York, 1990, The Free Press.
4. Mackay H: *How to swim with the sharks without being eaten alive*, New York, 1988, Ballantine Books.
5. Meyers GTC: *When it hits the fan: managing the nine crises of business*, Boston, 1986, Houghton Mifflin.
6. Mullis R, Shannon B: Building partnerships for the food marketing system: an expanding role for dietitians, *J Am Diet Assoc* 87:1622, 1987.
7. Naisbett J: *Megatrends: the new directions transforming our lives*, New York, 1982, Warner Books.
8. Owen AL: *Increasing our impact through building partnerships and collaborations*, speech to the building partnerships workshop at the University of Minnesota Heart Health Program, May 11, 1987.
9. Ries A, Trout J: *Positioning: the battle for your mind*, New York, 1982, Warner Books.

12 Public Policy and Legislation

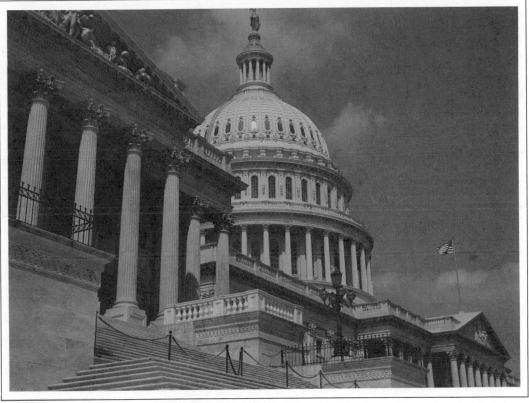

GENERAL CONCEPT

Nutrition policy exerts an overarching influence on the types of programs and services offered by dietitians and nutritionists in the community. It is essential that dietitians and nutritionists be familiar with the issues and the public policy process in order to provide leadership and direction to both nutrition programs and practice.

OUTCOME OBJECTIVES

When you finish this chapter, you should be able to:

- Define policy and discuss its importance in the field of community nutrition.
- Describe the policy-making process and steps at which informed advocacy on the part of dietitians and nutritionists can be effective.
- Compare and contrast the functions of the legislative, executive, and judicial branches of government in the policy-making process.
- Describe the major policy elements in nutrition, the programs now in existence, and the political and economic forces that may cause them to change in the future.
- Recognize the need for advocacy skills on the part of dietitians and nutritionists and discuss their role in shaping public policy.

PUBLIC POLICY

Policy provides a framework for decision making and a guide for making choices among alternative courses of action. Policy statements set the general tone for how an agency, a group, or even a government is to operate. Policies provide the guidelines for setting priorities among competing goals, the allocation of funds, selection of personnel, standards for program operation, and future direction. This chapter discusses the public policy process as it has affected the nutrition programs and services offered in the community.

Public policy guides the actions of governments, whether federal, state, or local. Public policies have significant impacts beyond the entity making the decision and usually involve the use of taxpayers' dollars in carrying out certain actions. Policies that guide governmental action are the means by which modern societies try to shape their futures in ways they consider acceptable. As Milio further shows,

> The important mutually evolving elements in [an] ecological view of policymaking are the social climate (the environmental conditions) and stakeholder organizations—including the policykeeper—and their agendas, priorities, resources, and perceptions of

timeliness, which affect the strategy and timing of the attempts to influence the shape of a policy.[37]

Policy-making is a dynamic process in which a number of participants—including influential organizations, interest groups, and legislators—work toward attaining mutually satisfactory goals by compromise and consensus. Public policy is shaped by groups who have deployed their resources to influence the form, pace, or direction of policy-making in ways that will enhance—or at least not harm—their own interests. The business of policy-making often involves an ongoing struggle among conflicting values, vested interests, and ambitious personalities. Even when interested parties share the same lofty goals, effective negotiation and trade-off skills must be employed in order to construct functional policy.

Public policy evolves out of a sound knowledge base, coupled with a supportive political climate (Fig. 12-1).[48] The knowledge base is derived from research data, program evaluations, or demonstration project results, that is, a convincing presentation of the "facts" behind the issue. A supportive political climate is necessary to make individual concerns apparent to others so that they will share in the goals for setting policy. Even the "right values" coupled with ample scientific evidence may not be enough to establish a policy. Setting policy always involves striking a balance between the scientific evidence and the values, priorities, needs, and concerns of stakeholders and constituents. Any enthusiasm for making new policy must be tempered by the realization that policy makers are always constrained by budget realities; maintaining the status quo is usually much less costly than changing policy or setting new policy directions. A complex balancing act is required to satisfy consumer concerns, industry interests, scientific principles, and budget realities.[10] Members of the nutrition community must be prepared to work with other professional organizations and interest groups with related agendas who, together with policy makers, can develop a set of workable, coordinated policy guidelines.

What has been described is the rational, "ideal" model for policy-making. All too often policy-mak-

POLICY FRAMEWORK

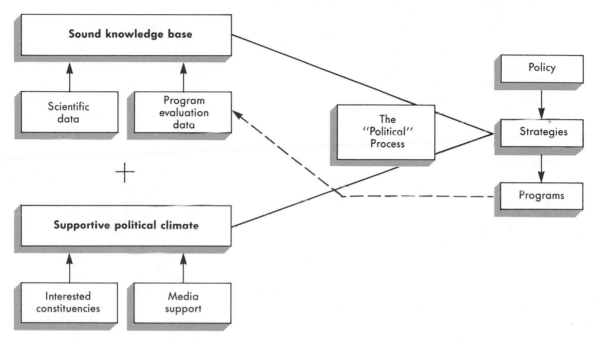

Figure 12-1. Basis of public policy formulation.

ing depends on raw—both positive and negative— emotion. Lobbyists know that if a legislator cares "passionately" about their issue, they will harness that extra measure of energy to capture yet another vote. This, then, is what policy-making is all about—bringing together those individuals and groups, even the media, who together want and will work to change the status quo in the direction they deem desirable. For us in the nutrition community, it means bringing together those forces who have the time, the resources, the expertise, and the intensity to work on public issues that will improve the nutritional status, and thus the health, of the American population—the fundamental goal of nutrition policy.

THE POLICY PROCESS

Setting the Agenda

The process by which issues compete—successfully—for governmental attention is called *agenda setting*. In applying this model to the issues of health and nutrition, Sims examined the process by which nutrition emerged as a viable public issue in the late 1960s, how the issue was legitimatized and institutionalized by a proliferation of programs and initiatives during the early and mid-1970s, and how in the early 1980s nutrition ceased to be a critical issue on the public policy agenda.[47]

In the late 1980s, nutrition emerged yet again as a salient public policy issue, aided by the publication of two landmark reports: *The Surgeon General's Report on Nutrition and Health*[53] and the National Research Council's *Diet and Health: Implications for Reducing Chronic Disease Risk*.[39] Although many reports had long supported the notion of the relationship between diet and health, the scientific credibility of these two reports legitimized the proposition that diet and nutrition were linked to six of the ten leading causes of death in the United States[53] and proposed dietary modifications to reduce the risk of these diseases. Spurred on by the power of these two reports, nutrition competed—successfully, this time—for governmental action, resulting in the passage of two major pieces of legislation in the 101st Congress in 1990: the Nutrition Monitoring and Related Research Act (PL 101-445) and the Nutrition Labeling and Education Act (PL 101-535), both of which had been under consideration by Congress for a number of years.

Influencing the Process

How did this happen? What went on? Who was involved? As presented earlier, public policy evolves when a sound knowledge base is coupled with a supportive political climate before being subjected to the policy-making process (Fig. 12-1). A number of converging forces contribute at each phase of the process; these forces include scientific organizations, the food industry, health professional associations, or voluntary health organizations who might provide data or evidence to contribute to the knowledge base surrounding the issue, as well as consumer advocacy groups, the media, or influential constituents who contribute to making the political climate supportive of the issue under discussion. Indeed, nutritionists may make important contributions at any point in this process, either by providing scientific evidence or data to strengthen the knowledge base or by sharing experiences that garner political support for the issue. Individuals can successfully influence the policy-making process if they develop a positive working relationship with public officials, are savvy and sensitive about the political environment, and provide knowledgeable input (both support and criticism) for a legislator's policy efforts.

Elected officials are in Washington or their state capitals to represent their constituents' views. Because of this fact, nutritionists have two positions of access and influence: first, they are tax-paying voters who are constituents of a particular congressional district; second, they have information to assist the legislator in supporting worthwhile legislation, the goal of all policy makers. Constituent support greatly affects a bill's chances of being en-

BUT WHAT CAN I *DO*?

Here are eight steps to help you lobby your legislators:

1. Begin by establishing contact with your state's congressional delegation, whether or not your senators and representatives sit on key authorizing or budget committees. Turn these contracts into relationships. Do not wait until you are angry to let them hear from you—your job is to educate.
2. Find out which members of the staff handle such issues as food, nutrition, trade, environment, and consumer affairs. Very often only one or two people will be in charge of all these issues.
3. Write to the appropriate members or staff; introduce yourself; explain your interest and the services you provide, and let them know what a vital role you or your interest plays in your community.
4. Follow up with a telephone call to make sure that the appropriate staff member received your letter and to answer any questions they might have.
5. Find out when they will be in the home district or tell them you are planning a trip to Washington, D.C. Make an appointment to meet either the staff or your legislator—or both.
6. Prepare exhaustively for that meeting. If you plan to discuss a particular piece of legislation, learn the vocabulary of that legislation and where it stands in committee (a call to the staff of the relevant committee can help here). You will also need to educate the member about your interest. Whether you are a food professional in an institution, a manager of a food bank, or an academic with a flair for consumer rights, promote your agenda in a manner that leaves the member with a feeling that he wants to help. One effective method of education is to invite the member to tour your workplace to see firsthand the societal benefits your interest foster.
7. Prepare some brief written materials—written in lay language—to distribute at your meeting.
8. After your visit, be sure to send a thank-you note summarizing the key points of your visit. Keep in touch with the office on a regular basis at least every other month.

From Community Nutrition Institute: *Nutrition Week*, March 13, 1992.

acted into law. The preceding boxes provide important tips for lobbying legislators and communicating with government officials.

A "winning" policy capitalizes on the policy makers' agenda, not the constituent's or the lobbyist's! To be sure, most legislators want respect from their colleagues on the Hill and desire to be respected, knowing that they have been responsible for passing "good policy."

Achieving a successful end to policy-making depends on choosing the right strategies. The following guides are offered to encourage nutritionists to get involved in the policy process and experience a successful outcome as a result.[11,33]

Be Well Informed

Be thoroughly knowledgeable about the issue, the need for the policy or legislation, and the arguments opponents may use against the issue. It is also crucial to be well informed about the legislative process and to use your knowledge of the stages of the policy process to your advantage.

Develop Broad Support

Forming active coalitions among diverse groups such as researchers, health professionals, educators, farmers, and consumer groups, as well as influential citizens, friends of decision makers, and respected community groups is the key to success. Such coalitions, often representing diverse points of interest on the issue, usually have greater political clout than individuals or organizations working alone. Currently the following coalitions of groups are focusing on affecting food and nutrition policies:[50]

Child Nutrition Forum. Organized to express a unified voice about support for child nutrition programs, its members include the Society for Nutrition Education (SNE), American Dietetic Association (ADA), American School Food Service Association (ASFSA), Food Research and Action Center (FRAC), National Parent Teacher Association (PTA), and the Community Nutrition Institute (CNI).

End Childhood Hunger. More than 100 different public health organizations including SNE, church groups, and trade associations joined FRAC in a national campaign to end childhood hunger.

The Food and Nutrition Labeling Group. Formed to discuss and lobby for nutrition labeling reform, it has a membership of more than 20 different groups, including American Dietetic Association, SNE, American Heart Association (AHA), the American Cancer Society (ACS), American Association for Retired Persons (AARP), Center for Science in the Public Interest (CSPI), and Public Voice for Food and Health Policy.

Task Force on Aging. Comprised of 60 member organizations that support elder care initiatives on health care, food assistance, and transportation.

Anticipate the Unexpected

Anticipate problems and develop alternative approaches or compromise positions. Learn to cooperate and collaborate without being compromised. Think about successful strategies that have worked for others, and adapt them to your situation. Murphy's Law will prevail—whatever can go wrong, will—but be creative in exploring and using other avenues to reach the same end.

Don't Get Discouraged

Many legislative initiatives require several sessions of Congress before they are passed. Remember that the Nutrition Monitoring bill, passed in 1990, was introduced in several Congresses, passed by the House and Senate, even vetoed by the president. In all, the whole process took more than 6 years before the proposed legislation actually became law.

The Framework

In the United States, separate and equal branches of government theoretically have primary responsibility for a particular phase of the policy process. Constitutionally, Congress is given the responsibility for policy formulation by the mandate of making laws. The president, as head of the executive branch, is mandated to "faithfully execute the laws." The judicial branch is required to interpret the laws as disputes arise and are litigated. In reality, each of the three branches performs most of the policy functions of formulation, implementation, and interpretation.[30]

The Legislative Process

Laws that initiate, modify, authorize, and appropriate funds for all programs and services administered by the federal government are passed by Congress, the principal arm of the legislative branch. Legislatures often assume three roles: a law-making role, a representative role, and a constituency service role. In the United States, these sometimes conflicting roles are all the responsibility of members of Congress.[30] The Congress is divided into two chambers: the House of Representatives and the Senate.

First and foremost, Congress is people. The members of Congress—100 senators and 435 representatives—are certainly the best known because they have stood for election to office. Each member of the House of Representatives is chosen by election every 2 years in all 50 states. The membership of the House remains constant at 435, with the number of representatives from each state determined by that state's share of the national population. Each member represents the state congressional district from which he or she was elected, with district lines redrawn every 10 years based on the most recent census results. The redistricting process can be highly political, in and of itself, because both parties hope to increase their advantages and incumbents want to ensure stability. Each member of the House represents an average of 500,000 people. Two senators are elected from each state, and each serves 6-year terms. These terms are on a staggered basis; one third of the Senate is up for reelection every 2 years.

In addition to the members of Congress, there are nearly 12,000 staff assistants who work for the members and for the many committees and subcommittees in both houses. They assist members with scheduling their time, keeping in touch with constituents, and keeping in touch with current issues.

Making Laws

In any given year, between 10,000 and 15,000 bills are introduced. Because of the volume of work and the potential for chaos in such a large legislative body, certain rules and procedures—as well as personalities—influence the process. Party leadership, the committee structure, and procedural rules all greatly affect legislative affairs. Thus the chances of any particular piece of legislation being passed do not depend solely on the number of members who support it. The ability of a bill's sponsors to propel it through complicated committee and floor procedures and their expertise in the topic of the bill are both important in ensuring passage.[4]

The general sequence of stages or steps through which a bill passes on its way to becoming a law is shown in Figure 12-2. Actually all steps can be recombined into six major phases, as indicated below.[13] Concerned professionals can take the appropriate actions if they know the steps in the legis-

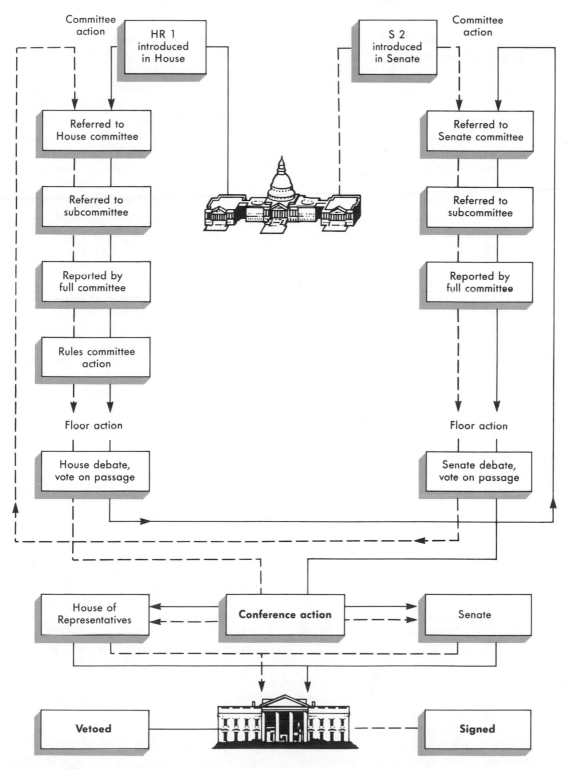

Figure 12-2. How a bill becomes law.
From Wormser MD, editor: *CQ's Guide to Congress*, ed 3, Washington, DC, 1982, Congressional Quarterly; p. 413.

lative process as well as the key decision makers and their responsibilities at each step of the process.

I. Introduction

1. The bill is introduced in one chamber, either the House or Senate. (In practice, most bills begin as similar proposals and are introduced in both houses.) Every member of Congress has the power to introduce legislation. In addition, the Constitution gives the president the authority to recommend legislation to Congress, either in an oral message to a joint session of Congress or through written messages to one or both chambers.

II. Committee Action

2. The bill is referred to the appropriate committee having jurisdiction over the subject matter. The most distinguishing characteristic of the legislative branch is the predominant role played by the committee system. Here the "real work" is done as committees have their own operating rules with the authority to draft, amend, and vote on legislation. The committees and subcommittees have been described as "the political nerve ends, the gatherers of information, the sifters of alternatives, the refiners of legislative detail."[17]

To make the workload more manageable, each committee is given responsibility for a specific area of public policy. However, because many bills are written so that they could be referred to more than one committee, the speaker of the House must decide which committee has jurisdiction; he can also issue joint or sequential referral to committee. The House has 21 standing (or permanent) committees and nearly 150 subcommittees. Food, nutrition, and health issues are generally considered by several committees. In the Senate, they include the Committee on Agriculture, Nutrition, and Forestry and the Committee on Labor and Human Resources, among others. In the House, most nutrition bills are sent to Agriculture, Education and Labor, or Energy and Commerce. Committees having jurisdiction over specific food, nutrition, and health issues are listed in the box on p. 295.

When needed, special or select committees may be created on a temporary basis for a limited and specific purpose. Although helpful for calling public attention to an issue or for information gathering, these committees do not have the authority to authorize or appropriate funds for programs. The Senate Select Committee on Aging and the House Select Committees on Children, Youth, and Families and on Hunger are currently active.

Committee chairmanship is held only by those in the majority party. This is an extremely powerful position as the committee chair has full authority to decide which matters the committee will act on, or even consider, during the course of a congressional session. This person may also be important in guiding the bill through passage by the full chamber.

Subcommittees are assigned responsibility for specific portions of the legislative jurisdiction of the full committees. Subcommittees also exercise oversight power over the federal agencies, boards, and departments that regulate matters within their subject areas. During discussion by the subcommittee, legislation undergoes the most intensive study and most extensive changes. Senior committee members are frequently given subcommittees to chair, so their expertise in the particular area is usually well established.

Committees and subcommittees can choose to take no action, thus killing a bill, or they can take action on it through such procedures as hearings and markups.

3. In further action, the bill becomes the subject of committee hearings, where pro and con arguments are presented and discussed. Hearings are called by the committee chair to gather public and expert testimony on whether legislation is needed and, if so, what form it should take. The committee may even hold field hearings outside Washington to gain grassroots support for a measure. Hearings are also used to establish a public record of the history and controversy surrounding a particular piece of legislation. They may be used to form or affect public opinion, especially when testimony is presented by celebrities. Hearings may be held to delay action on the legislation or to pacify a particular interest group. The information gathered

CONGRESS IN COMMITTEE

Members of Congress conduct most of their legislative work in committee. Each committee is broken down into subcommittees, which exercise jurisdiction over a specific program or issue. A committee can report out a bill, amendments to a bill, introduce a substitute bill, or ignore a bill. Several committees and subcommittees formulate policy on the following food and nutrition programs and issues:

Annual Fiscal Year Budget Proposals: Senate and House Committee on Budget

Appropriations for the Department of Health and Human Services (DHHS): Senate and House Committee on Appropriations; Subcommittee on Labor, Health, Human Services, Education, and Related Agencies

Appropriations for International Health, Agriculture, and Education: Senate and House Committee on Appropriations; Subcommittee on Foreign Operations

Appropriations for U.S. Department of Agriculture (USDA), the Food and Drug Administration (FDA), Food for Peace Program: Senate and House Committee on Appropriations; Subcommittee on Agriculture, Rural Development, and Related Agencies

Child Nutrition Programs: Senate Committee on Agriculture, Nutrition and Forestry; Subcommittee on Nutrition; House Committee on Education and Labor; Subcommittee on Elementary, Secondary, and Vocational Education

Food Labeling, Food Safety, Public Health Issues: Senate Committee on Labor and Human Resources; House Committee on Energy and Commerce; Subcommittee on Health and the Environment

Domestic Hunger: Senate Committee on Agriculture, Nutrition and Forestry; Subcommittee on Nutrition, House Committee on Agriculture; Subcommittee on Domestic Marketing, Consumer Relations, and Nutrition

Elderly Programs: Senate Committee on Labor and Human Resources; Subcommittee on Aging; House Committee on Education and Labor; Subcommittee on Human Resources

Food Stamp Program, Extension Service, Commodity Distribution: Senate Committee on Agriculture, Nutrition and Forestry; Subcommittee on Nutrition; House Committee on Agriculture; Subcommittee on Domestic Marketing, Consumer Relations, and Nutrition

International Hunger Issues: Senate Committee on Foreign Relations; House Committee on Foreign Affairs

Nutrition Monitoring and Research: Senate Committee on Governmental Affairs; Subcommittee on Oversight Government Management; Senate Committee on Agriculture; Subcommittee on Nutrition and Investigations; and Senate Committee on Labor and Human Resources; House Committee on Science, Space, and Technology; Subcommittee on Science; House Committee on Agriculture; Subcommittee on Department Operations, Research, and Foreign Agriculture; and House Committee on Energy and Commerce; Subcommittee on Health and the Environment

Select Committees

Senate Special Committee on Aging; House Select Committee on Aging

House Select Committee on Children, Youth, and Families

House Select Committee on Hunger

From Society for Nutrition Education. *Call to action: a public policy handbook*, Minneapolis, MN, 1992. Reprinted with permission.

during hearings is used by the committee to draft new legislation, amend the legislation already before it (done in a markup session), or decide that no final legislative action is necessary.

4. The bill is amended by committee members in markup sessions. In these sessions, the subcommittee goes over the bill line by line and rewrites it to reflect the subcommittee's views. If the subcommittee determines that the bill needs considerable revision, it may be completely redrafted, given a new number, and responsored by the full committee. If the subcommittee approves the bill

by a substantial margin, the full committee generally agrees to support the bill with few or no changes.

5. The bill is favorably reported by the committee to the floor of the chamber. When the committee has taken a final vote on the legislation and all its recommended amendments, the committee staff writes a report that explains the committee's reasons for approving the bill, and the legislation is "ordered reported." This step directs the committee staff to compile the various drafts of the legislation and recommended amendments into the bill format.

This process can take one of two forms. In the first type, the committee may direct the staff to mark changes in the actual text of the bill before the committee to make it consistent with the committee's recommendations. This "reported bill" is reprinted with dashes marked through its original language where changes have been recommended and the suggested new language is noted in italic print. These recommended changes or "committee amendments" are the first order of business when the bill reaches the floor of the chamber. In the second form, the staff may be directed by the committee to draft a "clean bill" that incorporates the committee recommendations into a cohesive piece of legislation, which is then sent to the floor intact. This strategy is chosen when the committee wants to avoid floor votes on the committee amendments that were added to the original language of the bill. Clean bills are usually sponsored by the committee or subcommittee chair.[4]

III. Scheduling for Vote

6. The bill is then placed on the chamber's agenda of business for a particular day. After a bill is reported from committee, it goes (in the House) to the Rules Committee, where further hearings are held to determine the importance of the bill and whether it should be sent to the floor for consideration by the entire chamber. The bill is then either granted or denied a "rule." If granted, the speaker, in concert with the majority leader, schedules the bill for debate and floor vote.

IV. Decision

7. The bill is debated (and perhaps amended) on the floor of the chamber. The debate over the bill includes time allotted to supporters and opponents. If an open rule is in effect, amendments may be adopted by a majority vote. Finally, the bill is voted up or down.

8. The bill is passed in the first chamber.

Steps 9 through 16 are similar steps of introduction, referral to committee, hearings, markup, reporting out, placing on the agenda, floor debate, and passage, but in the other chamber.

V. Conference

17. If the House and Senate versions of the bill differ, a joint conference committee, composed of equal numbers of senators and representatives, is formed by the leadership to work out one acceptable version of the bill. This conference committee includes members of the relevant committees in each house as well as other interested members. If the conference committee creates a compromise bill, that bill then goes to each house for further action, which may include additional committee review and Rules Committee action prior to a final floor debate and vote.

VI. Executive Action

18. The bill, now an Act of Congress, goes to the president for signature. If the president signs the bill, it becomes law.

19. If the president declines to sign (vetoes) the bill, it is returned to Congress as "privileged business," usually accompanied by a veto message outlining the reasons why the bill was not signed. If both houses vote by a two-thirds majority to override the president's veto, then the act becomes law.

Although congressional procedures may seem overly complex, technical, and time-consuming, these very characteristics encourage parties to achieve consensus and compromise. Such procedures also serve to protect the interests of minorities by giving them the means to affect the course of legislative decision making, the very basis of democracy in action!

Federal Budget Process

Perhaps no better example exists of the inherent complexities of coordination of policy-making (by Congress) and policy execution (by the executive branch) than the budget process. Fiscal power—including both the power to raise revenues through taxes and the power to spend money through appropriations—is a fundamental power of the legislative branch. However, it is clear that the essence of budgetary debate and decision making on Capitol Hill is shaped by what the president chooses to emphasize in his original budget message to Congress each year. By approving, modifying, or disapproving proposed legislation, Congress can change the level of program funding, eliminate programs, or add programs not requested by the president; it can also enact legislation to raise or lower various types of federal taxes or generate other sources of revenue.[19] A strong case can be made that the budget process makes the president the main initiator of policy—not only of fiscal policy but also of policy in every area requiring the expenditure of public funds.

The federal budget process presents a number of formidable challenges. First is the overall complexity of the process; there are a number of stages and considerable delays from when the legislature approves spending to when the agencies actually provide the services and the bills are paid. The massive growth in federal government activity in this century has further complicated the budget process. Yet another complication is the number of congressional committees with responsibility at various stages of the budget process. One set of committees—Ways and Means in the House and Finance in the Senate—determines revenue policy, whereas another set—the two appropriations committees—determines spending policy.[13]

In Congress, programs can be authorized by those committees that establish government programs. An authorization defines the scope of a program and sets a ceiling for the total amount that can be spent; however, authorizations provide no money. Appropriation legislation establishes the specific funding level for federal programs within the limits established in authorizations. Congress does not vote directly on the specific level of outlays, but rather on budget authority to incur obligations for immediate or future outlays of federal funds. The appropriation cycle begins in the House of Representatives. Once appropriations have been passed by the House, the bills are considered by the Senate. Differences between the House and Senate decisions on program funding are reconciled through a House-Senate conference committee. After the differences are reconciled, the appropriations bills are sent to the president, who signs or vetoes them.[19]

The Congressional Budget Act of 1974 attempted to deal with many of the difficult budget problems by creating a new annual budget timetable and establishing new standing committees on the budget in each chamber, as well as the Congressional Budget Office (CBO) to assist with budget analysis. This legislation also required that current services estimates be transmitted to Congress, along with the budget request, to provide a basis for reviewing the president's budget recommendations. The current services estimates of budget authority and outlays are estimates of the funds required to continue federal programs and activities at their existing level during the fiscal year in progress. Current services estimates have been an important tool in efforts to maintain funding for the Special Supplemental Food Program for Women, Infants, and Children (WIC).[19]

The fiscal year is from October 1 to the following September 30. The president still presents his budget to Congress early in the calendar year; Congress has until October 1 of each year to finalize budget decisions. If Congress does not complete action on appropriations by the beginning of the federal fiscal year, Congress must enact a "continuing resolution" to authorize the affected federal agencies to continue paying their obligations up to a specified date or until the regular appropriations are enacted. (See box on p. 298.)

The Balanced Budget and Emergency Deficit Control Act of 1985 (better known as the Gramm-Rudman-Hollings Act) attempted to reduce federal

BUDGET TERMINOLOGY

The federal budget is the financial plan for the federal government. It accounts for how government funds have been raised and spent, and it proposes financial policies. It covers the *fiscal year*, which begins on October 1 and ends the following September 30.

The budget discusses *revenues*, amounts the government expects to raise in taxes; *budget authority*, amounts agencies are allowed to obligate or lend; and *outlays*, amounts actually paid out by the government in cash or checks during the year. Examples of outlays are funds spent to buy equipment or property, to meet the government's liability under a contract or to pay employee's salaries. Outlays also include net lending—the differences between disbursements and repayments under government lending programs.

The purpose of the budget is to establish priorities and to chart the government's *fiscal policy*, which is the co-ordinated use of taxes and expenditures to affect the economy.

Congress adopts its own budget in the form of *budget resolutions*. The *first budget resolution*, due May 15, sets overall goals for taxing and spending, broken down among major budget categories, called *functions*. The *second budget resolution*, due September 15, sets binding budget figures.

An *authorization* is an act of Congress that establishes government programs. It defines the scope of programs and sets a ceiling for how much can be spent on them. Authorizations do not actually provide the money. In the case of authority to enter contractual obligations, though, Congress authorizes the administration to make firm commitments for which funds must later be provided. Congress also occasionally includes mandatory spending requirements in an authorization to ensure spending at a certain level. Some authorizations, such as Medicare, are structured so that anyone who meets the eligibility requirements of the program may participate and enough funding must be made available to cover all participants; such authorizations are known as *entitlements*.

An *appropriation* provides money for programs within the limits established in authorizations. An appropriation may be for a single year, a specified period of years (multi-year appropriations), or an indefinite number of years (no-year appropriations). Appropriations generally take the form of budget authority, which often differs from actual outlays. That is because, in practice, funds actually spent or obligated during a year may be drawn partly from the budget authority conferred in the year in question and partly from budget authority conferred in previous years.

From Wormser MD, editor: *CQ's Guide to Congress*, ed 3, Washington, DC, 1982, Congressional Quarterly, p 138.

deficits by means of a complex and controversial mechanism—that of setting a series of deficit-reduction targets over a period of several years until the annual deficit was eliminated entirely. There have been two revisions to budget legislation since the Gramm-Rudman-Hollings Bill was originally enacted: the 1990 Omnibus Budget Reconciliation Act (OBRA) and the Budget Enforcement Act. This latter bill set new rules for how the budget works and established two funding categories: discretionary funds (a minor proportion of the total budget) are limited by spending caps set by the appropriations committees, and mandatory funds cover all entitlement programs. Under rules set by the 1990 budget summit, pay-as-you-go restrictions (the so-called PAYGO rules) cover tax cuts and mandatory spending, chiefly for entitlement programs such as

Medicare, Medicaid, and food stamps. Any changes must be "revenue neutral"; that is, any tax cut, new entitlement program, or change that increases spending in an entitlement program must be offset by a tax increase or cutbacks in entitlement spending.

Entitlement programs—those for which persons qualify because they meet certain income or other eligibility requirements—are funded out of the "mandatory" portion of the budget. Food stamps, Medicare, and Medicaid, as well as most other food assistance programs, are all entitlement programs. (Food assistance programs were first included under the 1977 Farm Bill in an effort to garner support from urban legislators for agricultural programs. This action essentially ties funding for food assistance to funding earmarked for price supports and other agricultural and food production programs.) Programs that are not entitlements compete for funds in the discretionary category, which are approved through the appropriation process. The Special Supplemental Food Program for Women, Infants, and Children (WIC) is a prime example of a program that depends on annual appropriations from Congress. One reason why the proportion of eligible recipients who receive service is less than 60% is that when appropriated funds are exhausted, none is left for program expansion, regardless of the number of eligible participants who have not yet received services.

The last stage in the federal budget process is budget execution. The Office of Management and Budget (OMB), in the executive branch, was created to compare spending budget priorities across agencies. This agency is charged with preparing the president's budget and is the only group authorized to determine spending limits. OMB allocates appropriations to each federal agency over the year and monitors activities to ensure that actual spending does not exceed that allocated. Whereas the "budget" arm of OMB has oversight responsibility for agency spending, the "management" arm oversees how governmental activities are performed. In addition, OMB's Office of Information and Regulatory Affairs performs regulatory review as well as review for government's requests for information from the general public through the auspices of the Paperwork Reduction Act; this latter function has enormous ramifications for survey researchers who rely on government agencies to collect census data or other food and health practices information.

Role of the Executive Branch

Once the legislation is passed and signed into law, implementation and enforcement of the law become the responsibility of the agency in the executive branch to which it is assigned. The executive branch is, of course, headed by the president. His 14 cabinet secretaries are political appointees, as are many of the "first line" administrators of these agencies. Most of the laws enacted that affect nutrition, food, and health are passed to the U.S.

Department of Agriculture (USDA) or the Department of Health and Human Services for implementation.

Congress grants the fundamental authority to an administrative agency to engage in policy-making either through rulemaking or adjudication.[38] Rulemaking is a process of setting, through established agency procedures, the rules or regulations that define the requirements for implementing the law. Adjudication is the process of determining by action of the judicial system an "order" for how the law will be carried out.

The most important activity of administrative agencies is rulemaking; rules are the mechanism by which agencies provide detailed restrictions and guidelines to congressional statutes that have been stated in terms of broad, less-defined goals. The interpretation of the intent and nature of the statute by the administrative agency through the administrative rules that the agency establishes both gives the statutory law some "life" and determines the extent and scope of impact. In the case of complicated legislation, such as Medicaid, the administratively developed regulations are usually much longer and more detailed than the enabling legislation.[30]

The enabling regulatory statute typically defines the scope of agency authority and describes any specific rulemaking procedures the agency must follow. Congress has also sought to control and expedite agency rulemaking by imposing statutory deadlines for completing rulemaking actions; this has been particularly true for laws pertaining to public health and the environment.

Regulatory tools include informal methods, rulemaking, and adjudication:

- Informal actions include inspections, meetings, recalls, and advisory opinions. The term *informal* may be misleading because these actions are informal only in a legal sense. To the agency and to the regulated industry, they can have the same impact as any formal action.
- In rulemaking, the agency issues a public statement of general or particular applicability and future effect. The rule may apply to products (e.g., food labels or standards) or to pro-

cedures to be followed by the regulated industry or the agency.

- An adjudication is basically a decision concerning a specific right based on specific facts, for example, a proceeding to suspend an emergency permit.[25]

Most significant agency policy decisions result from either rulemaking or adjudication. Apart from these two mechanisms of action, there are, of course, a variety of informal means by which administrative agencies articulate policy under a statute, including press releases, speeches, statements, letters, advisory opinions, and other types of communications. The use of such "informal rulemaking" was especially prevalent in the middle to late 1970s to resolve complex and complicated issues. The extent to which these informal means of articulating policy are binding on the public varies, but their effect is usually significantly less than that of a "rule" issued after rulemaking or an "order" after adjudication.

Some agencies, but not all, are considered to be regulatory agencies, that is, "a government body, other than a court or legislature, that exercises control or authority, subject to the rule of law, over certain private parties by establishing rules and/or making binding judgments that affect the rights of those parties."[25] There are two types of regulatory agencies: "independent" agencies and executive department agencies. Agencies that are considered independent include the Federal Trade Commission (FTC), which has regulatory responsibility for food advertising and truth-in-labeling laws; the Consumer Product Safety Commission; and the Federal Commerce Commission. Examples of executive department agencies are the Food and Drug Administration (FDA) in the Department of Health and Human Services (DHHS) and the Food Safety and Inspection Service (FSIS) and the Animal and Plant Health Inspection Service (APHIS) in USDA.

Regulations are written by the agency to carry out the intent of Congress; these statements issued by agencies in the executive branch carry the power of law and can be legally enforced with fines for noncompliance. How closely the regulations carry out the legislative intent may depend on whether the philosophy and policies of Congress and the agency officials coincide. When the president and the majority of Congress are of the same political party, there is usually some degree of unanimity. When they are of opposing parties, some discrepancies may be noted between the legislation and the proposed rules and guidance materials.[19]

Publications

Published daily, the *Federal Register* is the principal document that disseminates federal regulations. Items in the *Federal Register* are categorized by the type of action to be taken. A notice generally announces meetings or other items under agency review. A notice of proposed rulemaking (NPRM) announces an action that an agency is considering. Such notices precede the issuance of a proposed rule, and the response to an NPFM can affect the form and substance of a proposed rule. A proposed rule is a draft of a new regulation or a revision of an existing regulation. The public is invited to comment in response to both the NPRM and the proposed rules. The agency has discretion to set the length of the "comment period" to 30, 60, or 90 days, depending on the complexity of the proposed rule.

The agency then has responsibility for reviewing the comments received, seriously considering alternatives, revising when appropriate, and issuing what is called a final rule, which must also undergo approval at both the agency and the administration level. The final rule carries an effective date that can range from immediately to several years in the future. Corrections are issued to rectify problems with the content of regulations; generally, these are technical corrections such as dates, rates, and program formulas. Final rules are published as regulations for federal programs; the compilation of regulations is revised and published annually in the *Code of Federal Regulations* (CFR).

Petitions are also published in the *Federal Register*. A petition is a formal request made to an agency by an individual, firm, or organization that a certain action be taken or not taken or that a regulation or order be established, revoked, or revised. In the food, nutrition, and public health arena, most petitions are submitted to the FDA.[19]

One example of this process of interest to most dietitians and nutritionists was the action taken by the FDA after passage of the Nutrition Labeling and Education Act in November 1990. The statute specified that rules for its implementation had to be proposed by the agency within 1 year after its enactment; these were published in the *Federal Register* by FDA in November 1991, with a 90-day comment period allowed. On February 25, 1992, the comment period ended; FDA had received more than 30,000 comments in the 90-day period, 8000 on the last day! FDA has responsibility for compiling, sorting, and attending to all comments, so that final rules can be published in November 1992, with an effective date for implementation set for March 1993.

This illustration emphasizes that it is important for dietitians, nutritionists, and other parties interested in public policy to comment on proposals or other items of interest published in the *Federal Register* as much as it is important to communicate to Congress about pending legislation. When preparing comments on regulatory proposals, the comments should be accurately indexed to the regulatory citations (dockets) specified in the *Federal Register*. Comments should be stated succinctly; where appropriate, references from the scientific literature should be cited, and the identity and expertise of the respondent should also be included. Regulatory agencies need to receive informed comments in order to issue rules and regulations that are appropriate to meeting the needs of the public on these issues.

Role of the Judicial Branch

The judicial branch, including the Supreme Court and other federal court systems, has responsibility for legal oversight of the activities of both of the other branches of government. The judicial branch is not often involved in issues involving food and nutrition because most of the guidelines are governed by rules enforced by the regulatory agency in the executive branch. Involvement with the judicial branch generally occurs only when there is

evidence that legal authority has been violated and when legislative and executive branch (regulatory) options have been exhausted. One should never enter into cases involving the judicial system without thoroughly weighing the possibility of winning the case against the potential costs measured in terms of money and time. In 1973 and 1974, class action suits in the federal courts successfully forced the release of program funds for WIC that had been impounded by the president.[19]

NUTRITION POLICY

Despite a number of calls in the late 1970s to develop and implement a comprehensive national nutrition policy, none has yet evolved. Responsibilities for nutrition programs and policies in the United States are divided among a number of congressional committees, tens of federal agencies, and several major departments! This fractionation of effort characterizes the current debate over U.S. nutrition policy. At present, nutrition policy, in large measure, emanates from subpolicies set in a number of arenas—most notably agriculture and health—resulting in a number of distinct (related, but not necessarily coordinated) food, health, and social programs.

These disparate elements currently comprise nutrition policy, although the direction of the focus is changing. As Ostenso has noted, governmental involvement in nutrition policy has traditionally focused on providing some food-related information and educational programs; maintaining price supports on commodities such as milk, sugar, grain products, and animal foods; and regulating the quality and safety of the food supply.[41] Providing food and income assistance to the economically disadvantaged has also been encompassed in food and nutrition policy activities.

It is commonly assumed that nutrition policy is synonymous with food and agricultural policy. This conceptual pairing was fostered in the language of the 1977 Farm Bill, which gave "lead agency" responsibility for nutrition research to USDA. However, the view that "nutrition policy is food policy" is changing. Health policy, especially that portion that addresses disease prevention and health promotion, has embraced nutrition as a vital element because food consumption patterns are now seen as having a major role in chronic disease prevention. This view is certainly espoused by Spasoff, who has described nutrition as "an ideal area in which to demonstrate the principles of health promotion and healthy public policy."[51]

Elements of Nutrition Policy

The scope and goals for a natural nutrition policy have been discussed for some time. Each of the policy elements on which there has been relatively widespread agreement, as well as the programs we associate with them, are discussed in the following section.

Providing an Adequate Food Supply at Reasonable Cost

One of the basic tenets of nutrition policy is that adequate quantities of food must be produced and made available to consumers at reasonable cost. It has led to the conclusion that "farm policy has far greater consequences for health, intended or not, than current food and nutrition policy."[36] The types and amounts of food produced are directly affected by agricultural (i.e., farm) policy; this, in turn, affects the types, supply, and costs of foods available for the public to choose and consume.

The goal of agricultural policy, simplistically stated, is "cheap food" for consumers accompanied by the protection of farm income. Americans spend a smaller share of their budgets on food at home than any other country. Only 8.4% of total personal consumption expenditures were for food consumed at home in the United States, compared with Canada, the closest at 12.1%, or India, the highest at 54.2%.[45] This situation reflects not only our high average income level but also results from the efficiency of the U.S. food system in providing reasonably priced food. Thus we have the "historic bargain of American food and agriculture policy,"[44] the situation whereby consumers, who want low food prices, are brought together with farmers, who want control over their markets and an assurance of stable commodity prices.

American farmers are the most efficient producers of food in the world. Technology and judi-

cious use of science have advanced agriculture to the point where only 2% of the population is able to produce more than twice the amount of food that Americans can consume.[44] Such production efficiency has come with a hefty price tag. Scientists are now questioning the nutritive quality of the U.S. food supply and charging that this elaborate system of agricultural policy instruments, such as price supports and marketing orders, have fostered overproduction of high-fat commodities.[12] Moreover, others have charged that decades of agricultural chemical use (fertilizers, pesticides, and the like) have caused immeasurable damage to the quality of the soil, groundwater, and other environmental resources.[34] Articulating these issues and negotiating "win-win" solutions among competing interest groups remain a paramount challenge for nutritionists interested in agricultural policy in the 1990s.

Ensuring a Safe and Wholesome Food Supply

Food safety. Food safety includes issues as varied as environmental contaminants, pesticide residues, product tampering, nutritional imbalances, and microbial contamination. In recent years, consumers have developed a growing concern about the safety of their food and its impact on their health. Consumer advocates, the food industry, and even some government regulators have widely divergent views on food safety issues. Given these often conflicting perspectives, it is not surprising that some food safety concerns have become highly charged public policy issues.[46]

At the turn of the century in the United States, avoiding food spoilage and food adulteration were the primary food safety concerns, brought about primarily by technological advances in food preservation methods such as canning.[42] In addition to the public outrage created by Upton Sinclair's *The Jungle*, Harvey Wiley, chief of the Bureau of Chemistry in the USDA, was concerned with fraud, sanitation, and safety in the food supply. To test the safety of commonly used preservatives, he fed foods containing these substances to a group of volunteers (called the "poison squad"). The results from these feeding experiments helped to dramatize the need for federal legislation to protect the U.S. food supply and led to the enactment of the Federal Food and Drugs Act of 1906, as well as to the Federal Meat Inspection Act passed the same year. These simple and bold actions were credited with ridding the U.S. marketplace of food fraud.[24] More important, perhaps, is the fact that these laws established that the federal government had a responsibility and a legal right to ensure a safe and wholesome food supply.

The passage of the Federal Food, Drug, and Cosmetic Act in 1938 gave the FDA, for the first time, the authority to fine and imprison violators.[46] After the passage of this act, there was discussion about the need to regulate the food supply in terms of its contribution to human nutrition. Congress was concerned with preventing and controlling practices by unscrupulous food manufacturers that might harm the public health or mislead the public about the true nature and value of individual food products. The language of the 1938 act was sufficiently broad so that over the ensuing years FDA could use it to promote regulation of "general purpose" food (which includes both unprocessed and processed foods), special dietary foods such as vitamin and mineral supplements and fortified foods, and medical foods, those foods used primarily to treat specific disease conditions.[24]

Responsibilities for inspection and regulation of food and water are shared among FDA, USDA, and EPA. Food safety issues that have emerged as topics of current concern include the safety of pesticide residues, microbiological contamination, food additives, and seafood inspection.

Pesticides. Pesticide residues have become an issue for many consumers who are worried about food safety. The EPA is responsible for setting the permissible tolerance levels for pesticide residues. However, the monitoring and enforcement of those levels is under the authority of the FDA. The consensus among scientific experts is that the overall health hazard for consumers from pesticides used in accordance with good agricultural practices is small, especially in comparison with other major risk factors such as smoking. A far more serious health hazard is faced by farmers and other agricultural workers who are continually exposed to

pesticides from frequent and sometimes improper application of these chemicals.

Microbiological food contamination. The seriousness of the health problem posed by microbial food contamination should not be underestimated. Foodborne bacteria can cause two basic types of illness: infections, caused by consuming a foodborne microorganism that then infects the human body, and intoxications that result from eating something that contains a toxin that was produced by microorganisms growing in the food. The microorganisms *Salmonella, Staphylococcus aureus,* and *Clostridium perfringens* are currently responsible for the largest number of foodborne illnesses in the United States.[46] Between 1968 and 1977, meat and poultry were implicated in more than 50% of the reported foodborne disease outbreaks from known sources. Such findings suggest the inadequacy of the present meat and poultry inspection system, designed at the turn of the century to protect consumers from grossly visible evidence of microbial contamination, and now under the authority of the Food Safety and Inspection Service, a regulatory arm of the USDA. In 1985, a National Research Council expert panel concluded that current inspection methods are not adequate to detect *Salmonella* and *Campylobacter* and recommended major reform in the inspection system.[42]

Because most incidents of foodborne illness can be prevented by proper cooking and refrigeration, it is imperative for the general public to know the basic procedures that should be followed in home food preparation to minimize the risks. For example, cooking thoroughly at sufficiently high temperatures kills *Salmonella* in meat or poultry. In addition, proper sanitary food preparation procedures must be followed to prevent cross-contamination to other foods from contaminated countertops, cutting boards, knives, and even hands. The Meat and Poultry Hotline is staffed by FSIS to answer consumer questions and concerns about food safety.

Food additives. Food additives are substances added to foods in minor amounts, either intentionally to improve nutrition, quality, or shelf life or unintentionally as a result of production, processing, storage, or packaging. Over time, controversies have arisen over the use of additives such as saccharin, cyclamates, sodium nitrite, and several food dyes.

A major current issue concerns the adequacy of regulatory actions for establishment and enforcement of an acceptable risk standard. The law that serves as the current standard is the Delaney Clause, attached to the Food Additive Amendment of 1958 to the Food, Drug and Cosmetic Act; it states that "no additive shall be deemed to be safe if it is found to induce cancer when ingested by man or animal, or if it is found, after tests which are appropriate for the evaluation of the safety of food additives, to induce cancer in man or animal." The "zero tolerance" established by law in the Delaney clause appeals to much of the general public. However, the standard of zero tolerance has become less workable—and thus has created a policy dilemma—as technological advances have improved the ability to detect minute quantities of substances in food.[46]

Originally composed in 1958 when the Food Additive Amendment was passed, the GRAS (generally recognized as safe) list includes those substances that are nontoxic when "used in the food supply under normal manufacturing processes." This list has been modified, and some of the original additives have been banned because testing has shown that they did not pass the standard. Additives not on the GRAS list that are not known to be carcinogenic are evaluated on a risk-benefit basis and placed in the regulated food additives category for which the amounts that can be used are specified.[46]

Seafood inspection. Currently there is no mandatory federal inspection program for fish and other seafood as there is for meat and poultry. Data illustrating the number of cases of foodborne illness caused by uninspected seafood have been brought to the attention of Congress by consumer advocacy groups. Despite the current lack of law, legislation that sets up a comprehensive, mandatory seafood inspection program is expected to pass eventually. In the meantime, FDA and the National Marine Fisheries Service have stated their intention to start a joint voluntary, fee-for-service inspection program to enhance existing efforts, which cur-

rently inspect only about 25% of the seafood sold in the United States.

The present food safety policy presents unique challenges to revamp current laws and regulations so that they can adequately address long-standing issues such as uniformity of standards for food additives versus pesticides and detection of the complete range of significant chemicals and microbiological hazards of concern. In addition, food safety regulations now must extend to those actions needed to implement current diet and health recommendations. They include the need for uniformity in approaches to controlling microbiological contamination in food, assessing the range of significant chemical hazards and communicating the relative risks from various food products to the public, and addressing the regulation of new genetically engineered or formulated food products, such as "fat substitutes."[42]

Food fortification and enrichment. Between 1906 and 1930, the modern science of nutrition was born. The scientific discovery of vitamins and their role in human health precipitated what Hutt has called "one of the most difficult regulatory problems that FDA has had to confront."[24]

The first fortification (addition to a food of a nutrient not originally there) was in 1924 when the Michigan Department of Health and the Michigan Medical Society convinced salt manufacturers that goiter was such an endemic problem that they should add iodine to table salt at no additional cost to the consumer. Thus the basic principle of the first fortification policy was to correct a recognized deficiency of a nutrient in the diets of a significant number of individuals.[41]

As the nation moved from an agricultural base to one focused on an industrial-urban locale, the food supply needed to be transported from where it was produced to where it was consumed. This resulted in increased attention on the production and consumption of processed foods. Thus, as dietary habits changed, the second principle of fortification policy became the maintenance of the nutritional quality of the food supply.[41]

With this, nutrition emerged as a major marketing tool of the food industry and therefore as a major regulatory issue. When Congress enacted the Federal Food, Drug, and Cosmetic Act in 1938, there was, for the first time, explicit discussion about the need to regulate the food supply in terms of its contributions to human nutrition.[24] Under the standards of identity provisions, nutrients shown to be consumed in less than adequate amounts—iron, thiamin, niacin, and riboflavin—were added, in specified amounts, to "enriched" white flour and bread products.

In the early 1970s the proportion of processed foods in the diet continued to increase, and new nontraditional foods entered the marketplace. FDA sought to maintain the nutritional quality of the food supply through direct intervention by issuing regulations to encourage the development of modified products that might require nutrient additions to maintain nutritional quality similar to the products being imitated. At the same time, to ensure that factual information on the nutrient composition of foods was accurate and useful, FDA promulgated a regulation governing the format, content, and placement of nutrition labeling. These regulations will stand to govern food labeling standards until final regulations are issued to implement the Nutrition Labeling and Education Act, passed in 1990.

Thus, just as obtaining *enough* food was of concern in our early history, so was an early concern that the food supply must provide adequate amounts of micronutrients and macronutrients. Today, however, a major regulatory challenge affecting the FDA is the overabundance, rather than the undersupply, of these nutrients in the marketplace.[24]

Providing Food Access and Availability, Regardless of Income

Hunger and food security issues.* Policy options to meet the needs of the "hungry" depend,

*Hunger in the '80s and '90s: A Challenge for Nutrition Educators is a supplement to the January/February 1992 *Journal of Nutrition Education*. The supplement is a valuable resource for all interested in community nutrition for it includes research, reports, and viewpoints that document the problem of hunger in the United States, explore its causes and consequences, and suggest ways to work toward effective solutions. Copies may be obtained by writing the Society for Nutrition Education, 2001 Killebrew Drive, Suite 340, Minneapolis, MN 55425-1882.

in part, on the public perception of hunger and how it is defined. *Hunger* has frequently been defined in two ways.[15] The first defines *hunger* in terms of measurable forms of malnutrition, such as anemia, low birth weight, and infant mortality. *Hunger* may also be defined as a lack of "food security." This definition is an important tool for policymakers to "focus on food purchasing power and food availability to families in their community. This perspective makes it possible to detect and measure the extent of hunger, develop strategies to alleviate the problem, and monitor progress in its elimination."[5] *Food security* has been defined as "access by all people at all times to enough food for an active, healthy life, and at a minimum includes the following: 1) the ready availability of nutritionally adequate and safe foods, and 2) the assured ability to acquire personally acceptable foods in a socially acceptable way."[8] It follows, then, that potential consequences of food insecurity include hunger, malnutrition, and negative effects on health and quality of life, achieved either directly or indirectly by the lack of adequate food.

Results from the review of a number of hunger studies (based primarily on data collected at the state and local levels) provide evidence for the following conclusions about the state of food sufficiency in the United States.[40]

- Food insufficiency has become a chronic problem in the United States. Economic and social changes of the past decade have left large numbers of Americans unable to meet their daily food needs; in turn, this situation has increased pressures on food assistance programs.
- Food insufficiency is not due to food shortages. Hunger results from unequal distribution of economic resources, that is, poverty.
- People who lack access to a variety of resources are most at risk of hunger. When income is inadequate to meet the costs of housing, utilities, health care, and other fixed expenses, these items compete with and may take precedence over food.
- Hunger is a chronic societal problem that no longer can be addressed in isolation from other correlates of poverty such as underemployment, inadequate housing, or poor education.

Table 12-1. Selected events in the history of federal policies to address hunger in the United States

Date	Event
1930	USDA and Federal Emergency Relief Administration distributes surplus agricultural commodities as food relief through Federal Surplus Relief Corporation
1933	Congress creates Agricultural Adjustment Administration to control farm prices and production and Federal Surplus Relief Corporation to distribute surplus farm products to needy families
1935-42	Congress provides for continued operation of Federal Surplus Commodities Corporation which, under USDA, purchases commodities for distribution to state welfare agencies
1936-42	Amendments to Agricultural Act permits food donations to school lunches
1939-43	Federal Surplus Commodities Corporation initiates experimental food stamp program
1946	National School Lunch Program established
1954	Special Milk Program established
1955	USDA determines that average low-income family spends one third of after-tax income on food
1961	President Kennedy expands use of surplus foods for needy people at home and abroad and announces eight pilot food stamp programs
1964	Congress establishes national Food Stamp Program; Social Security Administration establishes poverty line at three times the cost of USDA's lowest-cost Economy Food Plan; since 1969, values are adjusted according to the Consumer Price Index
1966	Child Nutrition Act passes; School Breakfast Program initiated, becomes permanent in 1975; President Johnson outlines Food for Freedom program
1968-77	Senate establishes Select Committee on Nutrition and Human Needs to lead nation's anti hunger efforts.
1968-70	Ten-State and Preschool Nutrition Surveys and *Hunger, U.S.A.* report evidence of malnutrition among children in poverty
1969	President Nixon announces "war on hunger"; holds White House Conference on Food, Nutrition, and Health, USDA establishes Food and Nutrition Service to administer federal food assistance programs
1971	Results of Ten-State Survey released to Congress indicate high risk of malnutrition among low-income groups
1972	Congress authorizes Special Supplemental Food Program for Women, Infants, and Children (WIC); Older Americans Act authorizes Nutrition Program for Older Americans
1973	Amendments to Older Americans Act establishes congregate and home-delivered meals programs
1977	Food and Agricultural Act and Child Nutrition and National School Lunch Amendments passed
1981	USDA establishes a small demonstration project for commodity distribution, the Special Supplemental Dairy Distribution Program, which becomes institutionalized as the Temporary Emergency Food Assistance Program (TEFAP) in 1983
1981-82	Congress passed Omnibus Budget Reconcilliation Acts, Omnibus Farm Bill, and Tax Equity and Fiscal Responsibility Act, which eliminate, restrict, and reduce food and income benefits
1984	President's Task Force on Food Assistance finds little evidence of widespread or increasing undernutrition but concludes that hunger exists and is intolerable in the United States
1986	General Accounting Office finds that methodological flaws discredit findings of the Physician Task Force on Hunger that hunger is prevalent in counties with low food stamp participation rates
1988	DHHS publishes *Surgeon General's Report on Nutrition and Health*, which states that lack of access to an appropriate diet should not be a health problem for any American; Congress passes the Hunger Prevention Act increasing eligibility and benefits for Food Stamps, Child Care, and TEFAP programs
1989	House Select Committee on Hunger holds hearings on food security in the United States
1991	Mickey Leland Childhood Hunger Relief Act (HR-1202, S-757) introduced

From Nestle M, Guttmacher S: J Nutr Educ 24:22S, 1992. Reprinted by permission of the Society for Nutrition Education.

More than any other aspect of food and nutrition policy, food assistance programs are a form of governmental action directly tied to the nation's economic well-being. Table 12-1 showcases selected events in the history of federal policies to address hunger in the United States. Economic assistance, in the form of a variety of programs and strategies, must be provided by the government and, as stated previously, tied to the overall poverty problem are those of hunger, homelessness, underemployment, and poor education.

History of food assistance. Federal food assistance programs evolved as an outgrowth of farm support laws enacted during the Great Depression of the 1930s. A commodity distribution program was established that distributed surplus agricultural commodities directly to the needy; in 1939, 13 million Americans received such food assistance. In large measure, today's food programs have retained their original goals—to improve the nutrition of low-income people and other groups, while providing an outlet for surplus agricultural commodities from the farm programs.

In an attempt to increase the purchasing power of the poor, Congress authorized an experimental Food Stamp Program, which lasted from 1939 until 1943. In 1936, the first school lunch program allowed the donation of surplus commodities to state-supported educational institutions. The onset of World War II was accompanied by a tremendous demand for agricultural products, so there was less "surplus" food to distribute. Thus, when the National School Lunch Act was passed in 1946, one feature written into the law was that a considerable portion of federal assistance would be provided in the form of cash. During this era, food assistance programs remained relatively small and served principally as vehicles for the distribution of surplus agricultural commodities.[29]

After World War II and until the early 1960s, hunger and poverty received relatively little public attention.[40] Soon after taking office in 1961, President Kennedy outlined a program to expand food distribution and establish eight pilot food stamp programs in selected counties. Food stamps became available nationally after 1964, and the School Breakfast Program was initiated in 1966. During the late 1960s, the hunger and malnutrition issue burst onto the public scene and galvanized public attention. Independently, several groups, such as the Field Foundation and the Citizen's Board of Inquiry into Hunger and Malnutrition, conducted surveys to document the problem. The media also helped to focus public attention on the issue. The CBS documentary "Hunger in America," which first aired in 1968, provided graphic descriptions of starving children in the United States.[47]

Two "official" forces helped to place the hunger and malnutrition issue on the public policy agenda during the late 1960s. In 1968, the Senate Select Committee on Nutrition and Human Needs was formed, chaired by Sen. George McGovern. Then, in early 1969, President Nixon committed his administration to "putting an end to hunger in America itself for all time." One result of this presidential statement was the White House Conference on Food, Nutrition, and Health held in December 1969 and chaired by Jean Mayer. The recommendations from that conference, held more than 20 years ago, are still valid today.[47]

During the 1970s cash subsidies and vouchers increasingly replaced commodities in federal food programs as part of an evolving strategy to increase the purchasing power of the poor. This strategy included expansion of the Food Stamp Program, creation of the special Supplemental Food Program for Women, Infants, and Children (WIC) and other child food assistance programs, and development of nutrition programs for the elderly. From 1969 to 1977 annual federal expenditures for food assistance increased from $1.2 to $8.3 billion; by 1979 donated farm products accounted for less than 10% of the total federal expenditures on food programs.[40] By the late 1970s the positive effects of these efforts were evident. In 1979 representatives of the Field Foundation returned to the South to examine anew the problems of hunger and malnutrition. They returned to report that nutrition programs were working in fine order and that they could find nowhere near the extent of hunger and malnutrition that they had observed 10 years before.[47]

With the onset of the 1980s, national policies shifted a greater degree of responsibility for social programs from the federal government to the states and the private sector. In his 1982 State of the Union address, President Reagan proposed to devolve to the states the responsibility for administration and oversight of the food stamp, child nutrition, and WIC programs primarily by converting funds for these programs into block grants to the states. One of the hallmarks of the Reagan Administration was the mandate for government to spend less and to offer services only to the "truly needy." The issue becomes one of targeting services effectively to recipients who meet the objective criteria for program participation.[48] The Omnibus Reconciliation Acts of 1981 and 1982 instituted significant changes in the Food Stamp Program especially; these changes resulted in both a decrease in the number of persons deemed eligible for the program and a temporary reduction in benefits.[2] From 1980 to 1982 Congress reduced expenditures on food programs by one third as part of the effort to trim the federal budget.[10]

The consequences of these cutbacks soon became apparent. Concomitant with a reduction in benefits was the economic downturn of 1981, which caused significant unemployment and consequently increased the number of participants in food assistance programs. Emergency food and shelter providers began to report an increasing use of their services by the "new poor": children, unskilled and unemployed youth, families with insufficient resources, and the deinstitutionalized mentally ill.[40]

Although difficult to quantify, the problem of hunger affects millions of people in the United States. In 1984, the President's Task Force on Food Assistance reported that they could find little evidence of widespread or increasing undernutrition, but concluded that hunger existed and was intolerable in the United States. The Physicians' Task Force on Hunger in America conducted field investigations between 1983 and 1988; by their criteria, in which *hunger* was defined in economic terms, 12 million children and 8 million adults in the United States were said to be suffering from hunger.[6]

In recent years, both the White House and Congress have taken steps to improve access to and benefits of the food assistance programs. The Food Security Act of 1985 reinstated lost nutritional benefits for low-income households through changes in the Food Stamp Act and the Temporary Emergency Food Assistance Program (TEFAP). In 1986 Congress passed the School Lunch and Child Nutrition Program amendments that included increased funds for WIC and the School Breakfast Program and reauthorized the expiring Child Nutrition Program. Congress began to focus on the homeless by holding hearings and adopting legislation to extend food programs to this group.[10] The Hunger Prevention Act of 1988 provided federal matching funds to states to conduct outreach to households potentially eligible for the Food Stamp Program. In 1991, the Mickey Leland Childhood Hunger Relief Act (HR 1202, S 757), which represents the largest expansion of federal antihunger efforts since the 1970s, would make food assistance more accessible to families with children in need by strengthening the Food Stamp Program. Despite passage by both House and Senate Agriculture Committees, the president's budget for FY1993 failed to include funding to implement the bill. Therefore, it can only become law if it is paid for under the pay-as-you-go system, resulting from the 1990 budget summit. Proponents of the bill advocate full funding in the FY1993 budget.

The Medford Declaration to End Hunger in the United States was drafted over a period of several months by a committee of national hunger organizations and announced in April 1992.[35] The Medford Declaration calls for the elimination of hunger by 1995 and for a substantial reduction in poverty by the year 2000.

Food assistance programs. A number of food assistance programs exist*—all designed to meet the needs of the economically disadvantaged but in different ways. Each program is based on a different type of intervention strategy, and the effec-

*Perhaps the most complete guide to food assistance and other federal programs is the *Catalog of Federal Domestic Assistance*,[9] available at most public libraries that have federal government holdings.

tiveness of each must be judged on the basis of the extent to which it meets its specific stated objectives. Although such programs are all available to the economically disadvantaged, government officials point out that they are not intended to meet all needs. Most programs supplement earnings and other program benefits, including "welfare" and unemployment. Categories of food assistance are family nutrition programs, child nutrition programs, supplemental food programs, and food distribution programs.

Food stamp program. The family nutrition programs include the Food Stamp Program (FSP), the Nutrition Assistance Program for Puerto Rico, and the Food Distribution Program on Indian Reservations (Needy Family Program). The largest food assistance program is the *FSP,* originally established in 1964 and described as "the nation's single most important program in the fight against hunger."[23] The goal of the FSP, according to the Catalog of Federal Domestic Assistance, is "to improve the diets of low-income households by increasing their food purchasing ability."[9] Rather than a "family nutrition program," as the category implies, FSP actually employs an income transfer strategy because the food stamps provided to eligible recipients are actually a form of currency that can be used only to "purchase" food at participating grocery stores.

FSP is the only entitlement food program that is available to all who meet eligibility standards, regardless of their age or family composition. Eligibility is determined on the basis of both financial (income and resources) and nonfinancial (citizenship, work requirements, etc.) factors. To qualify, households must have gross incomes below 130% of the official poverty level; households with elderly and disabled members must have net incomes below 100% of the poverty line. Most households may have up to $2000 in assets. Fully 98% of food stamps go to households with incomes equal to or below the poverty line. Half of all food stamp participants are children, and 87% are children, the elderly, or women.[23,35]

The program is administered at the federal level by the Food and Nutrition Service, USDA, and at the state and local levels by welfare or human service agencies. The federal government pays the full cost of food stamps and at least half of the program's administrative costs, with states and local governments paying the remainder. Of all food assistance programs, FSP has led the way in program costs (Fig. 12-3). The program's overall costs to the government are determined by the participation rates and by the level of benefits, that is, the value of the food stamps. Because of the current economic situation and the level of unemployment, FSP reported its highest enrollments ever in January 1992, 25 million, almost 10% of the nation's population. Despite its size and cost, it is estimated

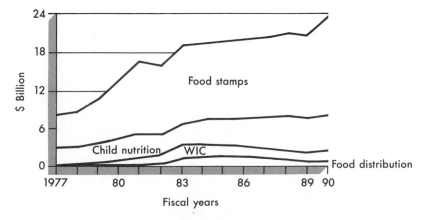

Figure 12-3. Food stamps have led the increase in food program costs.
From Community Nutrition Institute: *Nutrition Week,* June 14, 1991.

that only about half of all Americans who are eligible for food stamps actually receive them.[35]

Food price inflation has undoubtedly contributed to the program's overall costs as well. The Thrifty Food Plan (TFP) serves as the nutritional basis for calculating FSP benefits. The rate of food price inflation has a direct effect on the TFP, which in turn causes an increase in food stamp benefit costs. Currently these benefits provide an average of less than 70 cents a meal per person. The estimated funding for the program in 1992 is more than $22 million.

The current FSP has changed considerably from that established by the Food Stamp Act in 1964. Refinements have been designed to increase program benefits to recipients and encourage greater participation among those who are eligible. When the FSP was first conceived in the 1930s, it definitely had the focus of using farm surplus to feed the needy. When the current program was enacted in 1964, it included a purchase requirement as an "incentive" for the poor to use some of their own money on food purchases. This purchase requirement was eliminated in 1977, and electronic transfer (use of a credit card–like mechanism) is now being tested for use nationwide.

FSP is nearly 30 years old, yet surprisingly few studies have documented program impact. The basic premise underlying the program is that use of food stamps increases family food expenditures, which in turn improves dietary intake and ultimately improves health; the basic assumption is that more food equals more nutrition. Studies do indicate that food stamps result in somewhat greater food expenditures. However, because nutrient consumption in the United States is not highly responsive to changes in income, although income transfer programs like the FSP may positively influence nutrient intakes, the magnitude of the effect is likely to be small. FSP functions well as an income maintenance program and has been demonstrated to provide basic support during times of economic hardship. However, one must be cautious in concluding that FSP has actually improved the dietary status of its participants. Strengthening the nutrition education component

may enable participants to make better-informed food choices.[48]

Child nutrition programs. Five child nutrition programs are offered: the National School Lunch Program, the School Breakfast Program, the Child and Adult Care Food Program, the Special Milk Program, and the Summer Food Service Program.

The largest of these, and the one that has been in existence the longest, is the School Lunch Program. This program was permanently authorized in 1946 through the National School Lunch Act and was created as "a measure of national security, to safeguard the health and well-being of the Nation's children . . . and to encourage the domestic consumption of nutritious agricultural commodities and other food."[52] The National School Lunch Program is administered at the federal level by the Food and Nutrition Service (FNS) of USDA, at the state level by one of a variety of state agencies (usually the department of education), and at the local level by the school board.[23]

The School Lunch Program is an entitlement program, which means that federal funds must be provided to all schools that apply and meet the program's eligibility criteria. A three-tiered reimbursement system is used to calculate benefits: children from households with incomes at or below 130% of poverty receive free meals; those between 130% and 185% receive reduced-price meals; and those above 185% of poverty pay "full price," for which the school districts receive a small federal subsidy. In 1991, more than 24 million children were served lunch each school day in 87,000 schools. Approximately 41% of the lunches were served free, and 7% were served at a reduced price. In the 1990-91 school year, the cost of the program was $4 billion in cash and entitlement commodities.[32] USDA economists note that the costs of the child nutrition programs have not climbed as quickly as those of other food assistance programs, a fact they attribute to slower growth in the National School Lunch Program (NSLP) and declining school enrollment.[16]

In addition to direct funding from USDA, participating schools and residential child care institutions also receive a direct distribution of commodity products, thereby alleviating, to some extent, farm product surpluses. The value of the commodity products is said to be less than 20% of the total cash outlay for the NSLP. The continued use of surplus agricultural commodities has been a source of continuing controversy. Those who favor it cite economic reasons; if donated food commodities had not been used in 1987, the costs of the NSLP would have been $880 million higher than its actual cash costs. Those who oppose the use of commodity products in school meals reveal that the specific foods donated contribute higher levels of fat, cholesterol, sugar, and sodium than should be offered to children.[43]

Meals served in the NSLP must meet specific requirements in order for participating institutions to qualify for federal funds. Lunch must include:

½ pint fluid milk (whole milk must be one of the options offered)

2 ounces protein (meat, fish, 2 eggs, 4 tablespoons peanut butter, or 1 cup dry beans or peas)

¾ cup serving consisting of two or more vegetables or fruits or both (juice can meet half of this requirement)

8 servings of bread, pasta, or grain per week

This meal pattern reflects a standard that, over time, school lunches should provide one third of the Recommended Dietary Allowances. USDA studies have shown that low-income children depend upon NSLP for one third to one half of their total daily nutrient intake.

How effective is the National School Lunch Program? Surveys have documented that the food consumed makes an important dietary contribution to children's diets. An evaluation of the diets of children aged 6 to 11 years who participated in the NSLP found that the program had a significant positive impact on the nutrient consumption of participating children, particularly those from low-income families. These children had higher daily intakes of calcium, vitamin C, riboflavin, iron, vitamin A, and vitamin B_6.[1]

The School Breakfast Program provides assistance to schools and residential child care institutions that operate nonprofit breakfast programs. In 1975, amendments to the Child Nutrition Act of 1966 permanently authorized the program. The meal pattern requirements reflect a standard that, over time, school breakfasts provide one fourth of the RDA. In the 1990-91 school year, the program served 4 million children daily at a cost of $656 million. Most of those meals were either free or at reduced price.

The Child and Adult Care Food Program (CACFP) began in 1968 and is designed to assure nutritious meals for children to age 12, the elderly, and certain handicapped individuals who participate in a nonprofit, licensed, or approved day-care program.[23] Centers receive federal funds for two meals and one snack per participant per day plus one additional meal or snack if the child (or adult) is in attendance for 8 hours or longer. All meals in participating organizations are subsidized with federal funds. This program currently serves 1.5 million participants daily, only 1% of whom are elderly. In 1991 program costs were estimated to be $1 billion.[32]

The Special Milk Program provides milk in schools that are not participating in the National School Lunch Program. In 1990, 183 million half-pints of fluid milk were served at a cost of $19 million.[32]

The Summer Food Service Program provides funds and commodities for breakfast, lunch, and snacks free to all children under age 18 who attend the meal site of a sponsor organization, usually schools, residential camps, state or local governmental units, or private nonprofit organization locations. Peak participation in July 1990 was 1.7 million children. In 1991, the program was estimated to cost $180 million.

Supplemental feeding program. The most notable program, officially named the Special Supplemental Food Program for Women, Infants, and Children, is better known simply as WIC. This program was created as a pilot program in 1972 and then authorized as a national program in 1974. The program grew quickly in the 1980s and now includes special provisions under the Hunger Prevention Act of 1988 to reach the homeless.

Currently authorized through FY1994, WIC is

not an entitlement program like most of the other food assistance programs. Instead there is a cap on the amount of federal money allocated, which limits the number of participants who can be served. The U.S. House Select Committee on Hunger estimates that fewer than 60% of the eligible population received WIC benefits in 1991. It is estimated that to achieve full funding of the program—the amount needed to serve all eligible people by 1996—an appropriation in the range of $3 billion for FY93 would be needed.[35]

Because insufficient funds have been appropriated to provide services to all who have been determined to be eligible and in need of the program, coverage is provided on a priority basis. Local agencies maintain priority levels for eligible persons based on national guidelines. The highest priority group for service is pregnant women, followed by infants up to 1 year of age; the lowest priority is given to 4- and 5-year-old children who qualify on the basis of dietary risk only and who have no medical indication of risk such as poor growth or anemia. The first two priority groups typically receive complete coverage. It is true that fewer of those in the lowest-priority group are served, contributing, no doubt, to the alarming statistic regarding services to the eligible population. However, many government officials believe that if eligibility for WIC were to cap for children at age 3 or 4, the percentage of "coverage" for the total served nationwide would improve dramatically.[48]

For pregnant, postpartum, and lactating women, infants, and children up to age 5 who qualify, WIC offers supplemental nutritious foods, nutrition education, and access to health care. Participants must meet economic eligibility criteria (between 100% and 185% of the poverty level), must be certified by a qualified health professional to be at nutritional risk (which includes such medical problems as abnormal pregnancy weight gain, history of high-risk pregnancies, growth problems, iron deficiency anemia, or inadequate dietary pattern), and must meet state eligibility requirements. In addition, any individual who receives benefits from FSP, AFDC, or Medicaid is automatically deemed to meet the WIC income eligibility requirement.

WIC provides a monthly package of nutritious foods specifically chosen to provide protein, iron, calcium, and vitamins A and C, nutrients likely to be missing from the diets of low-income women and children. Authorized WIC foods are iron-fortified infant formula, infant cereal, milk, eggs, cheese, iron-fortified breakfast cereal, Vitamin C–rich juice, beans, and peanut butter. The total cost of the WIC food package averages $30 per person per month.

Offering nutrition education to participants is also a mandated component of the WIC program. These sessions are intended to help participants understand why they are nutritionally at risk and how eating the WIC foods will help them meet those risks.

The WIC program is administered at the federal level by the Food and Nutrition Service, USDA, which grants funds to state health departments and Indian tribal agencies. These state agencies in turn fund local sponsors such as health agencies, social service agencies, or other nonprofit agencies that are capable of providing nutrition and health services; currently more than 8000 local clinics are in operation throughout the nation.

Because data such as weight, height, hemoglobin, and/or hematocrit are *required* to be collected from program participants as part of program administration, there is no paucity of data on which to base reporting of program results. Indeed, these data have been well used to document the impressive results of the WIC program to Congress.

WIC is generally regarded as one of the most effective nutrition programs. Regardless of the type of research design employed, studies conducted since the mid-1970s consistently show the following results: increased weight gain of mothers during pregnancy, increased mean birth weight of infants, improved hemoglobin and hematocrit levels in children, longer gestational age of infants at birth, and decreased neonatal mortality rate. Most of the more positive results associated with program participation have been reported for pregnant women and infants, rather than for older children.

WIC has also been shown to be cost-effective. Data from several studies have demonstrated that by decreasing the incidence of low birth weight and the need for hospital care for these infants, medical costs are reduced. A 1990 USDA study showed that every $1 spent on the prenatal component of WIC was associated with savings of about $3 in Medicaid costs for newborns and their mothers during the first 60 days after birth.[35]

Food distribution programs. This category of programs, historically associated with the distribution of surplus commodities obtained through farm price supports, includes the Temporary Emergency Food Assistance Program (TEFAP), the Nutrition Program for the Elderly, and commodity distribution to charitable institutions. TEFAP was established in 1981 to reduce the level of government-held surplus dairy commodities and to provide foods as supplements to purchased food for low-income households. The focus of these programs can be shifted from commodity disposal to nutrition assistance with varying levels of government stocks.[16]

TEFAP is administered nationally by the Food and Nutrition Service (FNS) of USDA and at the state level by the state agency responsible for food distribution, which in turn transfers commodities to local agencies for distribution. According to an FNS-commissioned study, approximately 20,000 local sites distributed TEFAP commodities to 15 million participants in 1986. The foods distributed to households include egg mix, canned beans, canned pork, peanut butter, raisins, butter, flour, and cornmeal; prior to 1988, more packaged dairy products, such as cheese, butter, and nonfat dry milk, were distributed.[23] (The reason that distribution of such dairy products was halted was that the large quantities of surplus butter and cheese that TEFAP distributed displaced some commercial product sales.[16]) Provisions of the Hunger Prevention Act of 1988 earmarked the distribution of some TEFAP commodities to soup kitchens and food banks. In 1991, FNS spent $170 million on the TEFAP program and $32 million to purchase and distribute commodities to soup kitchens and food banks.[32] The difficulties encountered when large distribution programs and reduced government purchases of many commodities have depleted some product inventories and created competition among the food assistance programs for available supplies point out the inherent problems with basing food assistance policy on surplus government commodities.[16]

Senior nutrition programs. Nutrition programs for the elderly are designed to provide older Americans with low-cost nutritional meals, nutrition education, and an opportunity for social interaction. The Older Americans Act of 1965 authorized two programs: the Congregate Meals Program and the Home-Delivered Meals Program. USDA contributes to the senior nutrition programs through its Nutrition Program for the Elderly (NPE), which provides cash and commodities to local elderly nutrition centers for use in both programs. In 1991 NPE served approximately 260 million meals at 14,000 sites at a cost estimated to be $150 million.[32]

These programs are administered federally by DHHS' Administration on Aging. Federal funds are distributed to Area Agencies on Aging in the state, which contract with local organizations to provide the congregate and home-delivered meals to participating seniors.

Anyone 60 years or older may participate in the Congregate Meals Program; their spouse, regardless of age, may also participate. Congregate meals are usually served once a day, Monday through Friday, at a local site, such as a senior center, community center, or neighborhood church. Program participants enjoy a nutritious meal and the opportunity to socialize. Many centers also provide other services, including transportation to and from the center, information and referral for health and social services counseling, nutrition education, shopping assistance, and recreation.

Participants in the Home-Delivered Meals Program must be older than 60 years of age, live in the program's service area, and be unable to prepare meals for themselves. This program delivers nutritious meals to the homes of disabled elderly persons on a daily basis, Monday through Friday, and some make provisions for meals to be available for weekend use. This type of program provides invaluable assistance to the frail elderly who wish to remain in their community and avoid institutionalization.

In the past few years, the funding level for these programs under Title III-C of the Older Americans

Act has decreased. As the "graying of America" continues, no doubt the demands for the senior nutrition programs can be expected to increase, not diminish. In FY1991, $370 million was appropriated for the Congregate Meals Program and $90 million for the Home-Delivered Meals Program. The 1992 and 1993 funding levels are expected to maintain the current level of services.

The fundamental challenge facing food assistance policy makers in the 1990s is the need to hold down food program costs in the face of budget constraints while continuing to provide nutritional assistance to needy persons. Historically, federal approaches to nutritional problems have been categorical; most programs have focused on individual groups with specific problems or with special vulnerability to developing such problems. Traditional benefactors of nutrition programs have been the school-aged child, the poor, and, more recently, pregnant women, lactating mothers, infants, children, and the elderly. However, this approach may need to be reevaluated, especially in light of the increasing recognition that nutrition is an essential component of preventive health care. Implementation of a more effective federal initiative will require closer linkages between local, state, and federal activities, those undertaken by consumer and advocacy groups, and those supported by industry, foundations, or other funding sources.

In recent years, program growth and expenditures for food assistance have been limited by budget constraints, which have resulted in the development of tighter program eligibility requirements and new program management systems. Regulatory and legislative changes were partly responsible for lowering the growth rate of real (adjusted for inflation) program expenditures, particularly in the school lunch and food stamp programs. Actual expenditures for all food assistance programs have continued to increase despite the fact that the number of participants in the National School Lunch Program, School Breakfast Program, and WIC has remained relatively constant.

In contrast, attempts to increase food consumption of low-income people have expanded the scope of some existing programs and created new ones. The increased funding of both the Child and Adult Care Food program and WIC, the creation of TEFAP, and the rise in food stamp participation reflects efforts to expand, rather than reduce, food assistance programs. This goal is also shown in the gradual increase in food stamp benefits mandated in the Hunger Prevention Act of 1988, with future increases a possibility. The dilemma, however, is that in the face of existing budget limitations, additional expenditures on some programs may come at the expense of others.[15]

Providing Research-based Information and Educational Programs to Encourage Informed Food Choices

Dietary guidance policies have followed closely behind related scientific discoveries in nutrition. Since 1916, when USDA published its first dietary guidance plan, food guides have been developed to assist consumers in selecting nutritionally balanced diets.[32] Food guides such as the Basic Four Food Groups and its precursors, such as the Five Food Groups and the Basic Seven, were based on the concept of selecting from different food groups and maintaining a balance between the proportion of micronutrient-dense foods and energy-yielding foods.

In the past two decades, there has been a notable shift in the nature of the dietary guidance provided to consumers. Early food guides had advised consuming a particular number of servings from specific food "groups," the goal being to eat enough of specifically identified foods to provide the nutrients and energy required for "good health." The emphasis was on the quantity of foods to be selected, not on the quality of those food choices. All this changed when the Senate Select Committee on Nutrition and Human Needs was established in 1968 and the 1969 White House Conference on Food, Nutrition, and Health began to call public attention to the links between diet and chronic disease.

Then, in 1977, the Senate Select Committee on Nutrition and Human Needs, under the chairmanship of Sen. George McGovern, released *Dietary Goals for the U.S.*[54] A major milestone in dietary guidance policy, these guidelines set quantitative goals for the consumption of a diet lower in total fat, saturated fat, sodium, dietary cholesterol, and sugar, food components that were shown to be linked to the prevalence of certain chronic diseases. In the 6-year period of 1977 through 1982, government-related organizations issued six different versions of dietary guidance for the general public. The publication of these different documents sparked controversy among scientists, commodity and other special interest groups, and the agencies that had published the guidelines. The controversy centered basically on the benefits and therefore the advisability of recommending uniform reductions of saturated fat and cholesterol and increased fiber intake for the general public, versus providing targeted information to individuals identified as at risk for certain chronic disease.[39]

In an effort to quell the ensuing debate over dietary guidance, USDA and DHHS jointly published the first *Dietary Guidelines for Americans* in 1980. The language of these guidelines was qualitative rather than quantitative and followed the approach of advising the reader to eat more of certain dietary components and eat less of others. Revisions released in 1985 and again in 1990 closely followed the original language of the 1980 *Dietary Guidelines*. *Dietary Guidelines* currently serves as the official statement of federal policy on dietary guidance. Table 12-2 provides a summary of the dietary recommendations issued to the public from 1977 to 1990.[56]

Dietary recommendations now reflect general concern about the excessive consumption of certain dietary components, such as saturated fat and cholesterol, because these substances have been shown to be associated with the risk of certain chronic diseases. Consumers are now advised not only to make quantitative judgments to consume certain types of foods but also to make qualitative distinctions among foods, that is, to eat more of some foods and eat less of others.[49]

The debate about the nature of dietary guidance has largely subsided with the publication of the *Surgeon General's Report on Nutrition and Health*[53] and the National Research Council report *Diet and Health*.[39] Both reports reached similar conclusions and proposed similar modifications in the U.S. diet to reduce the risk of chronic disease. Issues that remain regarding dietary guidance include:

- The nature of the message. For example, will guidelines remain qualitative in nature or will quantitative targets, such as 30% calories as fat, be recommended?
- How can the same dietary guidance message be geared to individuals with different genetic profiles?
- How can dietary guidance be made more effective in actually changing dietary behavior?

Although the validity of the dietary recommendations is no longer in question, the critical issue that remains is how best to implement the recommendations.[42]

In 1991 the Food and Nutrition Board issued *Improving America's Diet and Health: From Recommendations to Action*.[14] Rather than relying on individual education to change dietary habits (the mainstay of most government intervention efforts), the committee recommended focusing on major sectors of society (such as government, the private sector [primarily the food industry], health care professionals, and educators) in order to increase the availability and accessibility of health-promoting foods to make such foods easily identifiable, economical, and appealing. As a practical guide for individuals and families interested in incorporating dietary guidelines into everyday life, the Food and Nutrition Board has published *Eat for Life*.[56]

Government-supported programs in nutrition education

Extension Homemaker Programs and the Expanded Food and Nutrition Education Program (EFNEP). The Extension Service of USDA administers a general food and nutrition education program for the public that was originally established by the Smith-Lever Act in 1914. Based on the extension delivery system, the program is designed to deliver research-based information through specialists based at land grant universities to agents located in each county throughout the country. Originally the home economics compo-

Table 12-2. Dietary recommendations to the U.S. public, 1977 to 1990

	Maintain appropriate body weight, exercise	Limit or reduce total fat (% kcal)	Reduce saturated fatty acids (% kcal)	Increase polyunsaturated fatty acids (% kcal)	Limit cholesterol (mg/day)	Limit simple sugars
U.S. Senate (1977)	Yes	27-33	Yes	Yes	250-350	Yes
Council on Scientific Affairs (AMA) (1979)	Yes	No	No	No	No	Yes
DHEW (1979)	Yes	Yes	Yes	NS	Yes	Yes
NRC (1980)	Yes	For weight reduction only	No	No	No	For weight reduction only
USDA/DHHS (1980, 1985)	Yes	Yes	Yes	No	Yes	Yes
DHHS (1988)	Yes	Yes	Yes	No	Yes	Yes
USDA/DHHS (1990)	Yes	Yes	Yes	No	Yes	Yes

NC, No comment; *NS,* not specified; *AMA,* American Medical Association; *DHEW,* Department of Health, Education, and Welfare; *NRC,* National Research Council; *USDA,* U.S. Department of Agriculture; *DHHS,* U.S. Department of Health and Human Services.
SOURCE: National Research Council: *Diet and health: implications for reducing chronic disease risk,* Washington, DC, 1989, National Academy Press.
From Woteki CE, Thomas PR, editors: *Eat for Life: The Food and Nutrition Board's guide to reducing your risk of chronic disease,* Washington, DC, 1992, National Academy Press, pp 18-19. Copyright © 1992, National Academy of Sciences. Reprinted with permission.

nent of the system was designed to deliver research-based information to "farm wives," and many of the programs were directed toward family resource management and food preservation. Recently, a national assessment of extension food and nutrition programs found that "health and wellness" was one of the three most frequently covered topics in the program.[27] Responsiveness to clientele needs in programming, continued efforts to enhance delivery methods, and strengthening linkages to the research base will all enable the extension program to continue to have a positive impact on the health and quality of life of its clientele.

Also administered at the federal level by USDA's Extension Service is the Expanded Food and Nutrition Education Program (EFNEP). Authorized by the Smith-Lever Act of 1970 with earmarked funds, EFNEP is designed to teach low-income families, especially those with small children, the skills needed to choose and prepare an adequate, varied, and balanced diet. Families receiving food stamps and WIC have been targeted for special attention through EFNEP. In this program, nutrition education programs are conducted by trained paraprofessional nutrition aides, who are often members of the local community who are able

Increase complex carbohydrates (% kcal from total carbohydrates)	Increase fiber	Restrict sodium chloride (g)	Moderate alcohol intake	Other recommendations
Yes	Yes	8	Yes	Reduce additives and processed foods
NC	NC	12	Yes	Consider high-risk groups
Yes	NS	Yes	Yes	More fish, poultry, legumes; less red meat
No	No	3-8	For weight reduction only	Variety in diet; consider high-risk groups
Eat adequate starch and fiber		Yes	Yes	Variety in diet; consider high-risk groups
Yes	Yes	Yes	Yes	Fluoridation of water; adolescent girls and women increase intake of calcium-rich foods; children, adolescents, and women of child-bearing age increase intake of iron-rich foods
Choose diet with plenty of vegetables, fruits, and grain products		Yes	Yes	Variety in diet

to work well with the homemakers in their own homes. Evaluations of the program, including a Senate-mandated study completed in 1981, have found that it improves the nutrition knowledge and food practices of the low-income homemakers who participate.

Nutrition Education and Training Program (NET). The Nutrition Education and Training Program (NET) was authorized in 1977, under amendments to the National School Lunch Act (PL 95-166). Thus, since its inception, NET has been integrally linked to school food programs. The goal of the program is to "provide nutrition education

training to teachers and school food service personnel so that they, in turn, can teach children the relationship between food and health and can encourage good eating habits."[23] Because of its ties to school feeding programs and school food service personnel, NET is unique; not only is it designed to teach children the concepts of food and nutrition but also the program is geared to put these concepts into practice in the lunchroom. In the early 1980s, a major study funded by USDA showed that, even in the initial years of NET, the program had effectively changed nutrition knowledge, attitudes, and practices among students, teachers, and food service personnel. In addition, evaluations of the program in California documented that plate waste had decreased by more than one quarter.

NET is administered at the federal level by USDA's FNS, which provides grants to state education agencies. The state, in turn, may distribute money to schools to provide nutrition education and training on the local level. Funding for NET is authorized through FY1994 with levels at $20 to $25 million.

Nutrition labeling. Although not identified specifically as a "nutrition education" program, providing nutrition information on the food label is a powerful tool for helping consumers make informed food choices. The Nutrition Labeling and Education Act of 1990 (NLEA; PL 101-535) instituted a sweeping set of changes in nutrition labeling to replace the voluntary system of labeling established by FDA regulations in 1973. The goal is to create a food label that the public can understand and count on that would bring them up-to-date with today's health concerns.[20] To implement NLEA, the FDA issued its initiatives in 23 documents in November 1991. After 90 days of review (the comment period), FDA must review all the comments received and issue final rules. A deadline of March 1993 for implementation of NLEA had initially been set by the Congress and endorsed by the president; however, this deadline may be postponed for up to 1 year if the agency determines that the timing of implementation would produce "undue economic hardship" for the food industry to comply with the requirements of the law.

Food labels have always been intended to help people make healthy diet choices. However, as dietary advice has changed, a newly designed label was needed to communicate this information. NLEA put the force of law behind a number of initiatives that will result in a truly new food label, one that will provide the consumer with accurate and useful information about the nutrient content of that product.

Coverage. The law requires mandatory nutrition labeling of virtually all processed foods regulated by the FDA and voluntary labeling of fresh produce and raw fish. (The voluntary program in existence since 1973 has resulted in only about 60% of all processed foods carrying the nutrition label.)

Content. Rather than presenting information on nutrients to prevent largely unheard-of deficiency diseases like beriberi or pellagra, the new label will provide information on the amount of cholesterol, saturated fat, complex carbohydrates, sugars, fiber, and calories from fat because today's health concerns involve these nutrients. FDA has proposed using the Reference Daily Intakes and Values (RDI/DRV), amounts of nutrients based on age-adjusted population means, to replace the 1968-based U.S. RDA as the standard by which to measure the amount of all nutrients listed on the label.

Serving size. Whereas food manufacturers used to have the freedom to determine the size of a serving and the units of measure, under the new rules there will be standardized reference amounts set for 131 food categories in quantities customarily consumed by individuals and expressed on the label in common household measures. For example, to determine the serving size for a loaf of sliced bread, a manufacturer would simply count the number of slices closest to the reference amount for bread (55 g), which would usually be two slices, but three or four for thinly sliced bread. Also, for single-serving containers, such as a 12-ounce can of soft drink, the serving size indicated on the label will be based on the assumption that it will be consumed in one sitting, not at two or three.

Descriptors. In the past, a variety of descriptors such as "low" or "reduced" could be used by the manufacturer to describe the level of calories or sodium in a product. In the proposed rules to implement NLEA, FDA has specified that every manufacturer will need to use the same "dictionary" of descriptors, which now contains nine core terms—free, low, light or lite, less, high, source of, more fresh, reduced—whose meaning has been defined by the FDA.

Health claims. Currently, there are no FDA-approved health claims. In order to provide some guidelines by which consumers can learn about the role of nutrition in disease risk reduction, FDA has proposed to approve, for the time being, several health messages linking specific nutrients and chronic disease conditions, such as fat and heart disease, fat and cancer, sodium and hypertension, and calcium and osteoporosis. The law requires approval of only messages for which there is significant scientific agreement and then only in a form most likely to give the consumer the full story.

Consumer education. NLEA also requires the secretary of DHHS to carry out activities that educate the consumer about the availability of nutrition information on the food label and the importance of this information in maintaining healthy dietary practices. Various coalitions consisting of representations from consumer groups, professional associations, and the food industry are already at work designing effective consumer information campaigns.

Not all foods under the jurisdiction of the FDA; the Food Safety and Inspection Service (FSIS) of the USDA has responsibility for labeling products containing at least 2% cooked (or 3% raw) meat or poultry. Although not specifically included in NLEA legislation, USDA has voluntarily proposed a mandatory nutrition labeling program for processed meat and poultry and voluntary guidelines for fresh meat and poultry products. It is important to consumers that there be harmonization of labeling efforts between FDA and USDA. It is equally important to coordinate food labeling policy with food advertising policy under the jurisdiction of the Federal Trade Commission (FTC).

Providing for an Adequate Science and Research Base in Food and Nutrition

Through the use of tax dollars, government has the means—and the responsibility—to conduct or support research. The federal government's involvement in nutrition research dates back to 1893, when USDA received the first appropriation to "conduct human nutrition investigations." Examples of research-based information needed for policy-making include data on human nutrition requirements throughout the life cycle, food consumption patterns, and the nutrient composition of food. Such information forms the scientific basis for policy decisions on food assistance programs,

food labeling, and dietary guidance. Other research results—especially epidemiological studies, clinical trials, animal experiments, and basic research—that delineate the nature of substantive relationships between diet and chronic disease have been used to justify requests for increased public funding for nutrition research.[10]

Recommended Dietary Allowances. The linkage between nutrition policy and research is dramatically demonstrated by the example of the Recommended Dietary Allowances. The National Academy of Sciences' National Research Council established the Food and Nutrition Board (FNB) in 1940 in response to concerns about widespread nutrient deficiencies noted among Americans at the start of World War II and a need for providing guidance on the nutrient adequacy of food supplies. FNB's first set of Recommended Dietary Allowances (RDAs) was published in 1943 to provide "standards to serve as a goal for good nutrition."[22] Because the RDAs are intended to reflect the best scientific judgment on nutrient allowances, the initial publication has been revised periodically to incorporate new scientific knowledge and interpretations. Revised approximately every 5 years, the tenth edition of the RDAs was published in 1989. RDAs are defined as "levels of intake of essential nutrients that, on the basis of scientific knowledge, are judged by the Food and Nutrition Board to be adequate to meet the known nutrient needs of practically all healthy persons."[22]

The blending of science and policy is achieved because of the research findings on which the RDAs are based and the policy uses to which RDAs are put. The scientific evidence on which the RDAs are formulated include nutrient balance studies, biochemical measurements of tissue saturation, nutrient intake studies of apparently healthy people, epidemiological observations, and, in some cases, extrapolation of data from animal experiments. The policy uses of the RDA are widespread and significant; as Palmer describes, "Since their origin, the RDAs have served as the primary dietary standard for federal food assistance programs and policies on vitamin and mineral supplementation, enrichment, and food fortification—policies that are credited with virtual elimination of deficiency diseases in the United States."[42]

Thus the RDAs have long been used as nutrition standards on which public policy has been based. Whether a single policy guide can be applied unilaterally is an issue that was brought into sharp focus when the FNB did not accept the revision prepared by the RDA committee in 1984. Rejection of the report stimulated discussion of the purposes and uses of the RDAs and the scientific and policy considerations for preparing them. This discussion resulted in written guidelines for use by future RDA committees, developed by members of the FNB with input from users of the RDAs, including both nutrition scientists and practicing nutritionists representing government agencies and industry.[21]

Research activities and support. USDA has traditionally had the responsibility for supporting research in the agricultural and food production system, up to and including food consumption and normal human nutrition needs. This role was strengthened by the language of the 1977 Food and Agriculture Act (also called the 1977 Farm Bill), in which USDA was identified as the lead agency in the federal government for food and agricultural sciences, including human nutrition.

Within USDA, a number of agencies conduct or support human nutrition research. The Agricultural Research Service (ARS) supports a program that is primarily intramural (i.e., conducted by scientists on its staff rather than by providing grants to outside scientists) in which the research is carried out at five geographically dispersed Human Nutrition Research Centers located in Massachusetts, Maryland, Texas, North Dakota, and California. USDA's Cooperative State Research Service (CSRS) supports research at state land grant universities and oversees the federal funds (the so-called Hatch Grants) that go to state agricultural experiment stations. CSRS also administers the Competitive Research Grants Program in human nutrition. The Human Nutrition Information Service (HNIS), which has USDA's primary role in nutrition monitoring, supports most of USDA's applied human nutrition research activity in the areas of food consumption, nutrient composition of foods,

and dietary guidance and education through a program of external contacts. Other USDA agencies have more limited research programs. The Food and Nutrition Service (FNS) supports research projects related to the evaluation of service delivery issues in the food assistance programs. The Food Safety and Inspection Service (FSIS) conducts research primarily related to the safety and inspection systems for meat and poultry. The Economic Research Service (ERS) conducts intramural research on economic issues related to food consumption and food assistance programs.

DHHS is responsible for studying the "causes, diagnosis, treatment, control and prevention of physical and mental diseases and impairments of man" under the Public Health Service Act. In DHHS, human nutrition research dealing with the metabolic effects of dietary consumption patterns, particularly as related to chronic diseases, has largely been in the domain of the National Institutes of Health (NIH). The research program at NIH consists mainly of extramural support provided to researchers at universities and medical school research facilities. FDA, an agency also in DHHS, conducts research related to food labeling and food safety issues.

The level and sources of federal support for nutrition research are of concern to most of the nutrition community because this is an indicator of the commitment of the government to food and nutrition. As Ostenso has noted, "Prior to 1950, the principal funding of human nutrition research was provided by three sources: the private sector, appropriated state funds, and USDA formula grants to Agricultural Experiment Stations in land grant colleges. Today, support for nutrition research has followed the public and Congressional interests in issues primarily related to the relationship between nutrition and health and disease."[41] Regardless of the source of funding, the federal contribution to nutrition research has kept pace neither with the rate of inflation nor with the percentage increase allocated by the government to basic research in most other disciplines.[41] The Human Nutrition Research and Information Management (HNRIM) system, a federal government–managed data base created to track human nutrition research activities, has reported data for FY1988, the last year for which such data are available.[26] In FY1988, federal nutrition research and training dollars totaled $385 million, representing an increase of 8% over that expended in FY1987. Of these funds 78% were expended by DHHS, 18% by USDA, 2% by the Agency for International Development (AID), and 1% each by the Department of Defense and the Department of Veterans Affairs. Of the total amount expended, 81% supported extramural research.

Nutrition monitoring. Nutrition monitoring is vital to policy-making and research.[18] Monitoring activities can contribute to a data base for public policy decisions related to food assistance programs; federally supported food service programs; nutrition education; public health nutrition programs; the regulation of fortification, safety, and labeling of the food supply; and food production and marketing, as well as providing a data base upon which to establish research priorities. Timely, complete, and accurate data are essential for developing nutrition policies and programs to meet the changing health needs of the nation.

Public interest in determining the nutritional status of the American population has usually peaked whenever testimonials are presented about the extent of hunger and malnutrition in the United States. One of the best known of these initiatives occurred in 1967, when there was congressional interest in documenting the existence of hunger and malnutrition in the United States, an interest that led to the Ten State Nutrition Survey. Further public interest was directed to the issue by the attention given to the discussion of hunger and malnutrition at the White House Conference on Food, Nutrition, and Health in 1969.

In 1979, a presidential directive called for the incorporation of the Ten State Nutrition Survey with the National Health Examination Survey; the result is what is known today as the National Health and Nutrition Examination Survey (NHANES), carried out by the National Center for Health Statistics (NCHS) in DHHS. USDA has long been involved in collecting data about the foods Amer-

icans consume. The Nationwide Food Consumption Surveys (NFCS) have been conducted by USDA agencies on an approximately decennial basis since 1935, with the most recent one conducted in 1987 and 1988. Other food consumption studies, such as the Continuing Survey of Food Intakes by Individuals (CSFII), are also conducted by USDA.

The executive branch has been working toward the implementation of a comprehensive, coordinated national nutrition monitoring system since the passage of the 1977 Food and Agriculture Act, which called for the establishment of such a system. In 1981 representatives from various agencies and departments prepared a document identifying all the ongoing nutrition monitoring activities carried out by the federal government and proposed an implementation plan to coordinate them. The primary components of this plan were the Nationwide Food Consumption Survey (NFCS), conducted by USDA, and the National Health and Nutrition Examination Survey (NHANES), conducted by DHHS. Despite these efforts, several scientific organizations, health groups, and antihunger advocacy groups joined to express their concerns to Congress that the system in place for nutrition monitoring was not effective in providing timely data or data that were useful for state and local planning efforts.[10] To address these concerns, nutrition monitoring legislation was first introduced in the Congress in 1984.

Introduction and defeat of several legislative efforts took place over the ensuing 6 years. On October 22, 1990, PL 101-445, the National Nutrition Monitoring and Related Research Act of 1990, was passed. In accordance with the requirements of the act, a 10-year comprehensive plan has been developed to "establish a comprehensive nutrition monitoring and related research program by collecting quality data that are continuous, coordinated, timely, and reliable; using comparable methods for data collection and reporting of results; conducting relevant research; and efficiently and effectively disseminating and exchanging information with data users."[18] As specified in the act, the secretaries of DHHS and USDA have joint responsibility for the implementation of the coordinated program; to perform this function, the Interagency Board for Nutrition Monitoring and Related Research, consisting of 21 federal agencies, has been established. In addition, a National Nutrition Monitoring Advisory Council was formed to provide input from users outside the federal government.

Activities associated with the National Nutrition Monitoring System (NNMS) are grouped into five measurement components:
- Nutrition and related health measurements
- Food and nutrient consumption
- Knowledge, attitudes, and behavior assessments
- Food composition and nutrient data bases
- Food supply determinations

Data derived from these components are used to assess the dietary, nutritional, and related health status of the population. Currently, more than 40 surveys and surveillance systems are operative. Integrating the results from these various systems will be a major challenge for the NNMS, but the rewards will be great.

Integrating Support for Nutrition Services as Part of the Health System

The delivery of food and nutrition services through the auspices of the health system is an area of nutrition policy that has proven to be of great importance for dietitians and nutritionists. Indeed, issues such as health care financing, credentialing of health services providers, and standards of practice for nutrition professionals have attracted policy attention over the past few years.

The overwhelming emphasis in health policy in the United States is on the delivery of personal health services. This strategy consumes more than 86% of all health expenditures and more than 90% of federal health spending.[36] As Milio's analysis reveals,

> [This] after-the-fact emphasis on health care policy, [which focuses on] ameliorating people's illness after it develops, shows the inflationary effects of present policy for financing health services. Basically, the policy sustains a delivery system that is dependent on energy-intensive and capital-intensive technologies to

deal with health problems. The cost effects spill over into the national economy with burdensome reverberations. They also reinforce the inequities that exist among Americans and, through their economic impact, serve to damage the prospects for the health of lower-income people.[36]

Within the bureaucracy, DHHS administers the majority of nutrition service programs, not including food assistance. The Health Care Financial Administration (HCFA), within DHHS, administers the Medicare (Title XVIII, Social Security Act) and Medicaid (Title XIX, Social Security Act) programs. Medicare provides insurance coverage for health services for older Americans. Medicare regulations cover nutrition and dietetic services in hospitals, nursing homes, home health agencies, hospices, and other facilities that meet the Medicare conditions of participation.[19] Medicaid establishes cooperative federal and state funding of health care for economically disadvantaged individuals and the disabled. Each state legislature sets its own state's eligibility standards and policies for health services within broad federal guidelines.

Primary care services. Primary care is "first contact care" or the basic level of medical care to ambulatory patients who come into the medical office or clinic.[28] Primary care should range from preventive services and anticipatory guidance to care for acute symptoms and management of chronic conditions and diseases. As part of primary care, nutrition services should be included in screening and diagnosis, health maintenance, health supervision, and health promotion. As Kaufman cogently points out, however, such integration of nutrition services into primary health care requires administrative support within the agency and linkages between nutrition personnel in the federal and state health agencies and the various free-standing primary health care programs, efforts that require resources as well as mutual respect among various health care providers.

Payment for nutrition services in primary health care has come, in part, through a series of federally financed DHHS block grant mechanisms. The Maternal and Child Health (MCH) Block Grant has routinely been used to pay for state and local public health nutrition personnel, local clinical nutrition services, and positions for dietitians in newborn intensive care units or specialty clinics such as metabolic disorders clinics. The Preventive Health and Health Services Block Grant has, in some states, funded state and local nutritionist positions to provide nutrition services as part of a health promotion program. In addition, the Primary Care Block Grant has financed Community Health and Migrant Health Center nutritionist positions and contracts for nutrition consultation from hospital dietitians and public health or private practice nutritionists. Other block grants that have been used to a more limited extent for nutrition services include the Social Services or Title XX Block Grant, which has, for example, provided for nutrition training of day-care personnel; the Alcohol, Drug Abuse, and Mental Health Block Grant, which has funded clinical nutritionist positions; and the Community Services Block Grant, which funds community food and nutrition programs, usually directed at emergency situations.[7]

Nutrition services as part of medical intervention and rehabilitation. Nutrition services, including screening and assessment, nutrition counseling, and nutrition support, have long been provided by qualified dietitians and nutritionists as an integral component of appropriate medical care. It is only of late that issues such as documenting the cost-effectiveness of nutrition services, third-party payment for nutrition services, and credentialing of dietitians and nutritionists have been of concern, particularly in the legislative and policy arena.

Providing documentation that nutrition services are cost-effective and efficient may lead to further reimbursement for nutrition and dietetics professionals. The American Dietetic Association, as part of its position statement on health care reform, has documented the following:

> Prenatal nutrition service helps reduce expensive neonatal intensive care unit charges, which can cost as much as $1500 per infant day.
> Among adults at risk for chronic disease, nutrition assessment and counseling by registered dietetic personnel has contributed to a decrease in the incidence of acute events and hospital admissions for heart dis-

eases (12.8-44.8% decrease), strokes (53-59% decrease), and diabetes mellitus (39.8% decrease).

The benefits of nutrition services for the elderly include delayed onset of chronic diseases and their complications, such as diabetes, heart and vascular disease, and certain forms of cancer. Provision of nutrition care for the elderly decreases the cost of medical and institutional care, surgery, and drug therapy.[3]

In recent years, third-party payment (i.e., reimbursement for nutrition services by public and private groups) has become an important source of financing for local nutrition services. Important sources of such payments include Medicaid, Blue Cross/Blue Shield, Supplemental Security Income, state programs for children with special health care needs, workers' compensation, and commercial carriers. Although coverage of nutrition services often varies from payer to payer and from state to state, some generalizations are useful. Nutrition services may be reimbursable if the following conditions are met: identifying those specific services that are or could be billable to the various third-party payers; having a documented physician referral or determination of medical necessity of the service; using acceptable terminology; using an appropriate provider number, often a physician or provider organization number; establishing fee schedules; and documenting that the service is provided.[7]

Credentialing of health service providers has assumed increasing importance as the reimbursement issue has surfaced and as the public has become better educated about what and from whom they are receiving health care services. The assumption underlying credentialing of nutrition service providers is that the consumer is protected from receiving inadequate care, misinformation, and inappropriate counseling. Two credentialing mechanisms exist in nutrition and dietetics: registration through the Commission on Dietetic Registration and licensure, now legislated in about half the states.[28]

To become a registered dietitian (RD) through the Commission on Dietetic Registration requires educational and experiential preparation for dietetics attained through routes approved by the

American Dietetic Association, followed by passing a standardized registration exam. Maintaining dietetic registration requires completing 75 clock hours of approved continuing education in each 5-year period.

As there is no federal program of licensure for nutrition and dietetics professionals, each state legislature must individually set up its own criteria for practice in the state and pass its own licensure laws. The criteria for licensure are generally the same or similar to those for dietetic registration. Satisfactory performance on the national dietetic registration examination is accepted by a number of states as the state's licensure examination.

SUMMARY

Policy has been defined as a set of guidelines that determine priorities, goals, and actions. Public policy governs the actions of governmental units. In the absence of a clearly defined nutrition policy in the United States, policy is set de facto by a number of programs, advisory groups, legislative actions, partnerships, and publications.

Six elements of nutrition policy have been identified and discussed in this chapter:

- Providing an adequate food supply at reasonable cost to consumers
- Ensuring a safe and wholesome food supply
- Providing food access and availability to all, regardless of income
- Providing research-based information and educational programs to encourage informed food choices
- Providing for an adequate science and research base in the area of food and nutrition
- Integrating support for nutrition services as part of the health system

Also included in this chapter has been a discussion of the public policy process, delineating the actors, structures, and groups active in this process. Is is essential for nutrition professionals to be knowledgeable about the process and adopt a proactive stance in advocating specific policies based on sound science that will be of benefit to the population. Appendix 12-1 lists specific resources as well as sources of information that will

be helpful to those who wish to pursue an active involvement in the nutrition policy process.

REFERENCES

1. Akin JS and others: Evaluating school meals, *Comm Nutr* 2:4, 1983.
2. Allen JE, Newton DW: Existing food policies and their relationship to hunger and nutrition, *Amer J Agric Econ* 68:1247, 1986.
3. American Dietetic Association: *White paper on health care reform*, Washington, DC, 1992, American Dietetic Association.
4. Blumer P: *How a bill becomes a law*. Paper presented at the legislative symposium of the American Dietetic Association, Washington, DC, March 1992.
5. Boisvert-Walsh C, Kallio J: *Reaching out to those at highest risk*. In Kaufman M, editor: *Nutrition in public health*, Rockville, Md, 1990, Aspen.
6. Brown JL: Hunger in the U.S., *Sci Am* 256:37, 1987.
7. Caldwell M: *Financing nutrition programs*. In Sharbaugh C, Egan M, editors: *Call to action: better nutrition for mothers, children, and families*, Washington, DC, 1990, National Center for Education in Maternal and Child Health.
8. Campbell CA: Food security: a nutritional outcome or a predictor variable? *J Nutr* 121:408, 1991.
9. *1991 Catalog of Federal Domestic Assistance*, Washington DC, 1991, Government Printing Office.
10. Chapman N: Consensus and coalitions: key to nutrition policy development, *Nutr Today* Sept/Oct 1987.
11. Chapman N: *Developing agency community and state nutrition policies* and *Advocating for national health and nutrition policies*. In Kaufman M, editor: *Nutrition in public health: a handbook for developing programs and services*, Rockville, MD, 1990, Aspen.
12. Clancy KL: Human nutrition, agriculture and human values, *Agric Hum Values* 1:10, 1984.
13. Clem AL: *Congress: powers, processes, and politics*, Pacific Grove, Calif, 1989, Brooks/Cole.
14. Committee on Dietary Guidelines Implementation, Food and Nutrition Board, Institute of Medicine: *Improving America's diet and health: from recommendations to action*, Washington, DC, 1991, National Academy Press.
15. Community Nutrition Institute: Food assistance programs reach 40 million Americans, *Nutr Week*, p 4, Sept 27, 1990.
16. Community Nutrition Institute: Food assistance programs serve tens of millions, *Nutr Week*, p 4, June 14, 1991.
17. Davidson RH, Oleszek WJ: *Congress and its members*, Washington, DC, 1981, Congressional Quarterly Press.
18. Department of Health and Human Services and Department of Agriculture: Ten-year comprehensive plan for the national nutrition monitoring and related research program; notice, *Federal Register* 56:55716, 1991.
19. Earl R: *Influencing federal health and nutrition legislation*

and regulations. Kaufman M, editor: *Nutrition in public health*, Rockville, Md, 1990, Aspen.

20. Food and Drug Administration: The new food label: your guide to better nutrition, *Nutr Today*, p 37, Jan/Feb 1992.

21. Food and Nutrition Board, National Research Council, National Academy of Sciences: Dietary allowances: scientific issues and process for the future, *J Nutr Educ* 18:82, 1986.

22. Food and Nutrition Board, National Research Council, National Academy of Sciences: *Recommended dietary allowances*, ed 10, Washington, DC, 1989, National Academy Press.

23. Food Research and Action Center (FRAC): *Fact sheets on the federal food programs*, Washington, DC, 1991, FRAC.

24. Hutt PB: National nutrition policy and the role of the Food and Drug Administration, *Currents* 2:2, 1986.

25. Hyman PM: The regulators: *Food Technology* 31:43, 1977.

26. Interagency Committee on Human Nutrition Research: *The human nutrition research and information management system, FY 1988, 7th progress report*, Washington, DC, 1990, The Committee.

27. Kaltreider DL, Sims LS, Brown JL: Extension food and nutrition programs: a national assessment, *Extension Review* 58:46, 1987.

28. Kaufman M: *Providing nutrition services in primary care*. In Kaufman M, editor: *Nutrition in public health*, Rockville, Md, 1990, Aspen.

29. Kerr NA: The evolution of USDA surplus disposal programs, *Natl Food Review* 11:25, 1988.

30. Kronenfeld JJ, Whicker ML: *U.S. national health policy: an analysis of the federal role*, New York, 1984, Praeger.

31. Light L, Cronin FJ: Food guidance revisited, *J Nutr Educ* 13:57, 1981.

32. Lilja JG: *Status of food assistance programs*, USDA Food and Nutrition Service, Unpublished, 1991.

33. Little L, Sims LS: *Let's get involved in the legislative process*. In Wright HS, Sims LS, editors. *Community nutrition: people, policies and programs*, Monterey, Calif, 1986, Jones and Bartlett.

34. McNutt K: Integrating nutrition and environmental objectives, *Nutr Today* p 40, Nov/Dec 1990.

35. *Medford declaration to end hunger in the U.S.* Press kit, Washington DC, April 1982.

36. Milio N: *Promoting health through public policy*, Philadelphia, 1981, FA Davis.

37. Milio N: *Nutrition policy for food-rich countries: a strategic analysis*, Baltimore, 1990, Johns Hopkins University Press.

38. Mintz BW, Miller NG: *A guide to federal agency rulemaking*, ed 2, Washington, DC, 1991, Administrative Conference of the United States.

39. National Research Council: *Diet and health: implications for reducing chronic disease risk*, Washington, DC, 1989, National Academy Press.

40. Nestle M, Guttmacher S: Hunger in the United States: rationale, methods, and policy implications of state hunger surveys, *J Nutr Educ* 24:18S, 1992.

41. Ostenso GL: Nutrition: policies and politics, 24th Lenna Frances Cooper memorial lecture, *J Am Diet Assoc* 88:909, 1988.

42. Palmer S: Food and nutrition policy: challenges for the 1990s, *Health Aff (Millwood)* 9:94, 1990.

43. Public Voice for Food and Health Policy: *Empty calories: the Reagen record on food policy*, Washington, DC, 1988, Public Voice.

44. Rapp D: *How the U.S. got into agriculture*, Washington, DC, 1988, Congressional Quarterly.

45. Senauer B: The food Americans buy: an economic perspective, *Food Nutr News* 64:11, 1992.

46. Senauer B, Asp E, Kinsey J: *Food trends and the changing consumer*, St Paul, Minn, 1991, Eagan Press.

47. Sims LS: The ebb and flow of nutrition as a public policy issue, *J Nutr Educ* 15:4, 1983.

48. Sims LS: *Nutrition policy through the Reagan era: feast or famine? Pew/Cornell lecture series on food and nutrition policy*, Ithaca, NY, 1988, Cornell Food and Nutrition Policy Program.

49. Sims LS: Government involvement in nutrition education: panacea or Pandora's box? *Health Educ Res* 5:517, 1990.

50. Society for Nutrition Education: *Call to action: a public policy handbook*, Minneapolis, MN, The Society, 1992.

51. Spasoff RA: The role of nutrition in healthy public policy, *Rapport* (published by the National Institute of Nutrition, Ottawa, Canada) 4:6, 1989.

52. U.S. Department of Agriculture, Food and Nutrition Service: *The national school lunch program: Background and development*, FNS-63, Washington, DC, 1971, U.S. Government Printing Office.

53. U.S. Department of Health and Human Services: *The surgeon general's report on nutrition and health*, U.S. Public Health Service Pub No 88-50210, Washington, DC, 1988, US Government Printing Office.

54. U.S. Senate Select Committee on Nutrition and Human Needs: *Dietary goals for the United States*, 2nd ed, Washington, DC, 1977, U.S. Government Printing Office.

55. Wormser MD, editor: *CQ's Guide to Congress*, ed 3, Washington, DC, 1982, Congresional Quarterly.

56. Woteki CE, Thomas PR, editors: *Eat for life: the Food and Nutrition Board's guide to reducing your risk of chronic disease*, Washington, DC, 1992, National Academy Press.

APPENDIX 12-1

Resources for further information

GOVERNMENT PUBLICATIONS

Government Printing Office (GPO): Publishes the *Congressional Directory, Congressional Record, Federal Register*, congressional bills, reports, hearings, and various other federal publications related to food and nutrition policy. Order by title or document number from GPO by calling 202/783-3228 or writing Superintendent of Documents, Attention: Inquiries, U.S. Government Printing Office, Washington, DC 20402.

House and Senate documents: For copies of House and Senate bills and documents such as committee reports and public laws, send a letter with request, accompanied by self-addressed, large, stamped envelope:

The Senate Document Room
Hart Senate Office Bldg.
Room B-04
Washington DC 20515

The House Document Room
226 House Annex I
Washington DC 20515

INFORMATION ON CONGRESS AND FEDERAL LEGISLATION

Almanac of American Politics (Macmillan): A complete listing of biographical sketches of congressional member's voting records, interest group ratings, and election percentages.

Congressional Directory (GPO): A complete directory of all government offices, congressional committees, and executive and judicial branch offices.

The U.S. Congress Handbooks (I & II): Complete directories that identify members of Congress, their committees, and staff, as well as cabinet members. Features special articles and key phone numbers (source: The U.S. Congress Handbook, McLean VA 22101).

Congressional Handbook: Annual directory of members of Congress (source: U.S. Chamber of Commerce, Legislative Action Department, 1615 H Street, NW, Washington, DC 20062).

Congress and Health: An Introduction to the Legislative Process and Its Key Participants (source: National Health Council, New York).

Congressional Insight Handbook: An Information Guide to the U.S. House of Representatives (source: Public Affairs Dept., National Association of Manufacturers, Washington, DC 20004-1703)

Congressional Quarterly Publications (Congressional Quarterly Inc., 1414 22d Street, NW, Washington, DC 20037):

Congressional Monitor: A weekly newsletter summarizing events in Congress, the White House, and the Supreme Court.

Congressional Record Scanner: A synopsis of the *Congressional Record* published daily when Congress is in session.

Campaign Practices Reports and Guide: A biweekly newsletter reporting on all significant campaign finance regulations, news, and trends.

Congressional Insight: A weekly newsletter analyzing the pressures, people, and politics that shape Capitol Hill decisions.

Congress in Print: A weekly notice that lists current published congressional documents.

The CQ Quarterly. A publication that summarizes current issues, organizes reference materials, and provides a bibliography of sources for further research.

The Congressional Record (GPO): A verbatim account of happenings on the Senate and House floors and scheduled committee meetings; issued daily when Congress is in session.

Congressional Yellow Book: A directory of Congress staff updated four times a year (source: The Washington Monitor, Inc., Washington DC 20004).

ORGANIZATIONS INVOLVED WITH DOMESTIC FOOD AND NUTRITION POLICY

Bread for the World
802 Rhode Island Ave., NE
Washington, DC 20018
202/269-0200

Center on Budget and Policy Priorities
777 N. Capitol Street NE, #705
Washington, DC 20002
202/408-1080

Center on Hunger, Poverty and Nutrition Policy
Tufts University School of Nutrition
126 Curtis Street
Medford, MA 02155
617/381-3223

Children's Defense Fund
122 C Street NW
Washington, DC 20001
202/628-8787

Community Nutrition Institute
2001 S Street NW, Suite #530
Washington, DC 20009
202/462-4700

Food Research and Action Center
1875 Connecticut Ave. NW, #540
Washington, DC 20009
202/986-2200

Public Voice for Food & Health Policy
1001 Connecticut Ave. NW, #522
Washington, DC 20036
202/659-5930

Nutrition Legislative News
P.O. Box 75035
Washington, DC 20013
202/488-8879

Second Harvest
116 South Michigan Ave., #4
Chicago, IL 60603
312/263-2303

Urban Institute
2100 M Street NW, 5th floor
Washington, DC 20037
202/833-7200

ASSOCIATIONS

American Dietetic Association
Office of Government Affairs
1225 Eye Street NW, Suite 1250
Washington, DC 20005

American Home Economics Assoc.
1555 King Street
Alexandria, VA 22314

American Institute of Nutrition
9650 Rockville Pike
Bethesda, MD 20014

American Public Health Assoc.
1015 Eighteenth Street NW
Washington, DC 20036

American School Food Service Assoc.
1600 Duke Street NW
Alexandria, VA 22314

Society for Nutrition Education
2001 Killebrew Dr., Suite 340
Minneapolis, MN 55425-1882

Managing Community Nutrition Services

13 Managing Successfully

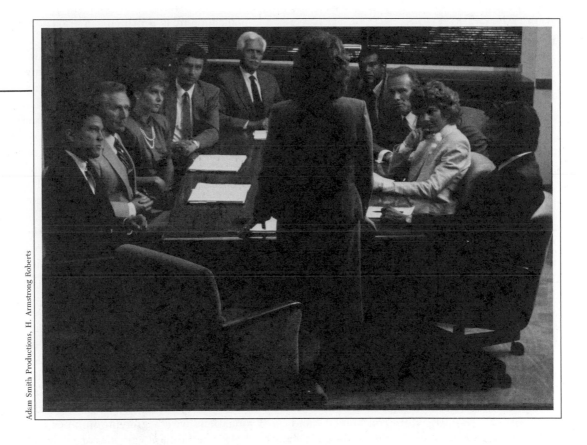

GENERAL CONCEPT

Enhancing the mangement effectiveness of the community dietitian or nutritionist may be the greatest challenge facing the profession in the 1990s. In order to assure high-level performance, the community dietitian or nutritionist must possess effective managerial skills. Addressing one's capabilities as the first step in the process of approaching the management role, the manager has a greater ability to succeed, because management is the art of getting things done through people. The changing business environment now includes social responsibility and managerial ethics as major components of a manager's work.

OUTCOME OBJECTIVES

When you finish this chapter, you should be able to:

- Define the qualities needed for personal success.
- Describe the interpersonal skills required to be an effective manager.
- Define the management process.
- Describe the manager's roles and responsibilities.
- Understand the implications of managerial performance.
- Discuss the issues involved in social responsibility and managerial ethics.

This chapter is about the job of the manager. It describes how men and women, dietitians and nutritionists, go about managing the people and activities of their organizations so that the goals of the organization, as well as their personal goals, will be achieved. Much has been written about management principles. Management is the process of getting things done through the efforts of other people.[14] This definition has not changed for many years but the methods for accomplishing this task have become more complex because of global competition, sophisticated consumers, and a shrinking American work force. To describe how management in America has changed, the following example makes the point quite aptly.

In the late 1960s, the French journalist Servan-Schreiber received considerable notoriety for his book *The American Challenge*.[18] In this book he warned Europeans that American industry was well ahead of the rest of the industrialized world and that the United States was widening its lead. He further suggested that the reason for this American supremacy was superior management. If Servan-Schreiber were to make the same assertions today, he would be regarded as a person completely out of touch with reality. In less than two decades the perception and reality of American industry have almost come full circle. The current concern is that the gap is being reversed. Japanese and European companies have gained dominance in many key industries and are challenging American leadership in others. Moreover, it is widely believed that poor management is a principal reason for the decline in American industrial might.

Clearly the situation is complex, and many factors affect it. Government policies, union attitudes, cultural factors, and natural resources have all played a role in the dramatic turn of events. Nevertheless, managers, because they make the decisions that shape the competitive posture of their firms and industries, must assume a major portion of the blame. In these difficult economic times community dietitians and nutritionists in leadership positions are being evaluated in terms of their managerial effectiveness. Technical skills are not enough; one must have managerial skills.

We see the world as becoming increasingly competitive. This is so not just in the business sector of the economy, where international competition has burgeoned in recent years, but also in the not-for-profit and governmental sectors, where many dietitians and nutritionists are employed. In the latter two sectors, organizations must compete with each other for scarce resources. Charitable and cultural organizations, for example, have to a great extent been cut off from government funding and find themselves competing vigorously for private donations with a growing number of rivals. Similarly, government agencies are fighting harder and harder for tax dollars. In such a competitive climate, the quality of management becomes a crucial determinant of success and even survival. For community dietitians and nutritionists much more emphasis must be placed on mastering management skills if we are to be recognized as effective.

With the present climate, responsibility for increasing employee performance is one of the most critical concerns of today's management. Managers who empower employees to higher levels of performance will be indispensable to their organizations. Managers who fail will be lost. But is there a common thread that is woven through such indispensable managers? Can specific habits be duplicated? According to Oechsli, the answer is an unequivocal yes.[15] Exhaustive management studies show that successful managers are as different as they are similar, yet close observation discloses five particular qualities. They are goal driven, have good communication skills, continually empower employees, act with a caring attitude, and embody total commitment. These qualities have become habits for indispensable managers. Because habits are acquired behaviors, they can be adopted by anyone. There is no major success formula.

This chapter addresses three important issues: personal success, management effectiveness in community nutrition, and, finally, the changing environment in management, which covers social responsibility and managerial ethics.

In this rapidly changing environment, we have initiated the management chapters with a discussion on personal success. The most recent literature on management stresses the importance of the "inside-out" approach. This approach starts with you first. By starting with your own assumptions, character, and motives, you have a much greater chance of being an effective manager than by starting with the organizational skills you need. Whether you are a new professional recently completing your education and working in your first job or have been a practicing dietitian or nutritionist for a long time, the approach is a very useful exercise. Taking another look at your own personality traits and how you manage people and resources should be a useful way to approach this complex area.

The second section on management effectiveness provides traditional information on management, including the manager's work and responsibilities, organizational performance, and the management process—how to get things done.

The third section addresses the changing environment that we now manage. With advancing technology and the fast pace of our society, we all know that change is affecting our lives. In this environment, social responsibility and managerial ethics are emerging as the issues of the 1990s.

PERSONAL SUCCESS

Heath, in his book *Fulfilling Lives, Paths to Maturity and Success*,[8] makes the following important observation:

> To grow up to succeed and be happy is to develop the mind and character necessary to satisfy our needs, achieve our goals, and fulfill our dreams. But what

needs and which goals and dreams? That is the first question we must answer. Only then can we seek to discover what kind of mind and character produce success and happiness.

Success is not just a matter of luck, family privilege, or society's program; it has become a matter of character and the way we use it, for example, learning how to be persons of integrity.

What does success mean to you? Try an exercise to initiate your thinking. Rank the following 12 goals that most people would like to achieve. Then you can compare your personal meanings to those of college-going adults who have similarly ranked their values. Rank your most important goal or value as 1, the next priority goal a 2, and so on. Try not to tie ranks. Discover just how clearly ordered your priorities are.[8]

——— Leadership; power
——— Happy marital relationship
——— High income
——— Competent and satisfied parenting
——— Psychological maturity; good mental health
——— Self-fulfillment; happiness
——— Religious or ethical ideals
——— Fulfilling sexual relationship
——— Competence in a satisfying vocation
——— Being a contributing citizen to the community or nation
——— Having a close friend of the same sex
——— Physical health

Heath compared the priorities of several thousand college-educated 30- to 50-year-olds. See how your priorities compare to this group. These respondents ranked the following as most to least important.

Self-fulfillment; happiness
Psychological maturity; good mental health
Physical health
Happy marital relationship
Religious or ethical ideals
Competent and satisfied parenting
Competence in a satisfying vocation
Being a contributing citizen to the community or nation
Fulfilling sexual relationship

Having a close friend of the same sex
Leadership; power
High income

Men and women really differ in a few of their priorities. Men value a fulfilling sexual relationship and high income more than women do. Women rank a close friendship with another woman and contributing to society more highly than men do.

If we are clear about our priorities, we now can ask what mind and character are necessary to achieve them. In an attempt to understand the mind and character necessary to succeed, Heath completed a longitudinal study of adult development. The study was undertaken to find out what successful and fulfilled people are actually like and how they got that way. The study participants' (65 men and 40 women who were partners of the men) own judgments were used about the strengths necessary to succeed in their principal adult roles as citizens, marital partners, parents, friends, and workers. They agreed that 11 core strengths are necessary.[8]

The most important strengths are caring and compassion, honesty and integrity, and a sense of humor. Every major adult role involves other persons; our success depends upon the quality of our relationships with them. When we care, we affirm to others that they count, are important, and are valued. When we speak honestly and act out of our hearts with integrity, we create trust. When we bring the perspective of humor to our relationships, we help each other transcend the pain of the frustration and anger that inevitably arise in our relations with others.

The next core strengths needed to succeed are openness, lack of defensiveness about sharing our feelings, tolerance, and acceptance of others' quirks and failings. Other strengths are dedication and commitment to fulfill our roles well. Without such commitment, work becomes sloppy, marriages are unstable, good parenting is unreliable, friendships are untrustworthy, and community contributions are ineffective. The men and women in the study then identified the interpersonal strength of understanding, respecting, and empathizing with others and rounded out the list with adaptability and self-confidence.

Heath did not anticipate that so many interpersonal skills would be critical for success in all of our adult roles.[8] Unless one is a hermit, strengths like caring, openness, tolerance, and honesty are essential. But what happens to the intellectual skills and knowledge that our society values so highly? They were *not* at the top of the list. They are important but are not even as important as patience.

In this research, it is ironic and unsettling that not one of the principal strengths that contribute to adult success is directly measured by the academic grades and the achievement and scholastic aptitude test scores that create so much anxiety in young people. Instead of measuring the likelihood of adult success, these tests humble our children, enhance self-centered competitiveness, and undermine their confidence in their ability to learn and educate themselves. It is not that the kind of intelligence that they measure is unimportant; grades and scholastic aptitude scores tell us how rapidly we can learn, particularly abstract ideas. It is just that they do not measure well the rich variety of skills and character strengths, particularly interpersonal and ethical ones like caring, empathy, and honesty, that contribute most to adult success.

Covey, in his book about powerful lessons in personal change, describes seven habits of highly effective people.[2] He, like Heath, describes in detail a principle-centered, character-based, inside-out approach to personal and interpersonal effectiveness. *Inside-out* means to start first with self, even more fundamentally, to start with the most inside part of self with your assumptions, your character, and your motives. The inside-out approach says that private victories precede public victories, that making and keeping promises to ourselves precedes making and keeping promises to others. It says it is futile to put personality ahead of character or to try to improve relationships with others before improving ourselves.

As Covey was completing his research, he scanned hundreds of books, articles, and essays in fields such as self-improvement, popular psychology, and self-help.[2] As he reviewed 200 years of writing about success, he noticed a startling pattern emerging in the content of the literature. He concluded that the success literature of the past 50 years was superficial. It was filled with social image, consciousness techniques, and quick fixes with social Band-Aids that did not really address acute and underlying chronic problems.

In stark contrast, almost all the literature in the first 150 years focused on what could be called the character ethic as the foundation of success—things like integrity, humility, fidelity, courage, justice, patience, industry, modesty, and the Golden Rule. The character ethic taught that there are basic principles of effective living and that people can experience true success and enduring happiness only as they learn and integrate these principles into their basic characters.

Shortly after World War I, the basic view of success shifted from the character ethic to what Covey calls the personality ethic. Success became more a function of personality, public image, attitudes and behavior, and skills and techniques that lubricate the processes of human interaction. This personality ethic took two paths. One was human and public relations techniques, and the other was positive mental attitude. Some of this philosophy was expressed in inspiring and sometimes valid maxims such as: "Your attitude determines your altitude," "Smiling wins more friends than frowning," and "Whatever the mind can conceive and believe, it can achieve."

Other parts of the personality approach were clearly manipulative, even deceptive, encouraging people to use techniques to get other people to like them, to fake interest in the hobbies of others to get out of them what they wanted, or to intimidate their way through life. Reference to the character ethic became mostly lip service; the basic thrust was quick-fix influence techniques, power strategies, communication skills, and positive attitudes.

Covey was not suggesting that elements of the personality ethic, personality growth, communication skills training, and education in the field of influence strategies and positive thinking are not beneficial. In fact, sometimes they are essential to success, but these are secondary, not primary, traits.

One of the basic flaws of the personality ethic is that it attempts to change outward attitudes and behaviors but does very little good in the long run

if we fail to examine the basic assumptions from which those attitudes and behaviors flow. The glitter of the personality ethic, the massive appeal, is that there is some quick and easy way to achieve quality of life—personal effectiveness and rich, deep relationships with other people—without going through the natural process of work and growth that makes it possible.

The more aware we are of our basic assumptions and the extent to which we have been influenced by our experience, the more we can take responsibility for these assumptions, examine them, test them against reality, listen to others, and be open to their perceptions, thereby getting a larger picture and a far more objective view.

REACHING EXCELLENCE

In dietetics and nutrition today, one of our major challenges is assuming leadership in the health care system and with consumers. Covey's[2] and Heath's[8] approaches to success, modeling the character ethic, the inside-out approach, is a starting point for the development of effective leaders and managers in dietetics. What are the general values for achieving excellence and leadership in our profession? Aristotle once said, "We are what we repeatedly do." Excellence, then, is not an act but a habit. Habits are powerful factors in our lives. Because they are consistent, often unconscious patterns, they daily express our character and produce our effectiveness or ineffectiveness.

Defining Habits

Our character basically is a composite of our habits. *Habit* is defined as the interaction of knowledge, skill, and desire. Figure 13-1 describes knowledge as the theoretical assumption, the what to do and the why. Skill is the how to do. Desire is the motivation, the want to do. In order to make something a habit in our lives, we have to have all three.

Covey provides a framework for developing effective habits. They move up progressively on a maturity continuum from dependence to independence to interdependence.[2] We begin life as an infant totally dependent on others. We are directed, nurtured, and sustained by others. Then, gradually, over the ensuing years, we become more

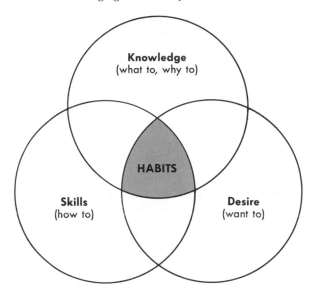

Figure 13-1. Effective habits. Internalized principles and patterns of behavior.
From Covey SR: *The seven habits of highly effective people: powerful lessons in personal change*, New York, 1989, Simon & Schuster.

and more independent—physically, mentally, emotionally, and financially—until eventually we take care of ourselves. As we continue to grow and mature, we become increasingly aware that all of nature is interdependent, that there is an ecological system that governs nature, including society. We further discover that the higher reaches of our nature have to do with our relationships with others, that human life is interdependent. Therefore, dependence is the idea that you take care of me; independence is the notion that I can do it, I am responsible; and interdependence is the we can do it, we can cooperate, we can combine our talents and abilities and create something greater together. The seven habits are based on the maturity continuum (Fig. 13-2).

Habit 1: Be Proactive

Proactivity means more than merely taking the initiative. It means that as human beings we are responsible for our own lives. Our behavior is a function of our decisions, not our conditions. We can subordinate feelings to values. We have the initia-

tive and the responsibility to make things happen. Responsibility is the ability to choose your response. Highly proactive people recognize that responsibility. They do not blame circumstances, conditions, or conditioning for their behavior. Their behavior is a product of their own conscious choice, based on values, rather than a product of their conditions based on feeling.

There are three central values in life: the experiential, or that which happens to us; the creative, or that which we bring into existence; and the attitudinal, or our responses in different circumstances, such as terminal illness. Covey believes that the highest of the three values is attitudinal. In other words, what matters most is how we respond to what we experience in life.[2]

Business, community groups, and organizations of every kind can be proactive. They can combine the creativity and resourcefulness of proactive individuals to create a proactive culture within the organization. The organization does not have to be at the mercy of the environment; it can take the initiative to accomplish the shared values and purposes of the individuals involved.

Listening to Our Language. Our language, for example, is a real indicator of the degree to which we see ourselves as proactive people. The language of reactive people absolves them of responsibility: "That's me." "That's just the way I am." "There's nothing I can do about it." Proactive people take responsibility: "Let's look at our alternatives." "I will."

Reactive Language	Proactive Language
There's nothing I can do.	Let's look at our alternatives.
That's just the way I am.	I can choose a different approach.
He makes me so mad.	I control my own feelings.
They won't allow that.	I can create and convincingly propose new approaches.
I have to do that.	I will choose an appropriate response.
I can't.	I choose.
I must.	I prefer.
If only.	I will.

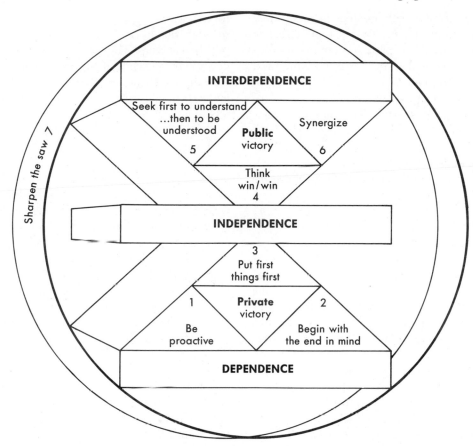

Figure 13-2. The seven habits paradigm.
From Covey SR: *The seven habits of highly effective people: powerful lessons in personal change,* New York, 1989, Simon & Schuster.

Circles of concern and influence. Another excellent way to become more self-aware regarding our own degree of proactivity is to look at where we focus our time and energy. We each have many concerns: our health, our children, problems at work, the national debt. We could separate them from things in which we have no particular mental or emotional involvement by creating a "circle of concern." As we look within our circle of concern, it becomes apparent that there are some things over which we have no real control and others that we can do something about by circumscribing them within a smaller "circle of influence." By determining which of these two circles is the focus of

most of our time and energy, we can discover much about the degree of our proactivity.

Proactive people focus their efforts in the circle of influence. They work on things they can do something about. The nature of their energy is positive, enlarging, and magnifying, causing their circle of influence to increase.

Reactive people, however, focus their efforts on the circle of concern. They focus on the weakness of other people, the problems in the environment, and circumstances over which they have no control. Their focus results in blaming and accusing attitudes, reactive language, and increased feelings of victimization. The negative energy generated by that focus, combined with neglect in areas they could do something about, causes their circle of influence to shrink. To expand our circles of influence, we need to make small commitments and keep them. Be a model, not a critic. Be part of the solution, not part of the problem.

Samuel Johnson observed: "The fountain of content must spring up in the mind and he who hath so little knowledge of human nature as to seek happiness by changing anything but his own disposition will waste his life in fruitless efforts and multiply the grief he proposes to remove."

Habit 2: Begin with the End in Mind

Let's take the business world as an example. If you want to have a successful enterprise, you clearly define what you are trying to accomplish. You carefully think through the product or service you want to provide in terms of your market target; then you organize all the elements—financial, research and development, operations, marketing, personnel, physical facilities, and so on—to meet that objective. The extent to which you begin with the end in mind often determines whether you are able to create a successful enterprise. Most business failures begin with problems such as underfunding, misunderstanding of the market, or lack of a business plan. In the field of dietetics, establishing a private practice is one good example of beginning with the end in mind. The dietitian or nutritionist who does not complete a business plan with the appropriate and correct data will be doomed to failure. If she develops an effective plan, she will have a successful enterprise.

"Begin with the end in mind" is based on principles of personal leadership. Leadership is not management. Management comes second, after leadership, which has to come first. Management is a bottom-line focus: How can I best accomplish certain things? Leadership deals with the top line: What are the things I want to accomplish? Management is efficiency in climbing the ladder of success; leadership determines whether the ladder is leaning against the right wall.

Covey presents a vivid example of the differences between leadership and management when he describes a group of workers cutting their way through the jungle with machetes. They are the problem solvers. They are cutting through the undergrowth, clearing it out. The managers are behind them, sharpening their machetes, writing policy and procedure manuals, bringing in improved technologies, and setting up work schedules. The leader is the one who climbs the tallest tree, surveys the entire situation, and yells, "Wrong jungle!"[2]

As individuals, groups, and businesses, we are often so busy cutting through the undergrowth that we fail to realize we are in the wrong jungle. We are more in need of a vision or destination and a compass and less in need of a road map. We often do not know what the terrain ahead will be like or what we will need to go through it; much will depend on our judgment at the time.

Efficient management without effective leadership is, as one individual phrased it, "like straightening the deck chairs on the *Titanic*."

Habit 3: Put First Things First

This habit embodies the principles of personal management. Practicing effective self-management requires discipline. Effective management is putting first things first. Whereas leadership decides what "first things" are, it is management that puts them first. Management is discipline, carrying things out. In other words, if you are an effective manager of yourself, your discipline comes from within and is a function of your independent will. Habit 3 deals with many of the questions addressed in the field of time management. The essence of the best thinking in time management can be captured in a single phrase: Organize and execute around *priorities*. Time management may really be a misnomer; the challenge is not to manage time but to manage ourselves.

We accomplish all that we do through delegation, either to time or to other people. Many people refuse to delegate to other people because they feel it takes too much time and effort and they could do the job better themselves. But appropriately delegating to others is perhaps the single most powerful activity there is. Delegation means growth for individuals and for organizations. If it is done correctly, it will generate a great deal of trust.

Trust is the highest form of human motivation. It brings out the very best in people. It takes time and patience, however, and it does not preclude the necessity to train and develop people so that their competency can rise to the level of that trust.

The most important ingredient we put into any relationship is not what we say or what we do, but what we are. If our words and actions come from superficial human relations techniques (the personality ethic) rather than from our inner core (the character ethic) others will sense that duplicity.

The techniques and skills that really make a difference in human interaction are the ones that almost naturally flow from a truly independent character. So, the place to begin building any relationship is inside ourselves, inside our circle of influence, our own character. As we become independent, proactive, and able to organize and execute around the priorities in our life with integrity, we then can choose to become interdependent—capable of building rich, enduring, highly productive relationships with other people. *Integrity* is defined as conforming reality to our words and actions, keeping promises and fulfilling expectations.

The emotional bank account. Covey uses the analogy of a financial bank account to discuss the emotional bank account. In a financial bank account we make deposits into it and build up a reserve from which we can make withdrawals when we need them. An emotional bank account is a metaphor that describes the amount of trust that has been built up in a relationship. If I make deposits into an emotional bank account with you through courtesy, kindness, honesty, and keeping my commitments to you, I build up a reserve. When the trust is high, communication is easy, instant, and effective. But if I have a habit of showing discourtesy and disrespect, overreacting, ignoring you, becoming arbitrary, and threatening you, then my account gets overdrawn. The trust level is very low.

When considering principles of personal management, remember, "Things which matter most must never be at the mercy of things which matter least."[2]

Habit 4: Think Win-Win

Win-win is not a personality technique. It is a total plan of human interaction. It comes from a character of integrity and maturity. It grows out of high-trust relationships. Win-win is a frame of mind that seeks mutual benefit in all human interactions.

Thinking win-win is the habit of interpersonal leadership. It involves the exercise of each of the unique human endowments—self-awareness, imagination, conscience, and independent will—in our relationships with others. It involves mutual learning, mutual influence, and mutual benefits.

The principle of win-win is fundamental to success in all our interactions, and it embraces five interdependent dimensions of life. It begins with *character* and moves toward *relationships*, out of which flow *agreements*. It is nurtured in an environment where *structure* and *systems* are based on win-win, and it involves *process;* we cannot achieve *win-win* ends with win-lose or lose-win means.

Habit 5: Seeking First to Understand, Then to Be Understood

This principle is the key to effective interpersonal communication. Communication is the most important skill in life. We spend most of our waking hours communicating. But consider this: you have spent years learning how to read and write, years learning how to speak, but what about listening?

"Seek first to understand" involves a very deep shift in our thinking. We typically seek first to be understood. Most people do not listen with the intent to understand; they listen with the intent to reply. They're either speaking or preparing to speak. They're filtering everything through their own assumptions, reading their autobiography into other people's lives.

When another person speaks, we're usually "listening" at one of four levels. We may be ignoring another person, not really listening at all. We may be pretending to listen with a response of "uh-huh, right." We may practice selective listening, hearing only certain parts of the conversation. We may even practice attentive listening, paying attention and focusing energy on the words that are being said. Very few of us ever practice the fifth level, the highest form of listening, empathic listening. Empathic listening gets inside another person's frame of reference. You look out through it, you see the world the way they see the world, you understand their assumptions, you understand how they feel.

Empathic listening involves much more than registering, reflecting, or even understanding the words that are said. Communications experts estimate, in fact, that only 10% of our communication is represented by the words we say. Another 30% is represented by our sounds, and 60% by our body language. In empathic listening, you listen with your ears, but you also listen with your eyes and with your heart. You listen for feeling, for meaning. You listen for behavior. Empathic listening is so powerful because it gives you accurate data to work with.

"Seek to be understood," that is, knowing how to be understood, is the other half of habit 5 and is equally critical in reaching a win-win solution. Seeking to understand requires consideration; seeking to be understood takes courage.

Habit 6: Synergize

Synergy means that the whole is greater than the sum of its parts. It means that the relationship the parts have to each other is a part in and of itself. Synergy is everywhere in nature.

The challenge is to apply the principle of creative cooperation, which we learn from nature, in our social interactions. Dietitians and nutritionists function as synergistic professionals. They have meaningful interactions with many groups— nurses, physicians, and media—to assist their patients to reach agreed-upon goals for their care. In a broader sense, networking with other groups provides the synergy needed to be an effective professional. The essence of synergy is to value differences, respect them, build on strengths, and compensate for weakness.

Habit 7: Sharpen the Saw

Habit 7 addresses self-renewal. It is preserving and enhancing the greatest asset you have: *you*. It is renewing the four dimensions of your nature: physical, spiritual, mental, and social-emotional. A

healthy, balanced life revolves around the four values. All four must be considered; none can be neglected. "Sharpening the saw" basically means expressing all four dimensions. It means exercising all four dimensions of our nature regularly and consistently in a wise and balanced way.

The physical dimension includes exercise, nutrition, and stress management. The spiritual dimension addresses values clarification and commitment, study, and meditation. The mental dimension includes reading, visualizing, planning, and writing. The social-emotional dimension deals with service, empathy, personal synergy, and intrinsic security.

In organizations, as well as in individual lives, if we neglect one of the four, it impacts negatively on the rest. In organizations, the physical dimension is expressed in productivity and economic terms. The mental or psychological dimension deals with the recognition, development, and use of talent. The social-emotional dimension has to do with human relations, with how people are treated. The spiritual dimension deals with finding meaning through purpose or contribution and through organizational integrity.

When an organization neglects any one or more of these areas, it negatively affects the entire organization. The creative energies that could result in positive synergy are instead used to fight against the organization and become restraining forces to growth and productivity.

The seven habits of highly effective people create optimum synergy in people. Renewal in any dimension increases our ability to live at least one of the seven habits. Although the habits are sequential, improvement in one habit synergetically increases your ability to live the rest.

The more proactive you are (habit 1), the more effectively you can exercise personal leadership (habit 2) and management (habit 3) in your life. The more effectively you manage your life (habit 3), the more renewing activities you can do (habit 7). The more you seek first to understand (habit 5), the more effectively you can go for synergetic win-win solutions (habits 4 and 6). The more you improve in any of the habits that lead to independence (habits 1, 2, and 3), the more effective you will be in interdependent situations (habits 4, 5, and 6). And renewal (habit 7) is the process of renewing all the habits.

Rewriting the Script

After renewing the seven habits, we may need to rewrite our scripts. Change, real change, comes from inside out. It does not come from hacking at the leaves of attitude and behavior with quick-fix personality techniques. It comes from striking at the root—the fabric of our thought, the fundamental, essential assumptions that give definition to our character and create the lens through which we see the world.

Based on this discussion of Covey's seven habits, dietitians and nutritionists are more in need of a vision or destination and a compass (a set of principles or directions) and less in need of a road map.[2] Keep in mind: leadership first, management second.

MANAGEMENT EFFECTIVENESS IN COMMUNITY NUTRITION

Community dietitians and nutritionists are expected to provide strong management in their area of professional responsibility. Because of the environmental challenges facing our profession, intensifying managerial effectiveness may emerge as the issue of the 1990s. Many of the issues we face require strong leadership and management. The following vivid examples express our concerns.

Over the past decade, Americans have become obsessed with the nutritional value of the food they eat. Time and again nutrition ranks high among consumer concerns, along with food safety, convenience, quality, and value. Moreover, both demographic trends and market analysis indicate that their concern with food and diet will continue to grow well into the future.[16] It will take skillful management of resources and innovative approaches to capture this important market for services.

Another example of where strong management is needed is the American health care system. Today, health care is in the throes of what has justifiably been described as a revolution. This has led

to a highly charged environment in the health care field. New delivery systems, advanced technology and treatment, changing demographics, the wellness movement, the graying of America, and especially escalating costs are creating a present—and future—fraught with challenges and opportunities. At the core is who will pay for health care now.[5,6]

While payers—government insurers and corporate America—move to center stage in the new health arena, dietitians and nutritionists must develop and implement strategies that will position them to capture new opportunities.[6] We must use a full range of management skills, including the ability to market and sell ourselves and our profession.

In public health, dietitians and nutritionists must take a leadership role in assuring that comprehensive, community-based nutrition services are available to promote optimum nutrition to the American public. After a decade characterized by reductions of federal mandates and funds, nutritionists face management challenges in the 1990s.

The real challenge will be to provide a high level of services cost-effectively in a competitive environment and under considerable economic pressure.

In this section, emphasis will be placed on community dietitians and nutritionists as managers. The management process will be discussed in detail in subsequent chapters. Figure 13-3 describes the management process that will be used as the basis for each of the sections on management.

Defining Management

Management has been called "the art of getting things done through people." This definition calls attention to the fact that managers achieve organizational goals by arranging for others to perform whatever tasks may be necessary, not by performing the tasks themselves.[19]

Management is that, and more—so much more, in fact, that no one simple definition has been universally accepted. Moreover, existing definitions change as the environments of organizations continue to change. Our discussion will start with a

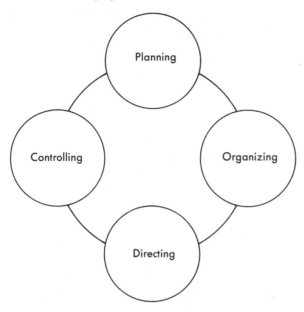

Figure 13-3. The management process.

1. Planning implies that managers think through their goals and actions in advance. Their actions are usually based on some method, plan, or logic, rather than on a hunch.
2. Organizing means that managers coordinate the human and material resources of the organization. The effectiveness of an organization depends on its ability to marshal its resources to attain its goals. Obviously, the more integrated and coordinated the work of an organization, the more effective it will be. Achieving this coordination is part of the manager's job.
3. Directing describes how managers lead and influence subordinates, getting others to perform essential tasks. By establishing the proper atmosphere, they help their subordinates do their best.
4. Controlling means that managers attempt to assure that the organization is moving toward its goals. If some part of their organization is on the wrong track— if it's not working toward stated goals or is not doing so effectively—managers try to find out why and set things right.

fairly complex definition, so that we may call attention to additional important aspects of managing: "Management is the process of planning, organizing, leading, and controlling the efforts of organizational members and of using all other organizational resources to achieve stated organizational goals."[12]

A process is a systematic way of doing things. Management is defined as a process because all managers, regardless of their particular aptitudes or skills, engage in certain interrelated activities in order to achieve their desired goals. The box above categorizes and describes the four basic functions in which managers are typically involved. You will also notice that the definition indicates that managers use all the resources of the organization—its finances, equipment, and information as well as its people—to attain their goals. People are the most basic resource of any organization, but managers would be limiting their achievements if they did not also rely on the other available organizational resources.

Finally, the definition stresses that management involves achieving the organization's "stated goals." This means that dietitians and nutritionist managers

of any organization try to attain specific ends. These ends are, of course, unique to each organization. The stated goal of the public health nutrition program may be to raise the nutritional status of their clients through the provision of high-quality nutrition services. If, however, the program succeeds only in handing out leaflets at a health clinic to all clients entering, the system may be serving all clients, but regarding its goal or end result, it may not be effective. Whatever the stated goals of a particular organization, management is the process by which the attainment of those goals is enhanced.

The Key Attributes of Managerial Responsibility

Our working definition describes managers as organizational planners, organizers, directors, and controllers (Fig. 13-4). Actually every manager, from the nutrition director to the commissioner of health, takes on a much wider range of roles to move the organization toward its stated objectives. In this discussion of the more detailed aspects of what managers do, what managers are will also be examined.

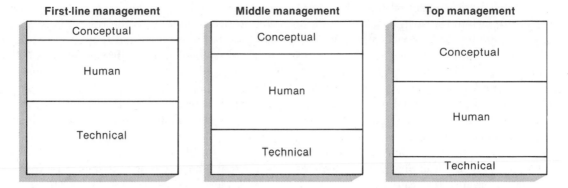

Figure 13-4. Relative skills needed for effective performance at different levels of management.

Managers work with and through other people. The term *people* includes not only employees and supervisors but also other managers in the organization. "People" also includes individuals outside the organization: patients, clients, suppliers, union representatives, and so on. These people and others provide goods and services to the organization or use its products or services. Managers, then, work with anyone at any level within or outside their organizations who can help to achieve unit or organizational goals. In addition, in working toward goals, managers work to achieve personal goals.

Finally, managers in any organization should work with each other to establish the organization's long-range goals and to plan how to achieve them. They should also work together to provide one another with the accurate information needed to perform tasks. Thus, managers act as channels of communication within the organization.

Managers are responsible and accountable. Managers are in charge of seeing that specific tasks are done successfully. They are usually evaluated on how well they arrange for these tasks to be accomplished. Managers are also responsible for the actions of their employees. The success or failure of employees is a direct reflection of managers' success or failure. Naturally, all members of an organization, including those who are not managers, are accountable for their particular tasks. Managers, however, are held responsible, or accountable, not only for their own work but also for the work of others.

Managers balance competing goals and set priorities. At any given time, every manager faces a number of organizational goals, problems, and needs—all of which compete for the manager's time and resources (both human and material). Because such resources are always limited, each manager must strike a balance between various goals and needs. Many managers, for example, arrange each day's tasks in order of priority; the most important things are done right away, and the less important tasks are looked at later. In this way managerial time is used more effectively.

Managers must think analytically and conceptually. To be an analytical thinker, a manager must be able to break a problem down into its components, analyze those components, and then come up with a feasible solution. Even more important, a manager must be a conceptual thinker, able to view the entire task in the abstract and relate it to other tasks. Thinking about a particular task in relation to its larger implications is no simple matter, but it is essential if the manager is to work toward the goals of the organization as a whole as well as toward the goals of an individual unit.

Managers are mediators. Organizations are made up of people, and people within the same organization often disagree about goals and the most effective way of attaining them. Disputes within a unit or organization can lower morale and productivity, and they may become so unpleasant or disruptive that competent employees decide to leave the organization. Such occurrences hinder work toward the goals of the unit or organization; therefore, managers must at times take on the role of mediator and resolve disputes as they occur. Settling quarrels requires skill and tact; managers who are careless in their handling of disputes may be dismayed to find that they have only made matters worse.

Managers are politicians. Managers must build relationships, use persuasion, and compromise to promote organizational goals, just as politicians do to move their programs forward. Managers should also develop other political skills. All effective managers "play politics" by developing networks of mutual obligations with other managers in the organization. They may also have to build or join alliances and coalitions. Managers draw upon these relationships to win support for proposals or decisions or to gain cooperation in carrying out various activities.

Managers are diplomats. They may serve as official representatives of their work units at organizational meetings. They may represent the entire organization as well as a particular unit in dealing with clients, customers, contractors, government officials, and personnel of other organizations.

Managers are symbols. They personify, both for organizational members and for outside observers, an organization's successes and failures. As symbols, managers may be held accountable for things over which they have little or no control. This accountability links managers to the goals and commitments of the organization.

Managers make difficult decisions. No organization runs smoothly all the time. There is almost no limit to the number and types of problems that may occur: financial difficulties, problems with employees, and differences of opinion concerning organization policy, to name just a few. Managers are expected to come up with solutions to difficult problems and to follow through on their decisions, even when doing so may be unpopular.

These brief descriptions of managerial roles show that managers must "change hats" frequently and be alert to the particular role needed at a given time. As a rule, a manager is a peer, a superior, and an employee at one and the same time. The ability to recognize the appropriate role to be played and to change roles readily is one mark of an effective manager.

Managerial and Organizational Performance

How successfully an organization achieves its objectives, satisfies social responsibilities, or both depends on how well the organization's managers do their jobs. If managers do not do their jobs well, the organization will fail to achieve its goals. Just as managers function within the organization, organizations function within the larger society. The performance of its organizations is a key factor in the performance of a society or a nation.

How well managers do their jobs—managerial performance—is the subject of much debate, analysis, and confusion in the United States and many other countries.[19] How well the organizations of a society do their "jobs"—organizational performance—gives rise to an equally lively debate.

Drucker has argued that a manager's performance can be measured in terms of two concepts: efficiency and effectiveness. As he puts it, efficiency means "doing things right," and effectiveness means "doing the right thing."[4]

Efficiency—that is, the ability to get things done with minimum resource consumption—is an input-output concept. An efficient manager is one who achieves outputs, or results, while controlling the inputs (labor, materials, and time) used to achieve them. Managers who are able to maximize output while minimizing cost of the resources they use to attain their goals are acting efficiently.

Effectiveness, in contrast, is the ability to choose and then achieve appropriate objectives; an effective manager selects the right things to get done. A manager who selects an inappropriate objective is an ineffective manager. No amount of efficiency can compensate for lack of effectiveness.

A manager's responsibilities require performance that is both efficient and effective. Although efficiency is important, effectiveness is critical. For Drucker, effectiveness is the key to the success of an organization. The manager's need to make the most of opportunities, says Drucker, implies that effectiveness rather than efficiency is essential to business.[4] The pertinent question is not how to do things right, but how to find the right things to do, and to concentrate resources and efforts on them.

The Management Process

It is easier to understand something as complex as management when it is described as a series of separate parts or functions that make up a whole process. Descriptions of this kind, known as models, have been used by students and practitioners of management for decades. A model is a simplification of the real world used to convey complex relationships in easy-to-understand terms. In fact, we used a model—without identifying it as such—when we said earlier that the major management activities were planning, organizing, directing, and controlling (Fig. 13-3).

Planning

Plans give the organization its goals and objectives and set up the best procedure for reaching them. In addition, plans become the guides by which (1) the organization obtains and commits the resources required to reach its objectives, (2) members of the organization carry on activities consistent with the chosen objectives and procedures, and (3) progress toward the objectives is monitored and measured, so that corrective action can be taken if progress is unsatisfactory.

The first step in planning is the selection of goals for the organization. Then objectives are established for the subunits of the organization—its divisions, departments, and so on. Once the objectives are determined, programs are established for

achieving them in a systematic manner. Of course, in selecting objectives and developing programs, the manager considers their feasibility and whether they will be acceptable to the organization's managers and employees and to its customers.

Community dietitians and nutritionists are expected to develop a plan for their portion of the services.

Organizing

Once managers have established objectives and developed plans or programs to reach them, they must design and staff an organization able to carry out those programs successfully.

Organizing is the development of a work structure, a framework within which the necessary tasks are carried out to reach the organization's objectives. The effectiveness of an organization depends on its ability to marshal its resources to attain its goals. Organizing includes assigning activities, dividing work into particular jobs, and defining the relationships among them. It also involves delegation of authority necessary to complete the tasks. Authority is the key to the manager's job. Community dietitians and nutritionists are often involved in the organizing aspects, while the total plan is left to someone else. Knowledge of only one piece of the plan can lead to disillusionment and negative attitudes. It is important for the community dietitian or nutritionist to review the organizational chart and planning documents of the health agency and be informed about where the nutrition staff fits into the overall plan of operation.

Directing

After plans have been made, the structure of the organization has been determined, and the staff has been recruited and trained, the next step is to arrange for movement toward the organization's defined objectives. This function can be called by various names: leading, directing, motivating, actuating, coordinating, and others. Whatever the name used to identify it, this function involves getting the members of the organization to perform in ways that will help it achieve its established objectives.

Whereas planning and organizing deal with the

more abstract aspects of the management process, the activity of directing is very concrete; it involves working directly with people.

Controlling. Finally, the manager must ensure that the actions of the organization's members do in fact move the organization toward its stated goals. This is the controlling function of management, which involves four main elements:

1. Establishing standards of performance.
2. Measuring current performance and comparing it against the established standards.
3. Detecting deviations from standard goals in order to make corrections before a sequence of activities is completed.
4. Taking action to correct performance that does not meet those standards.

Through the controlling function, the manager can keep the organization on its chosen track, keeping it from straying from its specified goals.

A model of the management process has been presented, but the relationships described are interrelated more than the model implies. For example, although standards are used as a means of controlling employees' actions, establishing such standards is also an inherent part of the planning process and an integral factor in motivating and leading employees. Taking corrective action, introduced as a control activity, often involves an adjustment in plans. In practice, the management process does not involve four separate or loosely related sets of activities, but a group of interactive functions. Moreover, these four functions do not necessarily occur in the sequence presented. In fact, various combinations of these activities are going on simultaneously in every organization.

In addition, the existence of these distinct management functions does not imply that any manager has complete freedom to perform them whenever he or she wishes. Managers are generally faced with various limitations on their activities, depending on their role in the organization, their designated position in its hierarchy, and the kind of organization they work for. Some managers, for example, may find that limits are set on their dealings with subordinates—on what they can do to direct, guide, or motivate them—because their leadership style conflicts with the style that prevails in their organization. A manager may not be able to hire new staff to pursue a new set of objectives because the organization cannot carry the added expense of their salaries.

In spite of their limitations, models provide a useful approach to understanding, as long as we remember their shortcomings and that they are not meant to be exact descriptions of the real world. By analyzing the management process—that is, by separating it into distinct pieces that we call "management functions"—this model can improve our understanding of what managers do.

Management Level and Skills

Managers at every level plan, organize, direct, and control. They differ in the amount of time devoted to each of these activities. Some of these differences depend on the kind of time devoted to each of these activities. Some of these differences depend on the kind of organization in which the manager works, some on the type of job the manager holds.

Managers of small private clinics, for example, spend their time quite differently from the way the heads of large research hospitals spend theirs; managers of clinics spend comparatively more time practicing medicine and less time actually managing than do directors of large hospitals. The director of nutrition services spends her time differently than does the dietitian or nutritionist giving direct service in a WIC clinic. Yet both are first-line managers, and there will be important similarities in the jobs of all managers.

Other differences in the way managers spend their time depend upon their levels in the organizational hierarchy. In the next sections, we shall consider how management skills and activities differ at these various levels and look at the various roles that managers perform.

Katz, a teacher and business executive, has identified three basic kinds of skills: technical, human, and conceptual.[11] Every manager needs all three. Technical skill is the ability to use the procedures, techniques, and knowledge of a specialized field. Dietitians and nutritionists, engineers, musicians, and accountants all have technical skills in their respective fields. Human skill is the ability to work with, understand, and motivate other people, as individuals or in groups. Conceptual skill is the ability to coordinate and integrate all of an organization's interests and activities. It involves the manager's ability to see the organization as a whole, to understand how its parts depend on one another, and to anticipate how a change in any of its parts will affect the whole.

Katz suggests that although all three of these skills are essential to a manager, their relative importance depends mainly on the manager's rank in the organization[11] (Fig. 13-4). Technical skill is most important at the lower levels. Human skill, by contrast, is important for managers at every level. Because they must get their work done primarily through others, the manager's ability to tap the technical skills of his or her subordinates is more important than his or her own technical skills. Finally, the importance of conceptual skill increases as one rises through the ranks of a management system based on hierarchical principles of authority and responsibility.

In a study by Rinke, David, and Bjoraker,[17] Katz's skill model was applied to the four routes used to train dietitians: internship, coordinated undergraduate, traineeship, and advanced degrees. They considered that the four routes to professional preparation in dietetics appeared to provide more adequate preparation in technical skill than in either human or conceptual skill. This observation is significant because it implies that dietitians are prepared for their specialist roles but are falling short of the human and conceptual skills needed to advance to higher-level positions in an organization.

Management Roles

A functional manager is someone responsible for one organizational activity or one unit within the organization, such as the director of dietetics or the chief nutritionist. In a broad sense, a role consists of the behavior patterns expected of an individual within a social unit. For the purposes of managerial thinking, a role is thus the behavioral pattern expected of someone within a functional unit. Roles are thus inherent in functions.

Mintzberg made an extensive survey of existing research on the subject of managerial roles and integrated his findings with the results of a study of chief executive officers (CEOs).[13] In an effort to catalog and analyze the various roles of managers, the combined review covered all kinds and levels of managers—from street-gang leaders to CEOs. Table 13-1 shows that, according to Mintzberg, managers perform basically ten roles that can be grouped according to three main functions.

Mintzberg concluded that, to a considerable extent, the jobs of many managers are quite similar.[13] All managers, he argued, have formal authority over their own organizational units and derive status from that authority. This status causes all managers to be involved in interpersonal relationships with subordinates, peers, and superiors, who in turn provide managers with the information they need to make decisions. All managers thus have a series of interpersonal, informational, and decision-making roles that Mintzberg defined as "organized sets of behaviors"[13] (Fig. 13-5). Here, we will summarize Mintzberg's findings and theories about managerial roles.

Interpersonal Roles

Three sometimes routine interpersonal roles help managers keep their organizations running smoothly. The first is that of the figurehead who performs ceremonial duties: greeting visitors, attending subordinates' weddings, taking customers to lunch. Second, there is the role of leader: hiring, training, motivating, and encouraging. First-line managers, in particular, stress effectiveness in this role. Finally, managers must play the interpersonal role of liaison in dealing with people other than employees or superiors: peers within the organization, as well as clients outside it.

Informational Roles

Receiving and communicating information, Mintzberg suggests, are the most important aspects of a manager's job.[13] Managers need information to make intelligent decisions, and other people in their units or organizations depend on information received or transmitted through them.

Table 13-1. Mintzberg's managerial roles

Role	Description	Identifiable activities
Interpersonal		
Figurehead	Symbolic head; obliged to perform a number of routine duties of a legal or social nature	Ceremony, status requests, solicitations
Leader	Responsible for the motivation and activation of subordinates; responsible for staffing, training, and associated duties	Virtually all managerial activities involving subordinates
Liaison	Maintains self-developed network of outside contacts and informers who provide favors and information	Acknowledgements of mail; external board work; other activities involving outsiders
Informational		
Monitor	Seeks and receives wide variety of special information (much of it current) to develop thorough understanding of organization and environment; emerges as nerve center of internal and external information of the organization	Handling all mail and contacts categorized as concerned primarily with receiving information (e.g., periodical news, observational tours)
Disseminator	Transmits information received from outsiders or from other subordinates to members of the organization; some information factual, some involving interpretation and integration of diverse value positions of organizational influencers	Forwarding mail into organization for informational purposes, verbal contacts involving information flow to subordinates (e.g., review sessions, instant communication flows)
Spokesperson	Transmits information to outsiders on organization's plans, policies, actions, results, etc.; serves as expert on organization's industry	Board meetings; handling mail and contacts involving transmission of information to outsiders
Decision making		
Entrepreneur	Searches organization and its environment for opportunities and initiates "improvement projects" to bring about change; supervises design of certain projects as well	Strategy and review sessions involving initiation or design of improvement projects.
Disturbance handler	Responsible for corrective action when organization faces important, unexpected disturbances	Strategy and review sessions involving disturbances and crises
Resource allocator	Responsible for the allocation of organizational resources of all kinds—in effect the making or approval of all significant organizational decisions	Scheduling; requests for authorization; any activity involving budgeting and the programming of subordinates' work
Negotiator	Responsible for representing the organization at major negotiations	Negotiation

Source: From *The Nature of Managerial Work* by Henry Mintzberg. Copyright © 1973 by Henry Mintzberg. Reprinted by permission of Harper & Row, Publishers, Inc.

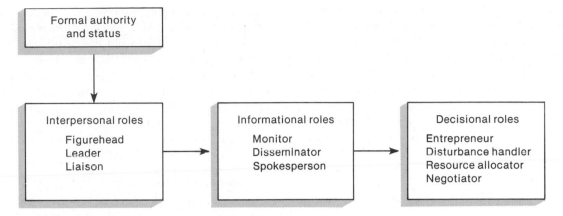

Figure 13-5. The manager's roles.
Reprinted by permission of the *Harvard Business Review*. An exhibit from "The manager's job: folklore and fact" by Henry Mintzberg (July/August 1975). Copyright 1975 by the President and Fellows of Harvard College; all rights reserved. Redrawn from James AF Stoner, *Management*, ed 2, 1982, pp 408, 593. Reprinted by permission of Prentice Hall, Inc., Englewood Cliffs, NJ.

Managers gather and disseminate information in three informational roles. The first is monitoring, whereby managers constantly look for useful information. They question subordinates and collect unsolicited information, usually through networks of contacts. The role of monitor usually makes managers the best-informed members of their groups.

In the role of disseminator, managers distribute to subordinates important information they would not otherwise know. Last, in the role of spokesperson, managers transmit information to people outside their own groups. Keeping superiors well informed is one important aspect of this role. Another is communicating with the world outside the organization.

Decision-Making Roles

So far, we have seen managers distributing information to others. Information is also the "basic input to decision-making for managers," according to Mintzberg,[13] who says that managers play four decision-making roles. As entrepreneurs, they try to improve their units. When, for example, managers receive a good idea, they might launch a development project to make it a reality. In this role, they initiate change of their own free will.

As disturbance handlers, they respond to problems beyond their control, such as strikes, bankrupt customers, breaches of contract, and the like. As resource allocators, managers decide how and to whom resources, including the managers' own time, should be given. Managers also screen important decisions made by employees.

The fourth and last decision-making role is that of negotiator. A company president might, for example, deal with a consulting firm; a production head might draw up a contract with a supplier. A dietitian or nutritionist may negotiate the price of foods provided in the WIC program. Managers spend a lot of their time as negotiators because only they have the knowledge and authority this role demands.

Mintzberg's work is particularly interesting because it calls attention to the uncertain, turbulent environment faced by managers in the real world.

THE CHANGING ENVIRONMENT, SOCIAL RESPONSIBILITY, AND MANAGERIAL ETHICS

Environmental Trends

Top-level managers are spending an increasing amount of their time dealing with environmental forces rather than internal operations. In 1969 only 1 of 127 CEOs rated public or environmental issues as being critical to the performance of the job. By 1980 a study showed that CEOs were spending between 20% and 75% of their time on external matters, with the mean being 50%.[7]

The environment facing business firms and other organizations is changing rapidly in many ways. To understand what is happening, it is useful to view the overall environment as a set of interrelated subenvironments in the technological, economic, sociocultural, governmental, and legal spheres.

Technological Environment

Everyone is aware of the rapidity with which technology is affecting and changing people's lives. Increasingly, technological changes directly reflect the vast effort and funds devoted to research and development. Technology has had, and will continue to have, a profound impact on business firms and other organizations.

Economic Environment

The economic environment has always been a major concern of management. Some firms' sales are highly correlated with the overall economy, whereas others are relatively immune to it. Firms in such industries as steel and automobiles are closely tied to the ups and downs of the business cycle. Firms in the baby food and motion picture industries, however, are relatively unaffected by recessions and booms.

Organizations such as state and local government agencies and public universities also tend to be affected by general economic conditions. During periods of recession, the revenues of state and local governments tend to go down, which translates into lower budgets for their dependent agencies. Dietitians and nutritionists are keenly aware of this phenomenon and must be creative in delivering services when there are economic downturns.

Today's economic environment has become especially significant for business firms because of its increasing complexity and turbulence. Three prominent trends are (1) the interrelationships among national economies, (2) the volatility of interest rates, and (3) fluctuating foreign exchange rates. A recent illustration of the interrelationship among national economies was the stock market crash of October 1987. During this period, the stock exchanges in Japan and Western Europe mirrored the downward spiral of Wall Street.

Currency exchange rates represent another economic dimension of monetary significance. Many economists believe that an overvalued dollar, coupled with an undervalued Japanese yen in the early and mid-1980s, was partially responsible for the huge American trade deficit.

Sociocultural Environment

The sociocultural environment consists of the prevailing values, attitudes, and customs of the society or culture within which the organization operates. Values have evolved and changed in American society in the recent past. One clear trend is the increased emphasis on improving the quality of life. There are persistent public demands for safer products, reduced pollution, less discrimination, and truthful advertising. As a result of these demands, federal and state laws have been passed and regulations imposed.

The quality of work life represents another emerging social trend. American workers, for the most part, are no longer satisfied with boring, repetitive jobs. They desire responsible positions that allow them to exercise creativity and participate in decisions that affect them.

A social trend of a different order is that more and more special interest groups are springing up to espouse social issues. This has resulted in what has been termed a pluralistic society (defined as a society composed of many autonomous and semi-autonomous groups through which power is diffused). Finally, changes in social values and attitudes can provide opportunities for new products and profit-making ventures. For instance, the growing preference for low-fat foods has motivated food companies to introduce new products such as low-fat cheese, cookies, and crackers. Further, the current fitness and health trend has led to a dramatic increase in the number of health clubs.

Governmental Environment

The range of interactions between business and government is vast. Profit and nonprofit organizations are affected by policies of federal, state, local, and foreign governments. These governments tax, subsidize, and regulate. Also, in many cases, they are important customers for companies' goods and services.

Federal government's regulation of business is perhaps the most dynamic area of business-government interaction today. The older model of regulations had its inception in the nineteenth century, when the focus of regulations was on industry-specific economic factors such as rates, markets, and services to the public.

The newer model regulatory agencies have been established for the most part during the past two decades to regulate business firms and other organizations in line with particular social concerns. Prominent among the bodies are the Environmental Protection Agency (EPA), the Equal Employment Opportunity Commission (EEOC) and the Consumer Product Safety Commission (CPSC). One example in the nutrition area is the labeling of foods, regulations for which will be put into effect by the FDA in 1993. These regulations will have far-reaching implications for food products and the education of the consumer. The authority of these agencies cuts across industries but is concerned with only a single organizational function, not with the entirety of the organization.

Legal Environment

The legal environment for business is also becoming increasingly complex and threatening. Today many legal issues consume both management time and corporate funds. Prominent among these are fair employment practices; product safety; work safety; air, water, and noise pollution; deceptive advertising; and stockholder grievances.

Corporate Social Performance

The notion of corporate social performance has, in recent years, become a prominent theme in management literature. Moreover, it has become an important issue within the social environment of business. Essentially, it is an extension of the concept of social responsibility. It has two major parts: (1) the traditional social responsibility dimension and (2) the newer concern for social responsiveness.

Social Responsibility

When a corporation behaves as if it has a conscience, it is said to be socially responsible. Social responsibility is the implied, enforced, or felt obligation of managers, acting in their official capacity, to serve or protect the interest of groups other than themselves.[14] When Johnson & Johnson chose to destroy millions of containers of Tylenol, the company surely suffered, at least in the short run. But the results of the *Fortune* "Most Admired Corporation" survey suggested that most respondents believed the company acted in a socially responsible way.

Many companies take action that tends to promote a corporate culture that emphasizes concern for moral issues. This is done through policy statements, practices, and programs of community involvement for their employees and managers. Some companies have programs of community involvement for their employees and managers. They cooperate with fund drives such as United Way.

It appears that the larger the number of stockholders a corporation has, the more committed management is to a sense of social responsibility.

During the 1980s, managers and the corporations they worked for were subjected to considerable criticism and received low levels of approval from the public. Hardly a week passed without news headlines of misconduct. On Wall Street, insider trading scandals have done much to lower the trust of the general public in the stock market. It is not surprising that a survey by Opinion Research Corporation found that 75% of the public agreed that business neglects the problems of society and that 65% believed business executives "do everything they can to make a profit," even if it means ignoring the public's needs.[9] Business executives were considered less ethical than doctors and lawyers, although more ethical than members of Congress. Clearly, the public had little confidence in the goodness of business in the 1980s.

Some experts believe businesses are increasingly willing to accept their societal responsibilities and that managers are becoming more ethical in the 1990s. They find that managers are more socially responsible and ethical than were their counterparts a generation ago.

According to social theorists, the demands made on business and the expectations of what is considered proper conduct have risen faster than the ability of business to raise its standards. It is believed that the ethical level of actual business practices will continue to rise, but not as quickly as society's expectations for business. Because of the discrepancy, the public's esteem for business will probably remain low while business actually becomes more and more socially responsible. In order to meet the expectations of society, future managers will need to strive to be more ethical and socially responsible.

Stakeholders analysis and the social contract

Most organizations, whether profit or nonprofit, have a large number of stakeholders. An organizational stakeholder is an individual or group whose interests are affected by organization's activities.[14] Protecting the diversity of stakeholders' interests requires answering such questions as these: During an economic downturn, should employees be afforded continuous employment, even if this will hurt profits in the long run? Should a company go beyond the requirements of the law in cleaning up the environment if competitors barely comply with the law?

Answering such questions is termed *stakeholder analysis*. One approach to stakeholder analysis involves consideration of the social contract.[3] The social contract is the set of written and unwritten rules and assumptions about acceptable relationships among the various elements of society. Much of the social contract is embedded in the customs of society. For example, in integrating minorities into the work force, society has come to expect companies to do more than the law requires.

The social contract concerns relationships with individuals, government, other organizations, and society in general.

Social Responsiveness

Social responsibility is concerned with the philosophical question of corporations' responsibilities. Corporations must decide, at least tacitly, whether they have any responsibilities beyond earning a good return for shareholders and staying within the law. Simply deciding that the firm does have additional social responsibilities, however, is no guarantee that these will be carried out. This requires planning and execution. Specifically, the company must determine the issues to be addressed, select the response strategies, and put the implementation plans into effect.

How do firms select which social issues to address? Some issues are chosen voluntarily; others are thrust upon them by government agencies, special interest groups, or other means. Holmes, in a survey of executives of large corporations, defined the five most prominent factors in the selection of areas of social involvement:[10]

- Matching a social need to a corporate need or ability to help
- Ranking the seriousness of the need
- Determining the interests of top executives
- Evaluating the public relations value of the social action
- Dealing with governmental pressure

Full-scale programs have been established by some large companies under the rubric of issues management. These programs seek to anticipate unfolding social issues and provide the organization with plans for constructive responses to them. Issues management programs vary from company to company but usually consist of three stages: issue identification, issue analysis, and response development.[7]

Although conventional wisdom suggests that reactionary values and attitudes of business leaders are the principal reason for poor corporate social performance, social writers have argued that a more critical impediment to effective social performance may be the inability or slowness of an organization to adapt to unfamiliar demands.

Managerial Ethics

Ethics is the study of moral values that guide rightness and wrongness. Managerial ethics is concerned with the rightness or wrongness of the actions and practices of managers. Managerial ethics is strongly related to corporate social responsibility in that both concepts are concerned with what ought to be done. The key distinction between the two is that social responsibility is concerned with the policies and activities of the organization, whereas managerial ethics focuses on the decisions and actions of individual managers.[1] Choices concerning a firm's social responsibility are, of course, made by managers and involve interactions with important stockholder groups or activities that may affect society as a whole. Their decisions have the possibility of compromising ethical issues. In fact, one category of social responsibility is specifically labeled *ethical responsibilities*.

Developing an Ethical Organizational Climate

Top management can take steps to create a more ethical climate within an organization. The first and probably most important step is simply to set a good example. The moral tone of an organization is established at the top.

A related step is to set realistic objectives at all levels. Obviously, this process must start at the top. When managers place undue pressure on subordinates to achieve results, they create an atmosphere conducive to unethical behavior.

Another step toward creating an ethical climate is to establish a code of ethics. Most large corporations and many smaller ones have such codes. Codes of ethics help clarify ethical thinking and encourage ethical choices. They are most effective, however, when they are backed by sanctions for violations. Without such accompanying sanctions, the codes tend to be just public relations gestures.

Still another step in creating an ethical organizational climate is a training program in business ethics. The pedagogical methods most commonly used for teaching ethics are corporate case studies, incidents, role playing, and the discussion of critical issues.[7] The benefits of ethics training include:

- Increasing managers' sensitivity to ethical problems
- Encouraging critical evaluation of priorities
- Increasing awareness of organizational realities
- Increasing awareness of societal realities
- Improving understanding of the importance of public image

SUMMARY

Community dietitians and nutritionists face great challenges as managers in the 1990s because of escalating health care costs, competition for scarce resources, and limited federal funds. In such a competitive environment, the quality of management becomes a critical factor in survival, as well as success. The most recent literature on management stresses the importance of knowing oneself first. By starting with one's own assumptions, character, and motives, a manager has a much greater chance of being successful. Interpersonal skills are most critical to the success of a manager. Personal strengths that managers in dietetics and nutrition require are caring and compassion, honesty and integrity, and a sense of humor. Some traits of highly effective people include being proactive, beginning with the end in mind, prioritizing (first things first), and thinking win-win.

Because management is the process of getting things done through the efforts of people, managers work in many significant roles to accomplish their objectives. For example, managers are accountable and responsible, balance competing goals, and set priorities. Managers are mediators, politicians, and diplomats. The classic managerial functions of planning, organizing, directing, and controlling are important elements for the community dietitian and nutritionist in today's health care system with quality and cost containment being the major focuses of management decisions. Managerial roles can be divided into three basic categories: interpersonal, informational, and decision making.

Corporate social performance has become an important issue within the social environment of business. Social performance has two major parts: the traditional social responsibility and the newer concern for social responsiveness. Managerial ethics is concerned with the rightness or wrongness of the actions and practices of managers.

REFERENCES

1. Cavanaugh GH, Molberg DJ, Velasquez M: The ethics of organizational politics, *Academy of Management Review* 6:363, 1981.
2. Covey SR: *The 7 habits of highly effective people: powerful lessons in personal change*, New York, 1989, Simon & Schuster.
3. Dobrzynski JH and others: Taking charge, *Business Week*, p 66, July 3, 1989.
4. Drucker P: *The effective executive*, New York, 1967, Harper & Row.

5. Finn SC: The decade of the dietitian: leadership can make it happen. *Topics in Clinical Nutrition* 6:3, 1991.

6. Finn SC, Martin G: The shifting balance of power: a new decade for dietitians, *Dietetic Currents* 18:3, 1991.

7. Gray ER, Smeltzer LR: *Management*, New York, 1989, Macmillan.

8. Heath DH: *Fulfilling lives, paths to maturity and success*, San Francisco, 1991, Jossey-Bass.

9. Hennessy EL Jr: Business ethics: is it a priority for corporate America, *Financial Executive*, p 14, October 1986.

10. Holmes SL: Executive perceptions of corporate social responsibility, *Business Horizon* 3:34, 1976.

11. Katz LR: Skills of an effective administrator, *Harvard Business Review* 52:23, 1974.

12. Mescon MH, Albert M, Khedouri F: Management: industrial and organizational effectiveness, ed 2, New York, 1985, Harper & Row.

13. Mintzberg H: The manager's job: folklore and fact, *Harvard Business Review* 68:163, 1990.

14. Mondy RW, Sharplin A, Premeaux SR: *Management concepts, practices and skills*, Boston, 1991, Allyn and Bacon.

15. Oechsli M: Managing successfully: strategies, *US Air Magazine*, July 1991.

16. Owen AL: The impact of future foods on nutrition and health, *J Am Diet Assoc* 90:9, 1990.

17. Renke WJ, David BD, Bjoraker WT: The entry-level generalist dietitian: II, employers' perceptions of the adequacy of preparation for specific administrative competencies, *J Am Diet Assoc* 80:139, 1982.

18. Servan-Schreiber JJ: *The American challenge*, New York, 1968, Atheneum.

19. Stoner JAF: *Management*, ed 4, Englewood Cliffs, NJ, 1989, Prentice Hall.

14 Planning and Decision Making

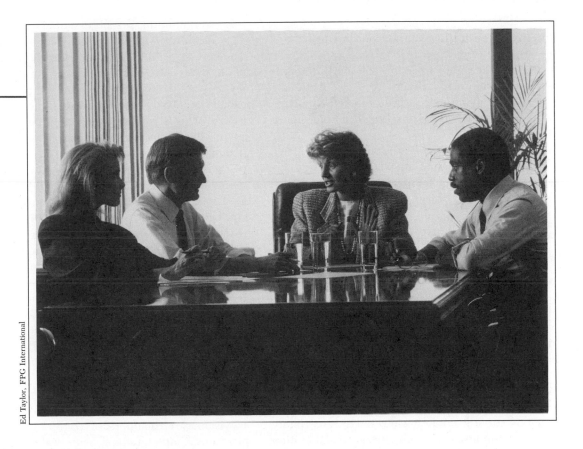

GENERAL CONCEPT

Planning is a forward-looking process through which uncertainty is reduced and action toward orderly results is initiated. Needs assessment is fundamental to planning. It provides information about health and nutrition problems, environmental and lifestyle factors, community values, and available resources. Complex, multifaceted problems require a systematic process for assessing needs, determining priorities, and selecting intervention alternatives. Decisions about how to address community problems are best made by those who are involved, including community members and program staff. Decisions should be made using objective criteria.

OUTCOME OBJECTIVES

When you finish this chapter, you should be able to:

- Explain the importance of strategic thinking in planning and management.
- Recognize planning as a future-directed activity.
- Identify five areas essential to community needs assessment.
- Use systematic processes for prioritizing problems and intervention alternatives.
- Define the steps of the problem-solving process.
- Write goals and objectives.

Dietitians and nutritionists must take a leadership role in assuring that comprehensive, community-based nutrition services are available and utilized. A coordinated system of nutrition services is necessary to promote optimum nutrition for all members of a community.

After a decade of declining federal mandates and funding for public programs and a shift to state and local priority setting, nutritionists face new challenges in the 1990s. The type and availability of nutrition services are being affected by uncertainty in the economic enviornment, greater collaboration between agencies in the public and private sectors, environmental consumerism, increasing health care costs, and a shift to self-care management. In this changing environment, dietitians and nutritionists must draw on knowledge and skills in community assessment, planning, strategic thinking, and decision making.

The report *The Future of Public Health*[6] identified the responsibilities of public health as:

1. *Assessment:* collection and interpretation of data, problems and causes, trend forecasting, evaluation of outcomes
2. *Policy development:* priority setting, policy leadership and advocacy, mobilization of resources, constituency building
3. *Assurance:* assure necessary personnel, educational, or environmental health services to reach agreed-upon goals by encouraging or requiring action by other entities or by provision of services directly, and guarantee

a minimum set of essential, high-priority health services

These responsibilities underscore the importance of dietitians' and nutritionists' involvement in policy or strategic planning, where the priorities are established and program directions are determined. This is in addition to their leadership responsibilities for implementation or operations planning, where intervention designs and program plans support optimum nutrition for community members. This is completed through efficient, effective, culturally sensitive, age-appropriate, and equitable nutrition programs. Dietitians and nutritionists can collaborate with nutrition-related service providers to establish nutrition service standards and protocols for available and acceptable-quality nutrition services.

By carrying out these responsibilities and being attuned to emerging trends, dietitians and nutritionists will contribute to the mission of public health: "The fulfillment of society's interests in assuring the conditions in which people can be healthy."[6]

This chapter and the following ones provide guidance to nutritionists and dietitians in their roles as visionaries, planners of community nutrition programs, implementers, and evaluators. Dietitians and nutritionists must be able to create a vision of ideal nutritional care for all community members. They must bring that vision to reality through the design and implementation of innovative community programs that have an impact on the needs and challenges of greatest priority. A clear vision expressed in a definitive plan for public health nutrition programs can result in nutrition-related programs and services that are coordinated throughout the food and nutrition and health care systems. The plan should guide accomplishments and define monitoring points used to assess achievement.

This chapter describes the strategic thinking and planning roles of the dietitian or nutritionist responsible for community nutrition programs. It presents the needs assessment processes and specific techniques that can be used to prioritize problems and intervention alternatives by using criteria commonly applied by public health agencies.

These techniques demonstrate the importance of using an objective decision-making process when complex problems are at stake. The chapter ends with some guidelines for writing goals and objectives.

STRATEGIC THINKING: DIRECTION SETTING

The definition of a strategy in terms of business is

"The pattern or plan that integrates an organization's major goals, policies, and action sequences into a cohesive whole. A well-formulated strategy helps to marshal and allocate an organization's resources into a unique and viable posture based on its relative internal competencies and shortcomings, anticipated changes in the environment, and contingent moves of intelligent opponents."[12]

Strategic thinking is a future-oriented and action-oriented process through which change is anticipated and initiated. Successful strategists consider a range of internal and external issues, trends, and opportunities; create a vision of a desirable future state; and establish a commitment to a course of action to bring their vision to reality.

According to Kotler,[9] strategic thinking is an inductive, direction-setting process. The focus on a direction or vision helps to clarify what kind of planning is essential. This requires information about patterns, relationships, and linkages and leads to a plan for how to achieve the vision over a period of time. Thinking strategically, creating a vision, and developing action plans that are driven by strategy are all essential to success in the 1990s.

PLANNING

Planning is an iterative process of foward-looking activities through which uncertainty is reduced and action toward orderly results is initiated. Planning is a part of the total management process and consists of planning, organizing (which includes staffing and budgeting), directing, and controlling (commonly referred to as monitoring and evaluation) (Fig. 14-1). It results in developing goals, objectives, and program activities. Planning focuses and directs effort, relates resources to desired goals, and sets benchmarks in the form of measurable objectives for evaluation. Formalized planning

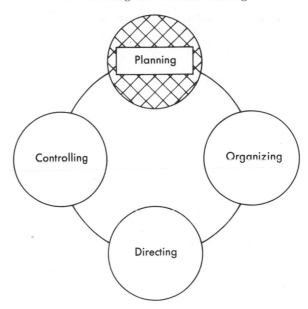

Figure 14-1. The management process.

efficiently focuses effort, commitment, and resources on priorities consistent with community values and needs and a desired vision of the future.

Defining the Planning Task

The planning task is determined by the organizational level of the planning effort, time horizon, and nature of the commitment. Time horizon is the period allowed for impact of the plan to be felt. Commitment is the description of the product of the planning effort. As illustrated in Table 14-1, the definition of the commitment is related to the time horizon and derived from a relevant information base. For example, organization goals express long-term commitments that are within the boundaries defined by the mission statement. These goals subsequently provide direction for intermediate and short-term programs and interventions. Thus, shorter-term plans evolve from longer-term commitments.

Strategic plans provide the basic framework or boundaries within which the organization operates to achieve its vision. By providing boundaries, a strategic plan provides a sense of coherence and

Table 14-1. Direction-setting and planning phases

Time horizon/organizational level	Information base	Nature of commitment
Direction setting		
Broad-based strategic thinking, 10-20 years	Review of dynamic environment Inductive review of relationships Patterns and linkages of data	Vision Establish strategies that shape or initiate change to reach idea Establish, review, and/or reaffirm mission statement
Policy planning		
Long-term planning, 5-10 years	Review of legal mandate, history and philosophy Environmental audit Social, political, economic, epidemiological, demographic, and technological trends	Broad organization goals

Intermediate planning, 3-5 years
Nutrition unit
	Community nutrition needs assessment
	  Nutrition needs by age, target group, geographic location, inventory of existing services
		Comprehensive nutrition plan
		  Goals and objectives
		Prioritization of programmatic focus areas

Implementation planning		
Short-term planning, 1-2 years Intervention design	Review of scientific basis for intervention strategies Market research Target population perception of wants and needs Formative evaluation	Outcome objectives Selection of specific interventions Process objectives Protocols Standards of performance

Sharbaugh C, editor: *Call to action: better nutrition for mothers, children and families,* Washington, DC, 1990, National Center for Education in Maternal and Child Health.

momentum to an organization's actions and decisions over time. As a first step in any planning, strategic planning involves establishment, revision, or reaffirmation of the organization's mission. The mission expresses organizational values and is usually fairly stable. Strategic planning is influenced by the internal culture and capabilities of the organization. It is also influenced by the public agenda, by the state of scientific knowledge, by the wants and needs of consumers, and by official positions of experts and professional groups. Hence, the greatest challenge for dietitians and nutritionists in doing strategic planning is to balance objectivity and creativity while accommodating the interests and priorities of constituencies and the political and value systems that determine those interests and priorities.

The strategic plan leads to broad organizational goals which guide action for a relatively long period (labeled *long-term planning* in Table 14-1).

Intermediate-term plans cover a period of 3 to 5 years. These plans define major priorities and focus departmental action on needs assessment. At this level of planning, alternative programs and their potential for impact on priority needs are identified and assessed.

Long-term and intermediate plans are reviewed periodically, usually annually, and only incremental adjustments are made. However, in these periods of review dietitians and nutritionists should proactively institute shifts in plans to redirect efforts to a new vision. Shifts in direction are most likely instigated and communicated in intermediate planning cycles. At these levels of planning, dietitians and nutritionists must anticipate specific actions necessary to redirect efforts. For example, major changes in emphasis or approach require time to educate and mobilize support (some call this "marketing"); develop new implementation or operational plans; recruit, train, and develop personnel; and secure the required funding base.

Short-term plans are usually tied to the budget cycle and identify specific programs and interventions to be implemented in the coming year. These plans define the operation of nutrition programs and services. They address where, when, how, by whom, and with what resources.

The longer-term strategic level of planning focuses on effectiveness (doing the right things), whereas shorter-term implementation or operations planning is concerned with efficiency (doing things the right way).

Dietitians and nutritionists will be better able to respond to the changing environment by utilizing strategic thinking to determine priorities for nutrition, and creating a vision for the future, and then carefully selecting programs and interventions that will lead to efficient accomplishment of the vision. Through participation and contributions at all levels of planning, dietitians and nutritionists can create innovative programs that anticipate and address emerging nutrition issues and problems experienced in a community.

Planning as a Shared Responsibility: Planning Teams within the Organization

Open planning processes help to accommodate different interests and values, foster orderly decision making, and enable development of realistic goals and objectives and feasible implementation plans. In determining the planning task, planners should make conscious decisions about what internal and external constituencies to involve at each stage of the process.

Planning is a responsibility that goes beyond the administrators, leaders, and program managers.

BENEFITS OF TEAM BUILDING

- The breadth of resources available enables a group to manage more complex situations
- Individuals working together build on individual strengths and compensate for any weakness
- Improves the quality of decisions and reduces risks of failure
- Increases the level of commitment to decisions made and programs developed
- Encourages achievement and activity that build motivation and momentum for the program
- If the team is well developed, it can increase performance and future skills of the organization

Adapted from Francis D, Young D: *Improving work groups: a practical manual for team building*, San Diego, 1979, University Association.

The planning process is strengthened by involving others, especially those who will be responsible for implementation. Personnel responsible for implementation bring practical knowledge of program operations and capabilities to the planning table.

Involvement in planning provides opportunities for professional growth and team building. Through the open planning process, an organization can produce successful plans that respond to the changing environment while effectively building a functioning team. Other benefits of team building are shown in the box above.

In contrast, there are also times when coalition building within an organization is not productive. Kanter outlines those conditions when it is clear that involvement of a team is not appropriate.[7] These conditions are listed in the box above.

Collaborative Planning Involving Outsiders

Planning for high-priority nutrition problems can also be improved by forming alliances with related constituencies in the service network. Collaborative planning by providers, advocates, and adversarial groups helps to assure that limited resources will be used efficiently. For external collaboration to succeed, each partner must contribute something distinctive. Hamel identified four other principles for beneficial external collaborations:[5]

- Collaboration is competition in a different

- When one person clearly has greater expertise on the subject than all others
- When those affected by that knowledge accept the expertise
- When there is a "hip-pocket" solution and the company already knows the "right answer"
- When someone has the subject as part of a job assignment and does not want to form a team
- When no one really cares about the issue
- When no important development or learning would be served by people's involvement
- When there is no time for discussion
- When people work more productively and happily alone

From Kanter RM: *The change masters: innovation and entrepreneurship in the American corporation*, New York, 1984, Simon & Schuster. Reprinted with permission.

form; organizations enter alliances with clear strategic objectives, and they understand how partners' objectives will affect their success.

- Harmony is not the most important measure of success.
- Cooperation has limits; confidential handling of specific information must be communicated to all involved.
- Learning from partners is paramount.

Effective collaborative planning bridges organizational and ideological boundaries, identifies mutual goals, and builds cohesion and capacity to act together. The activities of collaborative planning include:

1. Developing awareness of common problems and goals across organizational boundaries
2. Building cooperation around identified commonalities
3. Orchestrating planning activities to gain and maintain cooperation throughout planning and implementation
4. Assuring that constituents retain their own identity while developing ownership and recognition in collaborative activities
5. Using small successful collaborative efforts as potential areas for future collaboration.

The *process* of building collaborations is discussed further in Chapter 11.

WHAT IS A COMMUNITY?

Most public health professionals understand the term *community* as a group of individuals or families living together within a defined geographic boundary. *Community* can also be defined as a political entity (such as a city), a service area (such as a multicounty community health services area), a common interest (such as medical), or an ethnic or cultural background (such as Hispanic). Whatever the boundary, members within a community feel a sense of loyalty to the group and the values it represents. A needs assessment may cover the entire community defined in any of these ways, or, in some situations, the needs assessment may be narrowed to a specific target group within the community, such as the elderly or children with special needs.

Community Needs Assessment

In this chapter, broad guidelines for needs assessment will be identified. In Chapter 15, specific examples of how to apply this concept are given. Nutrition problems originate from complex interrelationships between environmental and social factors and the people in a community. In order to develop comprehensive nutrition plans, it is necessary to understand the full community assessment process. As commonly applied, a comprehensive community nutrition needs assessment:

1. Describes nutrition-related problems that exist in the community
2. Indicates the felt or perceived needs of the community and its desire for a solution
3. Establishes priorities and identifies resources that exist to deal with the problem.

Health planning customarily starts with demographic, socioeconomic, and epidemiological data to create indicators of health status. Data for indicators are compared to an ideal, such as state or national objectives for health; and discrepancies are identified as problem areas. Problems are then compared against an inventory of available public and private services to identify deficiencies in the

1. Internal organizational mission and competency to address community needs
2. Community characteristics related to health status of individuals and groups
3. Lifestyle and environmental factors
4. Availability and appropriateness of health service resources
5. Community values and health expectations

capacity of the service system to address identified problems. Nutrition-related problems and service gaps become priorities for action.

Other information-gathering methods can enrich the data base for planning. The environmental audit adds information on political and technological trends in the environment. Along with social, economic, demographic, and epidemiological data, this information expands the understanding of the context for nutrition problems and leads to more comprehensive intervention options, including citizens' views of the problems. In Chapter 15 needs assessment and a use of reference populations and classical measures of nutritional status are discussed, and specific examples are given. This provides practical information for developing a needs assessment for sound planning.

A broad base of information is essential for planning. Thus it is best to analyze the interrelated parts of the community structure. Areas (conditions) that provide a foundation for determining nutrition-related health problems and serve as the basis for developing a comprehensive nutrition plan (listed in box above) will be expanded later. Utilize the case study Vision City, USA, in this chapter's appendix to implement a needs assessment for this community.

Conduct a Community Nutrition Needs Assessment

The goal of any needs assessment is to obtain quantitative and qualitative information to identify nu-

trition-related problems and opportunities for reducing those problems. It requires interaction with the community or target groups to understand their values and behaviors, their perception of needs, and their feelings about acceptable interventions.

From this vantage point, an interpretation or diagnosis of the nutrition problems can be made, and community interest and support can be fostered to engage the community's involvement in efforts to change factors related to the identified problems.

For each of the five areas of essential information, it is necessary to make choices on what types of information (data elements) to gather and the best methods to use. No single approach or combination of information will work in every situation. Table 14-2 outlines the kinds of available data related to nutrition and where to find the information. It is designed to be an aid in identifying what information would provide relevant, time-efficient community nutrition needs assessment.

Assess Mission and Competency of Your Organization

A focus of the nutrition needs assessment should be within the scope of the mission statement of the sponsoring agency. Awareness of the mission and strategic directions of the organization is necessary to define the needs assessment and relevant collaborators. The community assessment must focus on nutrition-related factors and trends relevant to the organization. After nutrition-related problems are identified, an internal assessment should be initiated to explain the capabilities, resources, expertise, and willingness that exist within the agency to deal with the problems and potential solutions.

Identify Community Characteristics

Information used to define health status includes demographic, socioeconomic, geographic, and vital health statistics. Common indicators are described on Table 14-2.

Demography is the statistical study of human populations, especially with reference to size and density, distribution, and vital statistics. The U.S. Census tabulations are good source documents for

Text continued on p. 372.

Table 14-2. Sources of data related to nutrition

Condition	Data elements	Source of information	Demographic unit
Economic status	Median and mean income per household or family by family type: with no children under 18; married couple; female householder; no husband present with children under 6 years old	U.S. and special census data	State, county, census tracts, cities
	Per capita income	U.S. and special census data	State, county, census tracts, cities
	Occupation income and poverty status by ethnicity	U.S. and special census data	State, county, census tracts, cities
	Income by occupational unit: managerial and professional specialty occupations; executive, administrative, and managerial occupations; professional specialty occupations	U.S. and special census data	State, county, census tracts, cities
	Technical, sales, and administrative support technicians and related support sales and administrative support, including clerical	U.S. and special census data	State, county, census tracts, cities
	Service occupations, private household occupations, except protective and household	U.S. and special census data	State, county, census tracts, cities
	Farming, forestry, and fishing	U.S. and special census data	State, county, census tracts, cities
	Precision production, craft, repair	U.S. and special census data	State, county, census tracts, cities
	Operators, fabricators, and laborers, machine operators, assemblers, and inspectors; transportation and material moving occupation handlers; equipment cleaners, helpers, and laborers	U.S. and special census data	State, county, census tracts, cities
	Percent of population below poverty level 75%, 125%, 200% (by type of household; see above) 65 years or older	U.S. and special census data	State, county, census tracts, cities
	Unemployment rate	Employment Security Commission US Bureau of Labor Statistics	Region or county
	Major industries, business	Chamber of Commerce Planning Department, Public Information office	City County, city

From California Department of Health and Human Services: *Guidelines for nutrition services in local health jurisdictions*, ed 2, 1987, The Department.

Table 14-2. Sources of data related to nutrition—cont'd

Condition	Data elements	Source of information	Demographic unit
Vital statistics Population com-position Community re-sources	Age, sex, ethnicity, distribution of population	U.S. and special census data	County and census tracts
Housing	Number of units occupied by house-holds below poverty levels	U.S. and special census data	County and census tracts
	Low-income housing units	Housing authority	County, city
	Number of housing units lacking com-plete plumbing facilities	U.S. and special census data	County and census tracts
	Complete kitchen facilities	U.S. and special census data	County and census tracts
	Electricity, gas	Utility companies	Service areas
	Homeless: number of referrals for emergency shelter	Home health agencies	Service areas
		Social welfare agencies	Service areas
		United Way agencies	
Transportation	Public transportation system	Department of transporta-tion	State, county, regional Service areas
		Local and regional bus sys-tems	
	Special transportation services	Social welfare agencies	Service areas
	Highway conditions	Department of Transporta-tion	State, county, regional
		Chamber of Commerce, maps	City
Physical and rec-reational facili-ties Nutritional and health care programs	Access to physical recreational facili-ties	Parks and recreation depart-ments	County, city
Food assistance programs	Various food assistance programs	Department of Food and Agriculture	State
	Number of referrals to food assistance programs	Federal emergency food and shelter programs	Service areas
	Number and usage of soup kitchens and emergency food pantries	Nutrition programs	County
		United Way agencies	Service areas
	Number of expedited food stamps	Hunger Coalition	Service areas
	Number of expedited food stamps	Department Social Services	County
	Food stamp case load	Department of Social Ser-vices	County

Continued.

Table 14-2. Sources of data related to nutrition—cont'd

Condition	Data elements	Source of information	Demographic unit
Food assistance programs— cont'd	WIC	Local WIC program	County
	Number of free or reduced-price school meals (school lunch, breakfast)	School districts	School districts
	Number of food bank agencies	State Department of Education; Office of Surplus property; Hunger coalition; Second Harvest	State, county, or service area
	Number of meals served by food bank agencies per month	State Department of Education; Office of Surplus Property	State, county, or service area
		Second Harvest; Hunger Coalition	Defined area
	Congregate feeding for elderly	Office of Aging	County
	Home-delivered meals or meals on wheels	Office of Aging	County
Local nutritionists and dietitians	Number of available registered dietitians per population base	Local district dietetic association and local nutrition councils	Service areas
Primary care services	Number of available health care facilities in specific geographical areas of jurisdiction	Hospitals and outpatient clinics, private and public, including Veteran's Administration and Public Health Service	
		Prepaid health plans, health maintenance organizations, special clinics—rural, Indian, and farmworker clinics; neighborhood health centers	
		Health Department, clinic, community, and home-based services; skilled and intermediate care facilities, adult day health care	
		Home Health agencies, health planning agencies. Wellness centers, cardiac rehabilitation programs	Service areas
		Health personnel, physicians, public health nurses, dentists, midwifes, nurse practitioners, home economists	Service areas

Table 14-2. Sources of data related to nutrition—cont'd

Condition	Data elements	Source of information	Demographic unit
Other community resources	Number of available community resources in specific geographical areas of jurisdiction	Cooperative extension expanded food and nutrition education program; child care programs—day-care centers (public and private), Head Start; consumer advocacy groups; political organizations; local government officials; voluntary health agencies—American Heart Association, etc.	Service areas
		Nutrition groups—Dietetic Association local districts; Nutrition Council local chapters; School Food Service Association; National Council Against Health Fraud; Society for Nutrition Education	Service areas
		Food retailers—grocery stores, cooperative	Service areas
		Mass media—radio, television, newspapers	Service areas
Education system	Number of available classes in nutrition for specific targeted populations	School districts: Number of elementary and secondary schools (public and private); amount of nutrition education included in the curriculum, special NET projects	School districts
		Kinds of food available in vending machines	
		Colleges and universities—courses in nutrition, home economics, etc.	
		Other consumer education programs; adult education classes related to food, cooking, nutrition, etc.	
Food distribution system	Location and types of stores	Phone books (yellow pages) County Environmental Health	County
	Kinds of locations of restaurants	County Environmental Health	County

Continued.

Table 14-2. Sources of data related to nutrition—cont'd

Condition	Data elements	Source of information	Demographic unit
Food distribution system—cont'd	Cost of food	Retail grocer consumer services officers	
	Average retail prices of foods	USDA cost of food at home bulletins	U.S.
	Kinds of foods available: Low-fat milk products	Commodity brokers	Service areas
	Fresh fruit and vegetables Whole grains Enriched and fortified products (breads, iodized salt, etc.)	USDA bulletins Inventory for specific foods	State
	Types of food available in schools	Parent-Teacher Association, school food service and nutrition education personnel	School districts
	Number of school districts with food service menus conforming to U.S. Dietary Guidelines	Dental prevention program	County
	Number of restaurants with modified menus; availability of low-fat, low-sodium, and low-sugar foods	Local Heart Association chapter and ("Hearty Heart" or Creative Cuisine programs)	Chapter service area
Health statistics	Ten leading causes of death	County death records	County census tracts
	Birthrate	County birth records	County census tracts
	Gestational age	County birth records	County census tracts
	Death rate specific by age, disease, race, sex	County death records (special computer run)	County census tracts
	Maternal mortality rate	County death records	County census tracts
	Infant mortality rate	County infant death records	County census tracts
	Low-birth-weight infants (less than 2500 g) by ethnicity	County birth records	County census tracts
	Number of live births by age and ethnicity of mother	County birth records	County census tracts
	Days lost from school	School districts Vital and Health Statistics, series 10 No. 146*	School districts Specific cities, Regional U.S.
	Days lost from work	Vital and Health Statistics, series 10, No. 146* Employee records	Specific cities, Regional U.S. organization
	Bed disability days	Vital and Health Statistics, series 10, No. 146* Health: U.S. & Prevention Profile, U.S. Dept. of Health and Human Services, 1983	Specific cities, Regional U.S. Specific cities, Regional U.S.

*Vital and Health Statistics, U.S. Department of Health and Human Services, National Center for Health Statistics; series 10: data from the National Health Survey (Hanes); series 11: data from the National Health Survey (Hanes); series 13: data from National Hospital Discharge Survey; series 21: data from National Vital Statistics System.

Table 14-2. Sources of data related to nutrition—cont'd

Condition	Data elements	Source of information	Demographic unit
	Disability days	Vital and Health Statistics, series 10, No. 143 & 146*	Specific cities
	Days of restricted activity	Health: U.S. & Prevention Profile, U.S. Dept. of Health and Human Services, 1983	U.S. geographic regions
Nutrition-related diseases	Incidence of food poisoning	County communicable disease records	County
	Prevalence by age, sex, and ethnic distribution: heart disease, cancer, cirrhosis of liver, lead poisoning, dental caries, rickets, malnutrition	County health dept. records	Service area
	Rate of inpatients discharged from short-stay hospitals (diagnosis)	Hospitals admissions and discharges (Vital & Health Statistics, series 13, No. 101*)	Service area
	Food borne illness	Environmental health reports	County
		Disease registries	
	Blood lead levels	Vital and Health Statistics, series 1, No. 233*	City, rural
	Heart disease (with risk factors)	Vital and Health Statistics, series 11, No. 227*	Regional U.S.
	Blood pressure	Vital and Health Statistics, series 11, No. 226*	Regional U.S.
	Cancer	SEARS (Southeast Asian Refugees)	County
Nutritional disorders and high-risk conditions for nutritional inadequacies	Various anemias (Hb, Hct, iron intake)	Vital and Health Statistics, series 11, No. 232 and 229*	U.S.
	Anemia and pregnancy	Vital and Health Statistics, series 11, No. 229*	U.S.
		Birth records with county health dept./WIC	County
	Obesity	Vital Health and Statistics, series 11, No. 230*	U.S.
		County health dept.	County
	Cholesterol: intake and serum levels	Vital and Health Statistics, series 11, No. 231 and 227*	U.S.
	Number of teen births (not pregnancies)	County birth records	County
	Number of positive pregnancy tests at women's health clinics	County women's health program	County

Continued.

Table 14-2. Sources of data related to nutrition—cont'd

Condition	Data elements	Source of information	Demographic unit
Nutritional disorders and high-risk conditions for nutritional inadequacies—cont'd	Pregnant teens	Vital and Health Statistics, series 21, No. 42 and 41*	State and U.S. geographic division, school district
		School health records	
		CDC: nutritional surveillance system	
		Local Maternal and Child Health Office	County
	Pregnancies (less than 18 months apart)	U.S. and special census data (special computer run)	County census tract
		WIC	County
		CDC: nutritional surveillance system	
		Vital and Health Statistics, series 21, No. 42 and 41*	State and geographic division
	Hypertension	Preventive services for older adults, primary care clinics, family planning	Service areas
		School health records	School district
		Large medical laboratories	Service areas
		Clinics, nutritionists	Service areas
		Health maintenance organizations prepaid health plans	Service areas
		DRGs hospital discharges	Hospital service areas
		Vital and Health Statistics, series 11, No. 226*	Regional U.S.
		California Dept. of Health Services Hypertension survey: ages 25-74	State
		Other behavioral life factor surveys	
		Health and Human Services (Public Health Service): Health U.S. and Prevention Profile	U.S.
		Hypertension coordinating agencies	State
	Developmental disabilities	Regional centers for the developmentally delayed	Regional centers Service area
		California Children's Services	County
	Clinical manifestations of malnutrition	Private and public institutions	Service areas
	Inappropriate growth in children	Local Maternal and Child Health Office	County

*Vital and Health Statistics, U.S. Department of Health and Human Services, National Center for Health Statistics; series 10: data from the National Health Survey (Hanes); series 11: data from the National Health Survey (Hanes); series 13: data from National Hospital Discharge Survey; series 21: data from National Vital Statistics System.

Table 14-2. Sources of data related to nutrition—cont'd

Condition	Data elements	Source of information	Demographic unit
Dietary inadequacies, habits, and food and consumption patterns of individual and local subgroups of population	Consumption of particular (calories, nutrients, sugar)	Vital and Health Statistics, series 11, No. 209, 231 (By sex, age, and income status)*	U.S.
		Small- or large-scale nutrition services	County
	Per capita consumption of specific foods (e.g., eggs, meats, breads, salt, red meat)	USDA household food consumption surveys	U.S.
		Telephone risk factor prevalence survey	State
	Breastfeeding patterns Breastfeeding at hospital discharge	Local health dept.: newborn screening	County hospital
	Meals eaten in restaurants and fast-food restaurants	Environmental health inspectors, local restaurant association, marketing studies from Food Marketing Institute	County Service areas
	Expenditures for meals, snacks away from home (million$)	Food consumption prices and expenditures	U.S.
Smoking, drug, alcohol usage (substance abuse)	Smoking, drug, and alcohol usage	Treatment centers, county health dept. and mental health programs	Service areas
		MADD, SADD Prevalence survey Behavioral risk factor prevalence survey	Service areas CDC
	Cigarette smoked/day (20+ years) Frequency of use of marijuana and alcohol by high school seniors	U.S. Dept. Health and Human Services: Health U.S. and Prevention Profile Food consumption, prices, expenditures (USDA) 1960-1980	U.S.
Physical activity	Sales of alcoholic beverages (million $) Physical activity (minutes/day)	Behavioral risk factor prevalence telephone survey (CDC)	State

such data. Eight key determinants in census data are particularly useful for predicting health status:

- *Age:* Many disease conditions are age related.
- *Gender:* Disease conditions or injuries can affect males and females differently. Life expectancy is longer for females.
- *Race and ethnicity:* Race and ethnicity have been related to health problems. However, factors other than race may affect these outcomes more (e.g., differences in income, education, and occupations).
- *Residence and location:* Where people live can influence their health status and access to health care services. Location may increase exposure to certain environmental risks.
- *Family size:* The association of family size with health status is complex and varies by target group.
- *Household income and educational level of head of household:* Higher household income and educational levels are generally associated with higher levels of health status. Behavioral risk factors for chronic disease (such as tobacco use, poor eating habits, lack of physical activity) are associated with lower income and education levels.
- *Occupational level of head of household:* Blue-collar workers tend to experience a lower health status than white-collar workers. Some of this experience is related to risk-taking behaviors such as alcohol misuse or abuse, poor eating habits, and failure to use seat belts.[10]

Census information is available from the Office of the State Demographer within state planning agencies or at libraries designated as census depository libraries. See Table 14-2 for other aspects of the assessment of community health status. Apply this information to the case study Vision City, USA, in this chapter's appendix.

Observe and Record Lifestyle and Environmental Factors

Each community is unique in terms of its cultural traditions, lifestyle, and environmental factors. These factors can either protect people from or contribute to nutrition-related health problems.

Knowledge of the social and cultural factors impinging on eating patterns and health habits are crucial to the community nutrition assessment. Although some of these cultural factors are difficult to define and isolate, a community assessment should summarize the identifiable cultural traditions and values of the community.

Assessment of the local marketplaces, supermarkets, small grocery stores, food cooperatives, delicatessens, health food stores, and other food outlets provides information related to food availability and purchasing behaviors. Private organizations such as the Food Marketing Institute and government agencies also monitor food purchasing and food consumption trends.

Techniques of market research can be used to supplement the community nutrition needs assessment to gain an understanding of how community members perceive their own needs. Examples of market research techniques are the nominal group process and focus groups (see Chapter 16). Information from community members themselves, combined with experts' opinions and statistical data, will best guide the planning process to assure the development of programs that will be utilized by consumers.

Inventory Health and Nutrition Service Resources

The 1989 report of *Diet and Health* identifies voluntary health organizations and government agencies in the United States that have issued various dietary guidelines to promote good health in general or to prevent specific chronic diseases.[1] There is considerable agreement on general nutrition principles that promote good health. However, mechanisms to assure access to optimum nutrition for good health are not uniformly available. Health promotion and disease prevention services believed to be effective in reducing morbidity and mortality are not fully utilized because of barriers of accessibility, appropriateness, and availability.

An inventory of health and nutrition resources (type and volume of services) is crucial to a better understanding of nutrition-related services and networking in the community (Table 14-2).

Services to be included in the inventory are all health, human service, education, and voluntary programs involved in the provision of food or nutrition services. From the perspective of the consumer, these services might provide a basic need (such as housing or food), information and referral, outreach, advocacy, counseling, or individual case management. The agencies may include preventative, curative, or restorative services. Objective data recorded might be number and type of clients, number of visits, types of services provided, budget allocation to specific services, number of personnel, and underutilized capacity or unmet demands. Whatever information is collected should clarify what service delivery problems exist and must fall in line with the organization's service mission and competency.

The goal for the community is to have an effective service management system, which is defined by Kanter as "an integrated set of activities, methods, and technologies which maximize all available and potential resources to serve the population and sub-populations within the community."[7] Meeting the challenges of improving nutrition outcomes may involve utilizing a variety of health facilities, services, programs, or personnel. A successful inventory of resources should discover what is available and used to capacity, what is available but inappropriate or underutilized, and what gaps for nutrition-related services exist. Then planners will be in a position to work in concert with the community to fill unmet nutrition service needs. By involving all affiliated providers in the assessment, there will be a wider ownership of nutrition-related problems and better solutions put forth to address service gaps.

Identify Community Values and Expectations for Health

"Concern for people is the cornerstone of service strategy." Kotler goes on to state, "Many organizations are very clear about the needs they would like to serve but they don't understand these needs from the perspective of the customer."[9] These statements hold true for community nutrition. As mentioned previously, market research techniques can be used to understand the community's view of nutrition-related problems and what programs the community dislikes. Understanding the community's values, priorities, and expectations for health and health behavior is essential to planning effective programs that will be utilized by the target group.

What are values? Values provide a general "guidance system" for a person's behavior. They are different from attitudes in that values transcend specific objects, events, or people. *Values* may be defined as beliefs about what is "good" (freedom, justice, health) and what is "bad" (war, poverty, disease). Values are changing today because of the diverse cultures present in American society.

Changes in society reflect changing values. In our society, health is viewed as a resource that gives people the ability to manage and change their surroundings. This view of health as a resource gives individuals within a community the freedom to decide what behaviors to follow. Some decisions promote health; other decisions put health status at risk. Because values and behaviors are influenced by cultural traditions, belief systems, and social and physical environments, the value placed on health-promoting behaviors by community members may be in conflict with the values held by health professionals.

Values help to establish priorities and hierarchies of importance among needs and goals.[4] As discussed in Chapter 13, after determining your personal and professional values, you are responsible for expressing the organization's values and ensuring to the community that ethical values will be used in decision-making.

Joint value determination by professionals and the public should be used to create the objectives and acceptable methods of public service programs. As Drucker advises, "Non-profit people must respect their customers and their donors enough to listen to their values and understand their satisfactions. They do not impose the organization's own views and egos on those they serve."[2] This message is especially important now, when there is renewed appreciation for diversity. Ethnic and racial groups desire to retain their individuality rather than being assimilated into society. The opportunity for planning successful nutrition intervention programs rests with dietitians' and nutritionists' abilities to meet needs with "unassimilated diversity" and recognition of differing values for health and health behaviors.

Community needs assessment is an important and complex step in the planning process. Good plans require solid information on the health status, health behaviors, and values of the people in the community and knowledge of the availability of health services, including the competency of your own organization.

PRIORITIZE THE PROBLEMS

Data collection results in considerable understanding of problems; however, the essence of planning is prioritization of needs and actions in the face of constraints and uncertainties. Prioritization is an important step in selecting a manageable number of problems to address in the community. Methods for prioritization must be fair and objective and reflect community values. It is a systematic, perspective-taking process to understand another's viewpoint, as well as understand the problem. Methods such as the nominal group process that involve constituencies affected by the results have the added benefit of serving as a learning process for participants.[14] Four criteria for priority determination are widely used:

1. *Size:* uses rates at risk, and incidence or prevalence rates to compare number affected by problems
2. *Seriousness:* considers what happens if noth-

PRIORITIZATION OF PROBLEMS
(Reproduce this form for each problem identified)

Step 1:   **Define the problem** _____

_____

(A concise statement that describes the problem and who and how many it affects.)

Step 2:   **Rate importance of problem with specific criteria, using estimates.** (These estimates are based on your knowledge of the community and the health data obtained in your needs assessment process.)

	High Score 3	Medium Score 2	Low Score 1
a. Number of persons potentially affected by the problem • If the number of at-risk persons is a large proportion of the total population, enter a 3 in the "High" column. • If the number of at-risk persons is a moderate proportion of the total population, enter a 2 in the "Medium" column. • If the number of at-risk persons is a relatively small proportion of the total population, enter a 1 in the "Low" column. b. Number of at-risk persons actually affected by the problem • If almost all of the at-risk persons *are affected* by this problem, enter a 3 in the "High" column. If many of the at-risk persons *are affected*, enter a 2 in the "Medium" column. • If relatively few of the at-risk persons *are affected*, enter a 1 in the "Low" column.			

Adapted from Minnesota State Department of Health: *Guide for community health planning*, Minneapolis, 1988, Minnesota State Department of Health.

PRIORITIZATION OF PROBLEMS—cont'd

	High Score 3	Medium Score 2	Low Score 1
c. Amount of premature death and resulting family and social burden			

c. Amount of premature death and resulting family and social burden
  • If this problem leads to many premature deaths in the community, enter a 3 in the "High" column.
  • If it leads to a moderate number of premature deaths, enter a 2 in the "Medium" column.
  • If it leads to relatively few or no known premature deaths, enter a 1 in the "Low" column.
d. Severity (degree to which the problem limits persons' ability to live their lives)
  • If the problem severely limits life choices, enter a 3 in the "High" column.
  • If the problem moderately limits life choices, enter a 2 in the "Medium" column.
  • If the problem mildly limits life choices, enter a 1 in the "Low" column.
e. Economic burden to the community (lost productivity, high health care costs)
  • If the economic burden of this problem is high, enter a 3 in the "High" column.
  • If the economic burden of this problem is moderate, enter a 2 in the "Medium" column.
  • If the economic burden of this problem is relatively low, enter a 1 in the "Low" column.
f. Public perception of the problem
  • If the public views the problem as serious and requiring immediate action, enter a 3 in the "High" column.
  • If the public views the problem as moderate but not requiring urgent action, enter a 2 in the "Medium" column.
  • If the public views the problem as low with little or no sense of urgency, enter a 1 in the "Low" column.
g. Preventability (effective means to prevent the problem)
  • If the problem can be prevented from occurring, enter 3 in the "High" column.
  • If the problem cannot be prevented but can be detected early and stopped, enter a 2 in the "Medium" column.
  • If the problem cannot be prevented and cannot be detected before it becomes a problem, enter a 1 in the "Low" column.

Step 3:   **Subtotal columns**   _____ + _____ + _____

Step 4:   Sum the columns to identify the *problem importance index* ing is done based on urgency, severity, economic loss to family and society, and potential for involvement of others

3. *Effectiveness of intervention:* estimates probability of preventing or reducing the problem based on what is known about the efficacy of available interventions

4. *Political support:* considers propriety, economics, acceptability, resources, and legality.[14]

The State of Minnesota recommends a process for systematically rating the importance of the health problem.[10] Each problem is compared to other problems by completing the form in the box on pp. 374-375. In determining each problem's importance, seven criteria are evaluated:

1. An estimate of potential persons at risk
2. An estimate of at-risk persons *with* the problem
3. The number of premature deaths
4. The extent to which the problem limits a person's ability to live life as desired
5. Economic burden to the community
6. Public concern
7. Problem preventability

Before rating the final criteria, a problem's preventability, the following are identified: agent or cause (biological lifestyle, physical or social environment), the host (person suffering from the cause), and an effective means to break the link between the cause and the host. Raters are reminded that an estimate of preventability or any other criterion does not consider cost, political feasibility, or other factors. This caution prevents traditional barriers of cost and politics from influencing the prioritization of health problems.

Even though the process is objective, the scoring ultimately relies on the wisdom and ethics of the planning group. Explicit criteria and scoring are used to help raters override preconceived judgments. Raters are reminded to discriminate between what is actually of "high" importance and what is important but less "high." A number of people with a variety of skills and backgrounds are used as raters. Because the ratings are based on estimates, community and professional members who have knowledge about the community, who understand the health data obtained in the needs assessment process, and who appreciate the felt needs and values of the community should be involved. As a leader, it is important to consider these skills in selecting planning team members and determining the work group mixture and size.

Overall, the four steps involved in prioritizing problems (see the box on pp. 374-375) are:

Step 1: Define the problem(s).

Step 2: Rate the problem by using specific criteria.

Step 3. Sum the rating scores for each problem to obtain the problem importance index.

Step 4: Rank the problems in priority order according to the problem importance index (highest to lowest score).

FORMULATE NUTRITION INTERVENTION PRIORITIES

Setting priorities, according to Drucker, is the true test of leadership because doing so may mean abandoning problems that look important in order to focus resources to solve another problem.[2] Formulating nutrition intervention priorities is not implementing programs; rather, it is an approach to give you the ability to clearly state, in public health terms, why the problems identified should or should not be addressed.

Before proceeding, however, consider whether it is appropriate for your organization to be addressing a specific problem. Do the highest-priority problems (identified by the prioritization process) fall within the boundaries specified by your organization's strategy and mission statement? If the problems relate to your organization's purpose and fall within the boundaries of professional and organizational values, the next step is to use a systematic approach to make decisions about interventions to address problems.

Possible Intervention Approaches

This phase includes generating ideas for possible interventions. These ideas can include interventions that currently exist in the community or could exist in the future. A creative, nonjudgmental ap-

ORGANIZE PUBLIC HEALTH NUTRITION INTERVENTIONS FOR EACH PROBLEM

Step 1: **State the problem:** _____
            (As identified in the prioritization phase)

Step 2: **Identify target groups:** _____
            (Those persons for whom you would like to prevent or reduce the problem)

Step 3: **Classify all current and possible interventions:**
            (Ideas should be concrete, focused, and specific to target group)

Intervention type; prevention level	Primary prevention	Secondary prevention	Tertiary prevention
Individual-based: creating change in individuals			
Community-based: creating change in populations that have received some service			
Systems-based: creating change in organizations, policies, laws, and structures			

Step 4: **Circle those interventions in which your agency has or could have some direct involvement or responsibility.**
            (Do not circle those interventions provided by other providers if you are not involved or responsible)

Adapted from Minnesota State Department of Health: *Guide for community health planning*, Minneapolis, 1988, Minnesota State Department of Health.

proach will ensure that all possible ideas are considered. The more structured nominal group technique is preferred over simple brainstorming. The nominal group technique is generating information, ideas, and concepts relative to a problem or question. It is one of the most powerful designs for developing lists of unique ideas and concepts. With any approach, write down all ideas on either a flip chart or a tablet so that ideas are not forgotten. Participants in this stage should include community members as well as staff. Community members will have different creative ideas than staff. Involvement of people representing different perspectives

will expand options, help to clarify ideas, and expand ownership of the problem and its solution.

Once all of the ideas have been recorded, sort and organize the knowledge and information. The State of Minnesota uses a matrix to examine current and potential interventions for each specific problem (see the box above). This form is used to classify interventions into primary, secondary, and tertiary levels of prevention and individual-based, community-based, and systems-based intervention types. Definitions for each prevention and intervention level are given in the following box.

This matrix should reflect the entire system of

PREVENTION LEVELS AND INTERVENTION TYPE

Prevention levels

- Primary prevention interventions focus on preventing disease *before* it occurs or is diagnosed; it prevents a problem from affecting people in the first place. Examples include general nutrition education for health promotion; immunizations; and health risk appraisals (which include nutrition).
- Secondary prevention interventions focus on early detection and prompt treatment of an existing but often undetected problem; it prevents a problem from causing any serious or long-term effects to the individuals or from affecting others. Examples include cholesterol or cancer screening; sexually transmitted disease clinics; sexual abuse and neglect screening; water testing; food, beverage, and lodging inspections; early and periodic screening clinics.
- Tertiary prevention interventions focus on limiting further negative effects from a problem; it prevents an existing problem and its existing consequences from getting worse. Examples include home health visits for the chronically ill and disabled; reporting of abused and neglected children; referral to support groups; and supplemental feeding of growth-retarded infants.

Intervention type

- Individual-based interventions focus on creating changes (health status, knowledge, skills) in individuals, either singly or in small groups. They are typically seen as direct service to clients or residents. Examples include one-to-one counseling, classes, and home care visits.
- Community-based interventions focus on creating changes in populations. They are measured in terms of how much of the "community" (however defined) has received some service. The community could be children needing day-care services, the elderly receiving meals on wheels, or the entire community population. Examples include WIC clinics, media campaigns, community health events, screenings in school, lodging inspections, fitness trails.
- Systems-based interventions focus on creating change in organizations, policies, laws, and structures. The focus is not directly on individuals or communities but on the systems that serve them. Because these systems ultimately impact individuals, changing the system represents a cost-effective and long-lasting way to impact individuals. Examples include reducing fat in a school lunch program, establishing a wellness program at the work place, implementing regulations to monitor food served in day-care centers, and improving access to health care.

interventions related to the problem. It should include interventions your organization currently provides directly, those your organization coordinates or those to which it provides assistance, those services provided by other organizations in the community, and those that your organization could reasonably provide, coordinate, or assist in conjunction with another organization. The information in the matrix will also be helpful in the actual planning and implementation phases (see Chapter 16) to meet the goals and objectives established.

Improving the Quality of the Formulated Nutrition Intervention Plan

A well-formed nutrition intervention plan effectively and efficiently uses the systems in the community and the organization to prevent a nutrition problem or seek a permanent solution to a problem within a target population. It accomplishes this by addressing needs, wants, and capabilities of community members. Systematic approaches that use data rather than hunches and that identify root causes of the problem will improve the decision-making quality.

Identify the Root Causes of a Problem

Use of a risk indicator model is one method to examine the many factors that contribute to a nutrition-related health problem. Many causes often act together to create a complex pattern of risk factors (a "multifactorial etiology"). Such complex patterns mean that any intervention that focuses on only a single cause will limit the effectiveness for many of the individuals being targeted.

Risk indicator models examine problems by separating causes into four fields: lifestyle, environment, human biology, and health services. *Lifestyle* is the combination of decisions and actions taken by people that can affect their health or nutrition status, and over which they are generally believed to have control. *Environment* is both the physical surroundings and conditions and the social conditions to which people are exposed. Examples include air, water, noise, community norms, regulations, and level of nutrition information available. *Human biology* is an individual's genetic inheritance, something over which one generally has no control. Gender, body build, predisposition to chronic disease, and level of immunity are examples. *Health services* include the existence or absence of health care services and their accessibility, affordability, and acceptability to the community. They can also include the awareness, skills, and attitudes of health professionals. Insurance or other reimbursement sources can be a contributing factor, as can the lack or presence of coordination between providers.

Consideration of the root causes of a problem provides a more thorough understanding of what intervention approaches can be used to address the problem.

Determine Intervention Richness

The interventions listed for each problem in the box on p. 377 can be rated using public health principles. The box on p. 380 identifies five criteria used for systematic evaluation of the intervention richness for addressing each problem: (1) number of potential interventions, (2) number of intervention levels, (3) emphasis on primary prevention, (4) effectiveness of each intervention, and (5) overall efficiency of the intervention.

The rationales for using these criteria are:

1. It is more likely that an appropriate intervention can be selected to meet needs if there is greater flexibility among available choices (potential interventions).
2. Choices for interventions are broadened, and the potential for reducing the problem is enhanced. Simultaneous interventions of different types usually result in greater and longer-lasting change.
3. Interventions oriented toward primary prevention are usually more cost-beneficial.
4. Effective and efficient decisions seek permanent solutions rather than relying on personal interests or quick fixes.

MAKE A DECISION ON INTERVENTION PRIORITIES

For each nutrition problem, you have rated the importance (with the Prioritization of Problems box) and you have rated the number and scope of interventions to address that problem using public health principles (with the Intervention Richness box). The final step is to determine the relative importance of the various problems and the proposed activities to address the problems. This provides an overall ranking to aid in decision making. This phase has four steps:

1. Using the Prioritization of Problems box, divide the total problem index scores into two categories of "very important" and "less important."
2. Using the Intervention Richness box, divide the intervention richness index scores into two categories of "high richness" and "low richness."
3. For each problem, plot the rankings obtained from steps 1 and 2 in the appropriate quadrant on the grid in the Decision Matrix box.
4. Using the grid, determine the intervention priorities that are highly recommended.

How do you decide how to divide the index scores into two groups? Sometimes there is an obvious break point between high and low scores. At other times, it may be best to split the scores into roughly two equal groups (if the scores are evenly distributed). Then again, there may be another method that works best for your organization and provides a logical means to separate the groups.

The problems identified as "very important" and as having "high richness" are the ones that are highly recommended to be in the plan. These problems are in the top left quadrant of the Decision Matrix form and have four stars. The next set of

DETERMINE INTERVENTION RICHNESS

Step 1: Define the problem _____

Step 2: Rate intervention richness using criteria-specific public health principles

	High Score 3	Medium Score 2	Low Score 1
a. Number of potential interventions • If there are many *possible* interventions for this intervention, enter a 3 in the "High" column. • If there are a moderate number of possible interventions, enter a 2 in the "Medium" column. • If there are few possible interventions, enter a 1 in the "Low" column.			
b. Number of intervention types (i.e., individual, community, system) • If the possible interventions for this problem occur at *all three* levels, enter a 3 in the "High" column. • If the interventions occur at *two of the three* levels, enter a 2 in the "Medium" column. • If the interventions occur at only *one of the three* levels, enter a 1 in the "Low" column.			
c. Emphasize primary prevention • If the interventions for this problem focus more on primary prevention than on other levels of prevention, enter a 3 in the "High" column. • If the interventions focus on primary prevention only to the same extent or somewhat less than they focus on the other levels of prevention, enter a 2 in the "Medium" column. • If the interventions are very weak in primary prevention, focusing more or almost exclusively on other levels of prevention, enter a 1 in the "Low" column.			
d. Overall effectiveness of intervention* (Are you or would you be doing the right thing for the right people?) • If many of your current interventions are considered—through research, evaluation, or both—to be an effective means to reduce the problem, enter a 3 in the "High" column. • If your interventions include some effective interventions but also some relatively weak ones, enter a 2 in the "Medium" column. • If the current interventions include few or no effective interventions, enter a 1 in the "Low" column.			

*Keep in mind that knowledge of the effectiveness and efficiency of an intervention is derived through the research of others and through your objective evaluation of current and past programs. Preferably, both sources of information can be used in the rating.

DETERMINE INTERVENTION RICHNESS—cont'd

	High Score 3	Medium Score 2	Low Score 1
e. Overall efficiency of intervention* (Are you doing it or can it be done with minimum use of resources?) • If many of the interventions are considered to be an efficient means to reduce the problem, enter a 3 in the "High" column. • If the interventions include some efficient interventions but also some relatively inefficient ones, enter a 2 in the "Medium" column. • If the interventions include few or no efficient interventions, enter a 1 in the "Low" column.			

Step 3:   Subtotal columns _____ + _____ + _____

Step 4:   Total: richness index _____

DECISION MATRIX FOR RANKING PROBLEMS

Step 1:   Using the Prioritization of Problems box, indicate somewhere on the copy or a separate sheet of paper whether the problem score is "very important" or "less important."

Step 2:   Using the Intervention Richness box, indicate somewhere on the copy or on a separate sheet of paper whether the intervention richness is "high" or "low."

Step 3:   Enter *all* problems in the appropriate quadrant on the grid using *both* rankings.

	High importance	Low importance
High richness index	****	**
Low richness index	***	*

Step 4:   Identify those problems that are:
**** Highly recommended to be in plan (upper left quadrant)
*** Recommended to be in plan (lower left quadrant)
** Addressed in plan if possible (upper right quadrant)
* Continue surveillance; may not address (lower left quadrant)

problems to include in the plan are those ranked "very important" and "low richness" (bottom left quadrant). Those problems third in order are in the upper right quadrant ("less important" and "high richness"); they should receive continued surveillance but are not high priorities.

Effective managing demands the efficient use of resources. Optimum use of an organization's resources is the cornerstone of the management process. All managers, whether they are hospital administrators, directors of dietary departments, public health personnel, government officials, or business executives, are responsible for the property of others. Because resources are limited, managers cannot possibly take advantage of every opportunity.

Before a manager can act to use or withhold resources, opportunities must be identified and a process used to make a decision. *Decision making* is the deliberation about the alternative ways to use resources.[4] The process described in this chapter uses index ratings and a matrix to evaluate all problems within a community. It can be a time-consuming process, depending on the measures of the data, complexity of the problem, and the time horizon of the problem. Nevertheless, an accurate assessment of nutrition priorities can be achieved by competent community members and professionals. This approach enhances information exchange and social support among members and builds credibility in the community. Managers can accomplish significant tasks in a relatively short period of time. The matrix approach makes people act in a highly focused mode.

DECISION MAKING: SELECTING THE INTERVENTION

The planning process involves decision making at every juncture. Sound decisions emerge from an objective decision-making process. Decision making involves five distinct steps:

1. State the problem or situation requiring a decision.
2. Define criteria relevant to a "good" choice in the decision situation.
3. Brainstorm and suggest alternative solutions.
4. Assess each alternative with established criteria.
5. Select the most suitable alternative based on the objective assessment carried out at step 4.

These steps are followed by two more: implement the solution and evaluate the results.

The combination of creatively generated alternatives and clearly defined criteria to assess the alternatives leads to high-quality decisions. Through this process, those involved in decision making become aware of the strengths and limitations of various alternatives as judged against criteria relevant to the decision situation. Although no one best solution is possible, the process reveals the most preferred solutions to decision makers. Decision makers, then, have rational information to justify choices and can communicate the rationale for decisions to others. Using a concrete decision-making process avoids the pitfall of basing decisions on emotional reactions, past biases, and hunches. It also prevents powerful opinion leaders from dictating the decision process.

Great attention must be given to defining the criteria relevant to a "good" choice. Examples used earlier in this chapter had established criteria such as number affected, severity, and public perception (see the Prioritization of Problems box). In many decision situations, dietitians and nutritionists must define criteria relevant to a good solution to the problem. Criteria should be clearly stated, understood, and agreed upon by those involved in the decision-making process. Criteria reduce the complexity and subjectivity of the decision by separating complex factors into single characteristics that can be assessed independently. Criteria assure that each alternative is assessed consistently.

Processes presented earlier in this chapter for prioritizing problems and assessing intervention richness follow the decision-making process. Deciding which interventions to put into the nutrition plan is yet another application of decision making.

Potential criteria for selecting among intervention alternatives include:

- Available resources (personnel, money, equipment, knowledge, skill, and time)

DECISION MATRIX FOR SELECTING INTERVENTIONS BASE ON FEASIBILITY

Step 1: List the Problem: _____

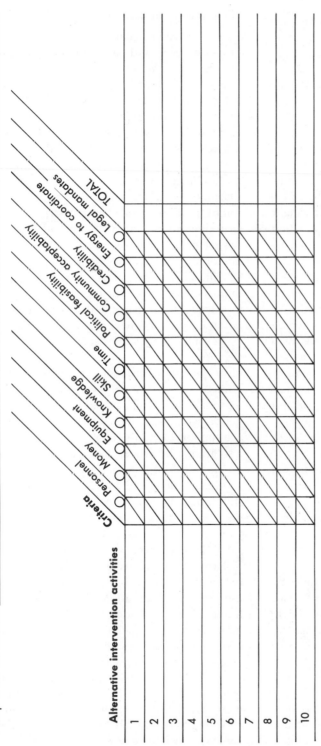

Step 2: Identify the criteria important to implementing possible interventions. (Add/delete from the criteria identified across the figure.)

Step 3: Weight the criteria on a scale of 1 to 10 where 1 is the least important criteria and 10 is the most important criteria. (Place the weighted values in the circle below the criteria.)

Step 4: Identify all possible intervention activities to address the problem. Write them in the appropriate rows.

Step 5: Based within each criteria, RANK each intervention activity where the highest number most favorably meets the criteria and the lowest number least favorably meets criteria. Place the rank number in the upper left-hand corner of the box. Complete the rankings for each intervention activity within each criteria by moving vertically down the column.

Step 6: After each intervention activity has been ranked within each criteria, multiply the criteria weight (Step 3) with the specific intervention ranking and place it below the diagonal line. This provides a weighting sum within each criteria.

Step 7: Sum all the criteria scores for each intervention activity, obtained in Step 6, by moving horizontally across each row to obtain a FEASIBILITY INDEX. Place in the appropriate "TOTAL" box.

Figure 14-2. Decision matrix for selecting interventions based on feasibility.
Adapted from Mullis RM, Snyder MP, and Hunt MK: Developing nutrient criteria for food-specific dietary guidelines for the general public, *J Am Dietetic Assoc* 90(46):847-851, 1990. Permission granted by the American Dietetic Association.

- Legal mandates requiring an organization to address a problem
- Political feasibility
- Community acceptability
- Reputation or credibility of the organization that is to address a problem
- Potential or available energy within the organization to address a problem

Dietitians and nutritionists can use Figure 14-2 for objectively selecting among possible interventions to address a high-priority community nutrition problem. This matrix adds a new dimension to the decision-making process by adding weights to criteria. This step should be used when all criteria are not of equal importance for making the final choice. In this more complex process, the weight of the criterion is multiplied by the rank of the alternative. The product (score) is totaled to produce a feasibility index for each alternative.

Note that all possible interventions for the high-priority problems were identified by using Table 14-1. The decision matrix in Figure 14-2 evaluates the feasibility of those interventions by using established criteria. This decision matrix can be used to select feasible interventions for each problem. The steps used to complete Figure 14-2 are:

1. List the problem.
2. Determine the criteria (standards) important to implementing the intervention.
3. Assign a weight to each criterion.
4. Identify all possible interventions to address the problem.
5. Rank each intervention action based within each criterion.
6. Multiply the weight of the criterion times the rank within each criterion to obtain a score.
7. Sum the score for each intervention activity (moving horizontally across the matrix) to obtain a feasibility index.

The relative "best choice" intervention can be selected by finding the highest feasibility index. It is never wise to select an intervention based on one conspicuous criterion. The objective process assesses each alternative in terms of all criteria.

Who Makes the Decision?

Group decision making is best when a high level of involvement and commitment by members will be needed to implement the decision.[3] At some point, however, it is important for a manager to fix some aspects of the process so that they are effectively removed from constant deliberations. For example, the forms illustrated in this chapter fix the criterion.

A group of individuals facing a complex but important decision often disagree. Decisions are multifaceted and there is no one right answer. It is critical to understand that opposition will exist and that the process of exploring and discussing opposing points of view usually improves the final decision. Using the decision-making process with specific criteria structures the discussion around important and relevant factors. An objective process leads to a defensible decision rather than one based on preconceived ideas and power tactics.

In some organizations and certain situations, the decisions will be made unilaterally by the supervisor, nutrition director, manager, or president. Unilateral decisions may be more efficient and even necessary in certain situations (e.g., in an emergency, when confidentiality is imperative, or when the support of others is not necessary to implement a solution). However, unilateral decisions may suffer from lack of information.

Management decisions may also be made with staff input. The manager may ask for others' opinions: "I'm thinking about doing it this way. What's your reaction?" The manager may or may not consider these staff opinions in making the decision.

Participatory decision making is more costly in terms of staff time, but a shared understanding of the problem, generation of creative alternative solutions, open consideration of the strengths and limitations of alternatives, and commitment to the final solutions are valuable payoffs.

Each of these approaches to decision making is appropriate for certain situations. Some are more efficient and less time-consuming. Others take more time, but when high commitment and involvement are needed, the extra time taken to involve others is essential.

ESTABLISH GOALS AND OBJECTIVES

Goals and objectives give meaning and direction to the work of the people associated with the organization. They are standards by which organizations can judge their performance.

Goals state what is to be achieved and may state when results are to be accomplished, but they do not state how the results are to be achieved. Objectives are subordinate to goals and are more specific and measurable. Both goals and objectives express desired results.

A goal is usually a statement of broad direction, general purpose, or wide interest. Goals tend to be broad, all-encompassing ideals because they are derived from values. The formulation of abstract goals is essential because many of the most important human goals can adequately and meaningfully be stated only in general terms. Goals may be somewhat unreachable. An example of such a goal statement is "to increase the health status and quality of life for the citizens of this state."

Objectives are more concrete, closer in time, and more measurable than goals. Although each problem may have only one goal, each goal usually has several objectives. Objectives are specific measurable statements of what one wants to accomplish by a given point in time. Objectives provide the main energizing and directive force for managerial action. Objectives are the focal point around which managers concentrate their efforts and mobilize available resources. Specific objectives serve as control points for evaluation.

Writing Goals

A goal is the "other side" of the problem. A written goal is a positive statement of what would exist if the problem was no longer there. For example, a goal might be "to reduce the number of premature deaths related to a high-fat diet." Goals should be future oriented, simple, easily understood, and broad.

Writing Objectives

The general guideline to formulating objectives for a person, unit, section, or department is to state the objectives in terms of expected results, not in terms of activities or processes and not in general terms. The objectives must be tangible and recognizable so they can be communicated to all those involved in planning and implementation.

Model state nutrition objectives have been developed to allow states to "identify their own target populations, focus on dietary intake and the food supply, and include objectives related to the delivery of service."[11] Objectives contain four common elements: (1) an indicator (the problem being addressed), (2) a target (who or what), (3) a time frame, and (4) the amount of change expected in either the indicator or the target. To be properly evaluated, an objective must be stated in numerical terms, indicate the present status of the objective, and indicate the status to be achieved.[8] For example, "By 1994, 48% (up from 20% in 1988) of Vision City adults will exercise at least three times per week. By 1994, Vision City adults will show a 28% increase (from 1988) in the number exercising at least three times per week." Two specific formulas for writing sound objectives are:

1. To *(action verb) (desired result) (time frame) (resource required)*.
2. By *(date)*, the following results will have been accomplished.

Outcome and Process Objectives

A common problem faced by people who are writing objectives is how to link what may be a long-term and rather unmeasurable goal with objectives that can be measured in a month, a year, or 4 years. Another challenge is to write objectives that not only tell you how you are getting from one point to another but also whether you are even going in the right direction. Bridging objectives and outcome and process objectives help to meet those challenges. All three types of objectives are important to effective program planning and implementation.

Outcome objectives define a desired future state via a unit of measure (indicator) at some point in the future. Indicators are often morbidity or mortality data or other health status data. Outcome objectives are *not* steps, processes, or actions to achieve that result. In the medical arena, outcome

Planning

Formulation ⎯⎯⎯⎯⎯⎯⎯⎯⎯⎯⎯⎯⎯→
(Deciding what to do) ←⎯⎯⎯⎯⎯⎯⎯⎯⎯⎯

Organizing/directing

Implementation
(Achieving results through
doing)

1. Needs assessment

2. Prioritize problems

3. Select intervention by determining the organization's material, technical, financial, and managerial resources

4. Personal values and professional responsibility to society

5. Determine goals and objectives

> Organizational Strategy/mission
>
> Pattern of purposes and policies defining the company and its business

1. Develop a clear definition of the technical aspects of the program and intervention strategies; balance with clients' needs and wants

2. Identify organization structure and relationships.
   Delegation of authority
   Coordination of divided responsibility
   Information systems

3. Organizational processes and behavior
   Managing conflict
   Managing organizational change
   Staff development

4. Directing
   Communicating
   Motivating
   Problem solving

> Leadership strategies, organizational, personal qualities

Figure 14-3. Leadership strategies, organization, personal qualities.
Adapted from Quinn J, Mintzberg H, James RM. *The strategy process: concepts, contexts, and cases,* Englewood Cliffs, NJ, 1988, Prentice Hall.

objectives are intended to define the desired health state.

Process objectives define benchmarks for how the intervention will be implemented. They express the "who will do what by when." Process objectives are used to guide and assess progress.

Intermediate objectives (or bridging objectives) are partial measures of the larger outcome. They bridge the gap between the specific activities planned (process objectives) and the long-term outcomes (outcome objectives). These objectives access certain measures that have a high probability of reducing the health problem. They can measure the impact of a specific intervention. Intermediate objectives usually measure changes in knowledge, attitudes, beliefs, values, skills, behaviors, and practices. Depending on the problem, it is often easier and less expensive to measure the short-term outcomes in individuals than the final outcome of a health problem in the community.

Can Goals and Objectives Change or Be Revised?

Goals reflect the basic principles and fundamental values of an organization, and thus they do not change substantially over time. Drucker challenges nonprofit organizations to set specific goals in terms of their service to people.[2] Drucker sees service organizations as "human-change agents" that need to raise goals constantly to increase performance expectations.

Priority public health problems are often emerging and complex. In new situations, the definition of realistic results and target timelines must be arbitrary and approximate. An assessment of the progress toward the 1990 objectives for the nation found that not all important objectives were measurable. But, with greater understanding of the problem, development of relevant indicators, and deliberate information gathering and evaluation, over time objectives can become more realistic and measurable in subsequent planning cycles.

Goals and objectives provide the basis for guiding, leading, and directing the organization and the work group.

SUMMARY

In these difficult economic times with a constantly changing environment, dietitians and nutritionists must have a strong knowledge base and skills in planning, community assessment, strategic thinking, and decision making. Dietitians and nutritionists must be able to create a vision for ideal nutritional care for all community members. This requires strategic thinking and planning for outcomes. The needs assessment processes, specific techniques that prioritize problems, and intervention alternatives using criteria are important tools to guide the planning process efficiently.

Planning focuses and directs efforts, relates resources to desired goals, and sets objectives to determine outcomes. The planning process is strengthened by involving others within the organization in the process, particularly those who will be responsible for implementation.

To make planning an effective process, a community needs assessment is necessary to obtain quantitative and qualitative information and to identify nutrition-related problems and opportunities for reducing these problems. With an understanding of the overall problem, it will be important to prioritize needs and actions in order to select a manageable number of problems to address in the community. Formulating priorities is not implementing programs; rather, it is an approach to give the planner the ability to state clearly why the problems identified should or should not be addressed. Generating ideas for possible interventions is important in order to determine how practical or impractical a program may be to manage.

The planning process involves decision making at every juncture. Sound decisions emerge from an objective decision-making process. Goals and objectives give direction to the work of the organizations. They are standards by which organizations can judge their performance.

FROM PLANNING TO IMPLEMENTATION

Planning makes the transition to implementation after the point of deciding which existing or new programs will be implemented to address the priority problems. The analysis of alternatives involves consideration of programmatic approaches for moving toward health goals and specific measurable objectives in light of priority needs, available resources, and existing constraints. Planning begins with the review of mission and strategies, moves through identification of issues and needs, and ends with a commitment to priority program areas and the specification of goals and objectives. The relationship among the key activities of formulation (planning) and implementation (organizing and directing) are illustrated in Figure 14-3. Both are connected to the overall strategy and mission: note that all phases of planning, organizing, and directing use strategic organization and personal lead-

PHASES OF PLANNING

Strategy (Direction setting)	Vision:	The organization will be recognized in the community and across the state for its leadership in addressing food and nutrition issues that impact the quality of life of people in this region.
	Strategy:	The organization will keep food and nutrition issues before the public and propose solutions that will improve the health and nutritional well-being of the public.
Policy planning (Prioritization)	Mission:	To assure the provision of high-quality nutrition services that achieve and maintain optimal nutrition status for all members of the population through the development of a comprehensive, accessible, community-based system of nutrition-related services in collaboration with other providers in the community.
	Problem priority:	The organization should initiate and take a leadership role in a program of coordinated activities that assures availability of adequate health-promoting foods to homeless children.
	Goal:	To assure that all children (aged 3 to 9) who reside in temporary shelters have access to foods consistent with their nutritional and developmental needs.
	Objective:	By 1995, all temporary shelters housing children will offer foods consistent with children's nutritional and developmental needs.
	Outcome objective:	By 1995, 100% of children aged 3 to 9 staying in temporary shelters will receive meals and snacks consistent with their nutritional and developmental needs.
	Process objectives:	By 1993, 100% (from 0% in 1990) of the temporary shelters with feeding programs will be exposed to information on low-cost foods to meet children's nutritional and developmental needs.
		By 1993, the four temporary shelters that house children and have no hot food service will be assisted in developing facilities for food storage, preparation, and service.
	Intermediate objectives:	By 1993, 80% (from 40% in 1990) of the temporary shelters will serve hot or cold meals consistent with children's nutritional and developmental needs.

ership qualities. The box shown above gives examples of the phases of planning and illustrates the increasing specificity as one moves down the organizational hierarchy. The implementation phase will be discussed in greater detail in the following chapter.

REFERENCES

1. Committee on Diet and Health, Food and Nutrition Board, Commission on Life Sciences, and National Research Council: *Diet and health implications for reducing chronic disease risk*, Washington, DC, 1989, National Academy Press.
2. Drucker PF: *Managing the non-profit organization*, New York, 1990, Harper Collins.
3. Fink A and others: Consensus methods: characteristics and guidelines for use, *Am J Public Health* 74:979, 1984.
4. Haimann T, Scott WG, Connor PE: *Management*, ed 4, Boston, 1982, Houghton Mifflin.
5. Hamel G, Yves D, Prahalad C: Collaborate with your competitors and win, *Harvard Business Review* 89:133, 1989.
6. Institute of Medicine, National Academy of Science: *The future of public health*, Washington, DC, 1988, National Academy Press.
7. Kanter RM: *The change masters: innovation and entrepreneurship in the American corporation*, New York, 1984, Simon & Schuster.
8. Klerman LV, Russel AY, Valadian I: *Promoting health of women and children through planning*, Washington, DC, 1982, Department of Health and Human Services.
9. Kotler P: *Strategic marketing for non-profit organizations*, Englewood Cliffs, NJ, 1987, Prentice Hall.
10. Minnesota Department of Health: *A guide for promoting health in Minnesota: a community approach*, Minneapolis, 1988, Minnesota Department of Health.

11. Model Standards Work Group: *Model standards: a guide for community preventive health services*, McLean Va., 1987, Association of State and Territorial Health Officers.
12. Quinn J: Strategy for change: logical incrementalism, Holmswood, Ill, 1980, R.D. Irwin.
13. Sharbough C, editor: Call to action: better nutrition for mothers, children and families. Washington, DC, 1990, National Center for Education in Maternal and Child Health.
14. Speigel AD, Hyman HH: *Basic health planning methods*, Germantown, Md, 1978, Aspen.

APPENDIX 14-1

Case Study, Vision City, USA

Vision City is an urban city located in the United States with a temperate climate and a mean temperature of 70° F. It has four distinct seasons. Its dominant geographic feature is the Heartland River, which borders the western side of the city.

DEMOGRAPHIC CHARACTERISTICS

The distinct characteristic of Vision City is that the proportion of elderly people and middle-aged working adults has increased in recent years. In fact, the elderly population has increased faster than the total population because of movement into the city. People have stated a variety of reasons for moving into the city, but the more commonly heard are access to many health services, availability of recreation, and lack of job opportunities in their former communities. The employment rate of the labor force has increased in most households. In some cases, however, employment has not provided enough income to prevent poverty. A significant number of households headed by women live in poverty.

Sex and Age Distribution

The population pyramid identifies the age distribution in Vision City (Table 14-A). Note the baby-boom generation population size and that there are more women ages 35 to 54 available to work than men. Moreover, the shift in the elderly population has changed the dependency ratio (Table 14-B). The *dependency ratio* is a rough measure of the number of nonworking persons who must be supported economically by the working population. For example, it is estimated that for every 79 nonworking people in Vision City, 100 working people are required to economically support them. Even though the youth dependency ratio has dropped from 10 years ago, it still remains greater than the aged dependency ratio.

Table 14-A. Sex and age distribution in Vision City, USA

	Total	Male (%)	Female
All ages (yr)	500,000	241,680 (48.0%)	258,320
< 5	35,893	17,049 (47.5%)	18,844
5-14	135,205	68,955 (51.0%)	66,250
15-19	26,623	14,643 (55.0%)	11,980
20-34	127,676	70,222 (55.0%)	57,454
35-54	95,473	38,189 (40.0%)	57,284
55-64	29,395	13,962 (47.5%)	15,433
65-79	41,735	15,860 (38.0%)	25,875
80+	8,000	2,800 (35.0%)	5,200

Table 14-B. Dependency ratio of persons younger than 15 years and older than 64 years per 100 people

Dependency ratios	1990	1980
Aged dependency ratio*	18	17
Youth dependency ratio†	61	76
TOTAL	79	93

*Aged dependency ratio is calculated as the ratio of population 65 and older to the population ages 15 to 64.
†Youth dependency ratio is calculated as the ratio of population younger than 15 years to the population ages 15 to 64.

Table 14-C. Race and median age distribution percentage of ethnic and minority groups in Vision City

Race	%	N	Median age
White	60	300,000	31.9
Black	17	85,000	25.0
Asian/Pacific Islander	10	50,000	28.7
Hispanic	5	25,000	23.2
North American/Eskimo/Aleut/Innuit	4	20,000	28.7
"Other"	4	20,000	N/A
TOTAL	100	500,000	

Race Distribution

Vision City has a variety of racial and ethnic groups (Table 14-C). In the case of Hispanics, specific neighborhoods are primarily Spanish-speaking. The median age distribution among the racial groups varies substantially.

Employment and Economic Income

In Vision City, 9% of the work force is unemployed. Seventy percent of women aged 15 to 55 years are employed. The median income for a family of four for the total population is $26,900. For low-income households of four persons, the median income is $15,000. Figure 14-A shows the sources of household income for the total and low-income population.

Figure 14-B identifies the types of low-income households. Of the total population in Vision City, 11% do not have health insurance. Of the low-income households, more than half of the adult members skipped at least one meal per month because of lack of money, and 20% of the households with children reported their children had involuntarily missed meals. Lack of money affects finding affordable, adequate housing, paying for basic necessities, and carying adequate medical coverage. These factors influence diet and health.

Factors affecting diet and health are complex. Low levels of educational attainment, subtle discrimination, and low income interfere with health-promoting behaviors. Table 14-D identifies some family characteristics in Vision City.

Table 14-D. Family characteristics of Vision City, USA

Characteristics	General population	Low income
Average family size	2.5	4
Educational attainment		
Completed HS or GED	91%	64%
College degree	25%	5%
Employment		
Full-time	57%	26%
Part-time	14%	21%
Low literacy	3%	10%

VITAL HEALTH STATISTICS

The birthrate for all women in Vision City is 14 births/1000 population. A substantial problem in Vision City is the high birthrate among teenage women (see Table 14-E). *Morbidity* can be defined as the number of sick persons or cases of disease in relationship to a specific population. Morbidity identifies health conditions that interfere with life activities. It is lost human potential. *Mortality* is the number of deaths in a given population. The infant mortality rate by race in Vision City and the United States are identified in Table 14-F.

The top five causes of death by life stages for Vision City are outlined in Table 14-G. The components of morbidity for life stages are described in Table 14-H.

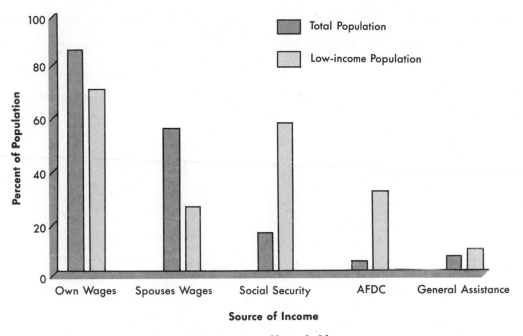

Figure 14-A. Sources of household income.

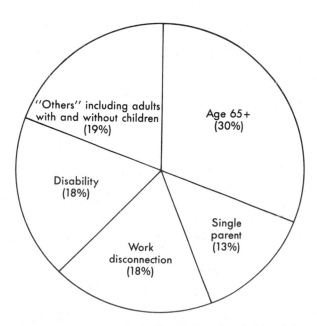

Figure 14-B. Types of low-income households. "Others" includes adults with and without children.

Table 14-E. Teenage birthrate among women of Vision City

Age (yr)	Birthrate/1000 population
10-14	1.2
15-17	31.8
18-19	80.2

Table 14-F. Infant mortality rates of United States and Vision City

Population	Infant mortality rate
United States (all races)	10.2
Vision City	
White	9.4
Black	18.4
Southeast Asian	N/A
American Indian	10.0

QUESTIONS FOR STUDY

Sex and Age Distribution

As a public health nutritionist,

1. Which age category would appear to be of highest priority? Why?
2. Where would you go to obtain additional information in a community nutrition needs assessment? (Please refer to Table 14-2 in this chapter.)
3. What additional sex or age information might be useful? (Hint: Note the age breakdowns. Do community members aged 35 to 54 have similar health needs?)
4. Note the baby-boom generation population size. There are more women than men aged 35 to 54 years available to work. What does this tell you about the kinds of jobs available in Vision City?
5. How would you motivate someone to return to work in order to be able to economically support nonworking dependents? (See Table 14-B.)

Race Distribution

1. Considering the race distribution in Vision City, is any ethnic group more advantageous to target with a nutrition intervention program? Why?
2. Considering the race distribution, what health risk behaviors are most important to address? Why? (Hint: Refer to Table 140-H, which lists risk factors.)
3. Why do you think Hispanics have the lowest median age? How would the median age of races affect access, availability, and appropriateness of health care services?

Employment and Economic Income

1. Is a 9% unemployment rate for Vision City higher or lower than the nation's unemployment rate? How would you find the national unemployment rate?
2. Define the difference between median income and mean income. Which income level is used to determine WIC eligibility?
3. What programs are available to those households that are skipping meals because of lack of money?
4. Who would be helpful collaborators in developing a program that addresses housing and health care insurance needs?
5. Brainstorm some ideas for programs that would target the low literacy populations.

Vital Health Statistics

1. What would be some nutritional goals and objectives for programs offering services to teenaged mothers? Who would be some effective collaborators? What programs might already be in place?
2. Study Table 14-F, the infant mortality rate of Vision City and the United States. Does any race have a greater need than other races? What are some nutrition intervention strategies that would reduce the mortality rate? What do you think the mortality rate of Southeast Asians is?
3. The federal government is offering a large block grant to reduce the number of deaths in Vision City. By studying Table 14-G, which cause of

Table 14-G. Top five causes of death by life stages in Vision City

Rank	Infants under 1	Children 1-14	Adolescents 15-19	Adults 20-34	Mature adults 35-64	Older adults 65-74	Older adults 75+	Total population
1	Birth-associated development problems	Accidental death by motor vehicle	Accidental death by motor vehicle	Accident	Heart disease	Heart disease	Heart disease	Heart disease
2	Congenital birth defects	Cancer	Suicide	Suicide	Cancer	Cancer	Stroke	Cancer
3	Ill-defined condition (SIDS)	Congenital birth defects	Cancer	Cancer	Accident	Stroke	Cancer	Stroke
4	Immaturity	Diseases of nervous system	Homicide	Heart disease	Diseases of digestive system	Diseases of digestive systems	Influenza and pneumonia	Accident
5	Infections and parasitic diseases	Homicide	Injuries undetermined	Homicide	Stroke	Influenza and pneumonia	Arterio-sclerosis	Influenza and pneumonia

Table 14-H. Vision City morbidity by life stages

Infants and children	Adolescents	Adults 20-34	Mature adults 35-64	Older adults 65 +
Components				
Child maltreatment	Depression		Dental disease	Limitations in activity due to chronic conditions
Learning disorders	Teenage pregnancy	Occupational injury	Diabetes	Physical disabilities; hypertension; cancer; accidents and falls
Handicapping conditions	Sexually transmitted diseases AIDS	Diabetes	Arthritis	Perceived health status needs
Communicable diseases	Acne	Dental disease	Cancer	Social isolation
Accidents and homicide	Overweight and underweight	AIDS; infectious diseases	Circulatory diseases	Dependency
Dental disease	Accidental injury	Alcohol and drug abuse	Hypertension	Depression
Developmental delay	Handicapping conditions	Hypertension; obesity	Alcohol and drug abuse	Drug misuse
Growth failure	Dental disease	Depression; cancer	Infectious diseases	Infectious diseases
Anemia	Eating disorders; anemia	Heart disease	Obesity	Obesity
AIDS	Alcohol and drug abuse			Inadequate nutritional intake

death would you recommend targeting? Are there any nutrition implications related to this cause of death?

Available Health and Nutrition Resources

1. For the morbidity by life stages in Vision City listed in Table 14-H, what nutritional behaviors would relate to their development?
2. What resources are available to improve the health status of the specific minority populations in Vision City?

Political Structure

1. Why is it beneficial to have Senator Jones a member of the Agricultural, Nutrition, and Forestry Committee?

2. Is it ethical to develop a community program for persons with Alzheimer's disease, knowing that Representative Smith has a personal interest? Discuss the pros and cons.
3. What government agency monitors day-care programs? What is the weakness of setting nutrition standards if there are day-care centers that are not licensed by the government? Who would monitor food served in nonlicensed day-care centers?
4. What are some health outcome indicators associated with good nutritional care of older adults in nursing homes?

Lifestyle, Environmental, and Social Structure

1. Brainstorm some possible interventions to ad-

dress the health, eating, and exercise concerns of Vision City. If a fast-food restaurant was willing to fund a program, how would this change your intervention?

2. Which group's behaviors would be more difficult to change: those who state they intend to exercise more or those who do not get regular exercise?

CHAPTER

15

Nutrition Assessment

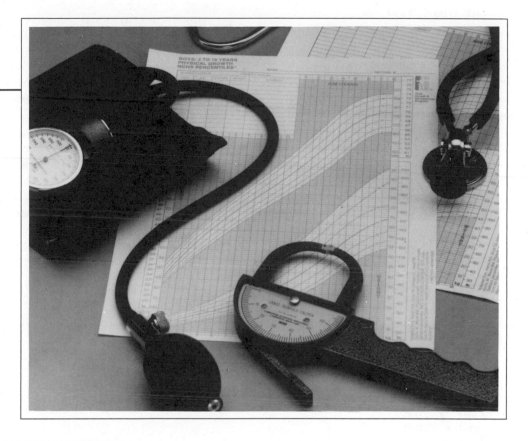

GENERAL CONCEPT

Knowledge of the community is essential to managing community nutrition services. Dietitians and nutritionists may find that their community is as large as an entire state or as small as a health maintenance organization. They may be charged with the vague responsibility to improve the nutritional health of the entire community or the precisely defined responsibilities within a federally mandated program. Some form of nutritional assessment will be part of managing nutrition services (see Chapter 13). Traditional measures of nutritional status are used in (1) assessing the needs of the community, (2) developing the program or nutritional service, (3) managing and monitoring day-to-day implementation of the program, and (4) evaluating the success of the program. The classical methods for nutritional assessment constitute a small part of the information needed to plan and provide nutrition services that truly meet the needs of the community. A general conceptual model of the role of food supply, sociocultural and economic factors, food choices, and nutrient intake in the nutrition-related health status of a population or community is shown in Figure 15-1. It is clear from the model that if nutrition programs and services are to have an impact on the outputs (nutritional status and health), they must modify the input boxes to the left of the diagram. The focus of nutritional assessment of the community is not only to identify the outputs in need of improvement but also to characterize the inputs most appropriate for modification. This means we must understand the food supply, food selection and preparation, social structures, and community contexts if we are to make appropriate interventions.

OUTCOME OBJECTIVES

When you finish this chapter, you should be able to:

- Use the classical measures of nutritional status for needs assessment, program development, program implementation, and program evaluation.
- Define and explain reference populations, nutrition screening, monitoring, and surveillance.
- Identify various resources such as nutritional guidelines, census data, zip code clusters, disease prevalence data, national nutrition surveys, and available nutrition services that can be used to characterize your community and its nutrition needs.
- List some approaches for collecting primary data on foodways, food consumption patterns, and perceived nutritional concerns of community members that can form the basis for program development and implementation.
- Gather bits and pieces of information into a form that allows you to identify the most pressing nutrition problems, the number of people needing service, and the most appropriate approaches to defining and implementing the service.
- Identify the measures of nutritional status to screen for individuals in greatest need of the nutritional service.
- Define the concepts of sensitivity, specificity, and the predictive value of a test, and explain how they are used to select nutritional status measures, appropriate cut-points, and combinations of measures to meet the objectives of the service you plan to provide.

NATIONAL FOOD SUPPLY ⟶ FOOD DISTRIBUTION ⟶ CONSUMPTION ⟶

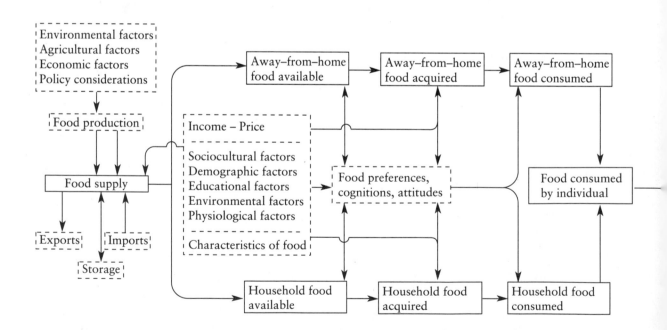

WHAT IS NUTRITIONAL STATUS?

The Joint Nutrition Monitoring Evaluation Committee describes "the nutritional status of an individual as the condition of his or her health as influenced by the intake and utilization of nutrients. Because nutritional status cannot be measured directly by any single test, assessment is dependent on the collective interpretation of relevant dietary and health data."[3] Therefore, nutritional status encompasses two types of measurements: measures of health and measures of diet. Health measures such as heights and weights, plasma cholesterol levels, or the presence of clinical deficiency symptoms alone are insufficient because they are outcomes that may have multiple causes, only one of which is diet. Likewise, measures of diet alone

may or may not indicate health consequences for a particular individual. We should be impeccable in our language when we speak of nutritional status and assessment so that the distinctions between health and diet measures are clear.

Measures of health and diet status fall into four categories:

1. Anthropometric: measurement of the size of body components (examples: height, weight, arm muscle area, body mass index).
2. Biochemical: measurement of the concentrations of substances in body fluids or tissues (examples: plasma cholesterol, urinary creatinine, red blood cell folic acid, glucose tolerance curves).
3. Clinical: assessment of characteristics asso-

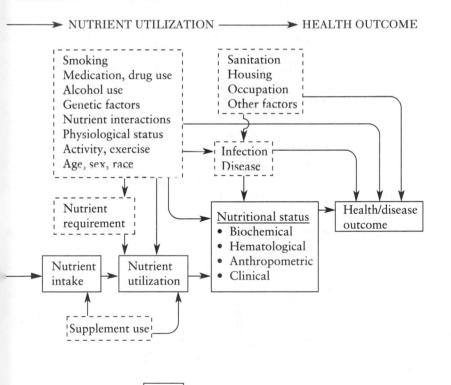

Figure 15-1. General conceptual model for food choice, food and nutrient intake, and nutritional and health status.
Source: DHHS, PHS, and USDA, FCS: *Nutrition Monitoring in the United States,* DHHS Pub (PHS) 89-1255, Washington, DC, 1989, US Government Printing Office.

ciated with nutrient deficiency or excess (examples: Bitot's spots on eyes, xanthomas, dull hair, bowed legs).

4. Dietary: assessment of nutrient intakes including food supply, foodways, preparation, and storage (examples: usual intake generated from food frequency tools, recent intake generated from diet recalls, food preparation such as frying, salting, and type of cooking utensils).

A fifth category shows promise:

5. Functional: measurement of performance on a physical or physiological test (examples: grip strength, memory, attention span, respiratory muscle strength).

We are limited to assessment measures with standards of evaluation that have been developed for populations similar to the community of interest. The dietitian and nutritionist generally work with very simple measures of nutritional status. Good textbooks that describe well-established measures of nutritional status and reference standards are available.[12,14] These texts are useful references for the dietitians and nutritionist. In addition, two excellent texts on food consumption methodology that cover all techniques, their uses, and interpretations have recently been published.[2,8]

Identification of a nutrition-related problem within a community is based on a number of abnormal values measuring different aspects of the problem because no one measure is adequate. For example, correct identification of iron deficiency anemia may require three different biochemical measures and indications that iron intake or bioavailability has been low.

A relatively new class of assessment measures has become prominent. Identification of risk factors for diseases with nutritional components can be useful for assessment purposes. Biochemical, anthropometric, and dietary factors can be used to measure risk for chronic diseases such as hypertension, non-insulin-dependent diabetes, cancer, and heart disease. The presence of the risk factor(s) rather than the disease itself triggers the development of appropriate nutrition services. This development has come with the understanding that chronic diseases take a long time to develop and that significant prevention can be achieved by the elimination of the risky behaviors. It is important to be clear about whether you are assessing a risk factor, the actual presence of poor nutritional status, or the chronic disease itself.

DEFINING TERMS COMMONLY USED IN LARGE NUTRITIONAL ASSESSMENT PROGRAMS

A number of terms are in current use among dietitians, nutritionists, and epidemiologists charged with monitoring the nutritional health of the nation. A *nutrition survey* is a study conducted over a relatively short time of a representative sample of a community by using a variety of measures of nutritional status, from which a numerical and descriptive picture of the nutrition problems of the community is developed. Surveys are generally expensive. They require an accurate enumeration of the population and skilled field personnel and data managers. The National Health and Nutrition Examination Surveys (NHANES) are recent examples. From these surveys comes the concept of reference populations. A *reference population* is an apparently healthy population for which measurements have been made for particular nutritional status parameters, and the distribution of values of the parameter are used as a reference for normality rather than a normal range. An example is the use of the 75th percentile of the NHANES I adult population as a cut-point for obesity rather than the Metropolitan Life weight-for-height tables.

Nutrition monitoring refers to the periodic observation and measurement of the nutritional status of a population. National nutrition monitoring collects, analyzes, and disseminates timely data on the nutritional and dietary status of the population, the nutritional quality of the food supply, food consumption patterns, and consumer knowledge and attitudes concerning nutrition. Monitoring activities identify high-risk groups and nutrition-related problems and trends in order to implement intervention activities.

Nutrition surveillance refers to the continuous collection of nutrition-related data on high-risk populations participating in nutrition programs. The monitoring of high-risk populations can alert planners to developing problems because more vulnerable populations often present with problems before the rest of the population.

NUTRITIONAL STATUS MEASURES USED IN PUBLIC HEALTH AND COMMUNITY NUTRITION PROGRAMS

Needs Assessment

The first part of this text discusses identification of nutrition-related problems. Familiarity with the national nutrition surveys, surveillance, and monitoring systems gives you insight into possible problems within the communities you serve. You will want to know how your particular community compares with the Year 2000 Objectives, the Dietary Guidelines, and other measures. We discuss in this chapter the resources available to you and how you can use them to assess the nutritional needs of your community. A clear understanding of the needs of your community and its subgroups is the foundation for effective programs. You also must describe the base where your community started if you are going to be able to describe what your program achieved. (See Chapter 14.)

Example

You are employed in the health department of a major Midwestern city with a sizable Hispanic population that is gaining political influence. Money becomes available from the mayor's office to start a highly visible nutrition project in the Hispanic part of the city. Budget limitations require it to be an education program rather than any sort of feeding program. The staff at the mayor's office say that they need the outlines of a possible program in a week.

By referring to the national data and consulting with dietitians, nutritionists, and other health professionals working in the community, you identify low consumption of fruits and vegetables as a major nutrition-related problem. You also identify the concerns of the community leaders that had generated the movement of money from the mayor's office.

In the proposal you must include data on the extent of the problem in the community and compare it to the national goals. How do you document the likely extent of the problem on such short notice? One of the national goals[6] is five or more servings per day of fruits and vegetables for an adult (the national estimate is only 2.5 servings per day). There is a high likelihood that the target Hispanic community is close to this estimate. WIC program diet assessments, diet records, and interviews with local dietitians and nutritionists can be used to estimate daily consumption rates of fruits and vegetables. Supermarkets and other food vendors in the community can give you an idea of availability and cost relative to surrounding communities. Accurate assessment of baseline values should be incorporated into the program you devise for program evaluation purposes. National data can be used to predict the effect of a number of health issues, from obesity to cancer, as the community reaches the national goal with respect to fruit and vegetable consumption. Identifying the nutritional needs of your community by using nutritional status measures is the foundation of any good program.

Program Development

Few programs are successful without built-in measures of success so that participants can assess their accomplishments. These measures must be easy to perform in terms of time, cost, and burden and yet be accurate. Therefore, the limitations of the assessment measures within the context of the community and the program to be developed have a bearing on the design of the intervention. (See Chapter 16.)

Example

You are an extension agent for a Louisiana parish. In your assessment of the needs of the community, you see that hypertension is a problem. You know that Louisiana is known for the highest per capita salt consumption in the United States. Because the extension's mission is to the entire healthy population, you enlist the help of other health organizations for a concerted effort. As a group, you contemplate the goals from *Healthy People 2000* regarding salt intake.[6] These goals are (1) that at least 65% of home meal preparers prepare foods without adding salt, (2) that at least 80% of the people avoid using salt at the table, and (3) that at least 40% of the adults regularly purchase foods that are lower in sodium. It is decided that these goals are overly ambitious for this community, and the group settles for the following goals: (1) salt reductions at the table and (2) use of lower-salt foods.

Past efforts using educational pamphlets alone met with minimal effect on salt intake and no change in the extent of hypertension in the parish. Therefore, you design a program with some excitement and payoff. The program involves a communitywide competition in which local organizations can earn money and prizes if their members succeed in obtaining the lowest salt intake. Clear plastic saltshakers containing a premeasured amount of salt are issued to participants. Flame photometers are set up in two major shopping malls with technicians available to run urine samples. Directions on collecting overnight urine samples as well as booklets on how to lower salt intake are made available in stores and other public places. Prizes, saltshakers, and the flame photometers are donated from local business organizations. Final prizes are awarded based on the sodium content of urine collections for each organization. Assessment is immediate for the participants because they see the salt disappearing from the saltshaker and can check their urine sodium output during the campaign. Technicians obtain the data on urine submitted during the campaign as well as the final competition. The final saltshaker weigh-in gives some idea of success in meeting the Year 2000 Goal in highly motivated groups. The nutritional assessment measures are an integral part of the program and the basis of program excitement. The program could be the "Talk of the Parish."

Monitoring Programs in Progress

Much can happen after a program is conceived and implemented. The goals of program monitoring are to maintain quality and make corrections when a program is falling short of its intended results. Program procedures and nutritional assessment mea-

sures should be included in the monitoring process, especially for large programs that are being implemented in a number of locations. These programs must have objective measures taken consistently to assure the quality of the program on a long-term basis. (See Chapter 18.)

Example

The WIC program has been considered a highly successful program, despite the necessity of operating in many locations under varying circumstances and contending with high staff turnover rates. How has it been so successful? Each clinic must report a number of different nutritional status measures both at baseline and at various times during a participant's program involvement. These measures include heights, weights, and hemoglobin levels of participants. These data are used as part of the national nutritional surveillance program and to assess the quality of each clinic's program. Early in the history of the WIC program, several clinics in one state appeared to have a preponderance of large weight for height babies, indicating a problem of overweight babies. Site visits to these clinics revealed that personnel were not properly obtaining the height of the babies because only one person was available to perform the measurements, a mandatory two-person operation (one person to fully extend the legs of an active baby and one person to hold the head and record the measurements). Without monitoring, it would have been difficult to identify clinics that were inappropriately reducing food prescriptions for inaccurately weighed infants. The anthropometric surveillance picked up the problem. Only with ongoing assessment can quality be maintained in any program.

Program Evaluation

The improvement of the nutritional status of a target community is the ultimate goal of most community nutrition programs. Therefore, it is imperative that a measure of nutritional status be incorporated into the evaluation of the program. It is unfortunate that many programs are developed and implemented without evaluation systems in place.

Evaluation is thought to be expensive and so when funds are limited it is often the first part of the program to be deleted. This is self-defeating because a convincing demonstration of the success of a program often brings more funds for its expansion or continuance. Evaluation usually involves the assessment of a status measure before and after intervention. Including a control group that did not receive intervention for comparison in the evaluation process is also very effective. This is often difficult and expensive but well worth including if possible. The selected measures should be objective, unambiguous, and easily performed. The measures should be easily interpreted and communicated to those who evaluate the program. This is often the public. Envision how you would communicate the success of the program to the public, and then incorporate the necessary evaluation measures. (See Chapter 18.)

Example

One of the major health status objectives of the nutrition section of *Healthy People 2000* is to reduce the incidence of overweight to no more than 20% of people aged 20 and older. Low-income and minority women have a higher prevalence of overweight (37% to 44%) than the general population. You are participating in the development of a community-based model program in a low-income African-American community in California. Your goal is to lower the percentage who are overweight of all adult women by 2% and the average weight of the overweight adult women in the community by 5 lb in one year. You have chosen a rather self-contained community of a large city served by two supermarkets. The community has many active social institutions including churches and a mosque. All are enthusiastic about program participation. The approach of the program is multifactorial and involves decreasing the fat and increasing the fiber, fruit, and vegetable intake of community members as a way to maintain and/or lose weight. The supermarkets will participate by featuring low-cost healthy choices. Restaurants will promote healthy menu items. Classes on choosing foods and modifying favorite recipes will be held at the churches and mosque. Demonstrations on how to prepare low-cost fruits and vegetables will be held in public places. Finally, weight reduction classes featuring behavior modification techniques will be made available for a nominal fee. The plan is to measure the heights and weights of the adult women in the community before and after the 1-year program. The percentage overweight and average weight difference of the overweight women will be calculated from this data. Most women frequent one of the supermarkets about once per week. While at the supermarket, they will be asked to have their weight and height measured in return for free food coupons (donated from food companies). The measurements at the supermarkets will use a randomized time sampling procedure and take place for an entire week. The hypothesis of the intervention is that although only 20% of the women will receive direct impact, 50% of the women will receive, either directly or indirectly, motivation and information. The success of the program depends not only on weight loss but also the failure to gain weight during the year.

In this example, a measure of nutritional status is used as the main evaluation for the success of a program. The measure is objective and inexpensive to implement, even on a communitywide basis. It is also easily understood by community members and public health planners as a measure of program success.

RESOURCES FOR ASSESSING NUTRITIONAL NEEDS

There is rarely enough money to perform classical nutrition surveys of a community, regardless of its size or constituency. How can the true needs of a specific community be identified so that scarce resources can be focused to the greatest need and the most appropriate programs?

Quite a bit can be accomplished by creatively using the resources at hand. Assessments made by looking at readily available information can allow you to estimate accurately enough for program development. Some valuable resources are discussed next.

Nutritional Goals and Guidelines

National nutrition goals and guidelines have been developed by assessing nutritional risk factors for various nutrition-related diseases and their prevalence in the United States compared with other parts of the world. The various dietary guidelines and Healthy People 2000 Nutrition Goals (see inside covers) are examples. They are generally in the form of dietary advice. Some of these guidelines are qualitative, using the terms "consume more" or "consume less." *Healthy People 2000*, the most recent and most comprehensive of the guidelines, gives quantitative dietary advice as well as baseline data for the population groups. For example,

2.5 Reduce dietary fat intake to an average of 30 percent of calories or less and average saturated fat

intake to less than 10% of calories among people aged 2 and older. (Baseline: 36 percent of calories from total fat and 13 percent from saturated fat for people aged 20 through 74 in 1976-80; 36 percent and 13 percent for women aged 19 through 50 in 1985).[6]

Such guidelines are the best starting point for your own exploration of the nutritional needs of the community you serve because they address the most prevalent nutritional needs in the United States. By determining whether your clients meet these nutritional goals, you can devise a plan of action for your community.

Example

You are responsible for providing nutrition advice and programming to the community of pregnant women surrounding a public obstetrics and gyne-

Table 15-1. Food and Nutrition Board, National Academy of Sciences—National Research Council Recommended Dietary Allowances,[a] Revised 1989. Designed for the maintenance of good nutrition of practically all healthy people in the United States

Category	Age (years) or condition	Weight[a] (kg)	Weight[a] (lb)	Height[b] (cm)	Height[b] (in)	Protein (g)	Fat-soluble vitamins Vitamin A (μg RE)[c]	Vitamin D (μg)[d]	Vitamin E (mg α-TE)[e]	Vitamin K (μg)	Vitamin C (mg)
Infants	0.0-0.5	6	13	60	24	13	375	7.5	3	5	30
	0.5-1.0	9	20	71	28	14	375	10	4	10	35
Children	1-3	13	29	90	35	16	400	10	6	15	40
	4-6	20	44	112	44	24	500	10	7	20	45
	7-10	28	62	132	52	28	700	10	7	30	45
Males	11-14	45	99	157	62	45	1000	10	10	45	50
	15-18	66	145	176	69	59	1000	10	10	65	60
	19-24	72	160	177	70	58	1000	10	10	70	60
	25-50	79	174	176	70	63	1000	5	10	80	60
	51+	77	170	173	68	63	1000	5	10	80	60
Females	11-14	46	101	157	62	46	800	10	8	45	50
	15-18	55	120	163	64	44	800	10	8	55	60
	19-24	58	128	164	65	46	800	10	8	60	60
	25-50	63	138	163	64	50	800	5	8	65	60
	51+	65	143	160	63	50	800	5	8	65	60
Pregnant						60	800	10	10	65	70
Lactating	1st 6 months					65	1300	10	12	65	95
	2nd 6 months					62	1200	10	11	65	90

[a]The allowances, expressed as average daily intakes over time, are intended to provide for individual variations among most normal persons as they live in the United States under usual environmental stresses. Diets should be based on a variety of common foods in order to provide other nutrients for which human requirements have been less well defined. See text for detailed discussion of allowances and of nutrients not tabulated.
[b]Weights and heights of reference adults are actual medians for the U.S. population of the designated age, as reported by NHANES II. The use of these figures does not imply that the height-to-weight ratios are ideal.

cology clinic, your base of operation. An economical approach to determining whether your pregnant women are obtaining adequate calcium is, rather than performing bone densitometry, to ask if they are consuming three or more servings of calcium-rich foods per day (one of the goals of the Healthy People 2000 Risk Reduction Objectives).

A caveat in using these guidelines rather than conducting a more extensive nutritional status survey is that your community may have more pressing problems than those addressed by the guidelines. You must know and understand the community you serve comprehensively if you are to accurately interpret the data obtained from dietary or nutritional assessment. (See Chapter 14.)

Example

After a quick community assessment, you discover that the chief problem in the rural area you serve is undernutrition brought on by a combination of low income, inadequate social services, and underutilization of the services available. Because most of the population is elderly, most of the *Healthy People 2000* objectives are not high priorities for your community.

The Recommended Dietary Allowances (RDAs) are a dietary guide in the form of quantities of nutrients that are likely to prevent deficiency diseases in most of the healthy population for various broad age and sex categories.[10] The RDAs for all nutrients, except kilocalories, are set two standard

Water-soluble vitamins						Minerals						
Thia-min (mg)	Ribo-flavin (mg)	Niacin (mg NE)^f	Vita-min B$_6$ (mg)	Fo-late (μg)	Vita-min B$_{12}$ (μg)	Cal-cium (mg)	Phos-phorus (mg)	Mag-nesium (mg)	Iron (mg)	Zinc (mg)	Iodine (μg)	Sele-nium- (μg)
0.3	0.4	5	0.3	25	0.3	400	300	40	6	5	40	10
0.4	0.5	6	0.6	35	0.5	600	500	60	10	5	50	15
0.7	0.8	9	1.0	50	0.7	800	800	80	10	10	70	20
0.9	1.1	12	1.1	75	1.0	800	800	120	10	10	90	20
1.0	1.2	13	1.4	100	1.4	800	800	170	10	10	120	30
1.3	1.5	17	1.7	150	2.0	1200	1200	270	12	15	150	40
1.5	1.8	20	2.0	200	2.0	1200	1200	400	12	15	150	50
1.5	1.7	19	2.0	200	2.0	1200	1200	350	10	15	150	70
1.5	1.7	19	2.0	200	2.0	800	800	350	10	15	150	70
1.2	1.4	15	2.0	200	2.0	800	800	350	10	15	150	70
1.1	1.3	15	1.4	150	2.0	1200	1200	280	15	12	150	45
1.1	1.3	15	1.5	180	2.0	1200	1200	300	15	12	150	50
1.1	1.3	15	1.6	180	2.0	1200	1200	280	15	12	150	55
1.1	1.3	15	1.6	180	2.0	800	800	280	15	12	150	55
1.0	1.2	13	1.6	180	2.0	800	800	280	10	12	150	55
1.5	1.6	17	2.2	400	2.2	1200	1200	320	30	15	175	65
1.6	1.8	20	2.1	280	2.6	1200	1200	355	15	19	200	75
1.6	1.7	20	2.1	260	2.6	1200	1200	340	15	16	200	75

^{c}Retinol equivalents. 1 retinol equivalent = 1 μg retinol or 6 μg β-carotene. See text for calculation of vitamin A activity of diets as retinol equivalents.
^{d}As cholecalciferol. 10 μg cholecalciferol = 400 IU of vitamin D.
^{e}α-Tocopherol equivalents. 1 mg d-α tocopherol = 1 α-TE. See text for variation in allowances and calculation of vitamin E activity of the diet as α-tocopherol equivalents.
^{f}1 NE (niacin equivalent) is equal to 1 mg of niacin or 60 mg of dietary tryptophan.

deviations above the estimated mean level needed for each particular age and sex group (See Table 15-1). For any one individual the RDAs are likely to be overestimates of their need, yet for 2% of the healthy population they are underestimates.

The RDAs constitute the only quantitative guidance available for estimating nutrient need. They have been used for a multitude of purposes in addition to those for which they were intended, the planning of diets and food supplies for groups of individuals such as armies and institutionalized communities. They have been used to set public policy for food stamp allowances, school food services, and congregate meals for the elderly. They are periodically reviewed by a panel of nutritional scientists whose commission is to assess new scientific evidence and new end points for establishing the average needs of various age and sex groups. Thus, the RDAs for nutrients change and will continue to change. Because public health programs are pegged to these requirements, these changes entangle public policy and science.

Example

The committee appointed to review the RDAs for the 1985 revisions proposed lowering the allowances for vitamins A and C in most age and sex categories. They based these decisions on new evidence concerning the amounts necessary to achieve body concentrations that prevent vitamin A and C–related outcomes in humans. Advocacy groups for federal food programs feared that reducing the RDAs for vitamins A and C would reduce the number of servings of fruits and vegetables (and therefore the total food allotment) used in setting the food stamp allowances, school lunch and breakfast programs, congregate meal programs for the elderly, and WIC. Advocates raised the issue that such a reduction in fruit and vegetable consumption would be occurring at the same time that many of the dietary goals and guidelines are advocating greater consumption of fruits and vegetables, mainly for the possibility that increased consumption would reduce the risk of selected cancers. In response, the Food and Nutrition Board did not accept the recommendations of the 1985

RDA Committee, and a new committee was appointed. The resulting RDAs were published in 1989 with vitamin A and C allowances no lower than the 1974 RDAs.

For better or worse, all these goals and guidelines are based on judgments that are a mix of science, practicality, and public policy. When using them for community assessment, be aware of the acceptability of the one you select for presentation to the committee that will promote, fund, or evaluate your program. Also resist the temptation to include the most current nutritional panacea, such as omega-3 fatty acids, oat bran, or the promising phytochemicals found in certain foods. These substances may be proved to be efficacious with further research, but their roles in the diet are uncertain. Research has not yet determined at what level they should be consumed or their importance in the diet.

An important proportion of any client community will fail to meet one or more of the dietary goals that now exist. You are on firm public policy ground when you use the national goals and guidelines to set your direction of action.

Using Goals, Guidelines and RDAs for Screening

In program planning, it is important to quantify the number of individuals at risk and in need of nutrition intervention services. This information determines the design and content of a program, as well as staffing needs.

The RDAs were never intended to be used for evaluating *individuals* but because there are no other guidelines for determining dietary adequacy they are often used for this purpose. The graph in Figure 15-2 refines the use of RDAs for assessment purposes.[1] The bell-shaped curve represents the distribution of nutrient requirements for any nutrient for a healthy population. Note the two lines below the graph of the curve. The first line indicates what the developers of this approach call the percent of recommended nutrient intake (RNI), which is merely the percentage of the RDAs. The second line assigns the probability that an individual's intake, expressed as percent of RNI, is below

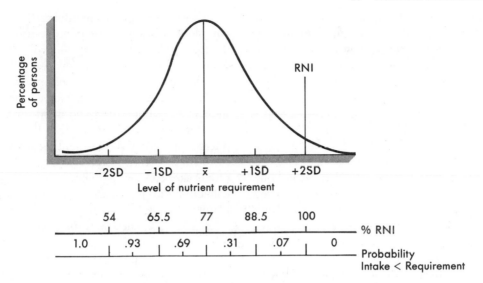

Figure 15-2. Assignment of "risk" or probability statements to observed intakes expressed as proportions of the recommended nutrient intake (RNI). Assumptions in the model are that the requirements are normally distributed with CV (coefficient of variation) = 15% and that the recommended intake is set at the average requirement +2 SD.
Source: Reprinted from Anderson GH, Peterson RD, Beaton GH: Estimating nutrient deficiencies in a population from dietary records: the use of probability analyses, *Nutrition Research* 2:409, 1982, with permission of Pergamon Press, Inc.

that individual's unique requirement. For example, a client whose usual vitamin C consumption is 67% of the RDAs would have almost an 80% risk for failing to meet vitamin C needs. Figure 15-2 is useful for choosing cut-points for assessing needs and program screening.

In the past we have used arbitrary cutpoints of two thirds or three quarters of the RDA to identify clients at risk. However, cutpoints for risk assessment and identification of clients often depend on available funds. If funds are limited, we would want to limit our services to those with the greatest risk, such as 50% of the RNI, which would mean that an individual consuming vitamin C at this level would be almost 100% likely to be consuming lower than required levels.

Quantitative guidelines such as those in *Healthy People 2000*[6] are useful for estimating the proportion of individuals in a community that fall short of

a particular goal. Guidelines that state outcomes in terms of "moderate use of alcohol" or "reducing sugar intake" must be converted to quantitative standards that can be assessed in prospective clients.

Example

It was determined that dental caries was a serious problem in a rural county in Virginia. Through interviews with dentists, assessment of food habits, and market research, a subset of the population was identified as having a high consumption of candy and other sweets. Funding was obtained for a pilot project aimed at changing the behavior of schoolage children with high sugar intakes. A quantitative definition of high intake, which was based upon scientific literature, was stated in terms of grams of simple sugars per 1000 kcal/day (i.e., sugar density). This had to be converted to easily measured behaviors in the form of a weekly sweets inventory along with sex, age, height, weight, and activity categories that could be quantified by computer spreadsheet using an optical scan reader to identify students who qualified for the behavior modification program.

Using Goals and Guidelines for Program Planning, Monitoring, and Evaluation

Use of preexisting goals and guidelines focuses your search for baseline data to establish need in your particular community and expected outcomes for your program. The more focus you can achieve early in the process, the greater the savings in time, effort, and cost. However, there are certain data that must be obtained for every community assessment, no matter how truncated the assessment is to be. You must define the population to be served and how they compare to the standards that you have set for improvement. Without a definition and quantification of the attributes to be changed, a proper evaluation of program effectiveness cannot be achieved. Without documentation of program effectiveness, worthwhile programs will not persist. (See Chapters 14 and 18.)

Resources for Defining the Community

Dietitians and nutritionists find themselves responsible for some surprisingly varied communities, ranging from an entire state to a very narrow subset of a geographically defined community such as elderly individuals within a municipality. The community could be confined to a particular corporation or HMO population. Although we discuss resources available for describing a community at large, the same principles can be applied to describing corporation employees or HMO subscribers.

Because the nutritional needs of a community and appropriate programs to address those needs depend on factors such as age, sex, socioeconomic status, level of education, housing, work, and family support structures, these data are the foundation of every community assessment. It is also imperative for the translation of national nutrition status information to the probable needs of your community.

Where do you find the information you need to complete a community demographic inventory? (See Chapter 14.) Census data broken down to the county and census tract level are available at your local library. Librarians can often assist you in locating the data you want. Census data give you most of the information you need for the community demographic inventory, but the census is conducted only every 10 years and the information may be too old to characterize your present community. Other agencies serving your community may have collected the information you need. Send your blank inventory with a request for leads to the various agencies. They may be able to provide the information you need.

With the advent of our information society and the need for identifying specific markets, the U.S population has been increasingly well characterized from our educational level to the food we purchase and the magazines we read. This information is available by zip code and zip code plus four, which identifies groups as small as one side of a street anywhere in the country. The availability of this information at a nominal cost from a variety of companies should revolutionize our ability to produce accurate needs assessments and appropriate programs for all sorts of communities. The story behind this possibility is described in *Clustering of America*.[13] Jonathan Robbin, a computer scientist, is credited with matching zip codes with census data and consumer surveys in 1974.[13] Performing cluster analysis by sorting the 36,000 U.S. zip codes, he identified 40 "lifestyle clusters" that would characterize the central tendency of the people living within each of these zip codes. These clusters (Table 15-2) are associated with age groups, buying habits, health problems by DRG, educational levels, socioeconomic groups, lifestyles, and beliefs on a whole range of subjects. A number of companies have sprung up to provide this information on ever smaller groups of people and wider ranges of attributes. Each has developed its own cluster names and description and, because populations and their attributes frequently change within a given zip code, the cluster names and descriptions are kept up-to-date. Most companies also provide 5-year projections. Large corporations purchase

Table 15-2. America's 40 neighborhood types

Cluster	Thumbnail description	Percent U.S. households
Blue Blood Estates	America's wealthiest neighborhoods includes suburban homes and one in ten millionaires	1.1
Money & Brains	Posh big-city enclaves of townhouses, condos and apartments	0.9
Furs & Station Wagons	New money in metropolitan bedroom suburbs	3.2
Urban Gold Coast	Upscale urban high-rise districts	0.5
Pools & Patios	Older, upper-middle-class, suburban communities	3.4
Two More Rungs	Comfortable multi-ethnic suburbs	0.7
Young Influentials	Yuppie, fringe-city condo and apartment developments	2.9
Young Suburbia	Child-rearing, outlying suburbs	5.3
God's Country	Upscale frontier boomtowns	2.7
Blue-Chip Blues	The wealthiest blue-collar suburbs	6.0
Bohemian Mix	Inner-city bohemian enclaves à la Greenwich Village	1.1
Levittown, U.S.A.	Aging, post–World War II tract subdivisions	3.1
Gray Power	Upper-middle-class retirement communities	2.9
Black Enterprise	Predominantly black, middle- and upper-middle-class neighborhoods	0.8
New Beginnings	Fringe-city areas of single complexes, garden apartments and trim bungalows	4.3
Blue-Collar Nursery	Middle-class, child-rearing towns	2.2
New Homesteaders	Exurban boom towns of young, midscale families	4.2
New Melting Pot	New immigrant neighborhoods, primarily in the nation's port cities	0.9
Towns & Gowns	America's college towns	1.2
Rank & File	Older, blue-collar, industrial suburbs	1.4
Middle America	Midscale, midsize towns	3.2
Old Yankee Rows	Working-class rowhouse districts	1.6
Coalburg & Corntown	Small towns based on light industry and farming	2.0
Shotguns & Pickups	Crossroads villages serving the nation's lumber and breadbasket needs	1.9
Golden Ponds	Rustic cottage communities located near the coasts, in the mountains or alongside lakes	5.2
Agri-Business	Small towns surrounded by large-scale farms and ranches	2.1
Emergent Minorities	Predominantly black, working-class, city neighborhoods	1.7
Single City Blues	Downscale, urban, singles districts	3.3
Mines & Mills	Struggling steeltowns and mining villages	2.8
Back-Country Folks	Remote, downscale, farm towns	3.4
Norma Rae-Ville	Lower-middle-class milltowns and industrial suburbs, primarily in the South	2.3
Smalltown Downtown	Inner-city districts of small industrial cities	2.5
Grain Belt	The nation's most sparsely populated rural communities	1.3
Heavy Industry	Lower-working-class districts in the nation's older industrial cities	2.8
Share Croppers	Primarily southern hamlets devoted to farming and light industry	4.0
Downtown Dixie Style	Aging, predominantly black neighborhoods, typically in southern cities	3.4
Hispanic Mix	America's Hispanic barrios	1.9
Tobacco Roads	Predominantly black farm communities throughout the South	1.2
Hard Scrabble	The nation's poorest rural settlements	1.5
Public Assistance	America's inner-city ghettos	3.1

Household percentages are based on 1987 census block groups and estimated to the closest 0.1 percent. Source: PRIZM (Census Demography), Claritas Corp., 1987.

From Weiss MJ: *The Clustering of America*, New York, 1988, Harper & Row. Reprinted by permission of HarperCollins Publishers, Inc.

this information to focus marketing campaigns; small companies wish to know, for example, whether a flower shop would be profitable in a certain neighborhood. You can obtain demographic information, 5-year projections, and information relative to eating habits and health programs based on the zip codes or the major cross-streets that mark the perimeter of your community. A few of the companies providing these services are:

Claritas CVNU Business Information Services, 701-683-8300

Donnelly Market Information Services, 800-866-2255 National Decision Systems, 800-866-6510

Example

In an example in the beginning of this chapter, you needed to come up with a fast proposal to take advantage of a politically inspired program for a Chicago Hispanic neighborhood. You call the Claritas Group of Alexandria, Virginia, and ask for the demographic data for the Pilsen neighborhood of Chicago, Illinois, 60608. They report that as of 1987 this neighborhood is characterized by the cluster "Hispanic Mix" ZQ 37. Hispanic Mix neighborhoods are found throughout the country, from Puerto Rican communities in New York City to Mexican-American sections in Los Angeles. They tend toward large families (20% of households have more than 5 residents), low incomes, rows of aging apartments or bungalows, and Spanish markets, bars, and restaurants. This cluster has the most recent immigrants and the highest concentration of foreign-born citizens. They have hopes of moving up and out of the neighborhood. Residents are above-average purchasers of Mexican food, tortilla chips, and canned chili as well as children's vitamins, cloth diapers, and baby shampoo. They also buy inexpensive foods such as rice, pancake mix, canned chicken, and spaghetti and exhibit concern for their health by purchasing above-average amounts of asthma remedies, throat lozenges, and first-aid products. The Hispanic Mix cluster has the least number of dieters. Therefore, a weight-control program may not have the same interest level as in other communities, although 38% of Hispanic

women are overweight compared to 27% for the entire U.S. adult female population. They watch 32% more boxing matches and the novella, which is Spanish soap opera. Democrats outnumber Republicans 2:1, but there is low voter turnout, in part because of a high number of illegal aliens and an historic distrust of the federal government. However, local issues such as housing, public safety, and parks can energize a community. Figure 15-3 shows a further breakdown of information about the Hispanic Mix cluster. This information, plus the specific demographic information on the Pilsen neighborhood and information from Pilsen community leaders and social service agencies, allows you to identify the preschool through elementary school child as the target of intervention. The intervention will be a Spanish-language booklet of simple questions and answers on nutrition for this age group. Questions will address vitamin pill usage, asthma, food allergies, food practices, and various concerns of the community. A nutrition hot line in Spanish and English will be operated during certain hous of the day, with an answering machine for off-hours. The telephone number will be prominently displayed on the front of the booklet, which will be distributed through public and parochial schools in the neighborhood. Effectiveness will be measured through a telephone survey of parents and the activity of the hot line. The booklet will be publicized on Spanish-language radio and TV programs. Because of the quick response of the Claritas Group, combined with your ability to obtain specific knowledge of the Pilsen neighborhood, you are able to respond with a complete proposal within the 1-week deadline.

This type of information is also available in the geography departments of universities. They often have access to these services as part of their teaching or research mission. Such community assessments may make appropriate undergraduate and graduate student projects for educational purposes.

Resources for Identifying Health Problems

A large number of health problems and causes of mortality are related to nutrition. An assessment of the incidence and prevalence of these problems

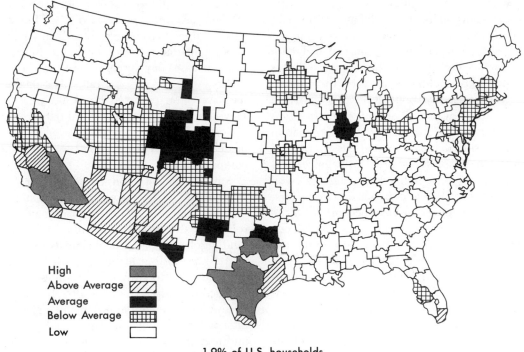

High	
Above Average	
Average	
Below Average	
Low	

1.9% of U.S. households
Primary age range: 18-34
Median household income: $16,270
Median home value: $49,533

Thumbnail Demographics
poor inner-city enclaves
multi-unit housing
predominantly Hispanic singles and families
grade-school educations
blue-collar jobs

Politics
Predominant ideology: moderate
1984 presidential vote: Reagan (51%)
Key issues: social programs, foreign-policy doves

Sample Neighborhoods
West San Antonio, Texas (78207)
East Los Angeles, California (90022)
Bushwick, Brooklyn, New York (11232)
Pilsen, Chicago, Illinois (60608)
Riverside, Miami, Florida (33135)
Hoboken, New Jersey (07030)

Figure 15-3. ZQ 37 Hispanic mix.
Source: Weiss MJ: *The Clustering of America*, New York, 1988, Harper & Row. Reprinted by permission of HarperCollins Publishers, Inc.

in your community is valuable in identifying nutrition-related problems. Some definitions of terms are helpful. Mortality, of course, refers to deaths and is generally reported per 100,000 in health statistics for the nation. Morbidity refers to illness and is reported by incidence rate (i.e., the number of *new* cases of disease/population at risk, over a *period* of time) or by prevalence rate (i.e., the number of *existing* cases of a disease/total population at a *point* in time). Incidence tells us the rate at which new illness occurs, whereas prevalence measures the residue of such illness existing at a given point in time. Prevalence depends on two factors: the number of people who have become ill in the past and the duration of their illnesses. Prevalence is used to assess morbidity from chronic disease such as cancer and diabetes, whereas incidence is used to assess morbidity from diseases of short duration such as measles or the common cold. Incidence rates for both acute and chronic diseases are indicators of disease risk in a community, whereas prevalence data indicate the number of individuals that might require a particular nutrition service. Prevalence data, more easily obtained because they require only a single time point, are tempting to use as a measure of incidence. However, high prevalence rates in a community could also indicate successful survival, such as well-controlled diabetes. In this case the high prevalence of diabetes in a community may falsely lead to a program of intervention where none is needed.

Because reporting of all births and deaths is mandated by law, these data provide reliable data bases for community assessment. Birth certificates report age and race of the mother and birth weight, sex, and gestational age of the infant. From this data you can identify the number of low- and very-low-birth-weight infants in your community compared to the city, state, or national average. By looking at death certificate data, you can also determine the extent of perinatal mortality in your community. This information, combined with nutritional status, demographic, and ethnographic information, can give you a picture of the extent and probable causes of the problems. Death certificates report both primary and secondary causes of death,

age, and sex. Because several of the major causes of death are nutrition-related (e.g., heart disease, cancer, hypertension, cirrhosis, and non-insulin-dependent diabetes mellitus), the mortality from these diseases in your community can be compared to city, state, or national rates. National and state data are often reported per 1000 or 10,000. You may need to convert your local data from number of deaths divided by the population to the number of deaths per 1000 or 10,000 to make the direct comparison.

State, regional, and city health departments publish yearly reports on morbidity statistics that may be helpful in identifying the major nutrition-related health problems in your community. Hospital discharge data by diagnosis-related groups (DRGs) are also available in most localities. Hospital data also identify other demographic characteristics of hospital admissions. Important inferences about the community using a particular hospital or group of hospitals can be obtained from this information. Care must be taken not to overinterpret this data with comparisons from other hospitals in other communities. There are variations in perceptions of illness that are based upon cultural, economic, and social variables that influence when and how often hospital services are sought. Generally the less life-threatening the illness, the greater the bias from these factors.

A number of health surveillance and reporting systems collect data from individual states and compile the data nationally. The Centers for Disease Control (CDC) has developed the Behavioral Risk Factor Surveillance System, which collects data on a representative sample of adults in each of the participating states. Interviews are conducted by telephone and data are collected on such health-related behaviors as seat belt use, physical activity, smoking, alcohol consumption, presence of hypertension, weights, heights, and weight-control practices. These data can be obtained through health agencies, and summaries are published in the CDC publication *Morbidity and Mortality Weekly Report*.[9]

The National Health Interview Survey is conducted annually by the National Center for Health

Statistics (NCHS) by administering to a representative sample of the U.S. population a core questionnaire that probes health status, use of health services, and a variety of health-related issues. Each year additional questions are asked concerning a variety of health-related issues. In the years 1988 and 1989 these issues included child health, alcohol consumption, diabetes, and digestive disorders.

The National Health and Nutrition Examination Surveys (NHANES I, II, III, and Hispanic HANES) (see Appendix 15-1) provide only nutrition information. However, participants in the national probability sample also undergo a physical exam, an extensive health interview, and a battery of biochemical tests, as well as anthropometric and dietary intake measures. Data from national samples are presented by age, race, gender, and income level. Ongoing reports from the current NHANES cycles are published in *Vital and Health Statistics, Series 11*. If you assume that groups in your community may be at risk, you may be able to infer at-risk populations by multiplying the number of individuals in a particular age and socioeconomic group by the national percentage for a given health problem. Such estimates are essential for needs assessment and program planning. You may find that although the problem you have identified is important there are not enough individuals at risk in your community to warrant services through a special program.

National and Regional Data on Nutritional Status

The federal government conducts many health, nutritional status, and food consumption surveys, such as:

1. Nationwide Food Consumption Survey (NFCS), USDA
2. Continuing Survey of Food Intakes by Individuals (CSFII), USDA
3. Second National Health and Nutrition Examination Survey (NHANES II), NCHS
4. National Health Interview Survey (NHIS), NCHS
5. Total Diet Study (TDS), FDS

6. Pediatric Nutrition Surveillance System (PedNSS), CDC
7. Behavioral Risk Factor Surveillance System (BRFSS), CDC

A full list of these surveys, their dates, populations, and data collected is contained in Appendix 15-1. Until the mid 1980s these data were not evaluated as a whole to obtain a more complete picture of the nutritional status of the United States. The Food and Agriculture Act of 1977 (Public Law 95-113) instructed the secretary of agriculture and the secretary of health, education, and welfare (now health and human services) to submit to Congress a proposal for the Comprehensive Nutritional Status Monitoring System to integrate the ongoing nutrition survey activities of both departments. After many recommendations, revisions, and denied requests for funding, the Joint Nutrition and Monitoring Evaluation Committee (JNMEC) was appointed in 1983 with two major objectives:

1. Achieve the best possible coordination between the two largest components of the system: the National Health and Nutrition Examination Survey and the Nationwide Food Consumption Survey
2. Develop a reporting system to translate findings from the two surveys, monitor activities, and report periodically to Congress on the nutritional status of the American population.

The first report, *Nutrition Monitoring in the United States*, appeared in 1986 and was a compilation and assessment of easily obtained data.[3] By 1989 the committee was reformed into the ad hoc Expert Panel on Nutrition Monitoring (EPONM) and charged with updating the dietary and nutritional status data as presented in the 1986 report and performing an in-depth analysis of the contributions of the National Nutrition Monitoring System (NNMS) to the assessment of the status of the population.

This resulted in the update report of 1989, *Nutrition Monitoring in the United States*.[3] Funding was finally approved for a permanent National Nutrition Monitoring System, and the periodic reports should become an ongoing library acquisition for you. In the pages of these reports you will find the philosophy, definitions, survey descriptions, and limitations, as well as assessments of nutrients of concern, the populations at risk, and the specific data to support these assessments. These reports will become a valuable source of nutritional status data for the dietitian or nutritionist. At this time the data are not available by state and region, so the subpopulation of interest to you may not be currently assessed. However, the data were collected by state, city, and region, and it should be possible at some point to request reports tailored to your specific needs if the monitoring program ever achieves sufficient funding. Here is a case for making your needs known to your government representatives at all levels. The Nutrition Monitoring and Related Research Act of 1990 expands the existing effort so that greater coordination between various federal and state agencies can be achieved. However, developing the infrastructure and the funding necessary to realize the goals of the bill lags behind the dream. Included in the plans for this project is the monitoring of populations such as migrant workers, homeless people, military personnel, the institutionalized, and Native Americans living on reservations, for whom we lack extensive data.

Community Services

An important part of community assessment is knowing the number of participants using nutrition services compared with the estimated need for the services. Emphasis should be placed on increasing the participation of those who qualify for federal or state nutrition programs such as food stamps or congregate meals. Another important consideration is what to do about the families who qualify for WIC but are not served because of inadequate funding. What can be done to identify and support these families? Interviews with staff members of local organizations such as food pantries, March of Dimes, and Catholic Charities will give you insights. Another good resource is the Food Research and Action Center, a nonprofit organization in Washington, D.C., whose mission is to end hunger in the United States. They produce numerous pertinent publications such as *Feeding the Other Half: Mothers and Children Left Out of WIC.*[4]

COLLECTING YOUR OWN DATA FOR ASSESSING THE NUTRITIONAL STATUS OF THE COMMUNITY

Local sources can give you an idea of the problems you are likely to encounter in your community. Although this information may be inadequate for truly assessing nutritional needs, it is important to identify the perceived needs of the community. If these needs are not addressed, effective programming will be difficult. Figure 15-4 presents a format for collecting subjective information from the community. Because these are perceived needs and problems, you are looking for repeating patterns rather than quantifiable data.

Focus Groups

When time and resources are short, meaningful data can be collected from community members, community leaders, agencies, schools, health professionals, and markets (see Fig. 15-4). Getting people together in groups to react to a single problem is useful. Such groups, recently called *focus groups*, have been used extensively in marketing research to identify motivations, rationales, and approaches that amplify the quantitative data obtained from marketing surveys. They can also be a useful tool for the dietitian and nutritionist because a number of key individuals can be interviewed at once. Also, the group forum format stimulates observations that may not have been evoked in an individual interview.

Example

Through existing data you have characterized your region of eastern Tennessee. It is dotted with small towns with single industries such as mills and packaging plants and with poor rural farms. The average income is low, and there are a lot of single-parent families whose mothers are employed in the mills. Family education levels are low, and school performance is below average for the state. Although school lunch is provided, none of the schools has taken advantage of the federal School Breakfast Program. You would like to know what proportion of the students have breakfast at home, what barriers exist to a school breakfast program, and the estimated participation rates at each school. Be-

	Perceived Health Problems	Perceived Nutrition Problems	Perceived Food Supply Problems	Perceived Food Preparation/ Storage Problems	Perceived Food Selection Problems
Community Members Men, Women, Elderly, Teens, Physically impaired, etc.					
Community Leaders Aldermen Clergy Organization leaders Newspaper editors					
Agencies Extension Aging ADC WIC Meals on Wheels United Way Red Cross Food pantries					
Schools Teachers Principals School food service					
Health Professionals Health educators Dietitians Nutricians Physicians Dentists Nurses Social workers					
Markets Supermarkets Food stores Cafeterias Restuants Street vendors Farmer's markets					

Figure 15-4. Nutrition problem community assessment inventory.

cause you do not have time to canvass all schools, you select representative schools, call the school principals, state your intentions, and request a meeting to include some selected teachers representing various grades and the heads of the school food service operations. You send the agenda for the meeting ahead of time so the focus group participants can be prepared, and you state the amount of time you will use. On the day of the meeting, you introduce yourself and explain the background of your request, giving a short exposition of the data that point to a possible problem and the availability of untapped resources. You assure the group that at this point you are still assessing the viability of the approach. You then ask your questions, starting from the most objective and easiest to answer and ending with the more probing and philosophical questions. The objective is to allow the group to develop its own discussion in response to the questions. You must learn to be comfortable with silences, especially at the beginning of the session. Your role is to ask the questions and record the comments of the group. You also ask them for their own questions and for observations that were not covered by your questions. Because such a group is acting as a partner in problem development and solution, a summary of what they have observed is often a useful ending. This approach also allows them to evaluate whether you have heard them correctly. You thank them and tell them when they are likely to know how you will proceed.

Participant Observation

Anthropologists have identified ways in which food operates to produce eating behaviors and foodways. Food is far more than what we eat. Food[7]:

1. Provides body energy and satisfies biophysiological hunger
2. Initiates and maintains interpersonal relationships with friends, kin, and strangers
3. Is a determinant of the nature and extent of interpersonal distance between people
4. Expresses social and religious ideas
5. Illustrates social status, prestige, and group achievements
6. Helps individuals cope with psychological stresses and needs

7. Rewards, punishes, or otherwise influences the behavior of others
8. Influences the political and economic status of a group
9. Detects, treats, and prevents social, physical, and cultural behavior deviations and illness manifestations

Anthropologists have often used the method of participant-observer to obtain this type of information. In classical anthropological research the participant-observer lives with the community for long periods of time and participates in the life of the community. If foodways are the focus, all aspects of food gathering, preparation, storage, eating, and disposal are observed, along with communications among community and family members. Questions concerning the reasons and meanings of behaviors are asked. Obviously the average dietitian or nutritionist cannot participate in this questioning. However, take every opportunity to get to know the community you serve by walking around in it, making friends, and observing food buying and eating behaviors. Individuals and families that are open to your friendship may invite you to spend time with them so that you can see their rhythm of living and food preparation.

Example

Ruth serves an Italian neighborhood in New York City that has a significant older population and a high prevalence of hypertension. Observation of markets and purchasing behavior and interviews with health professionals in the area do not identify obesity or high salt consumption as explanations for the excess cases. Ruth has gone out of her way to be of service to a number of her clients, and they have responded with their friendship. She invites herself to a few dinners and lunches at their homes and asks if she could observe how they cook such delicious food. Specific dates are set, and she observes the custom of a small hospitality gift. Her friends delight in showing her how to cook their favorite everyday dishes. In two different households, while helping to prepare the pasta, she is corrected for not adding enough salt to the pasta cooking water. Good pasta, it seems, requires a large handful of salt per pot of boiling water. This salt is taken up in the pasta as it cooks. Because pasta is central to two meals each day, it appears to be a hidden source of high sodium comsumption in this community.

DEVELOPING AND RANKING NUTRITIONAL NEEDS FROM QUANTITATIVE AND QUALITATIVE DATA: SCREENING

You have now collected quite a bit of data. Some of the data are specific for your community, and some are from national surveys. You have also identified the nutrition services already provided to the community and whether these services are adequate to cover the needs. How do you put this all together and come up with a simplified list that is sufficiently clear to make some prioritized decisions?

The community nutritional needs list in Figure 15-5 is a format that can help you form a gestalt (a configuration of ideas or material that is more than the mere listing of its parts) of the nutritional needs of your community. By providing information on the nutritional needs of your community, you clarify the information that supports your observations.

This is necessary documentation for gaining support for a program. You also have the data you need to make estimates of the numbers of people requiring nutrition services. In the process of filling in the community nutritional needs list, appropriate approaches to meet those needs will develop.

USING NUTRITIONAL STATUS MEASURES TO IDENTIFY CLIENTS IN NEED OF SERVICE

Unless you have decided on a communitywide educational campaign to meet a widespread nutritional need in the community, you will likely require some means of identifying those in a subpopulation who truly need services. This requires some screening measures that identify and then qualify an individual for program entitlement. The Consensus Conference of the Nutrition Screening Initiative defined *nutrition screening* as "the process of discovering characteristics known to be associated with dietary or nutritional problems. Its purpose is to identify individuals who are at high risk of nutritional problems or who have unrecognized malnutrition."[11] (See Appendix 15-2.)

This notion of screening identifies those with

Nutrition Problem	Population or Subgroup at Risk	Major Evidence for Need (Outputs)	Possible Causes for Problem (Inputs)	Existing Resources or Services and Numbers Unserved	Possible Approaches
Hypertension					
Heavy intakes of convenience foods					
Obesity					
Low-birth-weight babies					

Do not rank in order when listing problems. Quantify numbers at risk, numbers served and underserved, and evidence of need. The greater the quantification, the more accurate your assessment of the greatest benefit for program development.

Figure 15-5. Problem development list for community nutrition needs assessment.

nutritional problems as well as those at risk for nutritional problems. Figure 15-6 is a cartoon representation of how a screening program works. Characteristics for screening can include such factors as age, sex, socioeconomic group (SEG), disability, and nutritional status. The key points for a successful screening program are:

1. Locating people most likely to need the services. Many good programs fail because of inadequate effort toward finding possible clients and eliminating the barriers that prevent them from being screened. This is often due to concerns for staff convenience rather than participant convenience.

2. Choosing screening measures that are both cost-effective and sensitive enough to identify those who need the nutritional services (few false-negatives). Simple measures of nutritional status are often used at this point, such as total plasma cholesterol or weight for height.

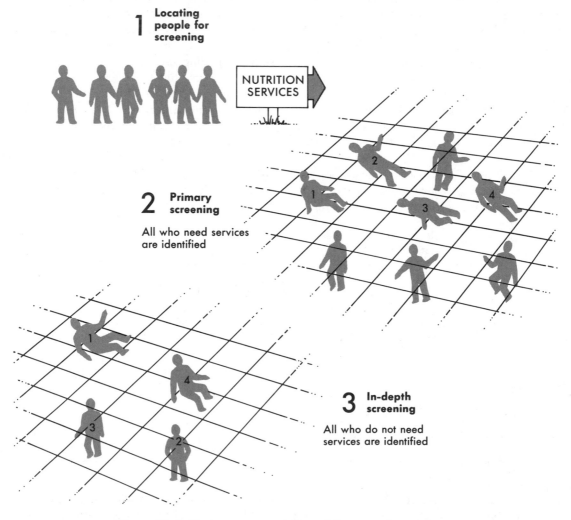

1 Locating people for screening

NUTRITION SERVICES

2 Primary screening

All who need services are identified

3 In-depth screening

All who do not need services are identified

Figure 15-6. Cartoon representation of the screening process.

3. Choosing in-depth screening techniques with high specificity to select individuals truly in need of services to be provided. These measures also identify the most appropriate interventions and may serve as baseline data to be used to assess the success of the intervention.

Selecting Appropriate Screening Tools: Understanding Sensitivity, Specificity, and Predictive Value

We used the term *sensitivity* when referring to preliminary screening measures and *specificity* when referring to in-depth or secondary screening measures. These terms have specific meanings and are powerful concepts in selecting measures and cut-points for qualification to receive nutrition services. A careful exposition of these concepts is presented in *Beyond Normality: The Predictive Value and Efficiency of Medical Diagnosis*.[5] The book addresses issues of selecting tests and characteristics that correctly identify individuals in need of treatment. The concepts are widely applicable and have the power to combine unquantifiable characteristics such as need for assistance in daily living activities with quantifiable measurements such as low blood hemoglobin values to qualify a person for a program.

By arranging the characteristics we want to use for screening into a test, we can define the sensitivity of that test by the number of true-positive results obtained when the test is applied to individuals known to have the disease (in our case poor nutrition or risk for poor nutrition).

$$\text{Sensitivity (Se)} = \text{TP}/(\text{TP} + \text{FN}) \times 100$$

where TP = true-positive (poorly nourished identified as poorly nourished) and FN = false-negative (poorly nourished but identified as healthy).

A sensitive test gives positive results in disease (poor nutrition or at risk for poor nutrition). It identifies those individuals who truly need nutrition services.

The specificity of a test is the incidence of true-negative results obtained when the test is applied to individuals known to be free of the disease (in our case, well-nourished individuals or individuals having no risk factors for poor nutrition).

$$\text{Specificity (Sp)} = \text{TN}/(\text{TN} + \text{FP}) \times 100$$

where TN = true-negative (well nourished and identified as such) and FP = false-positive (well nourished but identified as poorly nourished).

A good specific test gives negative results in healthy or well-nourished people (or having no risk factors for poor nutrition). It screens out people who truly have no need for nutrition services.

For a test to have positive predictive value and therefore be a good screening tool, we need to combine elements of each of these concepts. Ideally we want to identify all individuals who need the nutrition program, but we do not want to waste scarce resources on those who do not need the service. *Positive predictive value* is defined as the percent of positive results that are true-positive when the test is applied to a population containing both healthy and diseased individuals.

$$\text{Positive Predictive Value (PPV)} = \text{TP}/(\text{TP} + \text{FP}) \times 100$$

The positive predictive value of a test depends on the positivity of the test in disease and its negativity in health. A test with good positive predictive value correctly identifies all those who are poorly nourished and also correctly screens out those with good nutritional status.

The positive predictive value of a test used for screening is also dependent on the prevalence of poor nutrition in the community. The lower the prevalence, the poorer the positive predictive value. Table 15-3 shows that when prevalence of a condition is less than 0.1%, you have only a 1.9% chance of correctly identifying those with the condition, even when the sensitivity and specificity of the test are exceptionally good. However, when a large number of individuals in the community suffer from the condition, the efficiency of the test is increased.

Ideally, those people who have been identified by preliminary screening will be followed up with

Table 15-3. Effect of prevalence on predictive value when sensitivity and specificity equal 95%

Prevalence of the disease (percent)	Predictive value of a positive test (percent)
0.1	1.9
1.0	16.1
2.0	21.9
5.0	50.0
50.0	95.0

From Galen RS, Gambino SR: *Beyond normality: the predictive value and efficiency of medical diagnosis*. Reprinted by permission of Churchill-Livingstone, New York, 1975.

an in-depth screening (greater accuracy and greater cost). This system increases the prevalence of the disease (poor nutrition) in those seen for the secondary in-depth tests. The result is predictive values that may be 80% and above.

Other good reasons for having an estimate of the prevalence of nutrition problems in your community are to plan and evaluate nutrition programs, whether they are educational or clinical.

Changing Cut-Points as a Means of Changing Sensitivity, Specificity, and Cost of a Program

We can change the sensitivity and specificity of a test by changing the cut-point for a value that triggers qualification of an individual for a program. For example, would you choose 11 g/dl or 12 g/dl as a cut-point for the identification of iron deficiency anemia? If you choose 12 g/dl, you obtain higher sensitivity because true-positives increase and false-negatives decrease. However, specificity is reduced because true-negatives decrease and false-positives increase. Which is better: high sensitivity or high specificity for a screening test? A balance between sensitivity and specificity produces the best positive predictive value. However, the decision really rests with the program objectives. If resources are limited, a lower cut-point increases specificity, and only the most serious cases qualify for the program; if program objectives are to identify poor eating habits rather than full-blown iron deficiency anemia, then a higher cut-point is appropriate.

Example

Teenage girls are at risk for iron deficiency anemia because of their poor eating habits. Funding has been obtained for an Eating Beautiful project aimed at improving the nutritional status and general eating habits of teenage girls living in public housing in a Midwestern city. Of the estimated 1800 girls aged 11 to 19 years within this population, 80% are African-American and 20% are already served by the WIC program.

Healthy People 2000 reports that the prevalence of iron deficiency anemia among all low-income women of childbearing age is estimated to be 8% on the basis of a hemoglobin cut-point of 11 g/dl.[6] Using the mean corpuscular valve (MCV) model (a sum of several measures), *Nutrition Monitoring in the United States*,[3] reports that among girls living below the poverty line, aged 12 to 15 years, there is a 5.1% prevalence of true iron deficiency, and for those aged 16 to 19, a prevalence of 8.7%. You also find that hemoglobin is a poor test for African-Americans because they have a tendency for low hemoglobin concentrations that appears to be genetically based.

Blood hemoglobin concentrations can be obtained by a finger prick, and results are immediately available at the site of screening. Hemoglobin values are not intended to screen out those who are truly iron deficient; however, you will use them for qualification for program entry. If we use the 11 g/dl hemoglobin cut-point, we would estimate a maximum of 115 girls eligible for the program, subtracting those who are already participating in WIC. If we assume an optimistic 50% participation, the program would involve 57 girls. You have obtained enough funding to handle 100 girls in the program, so you decide to increase the hemoglobin cut point to 12 g/dl, which can be justified by CDC criteria.

In this example the sensitivity is increased at the expense of specificity, and the burden of the decision is based on program objectives and available funding. This example points out the importance of good demographic and prevalence estimates in program planning.

Combining Tests to Increase Sensitivity or Specificity

Single measures of nutritional status such as low serum albumin or low intakes of vitamin C are notoriously nonspecific in identifying a true nutritional deficiency. Dietitians and nutritionists have tried to overcome this problem by combining tests of varying types to identify individuals with overnutrition or undernutrition. The concepts of sensitivity and specificity are instructive in guiding us in designing screens from a combination of tests. For example, we have identified two tests with cutpoints derived from the nutritional assessment literature for screening iron deficiency anemia. Blood hemoglobin concentration (Hb) is a measure of hemopoietic activity that starts to drop once iron stores are depleted. Serum ferritin concentration

(Ftn) is a measure of iron stores and starts to drop at an earlier stage of iron deficiency. Suppose we perform both tests on the population to be screened. We can increase the specificity of our screen if we identify individuals as iron deficient only if a prospective client is below the cut-point for *both* tests.

$$Hb + Ftn = Iron\ deficiency\ anemia\ (high\ specificity,\ low\ sensitivity)$$

If we want to make sure that more individuals who are iron deficient qualify for a program, we could change the rules of qualification to state that a prospective client who is below the cut-point on *either* test would meet program qualifications. In this case we would be increasing the sensitivity and decreasing the specificity of the test.

MAJOR INDICATORS OF POOR NUTRITIONAL STATUS IN OLDER AMERICANS

Significant weight loss over time

- 5% or more of body weight in 1 month
- 7.5% or more of body weight in 3 months
- 10% or more of body weight in 6 months or involuntary weight loss of 10 pounds in 6 months

Significantly low or high weight for height

- 20% below or above the desirable body weight for that individual
- Including consideration of loss of height due to vertebral collapse, kyphosis, and deformity

Significant reduction in serum albumin

- Serum albumin of less than 3.5 g/dl

Significant change in functional status

- Change from "independent" to "dependent" in two of the activities of daily living or one of the nutrition-related instrumental activities of daily living (IADLs)*

Significant and inappropriate food intake

- Failure to consume the U.S. Dietary Guidelines recommended minimum from one or more basic food groups as well as sufficient variety of foods
- Failure to observe moderation in salt and sugar intake, to observe saturated fat limitation, or alcohol consumption above 1 oz/day (women) or 2 oz/day (men)

Significant reduction in midarm circumference

- To less than 10th percentile of NHANES standards

Significant increase or decrease in skinfold

- To less than 10th percentile or more than 95th percentile of NHANES standards

Significant obesity

- More than 120% of desirable weight or body mass index (BMI) over 27, or triceps skinfold above 95th percentile

Selected nutrition related disorders

- Osteoporosis
- Osteomalacia
- Folate deficiency
- B_{12} deficiency

From Nutrition Screening Initiative: *Report of nutrition screening 1: toward a Common View*, Washington, DC, 1991, reprinted with permission of Nutrition Screening Initiative.

*See also Disability classifications in: Berg RL and Cassells JS: *The second 50 years*, Institute of Medicine, Washington, DC, 1990; National Academy Press.

HB or Ftn = Iron deficiency anemia (low specificity, high sensitivity)

The Nutrition Screening Initiative has identified major indicators of poor nutritional status in older Americans (see the box on p. 421), along with cut-points for each test.[11] Note that the tests include anthropometric, dietary, biochemical, clinical, and functional components. Some are constructed from continuous variables such as serum albumin, whereas others, such as the test for independent living, are qualitative. Members of the Consensus Conference of the Screening Initiative suggest that it is the responsibility of dietitians, nutritionists, and other health care professionals to apply screens in every program where older Americans participate. How do we put these together for the purposes of identifying older Americans in need of nutritional programs? If we assess for all the suggested indicators and require that people be below the cut-points for every test, we will identify a very

NATIONAL FOOD SUPPLY ⟶ FOOD DISTRIBUTION ⟶ CONSUMPTION

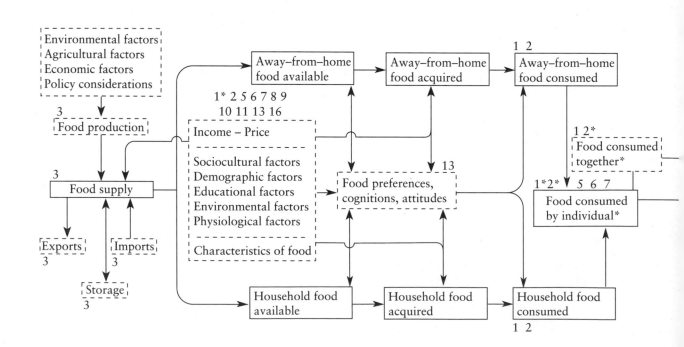

few individuals who truly are in great nutritional need. The panel would be highly specific but would miss a great number of individuals with poor nutritional status. An older American who falls below the cut-point for just one of the major indicators may not necessarily be poorly nourished. Some middle course, where sensitivity is balanced with specificity by using a cluster of tests, produces the best positive predictive values and improves the cost-benefit ratio of the intervention.

EVALUATING THE EFFECTIVENESS OF NUTRITION SERVICES

To select the appropriate measures for program evaluation, it is helpful to make a model of the nutrition service to be provided. Figure 15-1, in the beginning of this chapter, is an example of a model for nutrition monitoring. Based on experience and research, the model shows the inputs, the processes, their interrelationships, and the outputs.

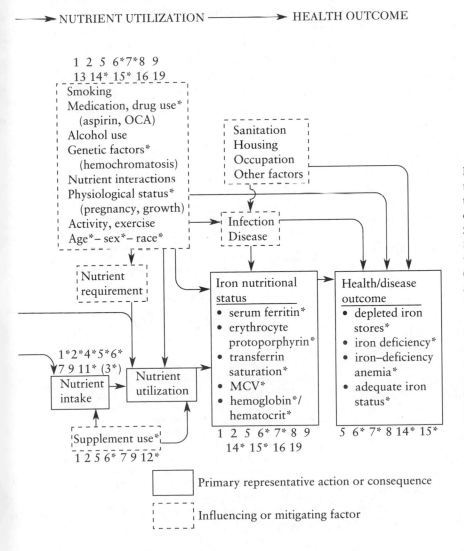

Figure 15-7. General conceptual model for iron status. National Nutrition Monitoring System and other data sources: 1 = CSFII, 1985-86, 2 = NFCS 1977-78, 3 = U.S. Food Supply Series, 4 = National Nutrient Data Bank, 5 = NHANES I, 6 = NHANES II, 7 = HHANES, 8 = NHEFS, 9 = NHIS, 10 = FLAPS, 11 = Total Diet Study, 12 = Vit/Min, 13 = Health and Diet Study, 14 = PedNSS, 15 = PNSS, 16 = BRFSS, 17 = U.S. Vital Statistics, 18 = AEDS, 19 = NHES. *Indicates data and data sources considered in this source.
Source: *Nutrition Monitoring in the United States.* DHHS Pub (PHS) 89 = 1255, Washington DC, 1989, US Government Printing Office.

Figure 15-7 shows how the conceptual model in Figure 15-1 has been adapted to assess iron status. The diagram identifies the data sources available, as well as where important data are missing. The model enables you to select the indicators on the input side and the output side that give the most information for the least cost.

Every program evaluation should include measures of the outputs, that is, improved nutritional or health status. However, nutrition intervention programs, whether educational or direct food aid, are slow to produce positive effects on health and nutritional status. This is why good nutrition as a primary public health measure has been overlooked for so many years. Effects were too slow and even unmeasurable in the ordinary time course of the typical public health program. Remember, it has taken 20 years for the beneficial effects of the Head Start Program to become apparent. How do you identify evaluation measures that point to effectiveness in a short period of time? Modeling the inputs, timelines for processes, and all the outputs again allows you to identify possible measures that are likely to change in the short run. The focus on risk factors rather than the development of chronic disease is an example of this approach. Heart disease may take 20 years to develop, but lowering plasma cholesterol levels can be evaluated in 1 month. The search for strong but reversible risk factors for various cancers is going strong, and the concept of intermediate end points of cancer itself appears to be a viable approach. For the most part, however, for community programs we must be satisfied with measurements of changes in inputs (eating behaviors, program attendance, nutrition message awareness). Again, a model that clearly shows how these inputs are linked to the outputs clarifies the most appropriate measurements and their interpretation. (See Chapter 18.)

SUMMARY

In this chapter we discussed the role of nutritional assessment in identifying the nutrition problems of the community, planning programs to meet those needs, identifying individuals who most require nutrition service through screening, and how

building models of the program process greatly aids in the identification of appropriate measurements for evaluation. Resources have been identified that can be used for all these activities and gave examples of how many of them can be used in a variety of community settings. The only way the ideas developed in this chapter will truly be of use to you is if you apply some of them to communities you have at hand. Gain experience in finding the data you need from census data and state and regional health status reports. Become familiar with finding data in the Nutrition and Food Consumption Surveys or the Nutrition Monitoring Reports. Model existing community nutrition services, and decide what might be the most appropriate evaluation tools for program effectiveness. Also, begin to collect a library of appropriate texts and government documents. Be aware of probable nutrition problems, the best nutrition status and dietary measures, and the standards for their evaluation. Learn by doing!

REFERENCES

1. Anderson GH, Peterson RD, Beaton GH: Estimating nutrient deficiencies in a population from dietary records: use of probability analyses, *Nutrition Researcher* 2:409, 1982.
2. Cameron ME, Van Staveren WA: *Manual of methodology for food consumption studies*, Oxford, 1988, Oxford University Press.
3. Department of Health and Human Services, Public Health Service, and US Department of Agriculture, Food and Consumer Services: *Nutrition monitoring in the United States*, DHHS Pub (PHS) 89-1255, Washington, DC, 1986 and 1989, US Government Printing Office.
4. Food Research and Action Center: *Feeding the other half: mothers and children left out of WIC*, Washington, DC, 1989, FRAC.
5. Galen RS, Gambino SR: *Beyond normality: The predictive value and efficiency of medical diagnosis*, New York, 1975, John Wiley & Sons.
6. *Healthy people 2000: national health promotion and disease prevention objectives*, US Department of Health and Human Services, Public Health Services, Washington, DC, 1990, US Government Printing Office.
7. Leinenger M: *Some cross-cultural universal and non-universal functions, beliefs, and practices of food.* In Dupont J, editor: *Dimension of nutrition*, Boulder, 1969, Colorado Associated University Press.
8. Macdonald I: *Monitoring dietary intakes*, Berlin, 1991, Springer-Verlag.

9. National Center for Health Statistics, Centers for Disease Control: *Reports on Mortality and Morbidity. (Monthly Vital Statistics Report* 37, 6 supplement; DHHS publications [PHS] 88-1120) Hyattsville, MD, 1988, Public Health Service.

10. National Research Council, Food and Nutrition Board: *Recommended Dietary Allowances,* ed 10, Washington, DC, 1989, National Academy Press.

11. Nutrition Screening Initiative: *Report of nutrition screening 1: toward a common view*, Washington, DC, 1991, NSI.

12. Simko MD, Cowell C, Gilbride JA: *Nutrition assessment*, Rockville, MD, 1984, Aspen.

13. Weiss MJ: *The clustering of America*, New York, 1988, Harper & Row.

14. Wright RA, Heymsfield S: *Nutritional assessment*, Cambridge, Mass, 1984, Blackwell Scientific.

APPENDIX 15-1

Sources of data from the National Nutrition Monitoring System considered in the EPONM report

Survey or study	Sponsoring agency	Date	Population	Data collected
Nationwide Food Consumption Survey (NFCS)	USDA	1977-78	Private households in the 48 conterminous states and the individuals in those households (all income and low income)	Household characteristics; foods used from home supplies (7 days); household income; name and description, quantity, form, source, and eating occasion for all food and beverages consumed by individuals (1-day recall, 2-day food records, 3 consecutive days); information on diet and health
Continuing Survey of Food Intakes by Individuals (CSFII)	USDA	1985	Women 19-50 years, children 1-5 years, men 19-50 years (all income and low income)	Household and individual characteristics, individual food intake (one to six 24-hour recalls, nonconsecutive days; 1 day only for men)
		1986	Women 19-50 years, children 1-5 years (all income and low income)	Household and individual characteristics, individual food intake (one to six 24-hour recalls, nonconsecutive days)
U.S. Food Supply Series	USDA	Each year since 1909	U.S. civilian population	Per capita disappearance of foods (levels of nutrients in food supply calculated)
National Nutrient Data Bank	USDA	Continuous	NA	Nutrient content of foods; basis of nutrient composition databases for other surveys
First National Health and Nutrition Examination Survey (NHANES I)	NCHS	1971-75	Civilian, noninstitutionalized population of the United States; 1-74 years	Dietary intake (one 24-hour recall), socioeconomic and demographic information, biochemical analyses of blood and urine, physical examination, body measurements
Second National Health and Nutrition Examination Survey (NHANES II)	NCHS	1976-80	Civilian, noninstitutionalized population of the United States; 6 months-74 years	Dietary intake (one 24-hour recall), socioeconomic and demographic information, biochemical analyses of blood and urine, physical examination, body measurements

Survey	Agency	Year	Population	Description
Hispanic Health and Nutrition Examination Survey (HHANES)	NCHS	1982-84	Civilian, noninstitutionalized Mexican-Americans in five southwestern states, Cuban-Americans in Dade County, Florida, and Puerto Ricans in metropolitan New York City; 6 months-74 years	Dietary intake (one 24-hour recall), socioeconomic and demographic information, biochemical analyses of blood and urine, physical examination, body measurements
NHANES I Epidemiological Follow-up Study (NHEFS)	NCHS	1982-84, 1986	Persons examined in NHANES I; 25-74 years old at baseline	Interviews of survivors and proxies for decedents; death certificate, hospitalization history, health status, food frequency
National Health Interview Survey (NHIS)	NCHS	1984	Civilian noninstitutionalized population; 55 years and over	Health and living conditions of elderly
		1985	Civilian, noninstitutionalized population of the United States; 18 years and over	Health promotion and disease prevention habits and knowledge
		1986	Civilian, noninstitutionalized children (2-6 years) and adults (18 years and over) in the United States	Use of vitamin and mineral supplements
Food Label and Package Survey (FLAPS)	FDA	1978, 1980, 1982, 1983, 1984, 1986	NA	Prevalence of nutrition labeling and declarations of selected nutrients and ingredients
Total Diet Study (TDS)	FDA	Annually since 1961	NA	Mineral and contaminant content of representative diets for various age-sex groups
Vitamin/Mineral Supplement Intake Survey	FDA	1980	Civilian, noninstitutionalized adults; 16 years and over	Supplement intake, attitudes, and behaviors (telephone interview)
Health and Diet Survey	FDA NHLBI	1982, 1984	Civilian, noninstitutionalized population; 18 years and over	Awareness, attitudes, knowledge, and behaviors regarding food and nutrition; health status and history (telephone interview)
	FDA NHLBI NCI	1986	Civilian, noninstitutionalized population; 18 years and over	Awareness, attitudes, knowledge, and behaviors regarding food and nutrition; health status and history (telephone interview)

Continued.

EPONM, Expert Panel on Nutrition Monitoring; *NA*, not applicable; *USDA*, U.S. Department of Agriculture; *NCHS*, National Center for Health Statistics; *FDA*, Food and Drug Administration; *NHLBI*, National Heart, Lung and Blood Institute; *NCI*, National Cancer Institute; *CDC*, Centers for Disease Control.
From Department of Health and Human Services, Public Health Service, and U.S. Department of Agriculture, Food and Consumer Services: *Nutrition Monitoring in the United States*, DHHS Pub No (PHs) 89-1255, Washington, DC, 1989, US Government Printing Office.

Sources of data from the National Nutrition Monitoring System considered in the EPONM report—cont'd

Survey or study	Sponsoring agency	Date	Population	Data collected
Pediatric Nutrition Surveillance System (PedNSS)	CDC	Continuous	Low-income, high-risk children (especially 1-5 years) in 36 states	Anthropometry, birth weight, hematological measures
Pregnancy Nutrition Surveillance System (PNSS)	CDC	Continuous	Low-income, high-risk, pregnant women in 12 states	Weight, health status, behavioral risk factors
Behavioral Risk Factor Surveillance System (BRFSS)	CDC	Continuous	Adults (18 years and over) in 35 states in households with telephones	Height, weight; diet practices; salt, alcohol, and tobacco use; cholesterol screening practices, awareness, and treatment

APPENDIX 15-2

The Nutrition Checklist is based on the Warning Signs described below. Use the word *DETERMINE* to remind you of the Warning Signs.

DISEASE

Any disease, illness or chronic condition which causes you to change the way you eat, or makes it hard for you to eat, puts your nutritional health at risk. Four out of five adults have chronic diseases that are affected by diet. Confusion or memory loss that keeps getting worse is estimated to affect one out of five or more of older adults. This can make it hard to remember what, when or if you've eaten. Feeling sad or depressed, which happens to about one in eight older adults, can cause big changes in appetite, digestion, energy level, weight and well-being.

EATING POORLY

Eating too little and eating too much both lead to poor health. Eating the same foods day after day or not eating fruit, vegetables, and milk products daily will also cause poor nutritional health. One in five adults skip meals daily. Only 13% of adults eat the minimum amount of fruit and vegetables needed. One in four older adults drink too much alcohol. Many health problems become worse if you drink more than one or two alcoholic beverages per day.

TOOTH LOSS/MOUTH PAIN

A healthy mouth, teeth and gums are needed to eat. Missing, loose or rotten teeth or dentures which don't fit well or cause mouth sores make it hard to eat.

Produced by The Nutrition Screening Initiative, 2626 Pennsylvania Avenue, NW, Suite 301, Washington, DC 20037. The Nutrition Screening Initiative is funded in part by a grant from Ross Laboratories, a division of Abbott Laboratories. Reprinted with permission from *J Am Diet Assoc*, 1992; 92(2):166. For more information, please refer to this issue of the J Am Diet Assoc.

ECONOMIC HARDSHIP

As many as 40% of older Americans have incomes of less than $6,000 per year. Having less—or choosing to spend less—than $25-30 per week for food makes it very hard to get the foods you need to stay healthy.

REDUCED SOCIAL CONTACT

One third of all older people live alone. Being with people daily has a positive effect on morale, well-being and eating.

MULTIPLE MEDICINES

Many older Americans must take medicines for health problems. Almost half of older Americans take multiple medicines daily. Growing old may change the way we respond to drugs. The more medicines you take, the greater the chance for side effects such as increased or decreased appetite, change in taste, constipation, weakness, drowsiness, diarrhea, nausea, and others. Vitamins or minerals when taken in large doses act like drugs and can cause harm. Alert your doctor to everything you take.

INVOLUNTARY WEIGHT LOSS/GAIN

Losing or gaining a lot of weight when you are not trying to do so is an important warning sign that must not be ignored. Being overweight or underweight also increases your chance of poor health.

NEEDS ASSISTANCE IN SELF CARE

Although most older people are able to eat, one of every five have trouble walking, shopping, buying and cooking food, especially as they get older.

ELDER YEARS ABOVE AGE 80

Most older people lead full and productive lives. But as age increases, risk of frailty and health problems increase. Checking your nutritional health regularly makes good sense.

16 Organizing Nutrition Services

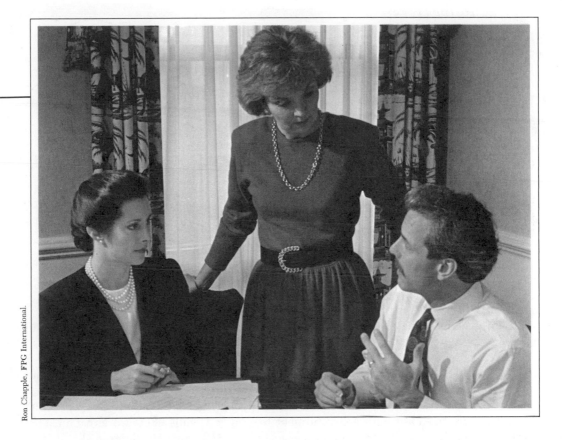

Ron Chapple, FPG International.

GENERAL CONCEPT

Organizing involves the division of work into manageable units and the assignment of responsibility and authority to individuals and work groups. Organizing also involves staffing the organization, defining lines of communication and coordination, and marshaling resources necessary to complete the work and achieve the goals and objectives of the organization.

OUTCOME OBJECTIVES

When you finish this chapter, you should be able to:

- Identify three types of organizational structure found in health departments.
- Differentiate between job classes of public health nutrition personnel.
- Recognize the sources of power.
- Discuss techniques of effective delegation.
- Outline the steps of the strategic marketing process for application in the design of nutrition programs.
- Appreciate the constructive role of conflict and identify principles of negotiation.

Planning makes a transition to implementation after the point of deciding which existing or new programs will be implemented to address high-priority problems (Fig. 16-1). The analysis of alternatives involves consideration of programmatic approaches for moving toward health goals and specific measurable objectives in light of priority needs, available resources, and existing constraints. Planning begins with the review of mission and strategies, moves through identification of issues and needs, and ends with a commitment to priority program areas and the specification of goals and objectives. The relationship among the key activities of formulation (planning) and implementation (organizing and directing) are illustrated in the Figure 16-2. Note how both are connected to the overall strategy and mission. The implementation phase is the focus of this chapter.

Planning defines expectations in the form of mission, goals, and objectives and determines which programs are needed to achieve them. Plans and programs are brought to reality through the management functions of organizing and directing. Organizing is setting up a formal structure of related activities to achieve goals and objectives. It is the division of work into manageable units and the assignment of responsibility and authority to individuals and work groups. Organizing also involves staffing the organization and defining lines of communication and coordination. Whereas planning identifies what to do, organizing begins the process

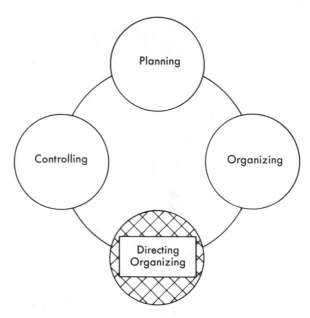

Figure 16-1. The management process.

of *doing*. Through the function of organizing, resources are allocated to structured activities so that work leads to desired outcomes.

Organizing is a multistep process that includes:

- Details all the work that must be done to attain the organization's goals
- Divides the total work load into activities that can be logically and comfortably performed by one person or by a group
- Marshals resources and staffs the organization
- Sets up a mechanism to coordinate the work of organization members into a unified, harmonious whole
- Establishes monitoring systems to track efficiency and effectiveness of the organization and trigger adjustments when necessary

Aspects of organizing and directing (or leading) in the implementation phase include organizational structure and relationships, organizational processes and behavior, and directing capabilities.

ORGANIZATIONAL STRUCTURE AND POSITION DESCRIPTIONS

Organizing involves determining the scope of work necessary to achieve the organization's goals and

Planning

Formulation ────────────────► Implementation
(Deciding what to do) ◄──────── (Achieving results through
doing)

Organizing/directing

1. Needs assessment

2. Prioritize problems

3. Select intervention by determining the organization's material, technical,
   financial, and managerial
   resources

4. Personal values and professional responsibility to society

5. Determine goals and objectives

```
┌─────────────────────┐
│ Organizational      │
│ Strategy/mission    │
│                     │
│ Pattern of purposes │
│ and policies defining│
│ the company and its │
│ business            │
└─────────────────────┘
```

1. Develop a clear definition
   of the technical aspects of
   the program and intervention strategies; balance
   with clients' needs and
   wants

2. Identify organization structure and relationships.
      Delegation of authority
      Coordination of divided
         responsibility
      Information systems

3. Organizational processes
   and behavior
      Managing conflict
      Managing organizational
         change
      Staff development

4. Directing
      Communicating
      Motivating
      Problem solving

```
┌──────────────────────────────────────────────────┐
│   Leadership: strategies, organizational, personal │
└──────────────────────────────────────────────────┘
```

Figure 16-2. From planning to implementation.
Adapted from Quinn J, Mintzberg H, James RM: *The strategy process: concepts, contexts and cases,*
1988.

the division of work into specialized activities and tasks so that each work group and individual in the organization is responsible for and performs a defined set of activities. Activities become viable programs through coordination, direction, and leadership.

As activities are determined, responsibility for their accomplishment must be assigned. Care should be taken to match qualifications and capa-

bilities of personnel with the activities for which they will be responsible. In some programs nutrition personnel are responsible for all activities. Other programs use members of a multidisciplinary team, collaborators across agencies, and volunteers. Organizational charts and position descriptions delineate responsibilities and define working relationships among personnel and collaborating agencies.

Organizational Models for Public Health Nutrition Services

Surveys of public health nutrition personnel reveal great disparity and inconsistency in the assigned responsibilities and qualifications required for positions having the same job title.[9] Organizational structures also vary considerably. The type of structure used in an agency may be the result of tradition, expediency, or political climate within or outside the agency. In most public service agencies, reorganization is a continuing process. The publication *Personnel in Public Health Nutrition for the 1990s*[3] provides a rational and consistent approach to organizing and staffing nutrition programs and services. Appropriate functions for each class of public health nutrition personnel are defined to assure that programs and services are provided by the appropriate and most cost-effective class of public health nutrition personnel.

Positions are classified into nine classes and grouped into three series—management, professional, and technical support—based on their major functions and focus. The positions are shown in Figure 16-3 along with the direction of their focus on population or client concerns. A detailed de-

scription of each class, including title, duties, job factors, and qualifications is provided in Appendix 16-1.

A position description must be written by the agency for every position in order to classify it and assign a pay grade. The position description is the official record of the work assigned to an employee. It is used to establish qualifications for hiring and promotion, orient new employees, develop performance standards, and determine training needs related to job functions. A sample position description for the public health nutritionist class is shown in Figure 16-4.

Each agency must determine the best placement for its public health nutrition personnel within its overall structure. Factors to consider include the basic structure of the health or human service agency, its mission, legislative mandates, funding sources, priorities, and service delivery systems.

The three most common organizational models for placement of nutrition services are centralized or hierarchical, matrix, and decentralized. They are illustrated in Figures 16-5 through 16-7. The advantages and disadvantages of each model are summarized in the next section. These models are fre-

Text continued on p. 440.

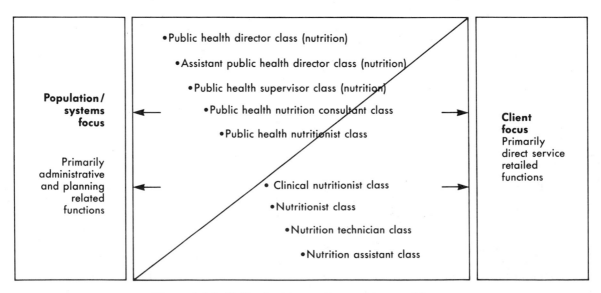

Figure 16-3. Public health nutrition positions and focus.

Position Class

PUBLIC HEALTH NUTRITIONIST

Job Title

Public Health Nutritionist

Major Duties

The public health nutritionist is employed in the county health department and is responsible for planning, managing, implementing, and evaluating the county's nutrition programs and services. The public health nutritionist advises the county health director as well as establishes joint programs with local health care facilities, food assistance programs, schools, child day-care services, meal programs for the elderly, and other human services and educational institutions in the community. Major functions for this position include: **Planning/Evaluation** Conducts community assessment of county's nutrition and diet-related health problems and resources to determine needs of the county's population; develops operational plan for nutrition service delivery using professional and consumer input; utilizes agency management and client information system to monitor and evaluate nutrition programs and to document activities and outcomes. **Education** Interprets and disseminates current scientific information regarding food, nutrition, diet, and health to professionals working in the county health department, related health and human service agencies, educational institutions, and the public; plans, directs, arranges, and evaluates educational programs addressed to professionals, paraprofessionals, volunteers, peer counselors, clients, and the public; speaks on nutrition and health through group programs, school programs, local newspaper, and radio and television stations; selects and/or develops, evaluates, and revises nutrition education materials for use in the county health department programs, assuring cultural, ethnic, educational, and literacy relevance of the materials to the county's population; utilizes available nutrition curriculum for training health and human service professionals, teachers, and students; supervises field training for students in public health, public health nutrition, and dietetics. **Consultation** Provides technical assistance on program development and nutritional care management to health agency care providers and professionals in local health care facilities; evaluates consultation to determine its effectiveness in accomplishing objectives. **Counseling** Counsels medically high-risk clients in the prenatal and pediatric clinics, usually on a demonstration basis as part of the case consultation and in-service education of county health department health care providers

Factor I Knowledge and Skills Requirements

- Broad knowledge of the theoretical and pragmatic principles and practices of nutrition, dietetics, and public health including health care ethics, case management, and care coordination.

- Specialized knowledge of the organization of health and nutrition services in the community with an advanced level of skill in conducting a community assessment and the ability to translate assessment data into a county plan for nutrition services.

Continued.

Figure 16-4. Sample position description: public health nutritionist.

Position Class
PUBLIC HEALTH NUTRITIONIST

- Advanced level of knowledge of current scientific information regarding nutrition, diet, and health and the ability to communicate this information to professionals and the public.

- Full range of knowledge and skill in using the consultation process both as consultant and consultee with advanced skills in interviewing, problem diagnosis, and evaluation.

- Full range of knowledge of principles of adult learning and principles of interdisciplinary teamwork with skill in using group process techniques.

- Full range of skill in presenting ideas orally and in writing in a clear, concise, and persuasive manner.

Factor II Supervisory Control

The public health nutritionist works independently under the general supervision of the county health director who reviews and approves the annual work plan, monitors monthly reports, and conducts an annual program review. Work is reviewed for achievement of objectives and compliance with county health department policies. Potential problems are discussed and solutions recommended, but there is a high degree of professional responsibility in program planning and in providing nutrition education, therapeutic diet counseling, and technical consultation.

Factor III Autonomy/Guidelines

Considerable independent judgement is required to adapt state and county health department policies, protocols, standards, and guidelines to new and changing situations in the community and to solve problems as they occur.

Factor IV Complexity of Work

This work requires the public health nutritionist to utilize in-depth knowledge of nutrition, dietetics, food science, and public health. Responsibilities are broad in scope, of substantial intricacy, involving many variables and unanticipated circumstances and situations with the constantly changing science and practice of nutrition and medicine and the dynamics of population needs for nutrition services.

Factor V Scope and Effect

Major contribution to the health and nutritional status of the county's population. Work involves authoritative application of county health department policies and practice to complex and important aspects of nutrition education to public health practice with particular attention to the needs of vulnerable populations.

Figure 16-4, cont'd. Sample position description: public health nutritionist.

Position Class

PUBLIC HEALTH NUTRITIONIST

Factor VI Types of Personal Contacts

County health director and professionals employed by the county health department including physicians, nurses, dentists, health educators, social workers, and staff of other agencies and faculty of educational institutions as well as the state health department administrators and consultants, general public, and health agency clients.

Factor VII Purpose of Personal Contacts

Contacts are used for community assessment, program planning, to receive and provide consultation, and to provide nutrition education and counseling.

Factor VIII Physical Demands

Relatively sedentary position, requires some walking in the county health department offices and clinics and in the community. May be required to carry some heavy audiovisual equipment when conducting educational programs in the community.

Factor IX Work Environment

Usually in the county health department offices and clinics or offices of other agencies and academic institutions with no unusual personal risks.

Qualifications

Minimum Education

Master's degree in public health nutrition or master's degree in nutrition with emphasis in public health or master's degree in applied human nutrition with core coursework in public health (biostatistics, epidemiology, health administration, and health planning).

Professional Credentials

Licensed dietitian (LD) or licensed nutritionist (LN) in state of employment.

Experience

One year of public health nutrition experience desirable.

Figure 16-4, cont'd. Sample position description: public health nutritionist.

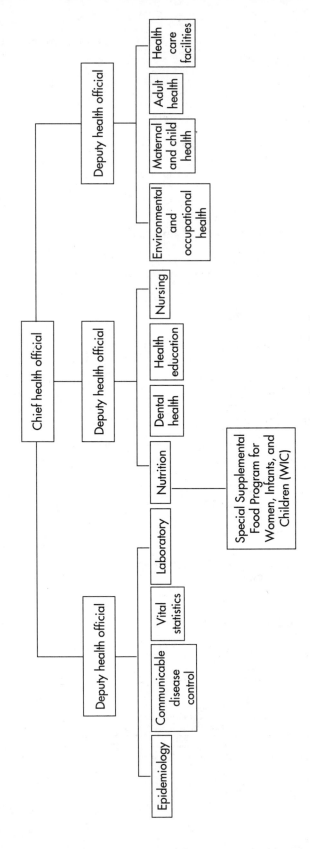

Figure 16-5. Public health agency with a centralized nutrition unit.

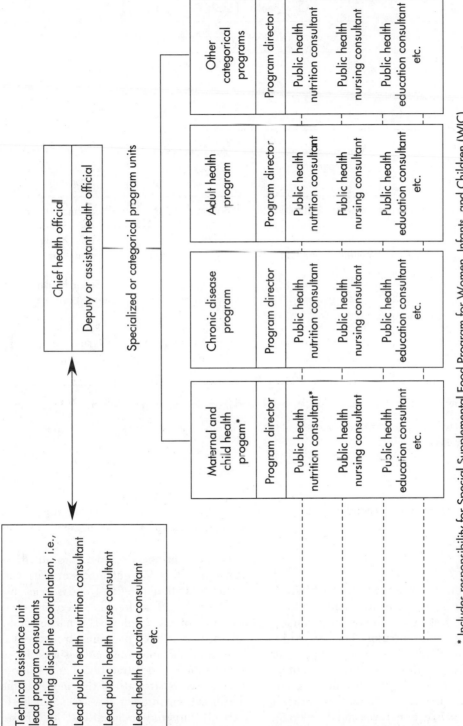

Figure 16-6. Public health agency with a matrix structure.
Adapted by M. Kaufman from Kaluzny AD et al: Management of health services. Englewood Cliffs, New Jersey, 1982, Prentice-Hall, with consultation from Dr. Kaluzny.

* Includes responsibility for Special Supplemental Food Program for Women, Infants, and Children (WIC).

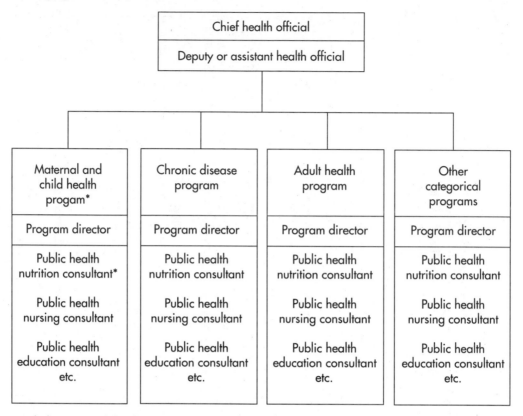

* Includes responsibility for Special Supplemental Food Program for Women, Infants, and Children (WIC).

Figure 16-7. Public health agency with nutrition consultants assigned to specialized programs (decentralized).

quently modified or combined to adapt to the needs and realities of individual agencies.

Centralized or Hierarchial Organizational Model

An example is a nutrition program unit with a director for nutrition services. In this model, all nutrition personnel employed in the organization are placed in an identifiable nutrition unit headed by a public health nutrition director who reports to the health officer. In this structure the public health nutrition director is responsible for conducting a nutrition needs assessment of the total population in the jurisdictional area and developing a program plan and budget for nutrition services as an integral part of the agency's overall health plan.

In the centralized model, the nutrition unit is the focal point for nutrition services within the agency nutrition program, and service needs are considered and included with the other health priorities of the agency. The participation of nutritionists in agency planning strengthens comprehensive health planning and assures the inclusion of nutrition in both traditional and emerging program areas. A strength of this model is that available fiscal and human resources can be more effectively targeted to identified high-risk populations. Personnel from the nutrition unit can be assigned to work on a full-time, part-time, or consultant basis, as needed by other agency programs that have, or should develop, a nutrition component. The public health nutrition director takes leadership in setting standards, coordinating, and establishing a quality assurance system, a data collection system, and a plan for personnel recruitment, continuing education, and career development.

Although this structure provides a focal point for nutrition-related activities and assures all health programs access to nutrition services, the nutritionists and dietitians may lack specific expertise in specialized program areas or may not be as readily accessible to assist other units of the organization to the degree that may be desired.

Matrix Organizational Model

An example is categorical nutrition program consultants with a lead public health nutrition consultant. In a matrix organization, the health agency is organized into categorical program units, each with a director and staff of specialized professional consultants, including a public health nutrition consultant. However, in a matrix organization, the agency officially appoints a lead public health nutrition consultant. The person in that position advises the agency director on nutrition policy issues, serves as the agency spokesperson on food and nutrition policy, assesses the nutrition needs of the community, assures nutrition content in agency health plans, coordinates agency nutrition services, and provides for technical guidance, continuing education, and career development for the specialized program nutrition consultants. In the matrix structure there is no separate nutrition unit or designated nutrition budget. The lead public health nutrition consultant does not have line authority over public health nutrition personnel in the agency and does not have control over the administration or evaluation of nutrition services.

The responsibilities delegated to the lead public health nutrition consultant must be clearly communicated to both the categorical program directors and the nutrition personnel on the specialized health teams throughout the agency. If this is not done clearly and with careful collaboration, uncoordinated and fragmented delivery of nutrition services may result.

In the agency using the matrix organizational structure, the public health nutrition consultants in the several specialized programs should have in-depth expertise in their specialized areas. The lead public health nutrition consultant should organize the specialized nutrition consultants into a coordinating council or committee that meets on a regular schedule to exchange information on nutrition programs and services, collaborate on work in areas of mutual concern, study unmet community needs, and make recommendations for improving the overall nutrition services in the community. For this to be an effective structure, the lead public health nutrition consultant must possess strong leadership skills yet be able to function collaboratively and diplomatically because the position lacks line authority over the categorical public health nutrition consultants.

Decentralized Organizational Model

An example is specialized program units employing public health nutrition consultants (Fig. 16-7). In this structure, the health agency is organized into categorical program units such as maternal and child health; children's special health services; chronic disease, adult health, health promotion, and risk reduction; and health care facilities. Public health nutrition consultants are employed independently to serve as full- or part-time members of the various specialized program consultant teams.

Such an organization facilitates interaction of public health nutrition consultants with other members of the specialized health program team. It allows each public health nutrition consultant to develop in-depth expertise and specialization in a designated program area but does not provide the agency with a visible focal point and central channel of communication for all nutrition services and activities. This model fragments nutrition services within the agency and may not provide for efficient use of resources during a time when block grants require greater program flexibility. This organizational model generally does not provide for nutrition input into all of the agency health programs or provide the support system needed by nutrition personnel to ensure their coordination and professional development.

In this structure there is not a public health director for nutrition assigned responsibility for conducting broad-based needs assessment, developing programs, or advising the chief health official on nutrition policy.

Staffing Public Health Nutrition Programs

Staffing patterns for nutrition programs and services depend on several factors:

- Size, age distribution, health, and nutritional status of the population
- Mix of community- or population-focused programs versus client care–focused delivery services
- Numbers and concentration of medically high-risk clients
- Availability of nutrition services provided by other health or human services agencies or related agencies in the jurisdictional area
- Number and type of related agencies
- Expectations of the public and health care providers
- Constraints imposed on service delivery by population disbursement, geographical and language barriers, and climate

Staffing for nutrition programs varies according to the organizational structure. The size and complexity of the overall public health program, the population, and the public health service delivery system all influence the staffing requirements. Guidelines for staffing nutrition programs are detailed in Figure 16-8. Staffing ratios recommended should be modified according to the factors listed previously. Figure 16-9 illustrates the organizational structure and staffing patterns for nutrition units in both a small local health agency and a large, complex agency.

Activities relating to staffing the organization should be specified in the implementation plan. All personnel must be adequately prepared for their responsibilities. Specialized projects may require procurement of technical assistance or consultation, recruitment of new personnel with the needed expertise, or in-service training and staff development.

Division of work and logical combinations of activities and tasks in organizations make coordination an important managerial activity. Coordination enables the activities and objectives of an organization's subunits to be harmoniously integrated so that the organization's goals can be achieved.

AUTHORITY AND DELEGATION

Authority

For an organization to function efficiently, a formal authority system must be supplemented by informal bases of power and influence. Unless managers have authority themselves and can give authority to subordinates to carry out work responsibilities, the structure has no meaning. The managers receive and assign authority; decentralization is the degree to which the authority is delegated throughout the organization. Managers use more than their official authority to obtain the cooperation of their subordinates. They also rely on their power, influence, and leadership abilities.[15]

Influence

Influence is defined as actions or examples that, either directly or indirectly, cause a change in the behavior or attitude of another person or group. For instance, a hard-working community dietitian or nutritionist can, by setting an example, influence others to increase their productivity. For example, a manager can use his or her influence to improve morale. This influence would not necessarily change behavior; it might simply bring about a change in employees' attitudes about their work.

Power

Power is defined as the ability to exert influence. To have power is to be able to change the behavior and attitudes of other individuals.

Formal authority is one type of power. It is based on the recognition of the legitimacy or lawfulness of the attempt to exert influence. The individuals

- A **public health director** (nutrition) is recommended for the large public health agency that employs five or more nutrition personnel plus support staff. The public health nutrition personnel may include a mix of public health nutrition consultants, public health nutritionist, public health supervisors (nutrition), nutritionists, nutrition technicians, and nutrition assistants. Many public health agencies will not be so large or complex as to require a position from the public health director class.

- One **assistant public health director** (nutrition) in addition to a public health director (nutrition) is recommended for the nutrition program in a public health agency serving a population of over 500,000 or that offers a complex public health nutrition program comprising a multiplicity of programs and services, manages a substantial nutrition program budget, and employs a large staff to serve medically high-risk populations.

- A **public health supervisor** (nutrition) to supervise subordinate nutrition personnel is needed by health agencies that provide significant amounts of one-on-one client nutritional care planning and counseling through clinical or home health programs. In general, one supervisor is suggested for every three to four subordinate nutrition workers.

- Public **health nutrition consultants** are generalists or specialists. Generalist public health consultants are employed by many local and state health agencies. The allocation of generalist public health nutrition consultants depends on the number and complexity of agencies and nutrition programs within the geographic area. In most states, a generalist nutrition consultant should be responsible for providing technical assistance to no more than three to four densely populated counties and/or municipalities or six to eight rural counties. Specialist public health nutrition consultants are usually employed on categorical program teams in state health agencies, in large complex city or county health agencies, or by special demonstration health projects or specialized voluntary health agencies.

- The **public health nutritionist** often functions as the one nutritionist working with other members of the public health team in a local health agency. For program development and evaluation with a community or population focus, one public health nutritionist per 50,000 population is generally suggested.

- The **clinical nutritionist** functions as case manager and/or care coordinator and nutrition counselor in clinical or home health programs serving large numbers of medically high-risk clients. The clinical nutritionist is supervised by the public health director (nutrition), public health supervisor (nutrition), or the clinic or home health program director.
  Staffing is based on an assessment of the size, risk level, and care needs of the target population, the amount of time required per encounter, the number of follow-up encounters required, and the amount of time required for care coordination and case management functions. A method of estimating direct care nutritionists is useful for estimating staffing needs for clinical nutritionists. Appendix 16-1 presents a formula
  Continued.

Figure 16-8. Staffing recommendations for nutrition programs.
Abstracted from Dodds J, Kaufman M: *Personnel in public health nutrition for the 1990s*. Washington, DC, 1991, The Public Health Foundation.

that can be used. Use of the formula requires careful estimation of the size of the specific target population of medically high-risk versus low-risk clients. Review of clinic and home health client records and hospital discharge data may provide data needed to use in the formula.

- **Nutritionists** plan, manage, and coordinate individual clients' nutrition care. This care includes individual patient/client nutrition assessments, care planning, management, and follow-up, and group education. This nutritionist is supervised by a public health supervisor (nutrition), clinical nutritionist, or in a small agency by a public health nutritionist. Staffing is based on an assessment of the size, risk level, and needs of the target client population, the time required per encounter, the number of follow-up encounters, the mix of services provided (e.g., individual counseling, small group education, computer-assisted instruction), travel time to sites, related duties, availability of computers, and availability of paraprofessionals and clerical support staff.

  A method for estimating the number of dietitians or nutritionists for direct client care is provided in Appendix 16-1. A rule of thumb suggested by the Association of State and Territorial Public Health Nutrition Directors for staffing ambulatory or home health programs serving a target population at high nutritional risk is one nutritionist or dietitian supervising two nutrition or dietetic technicians per 1000 registered clients. Other suggested staffing ratios vary from one direct service professional per 500 client population to one per 800 to 900 client population.

- **Nutrition technicians and nutrition assistants** from the technical support series can provide services that complement the professional skills of the nutritionist. Paraprofessional staff provide a cost-effective way of extending nutrition services. Staffing for technical support positions is recommended at a ratio to two nutrition technicians and/or nutrition assistants per one nutritionist in direct care services or per 1000 clients.

- **Clerical staff**—public health nutrition managers and professional workers will be more productive and cost-effective if one clerical position is provided for every one to four professional positions. Use of computers, fax machines, and telephone-answering equipment can maximize the productivity of both nutrition and clerical staff.

Figure 16-8, cont'd. Staffing recommendation for nutrition programs.

or groups attempting to exert influence are seen as having the right to do so within recognized boundaries. This right arises from their formal position in an organization.

The sources of power. Power does not simply derive from an individual's level in the organization hierarchy. Five sources of power have been identified, each of which may occur at any level of the organization:

1. *Reward power* is based on one person (the influencer) having the ability to reward another person for carrying out orders or meeting other requirements.

2. *Coercive power*, based on the influencer's ability to punish another person for not meeting requirements, is the negative side of reward power. Coercive power is used to maintain a minimum standard of performance or conformity among subordinates.

3. *Legitimate power*, which corresponds to our

Small Local Public Health Nutrition Unit

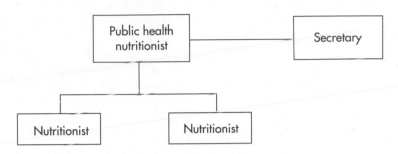

Complex Public Health Nutrition Unit

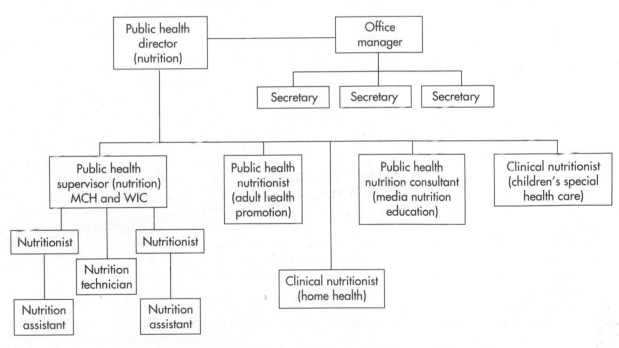

Figure 16-9. Organizational structures for small and large nutrition units.

term *authority*, exists when a subordinate or person being influenced acknowledges that the influencer has a "right" or is lawfully entitled to exert influence—within certain bounds. For example, the nutrition director has legitimate power to expect outcomes from staff in terms of patient care. The right of a manager to establish reasonable work schedules is an example of "downward" legitimate power. A security guard may have the "upward" authority to require even the chairman of the health board to present an identification card before being allowed to enter.

4. *Expert power* is based on the perception or belief that the influencer has some relevant expertise or special knowledge that the other person does not. When people accept advice from the community dietitian or nutritionist, they acknowledge his or her expert power. Expert power is usually applied to a specific, limited subject area.

5. *Referent power*, which may be held by a person or a group, is based on a person's desire to identify with or imitate the influencer. For example, a community dietitian or nutritionist manager has referent power if subordinates are motivated to emulate his or her work habits.

Characteristics of successful power users. What do managers do with their power? What specific techniques and styles are most effective? The following characteristics are common in managers who use their power successfully:

1. Effective managers are sensitive to the source of their power and are careful to keep their actions consistent with people's expectations.

2. Good managers understand—at least intuitively—the five bases of power and recognize which to draw on in different situations and with different people. They are aware of the costs, risks, and benefits of using each kind of power.

3. Effective managers recognize that all bases of power have merit in certain circumstances. They try to develop their skills and credibility

so they can use whatever method is needed.

4. Successful managers have career goals that allow them to develop and use power.

5. Effective managers temper power with maturity and self-control.

6. Successful managers know that power is necessary to get things done. They feel comfortable in their use of power and accept the fact that they must be able to influence the behavior of others to achieve goals. The power of a department of nutrition is evident when the dietitian or nutritionist is called to give expert testimony before a legislative committee on a nutrition issue such as food quackery. The dietitian or nutritionist has power because of his or her knowledge and position in the health department.

Power, then, is an important part of organizational life; it cannot be ignored. Managers must not only accept and understand power as an integral part of their jobs but also learn how to use and not abuse it to further their and the organization's goals.

Delegation

Delegation is the assignment to another person of formal authority and responsibility for carrying out specific activities. The delegation of authority by a supervisor to employees is obviously necessary for the efficient functioning of any organization because no supervisor can personally accomplish or completely supervise all the organization's activities and tasks.

The extent to which managers delegate authority is influenced by such factors as the type of the organization, the specific situation involved, and the relationships, personalities, and capabilities of the people in that situation.

How to Delegate

The first step in the delegation process requires that the manager has a clear understanding of what has to be done. The manager must establish the scope, depth, and framework of the responsibility and work demanded. For successful delegation, instructions must be specified clearly; the manager should explain the context of the assignment and define the expected output. After precisely defining the task, the manager must establish the framework for the work to be accomplished by:

- Soliciting the views of all team members about suggested approaches, expected schedules, and necessary resources
- Ensuring that team members have the authority, time, and resources (finances, people, equipment, training) to accomplish this assignment
- Knowing the capabilities of staff; if skills are not equal to the task, lost time, morale problems, and failure to meet deadlines will occur
- Establishing a clear understanding as to the time required for task completion

It is imperative that supervisors and employees work together and that communication between them be clear and consistent. The manager must be available to clarify issues and to help solve problems. Montana and Nash have compiled a list of delegation do's and don'ts.[13]

Do	Don't
Delegate as simply and directly as possible. Give precise instructions.	Do not threaten your staff. Effective delegation depends more on leadership skills than position power.
Illustrate how each delegation applies to organizational goals.	Do not assume a condescending attitude.
Mutually develop standards of performance.	Do not just give answers. Show an employee how to and why.
Clarify expected results.	Do not overreact to problems.
Anticipate what questions your employees may have and answer them in order.	Refrain from criticizing an employee in front of others.
Recognize superior performance.	Avoid excessive checks on progress.
Keep your promises.	

Effective Delegation

When used properly, delegation has several important advantages. The first and most obvious is that the more tasks managers are able to delegate, the more opportunity they have to seek and accept increased responsibilities from higher-level managers.

Several specific techniques have been suggested throughout the years for helping managers delegate effectively:

1. Establish goals and objectives. Managers must have good skills in planning, particularly in setting realistic, achievable objectives.
2. Define responsibility and authority. Team members should be clearly informed about what they will be held accountable for and what part of the organization's resources will be placed at their disposal.
3. Motivate team members. The challenge of extra responsibility alone will not always encourage subordinates to accept and perform delegated tasks. Managers can motivate team members by remaining sensitive to their needs and goals.
4. Require complete work. The manager's job is to provide guidelines, help, and information to all. Team members must do the actual delegated work.
5. Provide training. Managers need to teach subordinates how to improve their job performance.
6. Establish adequate controls. Managers should not spend all of their time checking on how well staff are doing. A reliable control system (such as weekly reports) should keep time spent in supervising to a minimum.

Barriers to Effective Delegation

Reluctance to delegate is a barrier to effective delegation. Managers offer a number of reasons why they do not delegate: "I can do it better myself." "My subordinates are not capable." These excuses are often used to hide the real reasons managers avoid delegation. Insecurity may be a major cause of reluctance to delegate. Managers are accountable for actions of their subordinates, and this may cause reluctance to take chances and delegate tasks. The manager may feel loss of power if a subordinate does too good a job. In addition, a manager may simply be too disorganized or inflexible to plan ahead and decide which tasks should be delegated to whom or to set up a control system so that subordinates' actions can be monitored. Lack of confidence in subordinates is another reason managers avoid delegation. Managers who lack confidence in their subordinates—perhaps because of an inflated sense of their own worth—will severely limit their subordinates' freedom to act.

STANDARDS AND MANAGEMENT INFORMATION SYSTEMS

The organizing function includes consideration of systems to monitor the activities of the organization. Beyond schedules of activities, most nutrition interventions require carefully defined protocols, standards of performance, or quality assurance criteria that delineate appropriate processes of the intervention. Quality assurance is discussed in Chapter 18.

Management Information Systems

Effective management requires timely information so that problems in resource availability, performance of activities, and volume of services can be identified early and adjustments made. Four kinds of information are needed for management of nutrition programs. Systems to document and monitor this information must be put in place in the organizing phase of the management process.

At the patient service level, *case management* requires a system for documenting and tracking patients through an appropriate sequence of service: screening and assessment, intervention, and follow-up. Case management information is used for quality assurance audits, is often linked to financial information, and may be used for efficiency studies.

At the program level, *service delivery information* is used to monitor units of service against service objectives. Based on appointment schedules and encounter records, it produces unduplicated head counts, service output reports, and descriptive measures of the population served. Service information is often required by administrators

and funders and is generally of interest to advocates and the public.

Financial information is needed to track the allocation of resources to planned programs and activities. This includes budgets, reports of expenditures and revenues, and records of billing and collections when fees are charged.

Evaluation information is gathered to assess specific indicators of program performance and client outcomes compared to established internal program objectives, as well as to state and national objectives.

Procedures and data systems that gather and summarize information for management decisions and evaluation are called *management information systems* (MIS). They provide data needed for program monitoring and evaluation. Most community agencies are implementing computerized systems to manage data. Data systems should be tailored to program and organization needs, as well as to reporting requirements of funders and of state and national nutrition monitoring systems. Standard health and nutrition status indicators that have scientific and practical significance to community health and nutrition programs should be incorporated into the MIS.

The internal MIS system may be supplemented with external data sets for overall program management purposes, such as needs assessment and assessing the program's contribution toward state and national health objectives.

In addition, the MIS of local health agencies should be designed to contribute data to state and national systems, which track information for a number of purposes:

1. To identify and track populations and geographic areas in need of service by poor rankings on health status indicators
2. To document types of services available and how well they are delivered
3. To determine accessibility and utilization of services by the population at risk
4. To measure intervening changes in behavior, knowledge, and risk status
5. To assess the effectiveness of existing services in improving health status

MARKETING: ORGANIZING WITH THE CLIENT IN MIND

Successful organizations in the 1990s are organized with their clients or customers foremost in mind. The public or not-for-profit sector, as well as the private business sector, have come to realize that it is essential to maintain a good fit between the organization's vision and goals and the wants and needs of the people who are served. This fit is the essence of marketing. Consumer-centeredness influences the way programs, products, and services are designed and the way employees throughout the organization behave.[12] This approach to management is called *strategic marketing*. The principles and process of strategic marketing are presented here.

If you were to ask several people what is meant by "marketing," most would say "selling" or "advertising." They would be only partially correct. Marketing is a process of creating, building, and maintaining beneficial exchange relationships with target audiences for the purpose of influencing behavior. A marketing mind-set, according to Kottler and Andreasen,[11] begins with the consumer. Through marketing, the organization systematically studies consumers' (target audience) needs, wants, perceptions, preferences, and satisfaction by using surveys, focus groups, and other means. This information is used to design services and products, to price them, to communicate (promote or advertise), and to deliver them to satisfy the target audience's needs and wants. The ultimate aim of marketing is to create a mutually beneficial exchange between the organization and its customers. A customer-centered organization is one that makes every effort to sense, serve, and satisfy the needs and wants of its clients and constituencies within the constraints of its budget.

Marketing Principles

1. Marketing seeks to bring about a voluntary exchange of value. The marketer seeks to formulate enough benefit for the target audience to produce a voluntary exchange.
2. Marketing involves segmentation of the community into subgroups or target audiences.
3. Effective marketing is consumer-oriented, not organization-oriented. Sensitivity to the target audience's needs and desires is a core component of effective marketing.
4. Marketing utilizes and blends a set of tools called the *marketing mix*, or the four *Ps*: product, price, promotion (communication), and place (distribution).

The not-for-profit sector offers challenging settings for the application of the marketing principles. Four characteristics of not-for-profit organizations require special attention:

1. *Multiple constituencies.* Not-for-profit organizations have at least two major constituencies: their clients and their funders. The former group poses the problem of resource allocation, and the latter the problem of resource attraction.
2. *Multiple objectives.* Not-for-profit organizations tend to pursue several important objectives simultaneously rather than only focusing on profits.
3. *Services versus physical goods.* Not-for-profit organizations frequently produce services rather than goods. In today's market, service is not an event; it is the process of creating a customer environment of information, assurance, and comfort. Ultimately, a service builds loyal customer relationships.
4. *Public scrutiny.* Not-for-profit organizations are usually subjected to close public scrutiny because they provide needed public services, are subsidized, are tax exempt, and in many cases are mandated into existence. They experience political pressures from various constituencies and are expected to operate in the public interest.

The ultimate objective of all marketing is to stimulate a specific behavior in the target audience.

The following examples illustrate the application of marketing principles to situations commonly experienced by dietitians and nutritionists working in a community nutrition setting: efforts to get individuals to change their food selection behaviors to reduce risk of cancer by substituting low-fat foods for those high in fat or by eating five fruits and

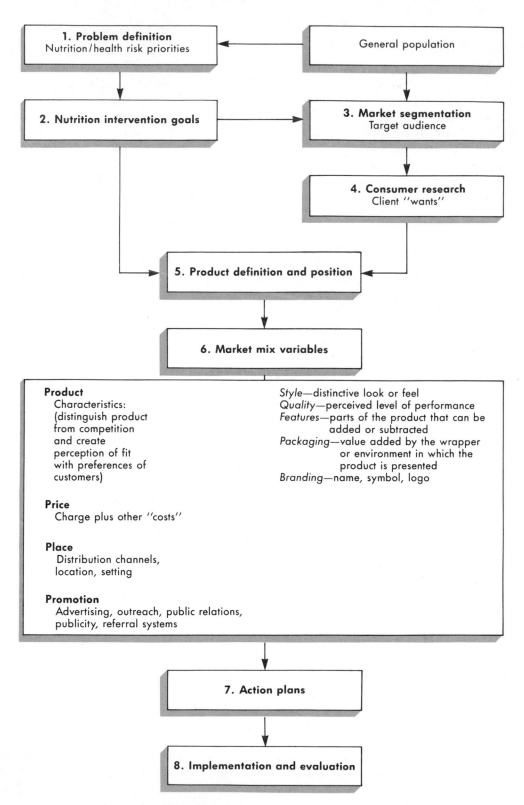

Figure 16-10. Strategic marketing applied to the design of nutrition programs.

vegetables a day; efforts to sell nutriton education materials to other agencies; efforts to secure funding from a foundation or payment from insurance companies; and efforts to enroll pregnant women in early prenatal care.

The Strategic Marketing Process

Organizations that adapt to a changing environment use strategic planning (see Chapter 14). Customer-oriented organizations use strategic marketing as a managerial process for developing and maintaining a strategic fit between the organization's goals and resources.

The process extends on the needs assessment and planning process. Eight steps summarized from the emerging literature on strategic marketing are illustrated in Figure 16-10. Note how the goals of the nutrition program fit the wants of the target audience through the strategic marketing process.

Step One: Problem Definition

Based on identified public health priorities and opportunities in the environment, define a potential area for change where a product, program, or service may reduce the problem and move toward the achievement of health goals. This step is accomplished through the needs assessment process described in Chapters 14 and 15.

Step Two: Goal Setting

Set measurable goals for separate segments of the population. This enables the program organizer to determine the scope of the plan and a budget. Goals also establish benchmarks for success.

Step Three: Target Audience Segmentation

Effectiveness is enhanced by tailoring programs to the specific subgroups within the overall population. At this step you select specific segments of the population on which to focus efforts. Segmentation is a process of dividing the total market or the total population into a smaller target audience or segment of people who have relatively similar wants. Segmentation is based on a number of observable factors such as geographic location, age, risk factor, socioeconomic status, attitudes and values, place of residence, or employment.

Step Four: Consumer Research and Analysis

This is the most crucial step. Considerable time and resources must be allocated to the challenge of understanding the consumers, their values and preferences, and their knowledge regarding the behavior you wish to change. Market research through telephone or mailed surveys, focus groups, observation, and existing data is used to determine the motivation and interest of the target audience, the characteristics of products and services they would be likely to use, their language and style preferences, and their knowledge and use of potential distribution channels. This step should result in a clear understanding of client "needs"—a desire that is *unexpressed* or not acted upon—and "wants"—things they desire to the point of being motivated to take some action to get them.

Step Five: Product Definition and Position

Information from the previous step is carefully considered in order to define the product concept. A product is anything that can be offered to a market to satisfy a need or want. It can be a physical object, service, person, program, policy, idea, or message. Also it is necessary to determine the market niche or "position" this product will have among competitors. Position is the image that customers will have of the product. For example, should it be positioned as innovative and on the cutting-edge, solid and dependable, conservative, elite, economical, or upscale? Care must be exercised to define the product and its niche or position in the marketplace in a way that will be most compatible with the target audience's preferences.

Step Six: Market Mix Variables

Market mix variables are factors that are directly under the control of those designing the product. They guide the development of the product and how it will be offered in the market place. This step provides the strategic opportunity to create a good fit between the wants of the target audience and the goals of the community nutrition program. The market mix variables are commonly known as the four *P*s—product, price, place, promotion. At this step each of the four *P*s is determined. The core product and its style, quality, features, packaging, and branding are determined. The price is the monetary cost plus anything else that must be given up by the consumer to receive the product. The price could be a fee, but it can also include travel and waiting time, embarrassment, or inconvenience. Place is the distribution channel. Although clinics are traditional sites, nutrition products can be creatively distributed through schools, worksites, mass media, grocery stores, and sports clubs. Promotion is the means by which the product is communicated to the target audience. It includes outreach, public relations, advertising, and other promotion efforts. Referral systems and word of mouth have been a commonly used means of making people aware of community nutrition services. More formalized communication activities

Table 16-1. Marketing strategy worksheet

Marketing process	Example
Target audience	1. Teenagers age 14-18 who become pregnant
Market mix variables	Prenatal dietary counseling offered by dietitian
Product	Objectives: 1. Modify snacking behavior to increase nutrient intakes of vitamins A and B_6, folic acid, calcium, and iron. 2. Gain adequate weight 3. Identify accessible food resources
Price	Miss class or after-school activities; no monetary charge
Place	School-based health clinic
Promotion	• School newsletter • Brochure in school nurse office • Planned Parenthood clinics • Community family planning
Competitive position	• Tailor counseling services to priorities of teens • Offer at school where pregnant students spend day • Integrate into prenatal program for academic credit

Adapted from Ward, Marcia, 1984. *Marketing Strategies: A Resource for Registered Dietitians*. Binghamton, NY: Niles and Phipps.

should be used for effectively connecting the target audience with the products designed to meet their needs and wants.

Together the selection of a target audience (market segment), the choice of a competitive position (market niche), and the development of the market mix to reach and serve the customers are called the *marketing strategy*. Table 16-1 illustrates the development of a marketing strategy for dietary counseling of pregnant teenagers.

Step Seven: Action Plan and Budget

Planning and scheduling activities. The action plan is a method of organizing that is familiar and useful to the community dietitian and nutritionist. It is a process that determines how each activity will be achieved. According to Craig,[2] an *activity* is defined as "a specific procedure or process, completed at a certain point in time and implemented by organization personnel as part of a plan for reaching the desired objective." A *task* is a specific procedure or process that includes what will be done, when, and by whom.

In the design of the action plan, a planning grid helps to organize all the key activities and tasks needed to reach a goal, such as designing a product and bringing it to the marketplace. Figure 16-11 provides a sample format for organizing efforts, including definitions of terms and tips for use.

The steps to creating a planning grid are:[16]

1. Specify the final outcome. How will you know when this project has been successfully completed?
2. Identify the final activity and its result.
3. Identify the starting point and its result.
4. Brainstorm a list of separate, distinct activities that will take place between the starting and ending points.
5. Refine the brainstormed list: clarify what is unclear, eliminate redundancy, subdivide tasks that are too large, and combine those that are too small.
6. Prepare the grid.
7. Arrange the list of activities in sequence down the left column of the planning grid. Use of self-stick notes is recommended so

Step number	Sequential steps activities tasks	Due date	Results	Responsibility	Whom to invite/contact	Budget and cost	Other categories

Definition of Terms Used in the Action Planning Grid

Step number

Simple numbering is used most frequently to indicate the sequence of events, but you may use some other code if you like.

Sequential steps/activities/tasks

Enter, in chronological order, each task that is part of this activity. For example, if the step involves "data collection," then the tasks might be: 1. Develop operational definitions, 2. Prepare checksheets, 3. Test and refine checksheets, 4. Train data collectors, 5. Collect data.

Result

Each discrete step results in some result, for example, a report, a tangible change, a decision, a phone call, a meeting. There is always something that indicates the completion of a step. Enter here a word or phrase describing what that completion sign is for this step.

Responsibility

Enter here the name of one or two people who are responsible for seeing that this task gets done. Note: They do not necessarily carry out the action themselves. They may just coordinate the actions of others.

Due data

The calendar data when this step should be finished.

Whom to involve/contact

If appropriate, enter here the names of people who should be part of the team working on this task, or who should at least be contacted and informed of progress or events.

Budget/cost

If funds have been allocated for this activity, or if there is a limit to expenditures, enter that figure.

Other catagories

Customers

This column lets you keep track of people who are particularly interested in or concerned about the successful outcome of this step or the project as a whole. Typically, this includes people whose work depends on what is assomplished at this step.

Limitations/specifications

Enter here any constraints under which the people involved with this step must operate, such as amount of time per week they can spend on the task, how many other people they can call on for help, the maximum time they can stop a process (if at all), and so forth. Note: You may also enter time and money limits here, though the categories of "budget" and "due date" usually indicate the same thing.

Hazards/pitfalls

Past experience with this activity may lead you to expect trouble in some form. Enter here any information that will help the team avoid pitfalls.

By-products

Many times a team will be given secondary objectives: "While you're at it, see if you can do this for another purpose." Although secondary purposes should not be allowed to interfere with the primary objectives of the activities, they should be allowed if they may lead to useful results without detracting.

Figure 16-11. Format for the action planning grid.
Source: Scholtes P. et al. The Team Handbook. How to use teams to improve quality. Madison, WI: Joiner Associates Inc. 1988.

that the steps can be easily rearranged until the sequence seems right.

8. Fill in the results column.
9. Enter a tentative date for each item. You need to complete this step before others because the time available for performing a task sometimes affects the nature of the project. ("Do what you can in the next 30 days!") Due dates also indicate when the person responsible for that item must be available. If you have an inflexible deadline, start at the end of the list and work backwards. Use prior experience and any knowledge about similar activities to set realistic deadlines.
10. If necessary, revise items.
11. Complete the remaining columns.

Another common technique for scheduling activities is Gantt scheduling.[2] In Gantt Scheduling (Fig. 16-12), a bar chart is used to reflect activities and their start and completion dates. Activities are listed in the first column on the left. To use the Gantt technique, one works from left to right, plotting activities as they must occur and establishing a completion date for the job. Horizontal dotted lines are drawn so that their lengths are proportional to the planned duration of each activity. Progress on each activity is monitored by drawing solid lines parallel to and below the dotted lines to show actual duration for activities underway or completed.

Planning resource needs. The action plan must include attention to resource needs and expenditure. If a financial reporting system is not in place, one must be established. What resources are needed to carry out the action plan? Where will these resources come from? Will the product generate revenue? The answers to these questions define the financial picture. Sources of money to finance community nutrition programs utilize public and private funding sources, including grants, contracts, third-party reimbursement, and payments for products and services.[4] Budgeting and financial control are discussed in the next chapter.

Step Eight: Implementation and Evaluation

Carry out the plan, introduce the product, and evaluate. This step documents the types of measurements, controls, and review procedures that will be used (see Chapter 18). It is important that the authority for evaluation, as well as decisions regarding adjustments, be clearly defined early in the implementation step.

In summary, this eight-step model can help you design a new product venture that meets the needs and wants of consumers. The customer orientation is essential to making community nutrition services relevant and accessible to members of the community.

Social Marketing

The term *social marketing* was first introduced in 1971 to describe the use of marketing principles and techniques to advance a social cause, idea, or behavior (such as a "five a day" to increase consumption of fruit and vegetables). Social marketing is the design, implementation, and control of programs that seek to increase the acceptability of a social idea or cause in a target program. It relies on concepts of market segmentation, consumer research, concept development, communication, facilitation, incentives, and exchange theory to maximize target group response.

The Process

The social marketing process consists of the following steps: (1) problem definition, (2) goal setting, (3) target market (audience) segmentation, (4) consumer analysis, (5) influence channel analysis, (6) marketing strategies and tactics including the four Ps, and (7) implementation and evaluation.

A social marketing approach does not guarantee that the intervention objectives will be achieved. However, social marketing that applies research from behavioral sciences to a process for design and implementation of programs for propagation of ideas increases the likelihood of success. It offers a useful framework for effective communitywide nutrition intervention at a time when more and more evidence links lifestyle habits with major

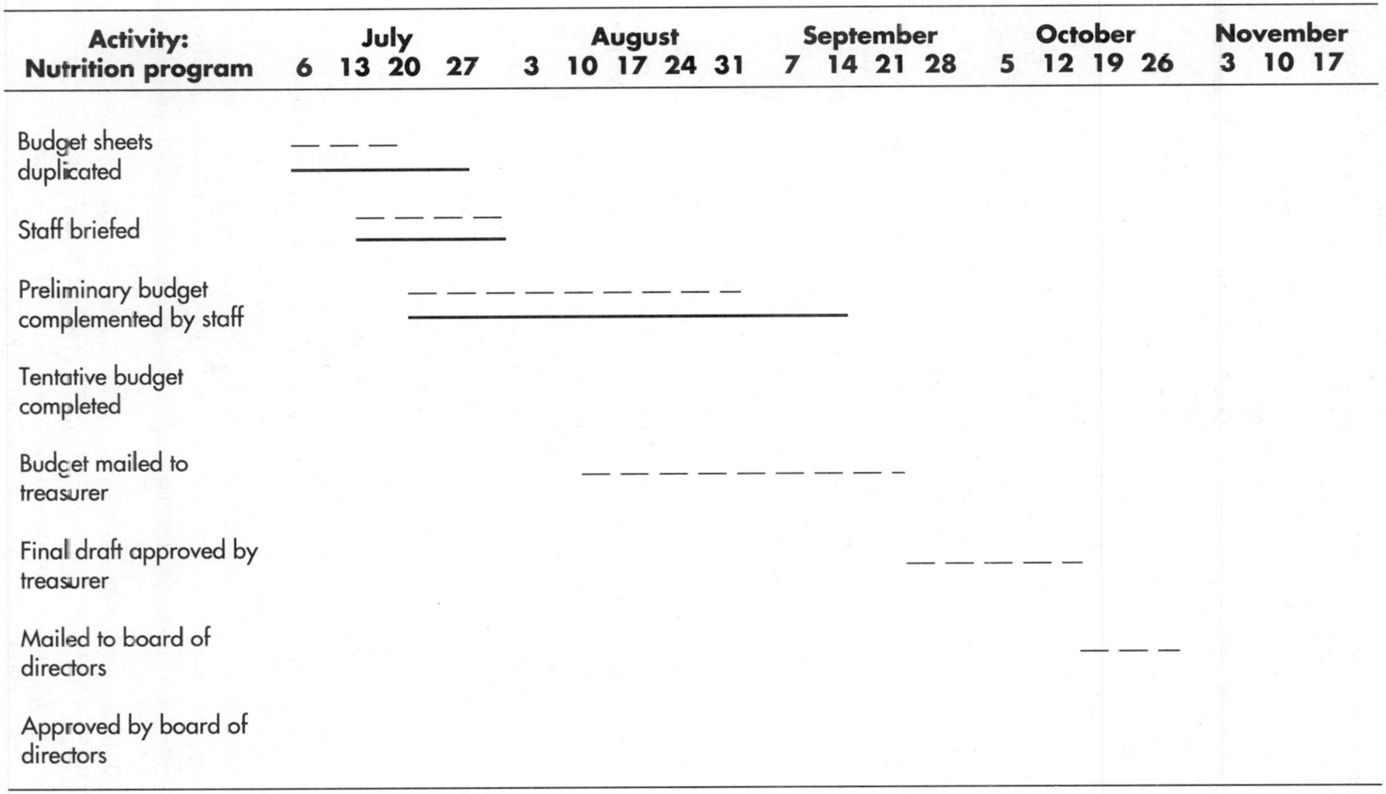

Figure 16-12. Gantt scheduling. Redrawn from Craig DP: *HIP pocket guide to planning and evaluation,* Austin, Texas, 1978, Learning Concepts, Inc.

chronic illness. Social marketing issues have become more relevant and critical.

A heuristic for identifying intervention approaches to address community nutrition problems is the four *E*s of public health: educate, enable, enact, and engineer.[17] These approaches, used alone or in combination, can be used to stimulate creativity and innovation in the design of nutrition programs, products, and services to stimulate a desired behavior in the target audience.

Educate. Education has been a traditional tool of public health and is the most responsive to social marketing. It is based on a belief in self-determination and personal freedom. Education is designed to increase individuals' awareness and knowledge of options, of benefits of particular options, and of reasons why certain practices are related to good health or well-being. It allows individuals to exercise free choice from a position of being fully informed; however, education can also take the negative form of persuasion or brainwashing.

Enable. Interventions that reduce social, physical, psychological, or economic barriers to action and make it easier for people to act according to the desired goal irrespective of knowledge base are enablers. For example, food assistance programs assist families in meeting basic nutritional needs, or child-care facilities near the workplace enable breastfeeding among working women. Enabling interventions relate to the four *P*s of the marketing mix (e.g., design of *product* to be culturally acceptable, location of clinic site [*place*] to reduce barriers to access, subsidized services to keep the *price* low, and tailoring of the *promotion* message to enable attention and acceptance).

Enact. Interventions in this category protect society by requiring or prohibiting certain actions through legislation or regulation. Legislative action may be initiated on behalf of vulnerable groups within the society (e.g., PL 99-457 to require services for handicapped children). Other examples are food safety and labeling regulations, mandated phenylketonuria (PKU) testing, and institutional food codes and nutrition care standards required for licensure.

Engineer. Science and technology can be used to ameliorate problems. Frequently, engineered interventions achieve health goals with no involvement or decision on the part of the individual (e.g., fluoridated water, air bags in automobiles, and milk fortified with vitamin A and D). Food engineering has responded to the need for lower-fat and higher-fiber food products. Social engineering through the use of community development approaches could also be categorized here.

MANAGING ORGANIZATIONAL CONFLICT

Conflict is not only inevitable but also necessary for organizations to survive. Conflict should lead to a search for solutions, and thus it is an instrument of organizational innovation and change. The role of managers is not to suppress or resolve all conflict but to manage it so as to minimize its harmful aspects and maximize its benefical aspects.

Organizational conflict is a disagreement between two or more individuals or groups arising from differences in opinion, fact, performance, or resources. The allocation of scarce resources and disagreements about roles and responsibility for activities are common sources of conflict. Conflict is also fueled by differences in status, goals, values, knowledge, or perceptions. Individuals and groups in disagreement attempt to have their own cause or point of view prevail over that of others.

Conflict Resolution

Conflict resolution is a skill needed by managers in the complex and often stressful changing environment of community nutrition. Managing in a multidisciplinary setting while working to meet the demands of many constituencies requires less autocratic control and more acting as "a coach to empower employees to participate in decision making."[14] Good communication and listening skills are needed to develop trust and cooperation when there is no way of avoiding conflict. Conflict and stress should be recognized as an opportunity to make changes within an organization that may be beneficial. Effective nutrition managers need to confront conflict and respond in a manner that leads to solutions so all parties can feel like winners.

The three basic conflict resolution approaches most commonly used are dominance and suppression, compromise, and integrative problem solving. These approaches form a hierarchy in the extent to which they yield effective and creative solutions to conflict and in the extent to which they leave parties in the conflict able to deal with future conflicts.[18]

Integrative Problem Solving

With integrative problem solving, intergroup conflict is converted into a joint problem-solving situation. Together, parties to the conflict try to resolve the problem that has arisen between them. Instead of suppressing conflict or trying to find a compromise, the parties openly try to find a solution they all can accept. Managers who give subordinates the feeling that all members and groups are working together for a common goal, encourage the free exchange of ideas, and stress the benefits of finding the optimum solution to a conflict are more likely to achieve integrative solutions.

The process used to achieve integrated decision making when conflict is present has been outlined by Filley.[5]

1. Review and adjust conditions in which the parties are related. They are primarily related to time, information, and power.
2. Review and adjust perceptions. This is "reality testing" to determine the facts relevant to the conflict situation.
3. Review and adjust attitudes, the use of reality testing of feelings and attitudes between parties.
4. Define the problem. Concentrate on the mutual determination of the depersonalized problem. It is important to not focus on solutions, people, or positions; rather, focus on the opportunities, needs, and wants.
5. Search for solutions. Generate many possible alternatives. Creative idea-generating techniques such as brainstorming, nominal group process, and delphi techniques can be used.
6. Reach a decision. Evaluate all alternative solutions and agree on a single solution.

An effective manager must demonstrate the energy and commitment to actively involve those affected by a conflict situation. Then, to arrive at a mutually agreed-upon decision, it is important that a manager can develop an atmosphere of trust and effectively lead the group. A manager needs to encourage active listening and open communication so that individuals' perceptions of the situation and attitudes about it are exposed for others' reactions. This reality testing moves beyond emotions to an understanding of what is actually the basis for the problem. Participation in integrative decision making becomes a training ground for improving communication and problem-solving skills.

Negotiation

Negotiation is defined as "an activity in which parties are trying to meet their needs."[1] It is an activity in which both sides feel a sense of accomplishment, respect, and fairness. They reflect how strongly people pursue their own concerns and how they work with others' concerns.

The Thomas-Kilmann model of negotiation styles examines the impact of two types of behavior on the resolution of conflict (Fig. 16-13).[10] The degree to which negotiators are assertive and cooperative produces five styles: avoiding, com-

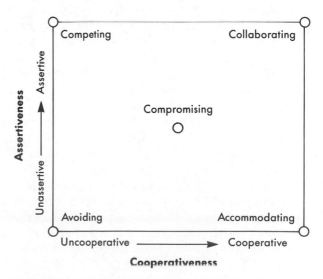

Figure 16-13. Negotiation styles.
From Killman R, Thomas K: *Thomas-Kilman conflict mode instrument*, Tuxedo, NY, 1974, Xicom Co.

promising, accommodating, competing, and collaborating.

Avoiding conflict is the result of being unassertive and uncooperative. The conflict is suppressed and not addressed. Although avoidance may provide immediate survival, it usually does not solve a problem or provide satisfaction for either party involved.

Accommodating results from a combination of unassertive and cooperative behavior. When accommodating, one neglects one's own concerns to satisfy the concerns of the other person. There is an element of self-sacrifice or "you win, I lose" in this approach. This form of selfless generosity does not provide acceptable solutions to the conflict.

In the Thomas-Kilmann model, *competing* is a power-play style. One party is assertive and uncooperative. The competitive party pursues his or her own concerns at the other person's expense. This is a power mode in which one uses whatever power that seems appropriate. These are tough battles in which the "winner" feels success and the "loser" feels hostility. The loser may initiate a rematch in which he or she can regain lost or damaged self-esteem.

Compromising is an intermediate approach to negotiation; it is between competing and accommodating. In compromising, each side settles differences by mutual concessions—each party must give up something. Although this approach is commonly used, it is viewed as "lose-lose" because both sides must give up something.

Collaboration combines assertiveness and cooperation. It leads to integrated problem solving and positive results. Collaboration is "a process through which parties who see different aspects of a problem can constructively explore their differences and search for solutions that go beyond their own limited vision of what is possible."[7] Collaboration has the greatest "win-win" potential of all the negotiation styles. However, collaborations can become ineffective if too much time is spent on insignificant parts of the problem, if people unfamiliar with the situation are asked for input, or if mutual trust is not present.

Principled negotiation, which was developed at the Harvard Negotiation Project,[6] is deciding the issues on their merits rather than on the power, position, or persuasion of either side. Its focus is mutual gains whenever possible while being hard on the merits but soft on the people. Principled negotiation has four principles:

1. Separate the people from the problem
2. Focus on interests, not position
3. Invent options for mutual gain
4. Insist on using objective criteria

MANAGING ORGANIZATIONAL CHANGE

Rapid societal changes as a result of advanced technological developments; blurring of boundaries between business, government, and labor; and shrinking of federal revenues for social programs places many demands on those who must manage the human component of an organization. Managers are confronted with a somewhat paradoxical situation. On the one hand, they must be responsive to demands for change in work environments. They must anticipate changes, and viewing their accountability broadly, they must exercise leadership in bringing changes to the organizations they manage. Managers must be change seekers, change agents, and change masters, adept at the art of anticipating the need for and of leading productive change.[8] On the other hand, managers must respond to the demands of stability in work environments. Thus managers are also stability seekers and stability agents. The paradox is a need for balance. Managers must create and maintain work environments that balance the demands of both stability and change. Nevertheless, organizational change is bound to occur, given the variety of forces for change that exists both within and outside an organization. There are two constructive ways that managers can deal with change: react to it or plan for it. The former is appropriate for the day-to-day decisions a manager must make; the latter approach is necessary when a major part or all of the organization needs to change.

The change agent is the individual who is responsible for taking a leadership role in managing the process of change. Change agents can be members of the organization, or they can be consultants

Table 16-2. Ways of overcoming resistance to change

Approach	Commonly used when	Advantages	Disadvantages
Education and communication	There is a lack of information or inaccurate information and analysis.	Once persuaded, people will often help implement the change.	Can be very time-consuming if many people are involved.
Participation and involvement	The initiators do not have all the information they need to design the change, and others have considerable power to resist.	People who participate will be committed to implementing change, and any relevant information they have will be integrated into the change plan.	Can be very time-consuming if participators design an inappropriate change.
Facilitation and support	People are resisting because of adjustment problems.	No other approach works as well with adjustment problems.	Can be time-consuming, expensive, and still fail.
Negotiation agreement	Some person or group with considerable power to resist will clearly lose out in a change.	Sometimes it is a relatively easy way to avoid major resistance.	Can be too expensive if it alerts others to neogotiate for compliance.
Manipulation and co-optation	Other tactics will not work or are too expensive.	It can be a relatively quick and inexpensive solution to resistance problems.	Can lead to future problems if people feel manipulated.
Explicit and implicit coercion	Speed is essential, and the change initiators possess considerable power.	It is speedy and can overcome any kind of resistance.	Can be risky if it leaves people angry with the initiators.

Reprinted by permission of the Harvard Business Review. Exhibit from "Choosing Strategies for Change" by John P. Kotter and Leonard A. Schlesinger (March/April 1979). Copyright © 1979 by the President and Fellows of Harvard College; all rights reserved. In James A.F. Stoner. Management, ed. 2, © 1982, pp. 408, 593. Reprinted by permission of Prentice-Hall, Inc., Englewood Cliffs, N.J.

brought in from the outside. The successful change agent is one who influences change by helping members of the organization and consumers understand and accept change. He or she must be sensitive to individuals or groups who are not supportive of the change and be able to redirect efforts to a collective goal. This can be a difficult and challenging role. Table 16-2 offers six highly situation-dependent ways of overcoming resistance to change.

Education and Communication

One of the most obvious ways to overcome resistance to change is to inform people about the planned change and the need for it early in the process. If the need for the change and its logic are explained—whether individually to subordinates, to groups in meetings, or to entire organizations through elaborate audiovisual education campaigns—the road to successful change may be smoother.

Participation and Involvement

If potential resisters are drawn into the actual design and implementation of the change, it may be better prepared and easier to effect.

Facilitation and Support

Easing the change process and providing support for those caught up in it are ways managers can deal with resistance. Implementing retraining programs, allowing time off after a difficult period, and offering emotional support and understanding may help.

Negotiation and Agreement

Another technique is negotiation with avowed or potential resisters. Examples include initiating union agreements, increasing an employee's pension benefits in exchange for his or her early retirement, or obtaining written letters of understanding from the heads of organization subunits that would be affected by the change.

Manipulation and Co-option

Sometimes managers covertly steer individuals or groups away from resistance to change. They may manipulate workers by releasing information selectively or by consciously structuring the sequence of events. They may co-opt an individual, perhaps a key person within a group, by giving him or her a desirable role in designing or carrying out the change process. Aside from the doubtful ethics of such a technique, this approach may backfire.

Explicit and Implicit Coercion

Managers may force people to go along with change by explicit or implicit threats involving loss of jobs, lack of promotion, and the like. Managers also dismiss or transfer employees who stand in the way of change. As with manipulation and co-option, such methods, although uncommon, are risky and make it more difficult to gain support for future change efforts.

Overcoming resistance to change involves using more than one of these six approaches. Which techniques to employ and how to translate them into effective actions depend on the specifics of the situation.

SUMMARY

Plans and programs become reality through the management function of organizing. Organizing sets up a formal structure to achieve goals and objectives. The organizational models for public health nutrition services provide a rational and consistent approach to organizing and staffing nutrition programs.

Five sources of power have been identified, and each may occur at any level of an organization. Delegation of authority by supervisors to their employees is necessary for the efficient functioning of any organization. The first and major step in the delegation process requires that the manager has a clear understanding of what he wants to have accomplished.

The organizing function includes a system to monitor the activities of the organization. Effective management requires timely information so that problems in resource availability, performance, and volume of services can be identified early and adjustments made.

Successful organizations are organized with their clients or customers in mind. Consumer-centeredness influences the way programs, products, and services are designed and the way employees behave. This approach to management is called *strategic marketing*. Four characteristics of not-for-profit organizations require special attention: multiple constituencies, multiple objectives, service versus physical goods, and public scrutiny.

Conflict resolution is a skill needed by dietitian and nutritionist managers in the complex, often stressful, changing environment of community nutrition. Good communication and listening skills are needed to develop trust and cooperation when there is no way of avoiding conflict.

Negotiation is defined as "an activity in which parties are trying to meet their needs." In negotiations, both sides should feel a sense of accomplishment, respect, and fairness.

Dietitian and nutritionist managers are both stability seekers and stability agents. The paradox is a need for balance. Managers must create and maintain work environments that balance the demands of both stability and change.

REFERENCES

1. Cohen H: *You can negotiate anything*, New York, 1980, Bantam Books.
2. Craig DP: *HIP pocket guide to planning and evaluation*, Austin, Tex, 1978, Learning Concepts.
3. Dodds JM, Kaufman M, editors: *Personnel in public health nutrition for the 1990s*, Washington, DC, 1991, The Public Health Foundation.

4. Egan MC, Kaufman M: Financing nutrition services in a competitive market, *J Am Diet Assoc* 852, 1985.
5. Filley A: *Interpersonal conflict resolution*, Glenview, Ill, 1975, Scott, Foresman.
6. Fisher R, Ury W: *Getting to yes*, New York, 1981, Penguin.
7. Gray B: *Collaborating: finding common ground for multi-party problems*, San Francisco, Calif, 1989, Jossey-Bass.
8. Kanter RM: *The change masters: innovative entrepreneurship in the American corporation*, New York, 1983, Simon & Schuster.
9. Kaufman M and others: Survey of nutritionists in state and local public health agencies, *J Am Diet Assoc* 86:1566, 1986.
10. Kilmann R, Thomas K: *Thomas-Kilman conflict mode instrument*, Tuxedo, NY, 1974, Xicom Co.
11. Kottler P, Andreasen AR: *Strategic marketing for nonprofit organizations*, ed 4, Englewood Cliffs, NJ, 1991, Prentice Hall.
12. McKenna R: Marketing is everything, *Harvard Business Review* 69:65, 1990.
13. Montana PJ, Nash DF: Delegation: the art of managing, *Personnel J*, 60:784, 1981.
14. Rinke W, Finn S: Winning strategies to excel in dietetics, *J Am Diet Assoc*, 91:935, 1990.
15. Scanlon BK, Atherton RM: Participation and the effective use of authority, *Personnel J* 60:697, 1981.
16. Scholtes PR and others: *The team handbook: how to use teams to improve quality*, Madison, Wisc, 1988, Joiner Associates.
17. Splett P: *Planning, implementation, and evaluation of nutrition programs*. In Sharbough CO, editor: *Call to action: better nutrition for mothers, children, and families*, Washington, DC, 1990, National Center for Education, Maternal and Child Health.
18. Stoner JAF: *Management*, ed 4. Englewood Cliffs, NJ, 1989, Prentice Hall.
19. Ward M: *Marketing strategies: a resource for registered dietitians*, Binghamton City, NY, 1984, Niles and Phipps.

APPENDIX 16-1

A method for estimating staffing needs for client nutrition care

STEP ONE

Establish the target populations for your agency's nutrition program and specify the type of service. Calculate for each target population:

L = the estimated length of time for each encounter

N = the total number of encounters needed per year (number of encounters multiplied by the number of clients or clients in a group)

Target Population 1

Clients with special nutrition needs because of their health status, for example, pregnant and lactating women, infants and children with identified nutrition-related health problems (e.g., WIC program), persons requiring therapeutic diets for chronic diseases.

- Type of encounter: individual counseling
- Length of encounter: 30 minutes = L_1 = ½ hour per client.

Adapted from Freeman RB, Holmes EM: *Administration of public health services*. Philadelphia, 1960, WB Saunders.

- Number of encounters per year = N_1 = 2 × number of clients seen in 1 year

Target Population 2

Persons identified at high nutritional risk through nutritional screening and assessment who are not also served as part of a high health risk population, for example, older children identified at high nutritional risk because of poor growth or abnormal biochemical assessment.

- Type of encounter: individual counseling
- Length of encounter: 30 minutes = L_2 = ½ hour per client
- Number of encounters per year = N_2 = 2 × number of clients seen in 1 year.

Target Population 3

Health care providers, educators, social workers, and child care staff providing nutrition care and food service to high-risk populations, for example, MCH nurses and nursing assistants.

- Type of encounter: group classes

- Length of encounter: 1 hour divided by 15 participants $= L_3 = \frac{1}{15}$ hour per person
- Number of encounters per year $= N_3 = 2 \times$ number of participants in 1 year

Target Population 4

School children, the elderly, or the general public involved in health promotion and disease prevention programs, for example, community congregate meal site for the elderly.

- Type of encounter: group classes
- Length of encounter: 1 hour divided by 30 participants $= L_4 = \frac{1}{30}$ hour per person
- Number of encounters per year $= N_4 = 2 \times$ number of participants for 1 year

STEP TWO

Estimate *K*, the effective hours per worker per year available. Total hours minus annual leave (an estimated average), holidays, sick leave (estimated based on average amount used in past), travel time, continuing education, and personal time, for example:

Total available working hours per year $(52 \times 40) =$	2080
minus annual leave $(8 \times 15) =$	-120
	1960
minus sick leave $(6 \times 8) =$	-48
	1912
minus travel time	-52
	1860
minus continuing education	-16
$K =$	1844

STEP THREE

Estimate *H*, the number of hours needed for adjunct activities per year, for example, planning and preparation, recording and reporting, consultation, meetings, and personal time.

STEP FOUR

Apply the formula:

$$\frac{L_1 N_1 + L_2 N_2 + L_3 N_3 + L_4 N_4 + H}{K}$$

$=$ number of direct service nutrition staff needed to serve program's target populations

Insert your program's figures in the following blanks:

$$\frac{L_1(\quad) \times N_1(\quad) + L_2(\quad) \times N_2(\quad) + L_3(\quad) \times N_3(\quad) + L_4(\quad) \times N(\quad) + H}{K(\quad)} = \underline{\quad}$$

Example

Estimating the Nutrition Direct Care Staffing Needs of One County Nutrition Program

Target population 1:

7000 clients at two 30-minute individual encounters per year.

6000 clients seen in group classes of 30 persons each class lasting 30 minutes and seen two times a year.

Target population 3:

In-service programs for nursing staff: 1-hour presentation, twice a year with 15 nurses and assistants attending each time.

K is calculated at 1844 hours

H is estimated at 400 hours

$$\frac{1/2 \times 14{,}000 + 1/60 \times 6000 + 1/15 \times 30 + 400}{1844}$$

$$= \frac{7502}{1844} = 4 \text{ direct care nutrition providers}$$

17

Leading to Achieve Goals

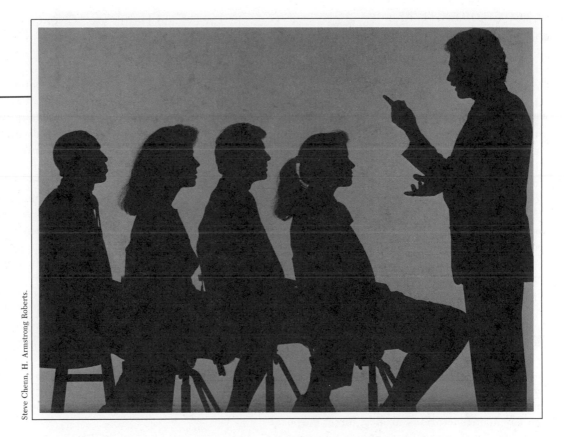

GENERAL CONCEPT

Leaders set direction by shaping both a vision and the strategies needed to achieve that vision. Management sets a plan into action by organizing efficient systems. The most appropriate leadership style is one that matches employees' abilities and helps them achieve satisfaction and accomplish goals. Dietitians and nutritionists need to define what leadership skills are needed in various professional situations; then they will be able to identify potential leaders as a prerequisite to leadership development.

465

OUTCOME OBJECTIVES

When you finish this chapter, you should be able to:

- Distinguish between the terms *leader* and *manager*.
- Identify trait, behavioral, and contingency approaches to leadership.
- Identify the issues concerning women as managerial leaders.
- Describe major approaches to leadership among dietitians and nutritionists, nurses, social workers, and physical therapists.

Abraham Lincoln, Franklin D. Roosevelt, Winston Churchill, and Gandhi come to mind when we think of great leaders, but many outstanding leaders are much less famous than these political figures. The importance of managerial leadership is demonstrated daily in the positions available section of any major newspaper. The advertisements for managerial positions are replete with phrases such as "strong leadership required," "must be a leader," and "an excellent opportunity for you to demonstrate your leadership skills." Leadership often connotes images of powerful, dynamic people who command victorious armies, direct corporate empires from atop gleaming skyscrapers, or shape the course of nations. Effective managers in any business organization, at all levels, must be leaders, too.

DIETITIANS AND NUTRITIONISTS: LEADERS OR FOLLOWERS?

A crisis in leadership is one of the greatest challenges facing our profession today. Within our health care system, we now have a work force of 60,000 dietitians and nutritionists in settings ranging from hospitals to private practice. Technological advances and a concomitant concern for cost containment have placed the health care delivery system in a state of turmoil and, as a result, our profession needs leaders who are competent, flexible, politically savvy, willing to accept diversity, and able to energize others to adapt to change.

To develop real change, we must begin with the individual and the inside-out approach described by Covey[8] and Heath[15] (see Chapter 13). In other words, we must begin with ourselves.

DEFINITION OF *LEADERSHIP*

What is leadership? Some people believe that the terms *leader* and *manager* are synonymous, but it is important that they be distinguished. According to Fiedler,[13] the *leader* is "the individual in the group given the task of directing and coordinating task-relevant activities." A *manager* is a person who occupies a designated role in an organized structure. Although this role gives the manager formal authority, some managers are totally incapable of leading. These managers will obviously have limited success in the organization. The phrase *managerial leadership* implies that both leadership and managerial skills are necessary.

A managerial leader must be able to direct and coordinate tasks with a group (Fig. 17-1). The focus of this chapter is on effective managerial leadership. The question addressed is, What is required for a person to be an effective leader in a managerial position?

In general, the literature suggests that leadership is epitomized by the statement "I have a

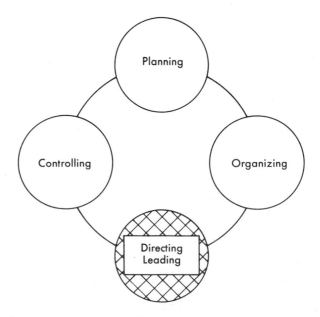

Figure 17-1. The management process.

dream," that is, by a sense of vision and the skill to construct a network to commit to that vision. Management, by contrast, is epitomized by the statement "I have a budget," that is, by the organization and skills to implement the vision.

Kotter asserts that leadership and management are two distinct, yet complementary functions, each of which is essential.[22] Leadership, in his opinion, is primarily about dealing with change, whereas management is concerned with complexity.

Leaders set a direction by shaping both a vision and the strategies needed to achieve that vision. They must be broad-based strategic thinkers who are also risk takers. Leaders must excel at aligning support for their visions as well. This includes working the appropriate networks extensively and credibly to spread the vision and to get people to buy into both its message and its likelihood of success. It also includes motivating and inspiring others by appealing to their basic values, needs for achievement, and self-esteem.

Management sets a plan into action by organizing and staffing efficient systems. Unlike leadership, it is concerned with planning and budgeting something concrete, not with bringing about change. This includes establishing control mechanisms to minimize deviations from goals and engaging in effective problem solving. Whereas leaders are involved in motivating people to take risks and bend to change, managers are interested in establishing fail-safe and risk-free systems.

Senge offers yet another view of the organizational leader. Leaders, in his opinion, must embrace learning. Both "generative" learning (about creating) and "adaptive" learning (about coping) are essential characteristics for a successful leader.[33]

First of all, such leaders need to be able to identify what their constituents really value. Then leaders must function as designers, teachers, and stewards to build organizations where people are always increasing their abilities to shape their futures.

As designer, the leader should construct concerns designing the governing ideas of purpose, vision, and core values. He or she must also design the policies, strategies, and structures to implement these concerns and the effective learning processes to ensure success.

As teacher, the leader's role is to help people define current reality with more accuracy, insight, and empowerment. By understanding the problems and advantages of current reality, people will be better able to shape a desirable future.

As steward, the leader must want to serve both his or her vision and the people who help to implement it.

On a more personal level, Smith defines leaders as people who know and understand themselves, know how to capitalize on their strengths while minimzing their weaknesses, are accomplished in a field and skilled in knowledge acquisition and problem solving, inspire trust, have moral courage, and are risk takers.[34] He also says that the manager focuses on systems and a short-range view, whereas the leader has a long-range perspective; the manager accepts the status quo, and the leader challenges it.

Bennis finds similar personal characteristics in leaders, who have a guiding vision; a passion for their vision; integrity growing from self-knowledge, candor, and maturity; trust; and daring and curiosity.[2]

Butera distinguishes leaders from managers by particular character traits.[6] For example, leaders are more visionary, greater risk takers, more self-confident, influential, adaptive, communicative, and organization-oriented. Above all, she states, being able to bend with both change and the needs of subordinates are the benchmarks of the most effective leadership style.

Moreover, according to Hyman, women managers have distinctive managerial styles. They show more warmth and concern than men, are more considerate and more production-oriented, have greater conflict-resolution skills, and show more concern for moving toward organizational goals and obeying rules and policies.[17]

Effective managers, in contrast, are defined by Garfield as people who have the skills and foresight to carry out plans, think ahead to line up resources, forge through stagnant periods, are risk takers, and have self-confidence and high self-esteem.[14]

Simply stated, Drucker defines *management* as doing things right and leadership as doing the right thing.[11]

In summary, although effective managers must portray substantial leadership qualities to motivate people, collect information, make decisions, and influence the boss, in general their primary responsibility is to *realize* an organization's vision. On a personal level, this translates into traits such as problem-solving skills, planning skills, assertiveness, self-knowledge, communication skills, a drive for task completion, and risk taking.

In contrast, effective leaders are charged with the mission of creating and driving an organization's vision. The personality traits most identified with this role include being visionary, risk taking, passionate, self-perceptive, and influential or persuasive.

If we were talking about a machine, we would say that managers are most concerned with the gear system, whereas leaders are focused on the effect of its movement.

THE DEVELOPMENT OF LEADERSHIP THOUGHT: TRAIT, BEHAVIORAL AND CONTINGENCY APPROACHES

Trait Approach to the Study of Leadership

One of the first theories of leadership held that great leaders were born with certain "traits" that made them great leaders; this is the so-called Great Man concept of leadership. Early researchers felt that if they studied the personality, intelligence, and attitudes of great leaders such as Joan of Arc, Napoleon, or Lincoln, they would find the combination of traits that made these people outstanding leaders.

Early attempts (between approximately 1900 and 1940) to identify the traits that characterize effective leaders were generally inconclusive. It was thought that leadership traits might include intelligence, assertiveness, above-average height, good vocabulary, attractiveness, self-confidence, and similar attributes.[13] But the research was inconsistent and generally disappointing. Researchers concluded that traits vary with the situation; however, many people still implicitly adhere to a trait approach.

Behavioral Approach to the Study of Leadership

What makes an effective leader? This question remains unanswered after hundreds of trait studies of leadership. The question gained importance during and immediately after World War II, when both the military and private industry recognized the need to identify and train potential leaders.

This need, coupled with the failure of the trait approach, led researchers to focus on the behavior, or style, of the leader. From the late 1940s to the early 1960s, intensive research in this area was conducted at Ohio State University and the University of Michigan.

The Ohio State University Studies

The goal at Ohio State was to identify the behaviors exhibited by leaders. Researchers hoped to learn how these behaviors affected employee satisfaction and performance. After an analysis of actual behavior of leaders in many situations, two important leadership behaviors were isolated: initiating structure and consideration.[35]

Initiating structure is defined as the extent to which the leaders structure and define the activities of subordinates so that organizational goals are achieved. Initiative structure is sometimes also referred to as a production or task orientation.

Consideration is the extent to which leaders are concerned with developing mutual trust between themselves and subordinates. It also measures respect for subordinates' proposals and concern for their feelings. Consideration is sometimes referred to as an employee or human relations orientation.

Extensive research conducted by the Ohio State investigators found that leaders who scored high in initiating structure and consideration (a "high-high leader") tended to achieve high subordinate performance and satisfaction more frequently than those who rated low on initiating structure, consideration, or both.

The findings were not consistent with other research, however. The high-style did not always result in positive consequences. For example, leaders' behavior characterized as high on initiating structure led to greater rates of grievances, absenteeism, and turnover and lower levels of job satisfaction. Enough exceptions were found to indicate that situational factors needed to be considered. The following situations clarify this point:

1. When subordinates are under a high degree of pressure because of deadlines, unclear tasks, or external threats, initiating structure increases satisfaction and performance. Structure is required because the employees are under stress and do not know what to expect.

2. When the task itself is personally satisfying, the need for high consideration and high structure is generally reduced. (An editor who enjoys writing should be able to function with less social-emotional support and less direction from the publisher.)

3. When the goals and methods of performing the job are clear and certain, consideration should promote subordinate satisfaction; structure should promote dissatisfaction. When subordinates do not know how to perform a job or the job itself has vague goals or methods, consideration becomes less important, and initiating becomes more important.

In summary, the leader high in both consideration and structure will not always perform better than other types of leaders. In some cases, one type of behavior or the other may be unhelpful or even damaging to subordinates' performance or satisfaction.

The University of Michigan Studies

At about the same time as the Ohio State Studies, another series of studies was being conducted at the University of Michigan's Survey Research Center. These studies had similar goals: to locate behavioral characteristics of leaders that appeared to be related to performance effectiveness.

The Michigan group identified two dimensions of leadership behavior, which they labeled employee-oriented and job-oriented.[19] Leaders who were employee-oriented were described as emphasizing interpersonal relations; they took a personal interest in the needs of their subordinates and accepted individual differences among them. The job-oriented leaders, in contrast, tended to emphasize the technical or task aspects of the job;

their main concern was in accomplishing their groups' tasks, and the group members were only a means to that end.

The conclusions of the Michigan researchers strongly favored leaders who were employee-oriented in their behavior. Employee-oriented leaders were associated with higher group productivity and high job satisfaction. Job-oriented leaders tended to be associated with low group productivity and lower satisfaction. Subsequent research, however, was inconclusive. In some cases, the units led by a person using an employee-oriented style were more productive, whereas in other situations the units led in a job-oriented style were more productive.

The situations in which the job-oriented leaders were effective could not be explained. Besides style, other factors must also affect a leader's effectiveness. Moreover, the leadership-style concept was one-dimensional, as depicted in Figure 17-2 on p. 470. A leader was either employee-oriented or job-oriented but seemingly did not possess the characteristics of both styles.

The Ohio State studies and the Michigan studies are quite similar. The major difference is that the Ohio State studies allow for two dimensions, whereas the Michigan studies do not (Fig. 17-2). In other words, a leader can exhibit characteristics of both consideration and initiating structure. In Figure 17-2, individual A is high on consideration and low on initiating structure. Individual D is high on both consideration and initiating structure. Thus we see that the leadership concept is two-dimensional in the Ohio State studies, as compared to the one-dimensional concept used in the Michigan studies.

The Managerial Grid

Blake and Mouton analyzed the deficiencies of the Michigan and Ohio State studies and applied conclusions from their own research to develop the Managerial Grid.[4] They constructed it by defining two dimensions of leadership behavior as concern for people and concern for production. These two dimensions are similar to the employee-oriented and job-oriented concepts, as well as to the concepts of consideration and initiating structure.

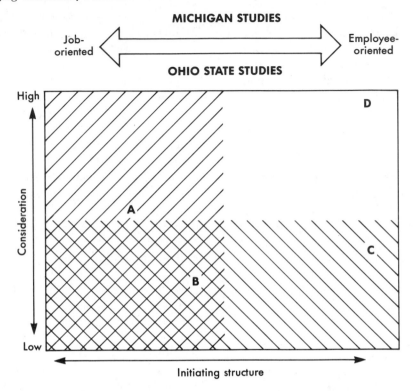

Individual A: high consideration, low initiating structure
Individual B: low consideration, medium initiating structure
Individual C: low consideration, high initiating structure
Individual D: high consideration, high initiating structure

Figure 17-2. Comparison of employer-oriented and job-oriented concepts with consideration and initiating structure concepts.
Adapted from Gray ER, Smeltzer LR: *Management: the competitive edge*, New York, 1989, Macmillan.

Blake and Mouton believed that leaders should be high in concern for people and production. Using a grid similar to that shown in Figure 17-3, they plotted leaders' styles of behavior. Two styles are depicted in Figure 17-3. Based on Blake and Mouton's assumptions, the 7,8 style would be more effective than the 3,4 style. The 9,9 style would be even more effective.

Although there are 81 possible positions on the grid, five of these are most commonly discussed.

(1,1) *Impoverished management*: Effective production is unobtainable because people are lazy, apathetic, and indifferent. Sound, ma-

ture relationships are difficult to achieve. Conflict is inevitable.

(9,1) *Task management*: Employees are a commodity just like machines. A manager's responsibility is to plan, direct, and control the work of subordinates.

(1,9) *Country club management*: Production is incidental. Lack of conflict and good fellowship receive more attention.

(5,5)*Dampened pendulum (middle-of-the-road) management*: Push for production but do not go all out. Give some but not all. Be fair and firm.

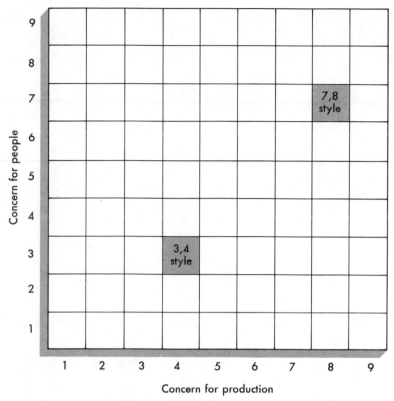

Figure 17-3. An illustration of a managerial grid.
From Blake RR, Mouton JS, Bedwell AC: Managerial grid, *Advanced Management-Office Executive*,
September 1962.

(9,9) *Team management*: production is from integration of task and human requirements.

Contingency Theories of Managerial Leadership

As the study of leadership became more sophisticated, the shortcomings of the trait and behavioral approaches of the 1950s and early 1960s became apparent. It became increasingly clear to those studying the leadership phenomenon that prediction of leadership success involved more than simply isolating a few traits or preferable behaviors. The failure to obtain consistent results led to a new focus on situational influences; that is, under condition I, style A would be appropriate, whereas style B would be more suitable for conditions II, and style C for condition III. But what were these

various conditions? It is one thing to say that leadership effectiveness is dependent on the situation and another to be able to isolate those situational conditions. The contingency approaches attempt to relate the appropriate leadership style to situational conditions.

Certain approaches to isolating key situational variables have proven more successful than others and as a result are more valuable to an understanding of the managerial leadership process. The following discussion considers four of these contingency theories or approaches to leadership.

Autocratic-Democratic Continuum Model

Tannenbaum and Schmidt wrote one of the most quoted articles ever to appear in the *Harvard Busi-*

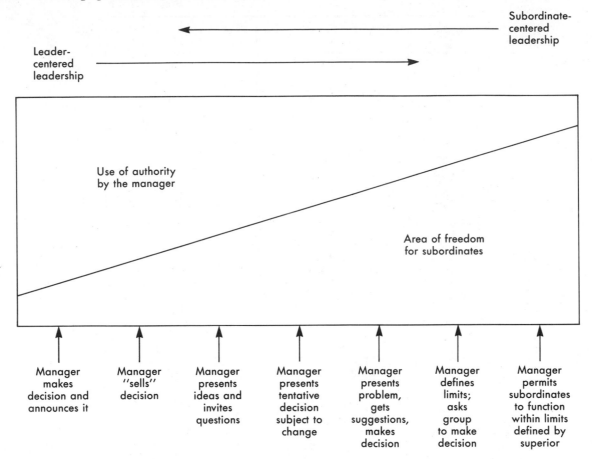

Figure 17-4. Autocratic-democratic continuum.
Tannenbaum R, Schmidt WH: *How to choose a leadership pattern, Harvard Business Review*, 38:96, 1958. With permission. Copyright 1958 by the President and Fellows of Harvard College; all rights reserved.

ness Review, "How to Choose a Leadership Pattern."[36] The model is presented in Figure 17-4. It has become known as the Autocratic-Democratic Continuum because, as depicted in the figure, there is a relationship between the degree of authority used by the manager and the amount of freedom available to subordinates in reaching decisions.

If autocratic and democratic behavior were viewed only as two extreme positions, this model would be correctly labeled as a behavioral theory. However, the behaviors are merely two of many positions along a continuum. At one extreme, the leader makes the decision, tells the subordinates, and expects them to carry out that decision. At the other extreme, the leader fully shares the decision-making power with subordinates, allowing each member of the group to carry an equal voice: one person, one vote. In contrast to the previous studies, there is no attempt to find one correct style.

Path Goal Theory

The Path Goal Theory first described by House in 1971 is one of the more recent attempts to find the key to effectiveness in managerial leadership.[16] The name is derived from leaders' attempts to influence subordinates' perceptions of goals and how to achieve them.

This theory links effective leadership to effective motivation, particularly when expectancy theory is used to explain motivation. Expectancies are the probability of obtaining goals, and valences are the value or attractiveness of those goals. Leaders may affect employees' expectancies and valences in several ways, for instance, by:

- Assigning workers to do tasks that they value and enjoy (valence)
- Supporting (e.g., providing information, training) employee efforts to achieve task goals (expectancy)
- Tying rewards such as a pay raise, recognition, and promotion to the accomplishment of task goals (expectancy)
- Providing consistent rewards (expectancy) that employees value (valence)

These actions by leaders increase effectiveness because they enable employees to reach higher levels of performance through increased motivation on the job. Hence, situations that allow leaders to exercise these behaviors can lead to greater effectiveness.

According to this theory, managerial leaders can choose among four styles of leadership:

1. Directive leadership is illustrated by a leader who informs subordinates what is expected of them, gives specific guidance as to what should be done, and shows how to do it.
2. Supportive leadership is characterized by a friendly and approachable leader who shows concern for the status, well-being, and needs of subordinates.
3. Participative leadership is demonstrated by a leader who consults with subordinates, solicits their suggestions, and takes these suggestions into account before making a decision.
4. Achievement-oriented leadership is characterized by a leader who sets challenging goals, expects subordinates to perform at their highest level, continuously seeks im-

provement in performance, and shows confidence that the subordinates will assume responsibility, put forth effort, and accomplish challenging goals.

The theory suggests that these four styles can be practiced by the same leader in various situations. To determine the correct style or combination of styles for a given situation, the manager must analyze two factors:

1. The subordinates' characteristics, particularly their abilities and the likelihood that their satisfaction will be enhanced by the leader's own behavior
2. The environment, which includes the subordinates' tasks, the formal authority system, and the primary work group

The correct leadership style is contingent on the particular situation. The most desirable leadership style is the one that matches an employee's abilities and helps him or her achieve satisfaction and accomplish goals. The leader can do this by increasing the number and kinds of rewards available to subordinates. The leader should also clarify how these rewards can be obtained. Subordinates should understand that expectancies are realistic and that goals are obtainable. For different employees and situations, these goals require different leadership styles.

As we have noted, the contingency theories are receiving extensive attention from leadership researchers at this time. These theories are important for managers because they offer a number of potentially useful managerial implications. The main message they are relaying is that there is no one best way to lead; the successful leader must be able to diagnose particular situations. One of the main questions that every manager is continually facing when diagnosing a situation is: Should influence be exercised in an autocratic or a democratic fashion?

The Autocratic-Democratic Decision

We have already discussed the autocratic-democratic continuum developed by Tannenbaum and Schmidt.[36] Unfortunately, the labels *autocratic* and *democratic* suggest analogies between dictatorial and democratic regimes. As a result, many managers are reluctant to admit that they operate in an "autocratic" manner, even though "democractic" may not be the appropriate description for the behavior of a leader of a group striving to achieve task goals.

A more appropriate term than *democratic* with an equally positive connotation is *participatory*. Part of this term's appeal is naturally a result of the high emphasis placed on the participative form of government in the United States. The human relations model stressed that responsibility felt by managers to motivate and make workers feel important. No doubt exists that participation accomplishes both of these objectives. "The person in the boat with you never bores a hole in it" is a phrase often heard in management discussions. Participation also increases employees' acceptance of decisions.

However, participation may have detrimental results at times. It may waste time and energy. A participative manager is out of place, for example, in the hospital emergency room! Some employees may not be receptive to partipation. When the leader is distrusted or the labor climate is poor, employees may resent "having to do management's work." There is also evidence that certain types of personalities may reject participative leadership. Even when subordinates are receptive, they may not know how to contribute effectively to decision making.

CONTEMPORARY PERSPECTIVES ON LEADERSHIP

Two current topics of interest to managerial leadership include the themes of women as managers and transformational leadership.

Women as Managerial Leaders

The Equal Employment Opportunity Commission guidelines have had a substantial impact on the number of women in leadership roles in business organizations. Managerial advancement for women had often been blocked by organizational tradition in the past, but Title VII of the Civil Rights Act of 1964 may be gradually removing this obstruction. Women increasingly have attained important lead-

ership positions in business; for instance, 7 of the 19 top officers of Boston's Baybanks are women, and the *Denver Post* employs women as the vice president, city editor, credit manager, and payroll manager. Ten years ago it would have been difficult to study similarities and differences among male and female leaders because too few women held management leadership positions. Although women in management remain a definite minority, these studies have recently become more common.

Two topics regarding women in leadership positions need to be addressed. The first concerns the skills and abilities necessary to lead: Are women more or less people-oriented than male leaders? Are women more or less job-oriented than men? The second question is related to employees' responses to male and female leaders: Will female leaders not be permitted to lead because of the stereotypes and biases of their employees?

There has been very little research on the first question. Some of the researchers involved in the Ohio State Studies found that there were no differences in the orientation of the two groups.[9] Two other researchers completed a scientific investigation of nearly 2000 managers (950 females and 966 males) to determine if they differed in how they administer the management process. Again, no differences were found between the female and male leaders.[10]

Another study relates to the second question, that is, addressing differences in how subordinates may relate to male and female leaders. In a study conducted by Jago and Vroom, females were found to have a more participative orientation than males.[18] Of greater significance, however, was their discovery that autocratic females were viewed much more negatively than autocratic males. This finding is particularly interesting because it shows that the traditional female stereotypes may still predominate in the managerial setting; women must be more permissive, less directive, and more concerned with others' feelings. According to this study, men need not be as concerned with these items as women. A related study found that female leaders who used directive authoritarian styles were less effective, and that male supervisors were generally perceived more favorably than female supervisors.

An initial summary may conclude that female leaders are not different but that they are perceived differently. However, this is only an initial summary. Educated women who will progress to leadership roles are joining the work force at an ever-increasing rate. As these women progress and receive leadership experience and training similar to that of men, it will be a more common occurrence to see women in positions of authority and responsibility. Thus, the perceived differences may gradually disappear. Unfortunately, women still face discrimination in the competition for management opportunities.

One heartening indication of the elimination of the perceived differences, however, is found in leadership training. During the 1970s, there was a proliferation of leadership-training programs for women. It appeared that women required different training than men; however, it gradually became apparent that female leaders really were no different than male leaders. Both faced the same type of problems and required the same training to be effective. During the 1980s, separate leadership training for women has been minimized.

Much of what has been said regarding women also applies to ethnic minorities in leadership positions. Once the "perceived differences" are eliminated, an effective minority leader will face the same challenges as any other effective leader.

Transformational Leadership

Can a leader change an entire corporation? Transformational or inspirational leaders attempt to change whole organizations from one "state" or "culture" to another. It is highly related to charisma, in which a leader develops strong feelings of trust and affection among subordinates toward himself or herself. In that way, the leader can encourage many transformations within the company's culture. In their description of transformational leadership, Bennis and Nanus maintain that transformational leaders are required to change America into a competitive information society from an industrial society.[3]

APPROACHES TO LEADERSHIP AMONG DIETITIANS AND NUTRITIONISTS

One issue concerning dietitians and nutritionists and leadership is that of professional image. Do they or others in the health care setting see Registered Dietitians and Nutritionists as administrators and leaders? Calvert's 1982 survey indicates that other health professionals are more likely to see them as leaders than the dietitians and nutritionists themselves: 50% of chief dietitians, but only 29% of nursing directors, thought dietitians and nutritionists will not perform administrative duties in the future.[7]

Calvert's study also found that dietitians and nutritionists thought they were negatively viewed more often than other health professionals; for example, 20% of dietitians and nutritionists thought their abilities were not understood and that they were not respected as professionals, and only 2% of nurses held similar opinions.

A more recent study by Ryan, however, showed a great increase in dietitians' and nutritionsists' self-image.[31] They now view themselves as positively— as competent, knowledgeable, professional, expert, respected, and directly involved—as other health professionals.

Although dietitians and nutritionists see themselves as professionals, do they have the leadership attributes necessary to stay in the professional arena? Schiller examines this question in a review of results from the Life Styles Inventory administered to approximately 500 dietitians.[32]

As a group, they scored higher in the affiliate style than in any other. This style stresses worker satisfaction more than productivity and can place too little attention on results. As Schiller points out, this leadership approach is not geared to the bottom-line orientation of today's health business.

Dietitians and nutritionists also scored above the 75th percentile in the Humanistic-Helpful, Conventional, and Dependence styles. These results indicate that they are largely considerate and supportive, follow the letter of the law, and are self-doubting, eager to please, and easily influenced.

Other less strong but predominant styles include Self-Actualization (the ideal model of fulfillment),

Table 17-1. Dietetic practice groups of the American Dietetic Association

Practice groups	Areas of expertise
Public Health Nutrition	Local, state, and federal government nutrition professionals who work with all age groups in the public health arena
Gerontological Nutritionists	Practitioners who work in congregate meal/home delivery programs, health care facilities, consulting/pritvate practice, or education/research to improve nutritional status of the elderly
Dietetics in Developmental and Psychiatric Disorders	Nutrition professionals whose work involves clients with physical and mental disabilities and developmental, substance abuse, and eating disorders
Vegetarian Nutrition	Nutrition professionals in community, clinical, education, or food service settings who wish to learn about plant-based diets and provide support to individuals following a vegetarian lifestyle
Renal Dietitians	Practitioners who work in dialysis facilities, clinics, hospitals, and private practice renal nutrition counseling
Pediatric Nutrition	Practitioners who provide nutrition services for the pediatric population in a wide variety of settings
Diabetes Care and Education	Practitioners involved in patient education, professional education, and research for the management of diabetes mellitus
Dietitians in Nutrition Support	Practitioners integrating the science of enteral and parenteral nutrition to provide appropriate nutrition support to individuals in the inpatient and outpatient settings
Dietetics in Physical Medicine and Rehabilitation	Practitioners who provide nutrition support, counseling, and education to clients undergoing rehabilitation in inpatient/outpatient centers, group homes, transitional living centers, and industry
Sports and Cardiovascular Nutritionists	Practitioners who assist well persons by providing sound nutrition principles for optimal health and athletic performance and who assist cardiovascular disease patients with therapeutic, rehabilitative, and lifestyle nutrition needs
Dietitians in General Clinical Practice	Practitioners who possess a mosaic of professional skills, provide and/or manage nutrition care in settings ranging from acute to long-term, and maintain working knowledge in many clinical areas
Consulting Nutritionists in Private Practice	Members who have nutrition counseling practices, nutrition products, and related services
Consultant Dietitians in Health Care Facilities	Practitioners typically employed under contract by skilled nursing and intermediate care facilities, and small hospitals
Dietitians in Business and Communications	Professionals employed by, seeking employment in, or self employed in the profit making organizations of the food and nutrition industry
ADA Members with Management Responsibilities in Health Care Delivery Systems	Food and nutrition care managers generally employed in institutions—includes directors of departments or facilities and administrative dietitians and technicians
School Nutrition Services	Food and nutrition care managers employed by school feeding programs, and directors of the child nutrition programs of these operations
Dietitians in College and University Food Service	Food and nutrition care managers who direct operations in colleges and universities
Clinical Nutrition Management	Managers of the clinical staff operation of health care facilities

Adapted from Flynn C: *Dietetic practice groups*, Chicago: 1991, American Dietetic Association.

Table 17-1. Dietetic practice groups of the American Dietetic Association—cont'd

Practice groups	Areas of expertise
Technical Practice in Dietetics	Focuses on the dietetic team (dietician and technician) in all practice settings, with particular emphasis on technician needs
Dietetic Educators of Practitioners	Educators of students enrolled in Dietetic Technician, Plan IV and V, Coordinated, Approved Preprofessional Practice (AP4), Internship and other programs
Nutrition Educators of Health Professionals	Practitioners involved in the education of health professionals in fields such as medical, dental and nursing
Nutrition Education for the Public	Practitioners involved in the design, implementation and evaluation of nutrition education programs for target populations
Nutrition Research	Members who conduct research in the various areas of practice and are employed in the different practice settings of dietetics

Approval (needing others' approval), Avoidance (avoiding conflict), and Achievement.

How will these leadership styles serve dietitians and nutritionists? The answer is that no one really knows. According to Kirk and associates, there is a great potential to employ many dietitians and nutritionists in business and industry, but they must prepare themselves with appropriate skills, attributes, and other qualifications.[20] Employers see an MBA as an asset, whereas dietitians and nutritionists do not rank that credential high on their list of priorities. Dietitians and nutritionists instead ranked registration status as important, but employers did not. Both agreed that communication skills are of paramount importance.

There were many discrepancies in personal and professional attributes as well. Business and industry employers ranked attributes such as strong work drive, problem-solving capabilities, and good timing considerably higher than did dietitians or nutritionists, who in contrast were more concerned with flexibility, self-discipline, aggressiveness, "chemistry" with the employer, research skills, and negotiation skills. It appears that dietitians and nutritionists need to become more in sync with workplace demands before they can lead in business and industry.

Dietetic Practice Groups

The American Dietetic Association practice groups are a vital part of the association. They are professional interest groups of ADA members who wish to network within their area of interest or practice (Table 17-1). They provide an important communication source, networking, and continuing education efforts for their members. The practice groups have consistently provided leadership for the profession in their respective areas of expertise.

The ADA practice groups were contacted in the summer of 1991 to provide demographic data on their members. Of the 15 practice groups that responded, 8 completed surveys of their membership, 5 sent information on their goals, and 2 had no data. Appendix 17-1 presents a summary of these data. One interesting observation is the diversity of approaches used by the groups to obtain data for their specific needs. It is clear from this information that the practice groups provide members with state-of-the art information in their specific areas. Members rank newsletters and practice group publications as the most important reasons for belonging to a practice group.

Approaches to Leadership among Other Health Professionals

Health care is undergoing a major reorganization of the service delivery system, primarily in response to limited funding. Many times these structural changes involve paring the middle-management layers. As a result, many health care workers find themselves with leadership responsibilities. To determine how health service professionals are approaching their newfound challenge of leadership, a review was completed of registered nurses, physical therapists, and social workers, and a comparison made of dietitians and nutritionists to the other three health care professions.

Registered Nurses

In recent times, nurses have found themselves with a crisis in leadership. In part, it is due to a severe national nursing shortage. Another contributing factor is the rapid and radical change in nursing responsibilities and duties; for example, many RNs are now heavily involved in the financial aspects of nursing operations in addition to participating in issues development and services marketing. Moreover, the nursing profession is diversified as never before, with RNs working in settings ranging from corporations to hospitals to private practice.[25] All of this represents a far cry from bedpans.

Nurses, then, need leaders who are familiar with modern technology, competent, flexible, politically savvy, amenable to diversity, and dynamic change agents. What is the profession doing to provide such leaders? For one thing, the nursing profession is researching the most important characteristics of leaders in its field to identify and educate potential candidates.[25,26]

Meighan's study among RNs concluded that being respected, experienced, knowledgeable, expert, and clinically competent were the most important leadership traits.[26] McCloskey and Molen found that the effective nurse leader has energy, commitment, and communication and change skills.[25] In particular, skills in the areas of decision making, communications, interpersonal relationships, conflict management, change, and risk taking are essential.

However, they also found that leadership effectiveness is largely related to situational variables; that is, workplace variables and personality and management traits must be matched to avoid role conflict and to foster job success.

In general, consideration and a participative style are considered most effective for nurses, as are warmth, assertiveness, and a positive view of self and others. A winning leadership style in nursing is clearly relationship-oriented. The nursing profession is also searching for ways to identify and develop people with leadership potential early in their careers. Studies among nurses suggest that personality traits such as dominance, aggressiveness, ambition, a high capacity to attain status, poise, self-confidence, tolerance for others' views, a high need to achieve, a well-ordered mind, sensitivity to others' needs, and flexibility distinguish leaders from nonleaders.[25]

Several studies indicate that it is vital to identify nurses with leadership potential, that is, who demonstrate professional commitment and appropriate personality traits, early in their careers. In this way, they can be educated to develop incipient leadership behaviors and to incorporate new leadership skills and performance models.[25] One regional health facility, in fact, established a program to do just that.[30] It instituted nurses assessment centers that evaluated referred RNs on their leadership strengths and development needs and implemented individualized development plans. Identifying and nurturing leadership talent were found to be critical if the profession was to retain its position of power and authority in the health field.

Leadership development is being implemented in the academic setting as well.[25] Although education does not predict leadership ability, educational programs can help nurses who are interested in leadership to build skills and goals consistent with the role. Studies indicate that schools should better prepare *academic* leaders, prepare nursing students to deal with conflicting values and expectations (the "school world" versus the "work world"), teach students how to develop life goals consistent with leadership, and develop flexible and astute nurses who can adapt to rapidly changing situational needs. Successful nurses have a different pattern of life goals than less successful nurses: they are more self-expressive, independent, and secure.[1] The successful nurse's life goals become more congruent with the leadership role itself. Based on these results, Baker recommended that educational programs be developed to help the nurse who is interested in a leadership role mold life goals that are consistent with that role.

The nursing profession values mentoring as a way to nurture leaders in the field.[5] An important function of mentoring is to guide an individual through the formal and informal power structures that can be a formidable barrier to career development. Studies show that one of the most crucial times for mentoring, if it is to become effective, is early in a nurse's career. Also, mentors must allow nurses to learn through experience, that is, to have the opportunity to make mistakes and to learn to deal with the consequences.

Boyle also reminds us that mentoring at the graduate and mid-management level is still essential to foster professional growth and development. Yet, in her study, only 34% of the nurses in mid-management positions reported currently having a mentor.

On-the-job leadership for nurses must involve the process of group work because they function in "teams." One approach, developed by a group of doctoral students in nursing, attempted to foster a team process that enables all participants to develop leadership skills with shared power and mutual growth.[21] This interactive model of leadership has the potential to empower all group members. Empowerment, in turn, reinforces the leader-member bond and enhances the leadership process. For example, if one person in the group develops a clear vision, she becomes the leader relating to the vision; however, the group as a whole becomes the seat of power. Because nursing is primarily a female profession (approximately 96%), the influence of gender on leadership has been examined as well.[12,21,24] Edwards points out that male nurses hold positions of leadership at approximately 17% of their number compared to approximately 5% for female nurses in the same employment categories.[12] She suggests that aspiring nurse leaders hone their communication behaviors to demonstrate both the "feminine" qualities of warmth and person-orientation and the "masculine" qualities of task-orientation and competence.

Kosowski sees a parallel between the process of power as empowerment as opposed to coercion and the "feminine" leadership approach.[21] She warns that adopting a definition of power that does not consider the power of caring abandons the values needed for "powerful caring and excellence."

Nurses should have six power qualities: transformative power, integrative caring, advocacy, healing power, participative/affirmative power, and problem-solving power.

There are several "feminine" traits, however, that do not bode well for nurse leaders. Manthey writes about this set of behaviors termed *co-dependency*, including thinking and feeling responsible for other people's feelings and actions, excessive empathy, anticipating other people's needs and expecting the same in return, trying to please others more than themselves, feeling insecure and guilty when others do give to them, and feeling bored or worthless without a crisis or someone in need of them.[24]

Nurses are advised to modify these behaviors by detaching themselves from unhealthy entanglements in other's lives. Nurse leaders are advised as well to learn when to own a problem and when to let it go.

Physical Therapists

Physical therapists (PTs) face a leadership crisis today as well. As with nurses, their profession is growing rapidly and faces expanded managerial, technical, and financial responsibilities. Consequently, future-oriented leaders with the vision to strengthen service and education are sorely needed.

There is another problem among the PT leadership. In one report, approximately 53% of PTs believed they were experiencing professional burnout, primarily in acute care hospital settings. The reasons for burnout were largely related to job dissatisfaction. Mueller postulates that poor PT leadership, seemingly preoccupied with departmental business details and oblivious to the growth needs of its professionals, is instrumental in creating burnout.[28] He suggests that PT leadership pay much closer attention to organization, administration, and professional satisfaction; that is, they need to provide professional values and growth as well as ensure fiscal stability.

Moore points out that PT leaders are frequently lost in the hospital hierarchy. As a result, they need to have better insight into the informal network of their organizations in order to participate in top-level decision making and get more visibility.[27]

As with the nurses, PTs see a need to identify, develop, and—most important—encourage young therapists to be active in leadership roles. There is more interest in the technical aspects of their jobs than in the administrative aspects. Little is done to expose PTs to interdisciplinary interaction or managerial or leadership skills and concepts, in spite of the fact that many PTs are now thrust into leadership positions.

Similar to RNs, the PT profession is female dominated.[1] In 1984 women made up 77% of the physical therapy work force, yet only approximately 35% of females in a poll were chiefs, compared to approximately 56% of male respondents. In addition, a study by Baker and McMahon demonstrated that female PTs earned an average of approximately 68% of male PTs' salaries for all managerial levels in 1987.

Unlike the nurses, however, PTs are not steeped in interpersonal relationship skills. The PT's job is primarily technical, not personal. The PT ranks, then, may not necessarily be full of practitioners who have readily transferable and definable leadership and people skills. In fact, a study by Lomastro and Fortin-Crosby found that PTs, as chiefs, are frequently involved in interpersonal activities requiring skills they were not in need of in the technical services.[23]

Moore points out that aspiring PTs with the desire and skills to be leaders should be actively recruited for PT study and then mentored carefully.[27]

In contrast to the nurses, there is little literature on leadership analysis and development among PTs.

Social Workers

Unlike the RNs and the PTs, social workers (SWs) are trained in interpersonal skills as an integral part or their profession. As Nielson points out, the primary job of the SW is to "lead" their clients to subscribe to a "new vision" of themselves by inspiring change and action.[29] In this way, most successful SWs, like successful leaders, are always engaged in planned change efforts—knowing who

will benefit from change, who needs to be influenced, and which alliances are necessary to bring about change.

Nielson asserts that social work practitioners can hone their leadership skills by becoming more conversant with their professional skills. Nevertheless, as with most health care areas, more education about management and leadership as professions must be available and encouraged. Moreover, the approach should be individualized, with every person aware of specific strengths and weaknesses.

Comparisons with Dietitians and Nutritionists

The social workers appear to be best trained for the leadership challenges facing most auxiliary health fields. As social workers, they function to lead people to realize a vision through appropriate action. Dietitians and nutritionists and physical therapists are considerably less involved in interpersonal interaction and more involved in technical tasks. As a result, they have further to go to develop person-oriented leadership skills. In addition, perhaps as a result of the technical nature of their fields, neither RDs nor PTs have fully investigated the basis or area for the leadership crisis they face. Nurses, by contrast, have gone well beyond first base and are fostering a team approach. Nurses have oriented their new roles to the business of health care and are now involved with the financial aspects and broad operational issues of health care. They are now defining what leadership skills are needed in various situations and are able to identify potential leaders as a prerequisite for leadership development.

SUMMARY

The dietitians and nutritionists of the future must be able to lead and manage effectively. Leadership and management are two distinct yet complementary functions, each of which is essential. Leadership is primarily about dealing with change, whereas management is concerned with complexity. Leaders set direction by shaping both a vision and the strategies needed to achieve that vision. Management sets a plan into action by organizing and staffing efficient systems.

The development of leadership through trait, behavioral, and contingency approaches provides the background necessary to understand how leadership styles and interpretations have changed throughout the years.

Two issues are addressed concerning women in leadership positions. The first concerns the skills and abilities necessary to lead, and the second issue is related to employee response to male and female leaders.

To determine how health professionals are approaching their newfound challenge of leadership, dietitians and nutritionists, registered nurses, physical therapists, and social workers were reviewed. A comparison was made of dietitians' and nutritionists' leadership knowledge and skills with the other health professionals.

REFERENCES

1. Baker CL, McMahon JD: Salary, education and managerial-level differences of physical therapists in Maryland, *Physical Therapy* 69:27, 1989.
2. Bennis W: Leaders invent themselves, *Executive Excellence* 6:3, 1989.
3. Bennis W, Nanus B: *Leaders: the strategies for taking charge*, New York, 1985, Harper & Row.
4. Blake RR, Mouton JS: *The managerial grid*, Houston, 1964, Gulf Publishing.
5. Boyle C, James SK: Nursing leaders as mentors: how are we doing? *Nursing Administration Quarterly* 15:44, 1990.
6. Butera AM: The leader versus the manager of today, *Retail Control* 55.22, 1987.
7. Calvert S, Pauish HY, Oliver K: Critical dietetics, forces shaping its future, *J Am Diet Assoc* 80:350, 1982.
8. Covey SR: *The seven habits of highly effective people*, New York, 1989, Simon & Schuster.
9. Day PR, Stogdill RM: Leader behavior of male and female supervisors: a comparative study, *Personnel Psychology* 25:353, 1972.
10. Donnel S, Hall J: Men and women as managers: a significant case of no significant difference, *Organizational Dynamics* 8, 1980.
11. Drucker P: *The new realities*, New York, 1989, Harper & Row.
12. Edwards JB, Lenz CL: The influence of gender in communication for nurse leaders, *Nursing Administration Quarterly* 15:49, 1990.
13. Fiedler FE: *A theory of leadership effectiveness*, New York, 1967, McGraw-Hill.
14. Garfield CA: The right stuff: a distinct combination of "learnable" qualities places excellent managers ahead of the pack, *Management World* 13:18, 1984.
15. Heath DH: *Fulfilling lives, paths to maturity and success*, San Francisco, 1991, Jossey-Bass.
16. House RJ: A path-goal theory of leadership effectiveness, *Administrative Science Quarterly* 5:321, 1971.
17. Hyman B: Responsive leadership: the women managers' asset or liability? *Supervisory Management* 25:40, 1980.
18. Jago AG, Vroom VH: Sex differences in the incidence and evaluation of participative leader behavior, *J Appl Psychol* 67:315, 1982.
19. Kahn RL, Katz D: *Leadership practices in relation to production and morale*. In Cartwright P, and Zander A: *Group dynamics: research and theory*, ed 3, New York, 1968, Harper & Row.
20. Kirk D, Schanklin CW, Gorman MA: Attributes and qualifications that employers seek when hiring dietitians in business and industry, *J Am Diet Assoc* 89:494, 1989.
21. Kosowski MM and others: An interactive model of leadership, *Nursing Administration Quarterly* 15:36, 1990.
22. Kotter JP: What leaders really do, *Harvard Business Review* 68:103, 1990.
23. Lomastro JA, Fortin-Crosby P: An analysis of the managerial roles of chief of physical therapy services, *American Archives of Rehabilitative Therapy* 28:17, 1980.
24. Manthey M: The nurse manager as a leader, *Nursing Management* 21:18, 1990.
25. McCloskey JC, Molen MT: Leadership in nursing, *Annual Reviews in Nursing Research* 5;177, 1987.
26. Meighan MM: The most important charcteristics of nursing leaders, *Nursing Administration Quarterly* 15:63, 1980.
27. Moore ML: Building winning teams, *Phys Ther* 58:1338, 1978.
28. Mueller MJ, Rose SJ: Physical therapy director as professional value setter, *Phys Ther* 62:1389, 1987.
29. Nielson SK: Administration: getting the right things done, *Soc Work Health Care* 12.59, 1989.
30. Rothwell C: Leadership: promoting potential, *Nursing Times* 87:28, 1991.
31. Ryan AS, Foltz MB, Calvert-Finn S: The role of the clinical dietitian. II, staffing patterns and job functions, *J Am Diet Assoc* 88(6):672, 1988.
32. Schiller MR: Looking for a few leaders, *Performance Page, Ideas for Pacesetters in Dietetics* 1:1, 1988.
33. Senge PM: The leaders' new work: building learning organizations, *Sloan Management Review* 31:7, 1990.
34. Smith AK: Good leaders, *Business and Economics Review* 10:10, 1990.
35. Stogdill RM, Coons AD, editors: Leader behavior: its description and measurement, research monograph 88, Columbus, 1951, Ohio State University Bureau of Business Research.
36. Tannenbaum R, Schmidt WH: How to choose a leadership pattern, *Harvard Business Review* 38(3):162, 1973.

APPENDIX 17-1

Dietetic practice groups

The American Dietetic Association Practice Groups are a vital part of the association. They are professional interest groups of ADA members who wish to network within their area of interest or practice (Table 17-1).

The ADA practice groups were contacted during the summer of 1991 to provide demographic data on their members. Fifteen practice groups responded. Eight groups completed surveys of their membership, five groups sent information on their goals, and two groups had no data.

1. PUBLIC HEALTH NUTRITION PRACTICE GROUP
M. ELIZABETH BRANNON, MSRD
BETSY HAUGHTON, EdD, RD

In 1990 the Public Health Nutrition Practice Group, in conjunction with the University of Tennessee, Knoxville, conducted an assessment of members' continuing education needs. More than 700 respondents returned the surveys, resulting in a 55% response rate from the 1312 members of this practice group. Academically, most respondents (62%) had completed masters degrees, 7% had completed doctorates, and 30% had completed bachelors degrees. More than 90% of the respondents were registered dietitians, 2% were dietetic registration eligible, and 5% were not registered. Most respondents classified their primary position as direct care service provider, administrator-manager, or both. Based on the findings, it was concluded that primary areas of continuing education needs relate to public health knowledge and skills, with particular emphasis on financial management and funding, data management and research, and policy development and planning.

Respondents reported they are less knowledgeable in public health and that they use this knowledge to a more limited extent in their jobs. Those in leadership positions use public health competencies more than those in direct care positions. Secondary continuing education needs to relate nutrition to social and behavioral sciences and education.

2. GERONTOLOGICAL NUTRITIONIST PRACTICE GROUP
LINDA R. SHARP, PhD, RD, LDN

Membership in this practice group is 1966 members. The purpose of the Gerontological Nutritionist Practice Group is to promote the optimal health and nutritional status of older people through high-quality dietetic practice, education, and research.

3. DIABETES CARE AND EDUCATION PRACTICE GROUP
ANN DALY, MS, RD, CDE

A recent survey (March 1991) of the Diabetes Care and Education Practice Group (DCEPG) indicates that the total membership is 2696. This represents a significant increase in membership since 1989, when the membership total was less than 2200 members. According to the survey (591/2670 = 22%), the percent of time spent in diabetes varies widely. The majority of respondents had 5 to 10 years experience in diabetic education and care, yet the majority of these respondents had been members less than 5 years. The largest primary practice setting was hospital inpatient, followed by hospital outpatient. Members listed 67 different ethnic groups they work with; the four most common groups (in order) were African-American, Puerto Rican, Chinese, and Vietnamese.

Forty percent of respondents were certified diabetes educators. Thirteen percent (72 respondents) were affiliated with recognized diabetes education programs, which means approximately half of all recognized programs were represented among respondents.

The two primary reasons for joining DCEPG were (1) that diabetes is a significant practice area, but not primary practice area; and (2) the newsletter. The most helpful service, by far, was the DCEPG newsletter, followed by the DCEPG publications, and then a network of diabetes-focused RDs.

4. DIETITIANS IN PHYSICAL MEDICINE AND REHABILITATION PRACTICE GROUP
CAROL HARTLAGE, MS, RD

This practice group has 418 members. Results of an August 1990 survey by the practice group include:

- Seventy-eight percent of members work in inpatient programs, 4% function in outpatient, and 6% in extended care facilities.
- The mean number of rehabilitation patients in member facilities is 40 per week, ranging from 7 to 90 patients per day.
- Forty-seven dietitian or nutritionist hours per week are budgeted for rehabilitation patients.
- Thirty-two dietitian hours per week are provided to the clinical care of rehabilitation patients.
- Major areas of practice and expertise of practice group members include dysphagia, stroke, amputee, traumatic brain injury, spinal cord injury, heart disease, and geriatric disorder.

5. SPORTS AND CARDIOVASCULAR NUTRITIONISTS
KAREN REZNIK COLINS, MS, RD

Sports and Cardiovascular Nutritionists (SCAN) group members have skill, knowledge, and practice in the fields of sports nutrition, cardiovascular disease, and health and wellness promotion. There are approximately 3500 SCAN members.

Major findings from SCAN member research (sponsored by Ross Laboratories) include:

- On average, members of SCAN have been practicing for 10 years.

- Thirty percent have obtained a masters degree.
- Seventy-seven percent of members are currently practicing in the area of wellness and health promotion, sports, and cardiovascular nutrition.
- One of four members (25%) acts as a consultant in a private practice.
- Sixty-one percent of members say that work experience has helped them develop expertise in wellness and health promotion.
- Eighty-two percent of members indicated that they planned to stay in the field of wellness and health promotion.
- Approximately 40% of members are employed in a hospital setting and work full-time.
- About 14 hours per week are dedicated to the field of wellness and health promotion.
- Almost 50% of the hours worked per week are in obesity and weight-loss management.
- Approximately three of four members (75%) recommend specialty food products to their clients.
- To keep current, the majority of members (approximately 87%) use newsletters and scientific literature.
- For professional development, members indicate that they would like more information on specific fitness problems, such as sports injuries, drugs and steroids, and high cholesterol intake.
- Most members are white (97%), 30 to 40 years of age (57%), and female (96%).

6. DIETITIANS IN GENERAL CLINICAL PRACTICE PRACTICE GROUP
SHARON CRISPIN, MS, RD

Dietitians in General Clinical Practice (DGCP) practice group has more than 2500 members. Members are found in all areas of dietetics, including generalists, specialists, and technicians. The DGCP practice group strives to keep today's practitioners informed by addressing the latest trends, challenges, and opportunities in the field of clinical nutrition services and management. Their goals are directed toward the practitioner who must apply a broad knowledge base in daily practice. Members are employed in a variety of settings such as acute care hospitals, long-term care facilities, private or public clinics, home health, educational institutions, and private practice.

7. CONSULTING NUTRITIONISTS AND DIETITIANS IN PRIVATE PRACTICE
LINDA McDONALD, MS, RD, LD

Consulting Nutritionists (CN) has a membership of approximately 2800 members. CN members are a diverse group of nutritionists who have established private practices or provide consultation to a variety of clients.

Demographic data, provided by a third-party reimbursement survey, indicates that CNs have been in private practice an average of 5 years, ranging from less than 1 year to 44 years. They spend an average of 20 hours per week doing individual and group counseling, with 58% of their referrals coming from physicians.

8. CONSULTANT DIETITIANS IN HEALTH CARE FACILITIES
SHARON BURNS, RD
CLARA GERWICK, RD

The Consultant Dietitians in Health Care Facilities (CD-HCF) is a practice group of the ADA that represents more than 5000 members. It is the oldest and largest practice group of the American Dietetic Association. Its members are committed to improving the nutrition health of the public and to providing cost-effective management of food service operations.

The purpose of CD-HCF is to:
- Promote and protect the health of the public by providing a qualified nutrition resource
- Encourage accessibility to safe food, nutrition resources, and nutrition services for the public
- Maximize private and public resources to maintain and/or restore nutrition health for medically at-risk individuals.

Consultant dietitians serve as valuable management tools by controling food service costs. Food service represents the second highest cost center

in health care institutions. In addition, Consultant Dietitians serve as educators in the field of preventive health care. Good nutrition promotes health and aids in the prevention of many diseases.

Eighty-two percent of consultant dietitians work in nursing homes and 24% in hospitals. In addition, they function in retirement centers, physicians' offices and clinics, home health and health care agencies, child and adult day-care centers, developmental disability facilities, rehabilitation centers, psychiatric centers, alcohol and substance abuse centers, correctional facilities, food companies, school food service, and dietetic, medical, dental, and nursing education programs. Forty percent have been in practice for 11 to 20 years, 10% for 5 to 10 years, and 35% have been consulting for 5 years or less.

9. DIETITIANS IN BUSINESS AND COMMUNICATIONS PRACTICE GROUP
KAREN VARTAN, RD

More than 1500 members practice in food and nutrition and business. Members of this practice group are food and nutrition professionals who know how to translate nutrition into action for business needs.

10. ADA MEMBERS WITH MANAGEMENT RESPONSIBILITIES IN HEALTH CARE DELIVERY SYSTEMS PRACTICE GROUP
LINDA HARACE, RD

A needs assessment completed in September 1990 (125 members or 5% responded), revealed that of the four major goals established by the practice group, "to promote professional and personal development of persons with responsibilities in Nutrition and Food Service Management" ranked highest. The other goals included uniting members with similar interests, providing a means of communication among members and with other groups, and to promote visibility of, and career opportunities in, this field of practice.

Of the numerous activities designed to meet the objectives of the practice group, regular publications and distribution of the newsletter, *Market-*

Link, was deemed most valuable by the membership. Provision of meaningful programming at the annual meeting scored a close second.

The respondents stated that additional knowledge skills were needed in productivity analysis, cost-benefit analysis, tools for analysis, and quality assurance.

11. DIETITIANS IN COLLEGE AND UNIVERSITY FOOD SERVICE MANAGEMENT PRACTICE GROUP
JANET ROSELAND, LRD

This practice group (DICUFS) has 232 members. DICUF's members have expertise in the area of nutrition education, recipe development and testing, nutrition counseling, training employees, athletic nutrition, and special events planning.

Most members work on campus in a full-time, part-time, or consultative capacity. Most responsibilities center around provision of services to clientele, who are primarily college students. In recent years, however, the clientele base has "expanded" on some campuses to include nutrition programs for day care, senior citizens, and outside catering operations.

12. NUTRITION EDUCATION FOR THE PUBLIC PRACTICE GROUP
BARBARA K. PAULSEN, MS, RD

Nutrition Education for the Public has 1647 members who work in a variety of settings. The purpose of this group is to bring together individuals with employment or interest in the area of providing nutrition-related health promotion and disease prevention information to the public. The ultimate goal of the group is to enhance the ability of members to provide consumers with solid nutrition information and the skills needed to make healthy food choices.

13. NUTRITION RESEARCH DIETETIC PRACTICE GROUP
JANIS SWAIN, MS, RD

The goals of this practice group, having a current membership of 600, include:

- To support goals and policies of the American Dietetic Association
- To assess and plan for the continuing education needs of members
- To promote the visibility of nutrition research and communication between researchers and practitioners
- To promote original research activity of practice group members
- To provide a network for reviewing and exchanging information and educational materials relating to research
- To assist in establishing guidelines for nutritional care protocols and procedures for continuing research studies

Controlling Nutrition Services for Productivity

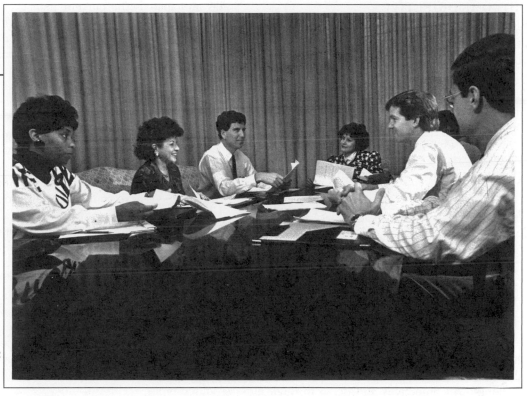

GENERAL CONCEPT

The nutrition program manager has the responsibility to assure that nutrition programs and services are operated in an efficient manner so that program goals, objectives, and standards for performance are achieved. The control and evaluation function incorporates processes that define standards, measure performance, compare with standards, and plan adjustments to improve productivity. This chapter presents the concepts, principles, and processes of managerial control, quality management, program evaluation, and budgeting, and the more complex evaluation techniques associated with effectiveness evaluation and cost-effectiveness and cost-benefit analysis.

OUTCOME OBJECTIVES

When you finish this chapter, you should be able to:

• Define the steps of the control process.
• Discuss recent trends in total quality management and continuous quality improvement.
• Identify distinct types of program evaluation appropriate to each phase of the life span of a nutrition program.
• Name three things that require special planning for designing more complex effectiveness evaluations.
• Distinguish between cost-effectiveness and cost-benefit analysis, and give an example of a situation in which each could be used.
• Identify specific productivity measures that could be used in assessing activities of nutrition programs.
• Describe the budgeting process and discuss its political nature.

MANAGERIAL CONTROL

The purpose of control is to maximize the probability that the organization will achieve its short- and long-term objectives and do so through efficient use of resources. Control is a means of assessing activities in order to take corrective action. During the execution of any plan, changes in the external environment, such as increasing unemployment or shifting political leadership and priorities, or changes inside the organization, such as staff turnover or equipment breakdown, are likely to occur. Such changes require new responses or adjustments in plans. Control systems are an intrinsic part of the management process because they help managers anticipate, monitor, and respond to changing circumstances in a timely manner. The control function enables an organization to adapt to changing conditions, limit the compounding of problems, and minimize costs.

The control process is closely linked with planning (Fig. 18-1). Management sets goals and objectives and puts in place monitoring systems for detecting deviations from goals and objectives and for ascertaining causes of the deviations. The control system tells the manager that things are going as anticipated (the current plan should be maintained), that things are not going as anticipated (the current plan should be modified), or that the situation has changed (a new plan should be developed). In small organizations operating in a stable environment, monitoring systems can be simple, perhaps including weekly staffing records, monthly service counts and expenditure reports, semiannual quality assurance audits, and an annual outcome evaluation and personnel performance review. Complex organizations with multiple goals and organizations operating in turbulent environments need more complex monitoring systems.

Areas of control include resource allocation and utilization (or costs) and program operations and goal attainment (production). Four types of resources that are controlled are physical resources including equipment and supply inventories and facilities; human resources including selection, training, and development, performance appraisal, and compensation; information resources including quality assurance systems and computerized data management systems; and financial resources that are integrally linked to the preceding three resource types.

The Control Process

The control process consists of four steps as illustrated in Figure 18-1. The first step is the establishment of standards. Standards are expressed in measurable terms and become the target against which subsequent performance is compared. A challenge in setting standards is deciding what behaviors or results can be observed, measured, and documented. These indicators of performance must be relevant to short- and long-term goals and objectives. For example, a meals on wheels program has a goal of providing hot, nutritious meals to home-bound disabled elderly people. A measurable, relevant indicator is the temperature of the food when it is delivered. A performance standard could be that the entrée of home-delivered meals will be at or above 145° F 100% of the time when measured at the participant's home. A comprehensive set of standards developed for the WIC program are included in Appendix 18-1.

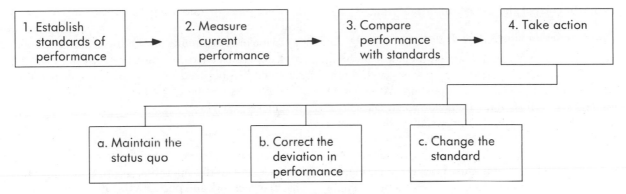

Figure 18-1. Steps in the control process.
Adapted from Griffin RW: *Management*, ed 3, Boston, 1990, Houghton Mifflin, p 604.

The second step is measuring performance. This is an ongoing activity that involves actual observation and documentation of relevant behaviors, actions, or results. Procedures must be developed and implemented for recording and summarizing indicators of performance. Client encounter records, checklists, audit forms, expense accounts, time sheets, and tickler files are examples of tools to aid documentation. Performance is commonly expressed in units of volume, quality indicators, or cost.

Objective data of actual performance is essential to the control process. Actual data fed back to employees can serve as a motivator to increase productivity or correct procedures to improve quality. Data can also serve as a reward and incentive to continue high-level performance. Valid data are essential to appropriate corrective action and good managerial control.

The third step involves the actual assessment. Current performance is compared with the standard on a regular basis, and a determination is made. The frequency of this assessment varies with the purpose of the standard. In the WIC program actual case load is compared with the agency's allocated number monthly. In a congregate dining program, food temperatures and dishwasher temperatures are compared with standards daily. A performance standard related to program outcome objectives, such as rates of anemia in the preschool population, may be assessed annually.

The fourth step involves the decision about what to do. Three courses of action may be followed: do nothing, change the performance, or change the standard. When performance is on track, no action is required. The assessment confirms earlier decisions and serves as a motivator to continue activities as planned.

Deviations, however, trigger required action. This should begin with further examination of the causes of the performance problem and should involve relevant staff in diagnosing causes and planning corrective action.

Sometimes comparing performance to standards leads to the conclusion that the standard for performance is too high or too low. When performance consistently exceeds the standard, the standard may be obsolete and should be upgraded. New conditions in the internal or external environment; different skill levels of personnel; changing expectations on the part of clients, society, or professionals; and advances in knowledge and technology may stimulate changes in performance levels defined in standards.

Other times examination of the cause behind performance problems leads to identification of specific correction action that must be taken. Several approaches can be used to initiate changes in order to correct the deviation in performance.

Approaches to Corrective Action

Approaches to corrective action include re-education and training, persuasion, power, facilitation, and structural change. Re-education assumes that people will adjust their behavior when factual information is presented. For instance, data from a quality assurance audit can signal the need for an adjustment in procedures to improve consistency of care. Feedback data must be specific enough to show what activity needs adjustment. People should participate in interpreting and using the data. This, in turn, serves as an internal motivator and results in personal goal setting. Targets for change should be meaningful, achievable, and connected with incentives or rewards for making the change.

Persuasion is biased structuring and presentation of message. It involves "selling" a concept through an influential person or using selected information to influence thinking in a desired direction. Persuasion is most useful in early stages of change. It can be used to increase expectations of what can be accomplished through a particular change, but expectations must be reasonable.

Power uses sanctions or influence to obtain implementation and compliance with change. Invoking and enforcing rules, procedures, laws, regulations, or accreditation standards are examples of the power approach to correction and compliance with change. This approach is useful when staff fail to perceive a problem in performance or simply refuse to deal with it. Use of this approach does not ensure acceptance and may, in fact, increase resistance and conflict and thus be counterproductive.

Facilitation is used to assist in the identification and implementation of corrective action. Team building and quality circles fall into this category, as does conflict management discussed in Chapter 16.

Structural change involves adjustments in staffing patterns or facilities. The recent trend toward "one-stop" social services is a structural change designed to improve coordination and cross-referrals between health, nutrition, and social service programs.

To make adjustments in activities following feedback of performance deviations, several approaches may need to be used in sequence to enhance the effectiveness of change and to avoid resistance or defensive behavior.

Forms of Control

Texts on management describe three forms of control relevant to the operation of programs: preliminary, screening, and postaction.[11] Preliminary control monitors the quality and quantity of inputs before they enter the production system, (in this case the nutrition unit or program). This is referred to as *feedforward*. For example, the nutrition director controls the knowledge and skill level of new employees entering the nutrition unit through careful recruitment, interviewing, and selection procedures. Nutrition education materials are assessed for technical accuracy and fit with target audience needs before they are purchased. Preliminary or feedforward control follows the principle of "get what you need to do it right the first time," rather than spending resources later to correct deficiencies. This is closely aligned with formative evaluation, which is discussed in the evaluation section of this chapter.

Screening control takes place during production or program operations. Ongoing performance assessment processes are put in place to provide regular feedback and catch problems early. It follows the principle of "test often, fail early (if you are going to fail), adjust fast." Screening control assigns responsibility to frontline personnel for identifying problems while work is in progress and then for participating in decisions regarding corrective action. Quality assurance systems common throughout health care are an example of screening control. Screening control is closely aligned with process evaluation.

Postaction control focuses on the output or results of the program or organization. This is related to outcome evaluation, in which the focus is on achievement of predetermined objectives. It follows the principle of "be accountable for your promises." Postaction control provides information about the effectiveness of past decisions and plans (feedback) and also provides information for future planning cycles (feedforward).

All three forms of control use the same steps of the control process (Fig. 18-1 on p. 489). They provide an information loop of continual assessment and improvement. This loop has been applied in organizations as continuous quality improvement (CQI) programs, which are an extension of quality assurance systems used throughout health care. Quality improvement programs work best when they are a part of total quality management. A discussion of total quality management, continuous quality improvement, and quality assurance follows.

QUALITY MANAGEMENT

In all organizations, top performance, high-quality products and services, and efficient utilization of resources ultimately depend on a commitment to total quality management at the highest level of administration. This commitment is then translated into systems and opportunities that involve personnel at all levels. Highly productive work units and organizations result from worker involvement in decisions about their work, assessment of their performance, and plans for corrective adjustments when needed. It is the responsibility of top administrators to make training, tools, and time available to enable employees to participate in defining and implementing quality improvement plans that assure the smooth operation of programs and achievement of performance objectives while staying within the budget.

This description captures the essence of total quality management (TQM), a management philosophy that was developed in Japan (by U.S. consultants) and has recently been adopted by high-performing U.S. organizations. The guiding principle of TQM is that quality must start at the top and have the total and continuing commitment of management. It must permeate the whole organization and become a way of life for all employees.

TQM is often implemented in the form of continuous quality improvement (CQI) programs. The commitment to quality goes beyond fault finding.

Rather, as in the 3M Corporation, every problem is viewed as a treasure—a newfound opportunity for enhancement of work processes, refinement of product or service details, or improvement of relationships with suppliers and customers.

Crosby,[6] Deming,[7] and Juran[13] are the "gurus" of the quality improvement movement, which has developed over several decades and now encompasses total quality management and continuous quality improvement. Deming has identified several principles of quality:

1. Management must accept ultimate responsibility for quality.
2. Direct resources to quality outcomes.
3. Focus on continuous improvement of product and service.
4. Continuously look for ways to improve the quality and productivity and thus minimize total costs.
5. Build quality in products and services in the first place (preliminary control), and decrease dependence on inspection (screening) to assure quality.
6. Make structural and management changes to improve productivity.
7. Institute training on the job.
8. Substitute leadership for management by numbers.
9. Support a vigorous program of education and self-improvement.
10. Institute leadership to help people and processes do a better job.
11. Break down barriers between departments.
12. Build cooperative work teams.
13. Instill pride in workmanship for all employees.
14. Empower all employees to contribute to continuous quality improvement.[18]

Quality depends on the constituency assessing it—provider, client, family, collaborator, payer, local community, state. Providers define quality in terms of technical processes and effectiveness, whereas clients are likely to assess it in terms of convenience, personal satisfaction, and having perceived needs met. Collaborators may judge in terms of professional competency, and funders or payers in terms of cost-effectiveness and appropriateness.

TQM recognizes that ultimate quality is in the eyes of consumers, and consumer satisfaction is a crucial part of performance. This was driven home by the 1985 publication of *Service America*, which featured successful corporations that put consumers first in their planning and operations.[1] This has lead to another trend in quality improvement—quality service management, in which the customer's needs and wants are first and foremost.

Deming and others have asserted that quality is 80% administration (leadership) and structural systems (organizing) and 20% performance by employees.[7] Performance and productivity are not only employee responsibilities, they are the responsibility of managers. According to Crosby,[6] performance problems are usually not the result of lack of will or skill of employees, but rather they are related to poor job design, failure of leadership, or unclear purpose.

Nutritionists and dietitians must be involved in defining and assuring quality of nutrition programs and services. High-quality management requires continuous attention. Standards must be updated regularly to reflect the current research in nutrition as well as state-of-the-art health and human service delivery systems. Monitoring and control systems should be used as resources come into the nutrition unit, throughout the processes of program operations, and at the end when program accomplishments are reviewed and reported and plans are made for subsequent planning cycles. Nutritionists and dietitians should recognize feedforward and feedback information loops as tools to identify opportunities for program enhancement. The control process should result in continuous improvements, which lead to accomplishment of the goals and objectives and satisfaction of consumer's needs and wants, while resources are used judiciously and efficiently.

QUALITY ASSURANCE AND CONTINUOUS QUALITY IMPROVEMENT OF NUTRITION SERVICES

In the past, quality assurance was focused on the *process* of care. Process is a fundamental element of quality care and cannot be ignored. However,

there is now a shift to outcomes measurement, with attention to the results or *outcomes* of care. Evaluation of the process and outcomes of nutrition care institutes continuous quality improvement (CQI) programs as an ongoing part of the nutrition program activities. By identifying the strengths and weaknesses in the care provided by dietitians and nutritionists, the nutrition program can become a stronger contributor to the overall organization and the health of its clients and the community.

In a quality assurance or CQI program, nutrition care is regularly or continuously documented and evaluated, and results are reviewed for the purpose of identifying needed action. If threshold criteria are met and desired outcomes achieved, providers and protocols are working and nutrition care is effective. Data showing that outcomes are achieved consistently over time should be presented to medical directors, administrators, funders, and legislators as support for the nutrition program. Less positive results should lead to program improvement through examining potential reasons for failure and then introducing procedural or protocol changes into the nutrition care. Subsequent assessment can verify whether the revised protocols are effective in prducing desired outcomes in most clients.

Before we continue, a clarification of terms is in order. Knowing the language of quality assessment and evaluation can help dietitians and nutritionists communicate the results of nutrition services in ways that are most useful to those they wish to influence. Table 18-1 presents a glossary of terms used in this chapter and in articles and discussions on the quality and effectiveness of health care.

The following section, adapted from Splett and Russo,[23] presents steps for the documentation and assessment of the process and outcome of nutrition care. It describes how assessments of process and outcome can be incorporated into ongoing program operations. It is followed by more detailed information on evaluation methods.

Evaluating Process and Outcome

Dietitians and nutritionists frequently cite their lack of time and knowledge about research methods as major obstacles to conducting evaluations in

Table 18-1. Glossary of terms used in quality assessment and effectiveness evaluation

Term	Definition
Clinical effectiveness	A change in clinical indicators that relate to the patients' risk or disease state as a result of implementation of the intervention (nutrition care)
Cost-benefit analysis	An approach to evaluation that converts outcomes to monetary terms (dollars) so that both costs and outcomes are expressed in economic terms
Cost-effectiveness analysis	An approach to evaluation that takes into account both costs and outcomes of two or more alternative methods of intervention for a specific purpose
Effectiveness	Desired outcome is achieved when the intervention is used under ordinary conditions (real-world rather than experimental controlled conditions)
Effectiveness evaluation	A systematic process for assessing the outcomes of health care
Indicator/criterion	A defined, measurable dimension of the quality or appropriateness of an important aspect of patient care; may address the structure, process, or outcome of care
Intervention	A purposefully planned action designed to achieve a defined outcome (e.g., nutrition counseling over a 12-week period to enable the patient to decrease caloric consumption and thereby reduce weight)
Outcome	An end result of the health care process; a measurable change in the patient's state of health or functioning
Protocol	Detailed guidelines for care that are specific to the disease or condition and type of patient
Quality assessment	An act of comparing present program structure, process, and outcomes with stated criteria for performance
Quality assurance	A systematic program for assuring excellence in health care; includes definition of indicators or criteria and thresholds or standards, devising methods for determining the degree to which standards are met, and mechanisms to identify and correct deficiencies
Threshold/standard	A precise specification of the level of performance that constitutes quality; the target against which performance is compared

their own settings. Believing that evaluation requires a sophisticated working knowledge of research design and statistical analysis, dietitians and nutritionists hesitate to get involved. Simko and Conklin[20] and Splett[21] have pointed out that these obstacles are real but surmountable. Many of the steps in conducting an evaluation are comparable to the steps involved in developing quality assurance (QA) studies. Time must be allocated to QA activities in every hospital department for accreditation and many federally funded community-based programs. QA studies should be incorporated into the ongoing operation of outpatient dietetic practices and community nutrition programs. The increasing volume of services delivered in outpatient settings makes quality assessment all the more important in those settings. Time allocated can have a valuable payoff in terms of improved

effectiveness and by generating data to share with payers and other decision makers.

Although knowledge of evaluation and research methods can help, evaluating the process and outcomes of nutrition care can be simplified into five phases. These phases form a cycle that provides feedback for continuous improvement of nutrition care. Attention to these phases helps to assure quality care while documenting results. The evidence of success that is produced by such a system will provide strong justification for internal allocation of funds to support nutrition services or external payment for care delivered. Figure 18-2 on p. 494 illustrates the phases as a feedback loop. Note their similarity with the steps of the control process (Fig. 18-1). A discussion of each phase follows, but first an example illustrates the practical application of quality assessment in a community nutrition program.

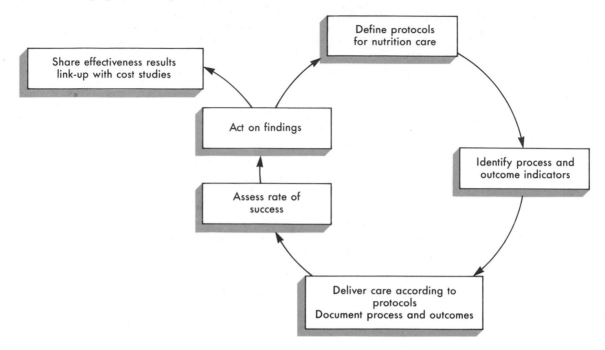

Figure 18-2. Feedback loop for evaluating the process and outcomes of nutrition care.

Figure 18-3 illustrates the integration of both process and outcome indicators in an example of quality assessment used in nutrition care for prenatal patients. Three process indicators are listed. However, the appropriate screening procedures for monitoring and specific guidelines regarding the content of counseling and recommendations for weight gain would be elaborated in other departmental documents defining protocols for nutrition care. Clear delineation of relevant, measurable patient outcomes focuses attention on assessing whether the process actually produces the desired outcomes. Consideration of process and outcome in tandem provides more useful data to guide future nutrition care than assessing process alone. Note in the example how current performance was compared to the performance standards (process and outcome criteria) and the conclusions lead to corrective action. A second cycle of the assessment verified that the corrective action cleared up the performance discrepancy.

Five Steps

1. Define protocols for nutrition care. Clearly define the level, content, and frequency of nutrition care that is appropriate for the specific disease or condition or prevention aim.

   Many nutrition programs have written guidelines specifying appropriate nutrition care for specific diseases, conditions, or prevention aims. These guidelines may be in the form of a diet manual, quality assurance standards, practice guidelines, or detailed protocols. In some cases, no written guidelines exist but dietitians and nutritionists carry in their heads a set of expectations for the type of care to be delivered to various clients under varying situations. Written protocols or practice guidelines are now essential. They define and guide appropriate and acceptable initial and follow-up care and help to assure consistency and quality of care across providers. Protocols establish minimum care that should be provided in order to expect that

Aspect of Care: Nutrition care of prenatal patients with low weight gain

Nutrition Care Indicators:

Process Criteria:

a. Community nutritionists monitor all prenatal patients to identify low weight gain. Threshold 95%.
b. When low weight gain is identified the patient receives counseling on adequate dietary intake. Threshold 95%.
c. A referral is made to WIC if indicated. Threshold 95%.

Outcome Criteria:

a. Weight gain by next visit. Threshold 80%.
b. Improvement in dietary intake. Threshold 80%.

Evaluation: Medical records of all prenatal patients who attended clinic during 1 month were requested and audited.

Process Assessment: Of a total of 100 patients, 25 had a weight gain that fell below the recommended weight gain curve. However, nutritionists had counseled only 15 of 25 (60%) of the cases, and referrals to WIC were made for only 3 of 6 (50%) women who were low income, not currently in WIC.

Outcome Assessment: Of the 15 low-weight-gain patients who were counseled, 12 (80%) achieved weight gain as demonstrated by measured weight at next visit; 13 (87%) had evidence of improved dietary intake. Outcomes could not be assessed for 2 (13%) due to transfer to another clinic for prenatal care.

Conclusions:

1. Many prenatal patients with low weight gain are not receiving adequate and appropriate nutrition care.
2. Those who receive nutrition care do achieve the established outcome criteria.

Actions: Brief interviews with staff showed a lack of knowledge about monitoring prenatal patients for low weight gain and processes for referral to WIC. The nutrition director scheduled a mandatory staff meeting to discuss the findings of the quality assurance audit. Because process was a problem, not outcome, the protocol for monitoring weight gain of prenatal patients was reviewed and a WIC referral form was developed. A repeat audit was scheduled in 3 months.

Improvement/follow-up: Data collected 3 months later showed improvement. Of 105 total prenatals, 28 had low weight gain. All 28 were identified and received counseling by a nutritionist (100%), evidenced by documentation in the medical record. Outcomes remained above 80% for both outcome critieria.

Figure 18-3. Quality assessment of nutrition care: process and outcomes.

desired outcomes can be achieved. They clarify the role of nutrition as a part of a health promotion and disease prevention aim or as a necessary aspect of medical management for specific risk conditions or diseases. Moreover, important for payment and reimbursement, written protocols can be used to communicate appropriate levels of nutrition care to funders and third-party payers. In addition, protocols are a basis for process and outcome criteria for quality assurance systems.

2. Identify outcome indicators. Specify the end re-

sult that nutrition care is expected to achieve. Express it in terms of measurable outcome indicators.

Outcomes are measurable changes in the client's state of health or functioning. They may be proximal outcomes that occur in a fairly short period of time, such as caloric or nutrient intake, weight gain, and serum cholesterol level, or intermediate outcomes, such as recurrent infections or weight maintenance. Outcomes may also be measured over the long term in more general terms such as disease incidence, disability, or death. Several considerations affect the choice of outcome indicators, including selecting indicators that are practical and feasible to measure and being sure that there is a definite link between the outcome and the nutrition intervention. For example, an infant could be born at a low birth weight (<2500 g) for a number of reasons. One cannot assume that nutrition intervention during pregnancy is the solo reason for reducing the rates of low-birth-weight infants in a community. However, the mother's amount and rate of weight gain during pregnancy is related to the infant's birth weight. Because nutrition intervention is directly linked to helping prenatal patients gain weight in pregnancy, total weight gain would be a good outcome indicator for nutrition care of prenatal clients. Because weight is routinely available, it is a practical measurement to use.

For many purposes, readily available biochemical and anthropometric measures can be identified as relevant outcome indicators of nutrition care. Specific clinical indicators are now being defined by practice groups of the American Dietetic Association and the joint Commission on Accreditation of Healthcare Organizations.[12]

3. Deliver care consistently according to protocols. Document both the processes and outcomes of care.

Once standard protocols are developed dietitians and nutritionists must deliver care according to those protocols consistently over time. Training may be necessary to assure that all staff understand and agree with the developed protocols and the charting or record keeping that is necessary to verify that care was delivered.

Because of time demands, documentation is frequently a challenge. Checklists, stamps, stickers, and other memory-aiding devices can be developed to remind clients of all aspects of care appropriate to a specific disease or condition. These devices can also facilitate regular and consistent documentation.

Documentation of outcomes is generally de-

pendent on follow-up visits or the ability to track clients over time. Follow-up visits provide an opportunity to check and support client compliance, and they make it possible to measure outcome indicators. Protocols should include follow-up visits, and clinic procedures should be structured to track and reschedule clients so that the outcomes of nutrition care can be measured and documented.

4. Assess the rate of success of nutrition services. Collect and summarize data from patients' records and evaluate the results.

Preestablished performance standards serve as standards or thresholds for performance. Recognizing that many, but not all, clients will benefit from nutrition intervention, standards define the rate of success dietitians and nutritionists expect to achieve in their practice for each specific type of care. The assessment phase allows dietitians and nutritionists to examine their performance over a period of time. Gathering data about performance may seem threatening, but it is an invaluable means of recognizing success as well as identifying problems that can be corrected.

It is critical that time be allocated to the tasks of reviewing records and summarizing data for the assessment of nutrition care. This activity is routinely done as part of quality assurance programs in most hospitals. However, it must be expanded to ambulatory and public health clinics.

5. Act on the findings. Utilize the results to report effectiveness results to others and to redefine protocols for improved outcomes in the future.

The final steps make the rest of the process worthwhile. The ability of dietitians and nutritionists to review the findings objectively and use them for expansion and continuous improvement of services is key to the evaluation process. Through this process dietitians and nutritionists not only accept accountability for the results of nutrition care but also have the information they need to justify the value of nutrition care in terms of clients' health outcomes. Further, when nutrition care is not found to be effective, data about the processes and outcomes can provide clues to corrective action.

EVALUATION ACROSS THE LIFE SPAN OF PROGRAMS

Evaluation is a process of formulating questions, collecting and summarizing data to address the questions, and interpreting the findings in order to guide decisions about action. Evaluation assesses past decisions, plans, and their execution and informs decisions about future action plans.

Evaluations is crucial to developing and maintaining effective community nutrition programs and services that meet the community's and clients' needs. The purpose and focus of evaluation efforts change over the life span of a program. The life span of a program can be divided into four stages: the idea stage, the formative stage, the implementation and maintenance stage, and the mature stage. Evaluation is important at every stage, but different types of questions guide the selection of evaluation methods to be used at each stage.

The Idea Stage

At the idea stage the evaluation aim is to identify the priority nutrition-related needs that should be addressed. This is accomplished through comprehensive community needs assessment or a more limited needs assessment focused on a high-risk target group or segment of the population. This process was discussed in detail in Chapters 14 and 15.

Needs assessment data at the idea stage are required to answer the question, What should we do? That is, what program, service, or product is needed by the community at large or by a target audience within the community? The result of the evaluation at this stage is a commitment to do something in the identified area. However, exactly what to do is not yet known.

The Formative Stage

The purpose of evaluation at the formative stage is twofold: (1) to determine the specific features of the program, service, or product to be offered; and (2) to develop and refine operational procedures (activities and intervention methods) for implementing it. At this formative stage it is absolutely essential to involve potential clients. The focus is to match the clients' perceived "wants" with the priority "needs" that were defined, usually according to health criteria, by health professionals directing the needs assessment. Market research as described in Chapter 17 is crucial in the formative stage. The method of data collection can include focus groups, surveys, interviews, and observation. By involving potential clients, the product, price, place, and promotion can be determined, and special features can be tailored to clients' preferences. The result of market research involving potential clientele is the design of a nutrition program that is acceptable and accessible to the target audience.

After the specific program is designed, it must be pilot tested. This small-scale preliminary trial can be used to evaluate the processes and procedures of operating the program. It allows for an evaluation of the recruitment and delivery methods and enables bugs to be worked out before full implementation. Final periods of the formative stage can also be used to measure preliminary outcomes. Often pilot studies, also called *demonstration projects*, are used as a method to evaluate the value of an idea before commitment is made to adopt it by funding full-scale implementation. For example, the WIC program funded demonstration projects in breastfeeding promotion for several years before directly allocating extensive resources to breastfeeding promotion.

Evaluation at the formative stage answers the question, How should we do it? In this stage the details of intervention program design necessary to match client needs and wants with the operational capacity of the sponsoring organization are developed and pilot tested. The result of evaluation at the formative stage is the development of a sound program.

The Implementation and Maintenance Stage

Following formative evaluation, the program is ready for the next stage: full implementation. During the early period of implementation, evaluation and feedback systems focus on process evaluation.

Process evaluation is important for documenting that the program is actually being implemented and delivered to the target audience as planned. It monitors the progress and quality of implementation activities by using financial and program records, quality assurance, and other reviews. Process evaluation is aided by a well-designed management information system (MIS). Quantitative information about participation and service delivery should be supplemented with periodic surveys of providers and clients to assess satisfaction with processes and services and to identify potential barriers to successful program operation and accomplishment of objectives. Personnel responsible for implementation of the program should review results of ongoing process evaluation and participate in decisions regarding corrective adjustments. Process evaluation questions at the implementation and maintenance stage include: Are the procedures and protocols for services being followed? Do they work smoothly? Are we reaching the desired clients? Are clients satisfied with services? Process evaluation is an essential prerequisite to outcome and effectiveness evaluation, which is examined later in the implementation phase.

At periodic points in program implementation and ongoing maintenance, evaluators take stock of performance in terms of meeting program objectives. Assessment of program objectives is called *outcome* or *summative evaluation*. Progress toward outcomes is assessed and summed up at the end of the program or at regular reporting periods, usually annually. Outcome evaluation compares the results of the program during a defined period of time with the specific, measurable outcome objectives that were established. It answers the questions, Did we achieve what we set out to achieve? Is there evidence that clients achieve defined outcomes? Systems of data collection must be in place throughout the year to make this possible. Outcome evaluation relies on a management information system that efficiently summarizes and organizes data regarding services delivered, clients' outcomes, and resources used. A challenge of outcome evaluation is tracking clients after their involvement with nutrition programs so that outcome indicators can be measured.

The result of process and outcome evaluation during the implementation and maintenance phase of programs is assurance that the program is doing what it was designed to do. Ongoing evaluations procedures should facilitate continuous quality improvement and enable incremental adjustments in the program. This should assure its efficiency and effectiveness, as discussed in other sections of this chapter.

The Mature Stage

When programs have reached maturity, ongoing process and outcome evaluation continues to be necessary to prevent deterioration of performance. In addition, needs assessment and marketing information should be gathered to assess the program's currrent fit with and relevance to current and future needs. When evaluation results indicate that the program no longer fits with priority needs, it may be time to dismantle the program and shift resources to higher-priority areas.

Goal-free evaluation, originally described by Scriven for education programs,[19] is a comprehensive evaluation approach that is appropriate for mature programs that require a substantial commitment of resources. Goal-free evaluation is a comprehensive examination of a program and its costs and consequences, both positive and negative, as seen by clients, providers, external stakeholders, and society. This type of evaluation is especially important for policy decisions and is often carried out by outside evaluators. It is most commonly used for mature programs when reauthorization decisions are pending and at times of agency reorganization or priority setting. Goal-free evaluation is closely aligned with policy analysis, where a broad range of criteria are examined, including ethical and equity considerations. Whereas other evaluation methods tend to accept the existence of the program as a given, goal-free evaluation asks, Is this really what we should be doing? How much of it should we be doing? How does the program impact on other aspects of the organization, providers, clients, and society? Goal-free evaluation uses available process and outcome evaluation results, but through interviewing and other methods a much broader description of the program and its consequences is developed. Goal-free evaluation draws heavily on the view of the broad constituency to develop a picture of the program's processes and practices and its direct and indirect consequences. Goal-free evaluation forces examination of accepted assumptions about programs, opens programs to wider scrutiny and wider visibility, and facilitates access to the advice of a range of experts. This can be a beneficial process that may lead to broader program support, modernization of assumptions and intervention techniques, authorization of needed resources, and reallocation of resources to more important or more effective programs. By using goal-free evaluation, nutrition program managers will be better equipped to integrate nutrition priorities and programs into the existing priorities of the organization and collaborating agencies.

PLANNING MORE COMPLEX EFFECTIVENESS EVALUATIONS

In-house evaluations of the results of nutrition care provide important feedback to improve nutrition services. They can also serve as a starting point for more elaborate effectiveness studies. With some additional time allocated, dietitians and nutritionists may be able to carry out special studies of clinical effectiveness. Steps to include in carrying out more complex effectiveness evaluations are shown in the box at right. Guidelines for planning studies on effectiveness and cost-effectiveness have been published by the American Dietetic Association.[22] They require attention to the proper design of the evaluation itself.

In complex studies, additional steps, such as selecting comparison groups and controlling for other factors that may also influence outcomes, are necessary to show a true causal relationship between nutrition care and patient outcomes. For some purposes, this level of complexity is necessary. The following example illustrates a study that incorporated controls and a comparison group.

Bruce and Tchabo studied the effect of nutrition counseling on underweight and failure to gain pregnant women in terms of weight gain in pregnancy and birth weight of the infant.[3] The specific question to be answered was, Does a nutrition intervention program that provides intensive nutri-

STEPS FOR EFFECTIVENESS EVALUATION

1. Select disease or prevention area
   Based on seriousness of consequences
   Nutrition has a role in its prevention or management
   Specify subcategory for evaluation
2. List factors that affect outcome indicators of disease
   Physiological changes
   Environmental factor
   Medical and pharmaceutical intervention
3. Specify questions to be answered
   Does nutrition care delivered according to protocol make a difference?
4. Select comparison groups
   Meaningful comparison
   Adequate sample size
   Random assignment if possible
5. Identify relevant indicators
   Available
   Consistently measured
   Relevant to disease outcome
6. Develop and pilot test data collection form
   Ease of use
   Accuracy of data
7. Collect data following standard instructions
   Consistency of time and between persons
   Training and supervision
8. Determine clinical and statistical significance
   Compare with medical norms
   Use appropriate statistical analysis
9. Determine costs for cost-effectiveness analysis
   Resource requirements
10. Report results
    Administrators
    Health director
    Professional peers
    Federal health policy agencies
    State payers and funders

Adapted from Splett PL, *Topics in Clinical Nutrition* 5:26, 1990.

tion education and follow-up improve maternal weight gain and infant birth weight?

Two groups of underweight, failure-to-gain women were studied: one that received intensive nutrition care from a nutritionist and a similar group of women, receiving prenatal care in the same clinic 1 year later, who received no nutrition care beyond routine advice given by the nurse or physician. The comparison group with no treatment allowed the investigators to assess the course of pregnancy among this high-risk group when specialized nutrition care was not included. The comparison between groups helps provide evidence that any change seen is, in fact, a result of the intervention and not caused by other factors in the environment. The outcome indicators selected by the investigators (weight gain and birth weight) were appropriate because they would be expected to improve as a result of the nutrition intervention and because higher weights suggest improved health status of the woman and infant, improved clinical management of pregnancy for practitioners, and a measure of success to the third-party payer. Recognizing that smoking, race, age, start of prenatal care, medical complications, and access to supplemental foods can affect these outcomes, the investigators also tracked these factors in the study and considered them in the analysis. The data collection procedures used had been tested for reliability and validity, and all data were collected following established procedures. After the data were collected and summarized, the results were compared between groups and to existing standards for weight gain and birth weight, and statistical tests were performed to make judgments about the statistical significance of differences between groups. The results, showing that the group receiving nutrition counseling had significantly higher weight gain (1.3 kg) and infant birth weight (300 g) than the no-treatment group, were reported in a widely read medical journal. This study represents a good model of an effectiveness study carried out in a clinical setting.

When a series of studies show similar results, a strong case is established for nutrition care in the disease or condition. Trouba[26] illustrates the use of published reports to justify the role of nutrition education and food supplementation in prenatal care.

EVALUATION DESIGN FOR EFFECTIVENESS EVALUATION

In the evaluation of nutrition programs and services, the ultimate questions is, Did it work? Did the specific intervention bring about the desired effect or outcome? This is a question of causation, which can be demonstrated only with carefully planned and controlled investigations. This section presents a discussion of evaluation designs and essential aspects of evaluation studies that can be used to determine whether an outcome is really achieved and if it can be attributed to the nutrition intervention.

The design of an evaluation involves determining three things: (1) how the sample will be selected, (2) definition of variables and their measurement, and (3) how the intervention will be delivered to experimental and control (or comparison) groups.

Sample Selection

The first point of sample selection is to study people and settings that directly match with the intent of the program. The sample must be drawn from the target population. For example, cholesterol screening and intervention programs desire to identify and reduce the cholesterol level of young adults at risk for future cardiovascular disease. However, the people most predominantly represented at many shopping center cholesterol screening clinics are elderly. Worksites or other locations may have to be used as places to enroll subjects who represent the actual target population of the cholesterol intervention program.

Adequate sample size is necessary to observe the true distribution of results within each study group. Most outcome indicators will have a range of normal variation. The challenge of evaluation is to detect a change that is so large that it indicates an effect of the intervention. A hazard of small sample sizes is that an effect may not be detected even in cases where the intervention has some effect. Sample size determinations are based on normal variation of the outcome indicator, a minimum value or threshold for a clinically meaningful change, and a prediction of attrition rates. In practical terms, many evaluations are carried out with as few as 20 to 40 in a group. In complex effectiveness evaluations, it is best to consult with a statistician regarding appropriate sample size.

Variables and Their Measurement

Three kinds of variables are specified in effectiveness evaluations: independent variable, intervening or confounding variables, and the dependent variable or outcome. The independent variable is simply exposure to or participation in the nutrition intervention. At times it is necessary to further define the intervention into amount, intensity level, or time period of participation. Data about the type and amount of intervention verify that in fact the intervention was delivered according to protocol, and these data also allow further investigation into the relationship between aspects of the program and degree of effect.

Intervening or confounding variables are other factors that could influence the effect of the nutrition program on the participant. For example, men may respond differently than women, so gender would be an important variable to document. Other examples include presence of risk factors, previous experience with the problem or intervention, concomitant participation in another similar program, educational attainment, and lifestyle factors. Data on intervening or confounding variables are used in the analysis to sort out the true effects of the intervention from other factors that could interfere with or mediate effects. Consideration of these variables leads to a greater understanding of how well the program works and for whom, and it may give clues as to why or when the program does not work.

The dependent variable is the specific indicator of effectiveness of the program or intervention. It must be directly linked to the intervention and is probably specified in an outcome objective of the program. A decrease in serum cholesterol could be the dependent variable of a cholesterol program, increase in a score on a nutrition knowledge test could be the measured outcome of a school-based nutrition education program, and an increased rate of breastfeeding would be an obvious indicator of success of a breastfeeding promotion program.

The next challenge is determining how to measure the variables. Each variable must be observed and recorded in a way that assures its validity, reliability, precision, and completeness. Validity is the degree to which the measure captures the essence of the phenomenon being observed. Reliability refers to the ability to obtain the same result with repeated measurement. Precision defines the extent to which the measurement can discriminate between differences in magnitude. Completeness is the extent to which the phenomenon of interest (total of all parts including scientific description) is assessed in totality rather than in part. Some variables can be determined from program records, some from special surveys or questionnaires, and others from biochemical or anthropometric techniques. Consider the challenges to measuring the following variables that could be included in the evaluation of a nutrition intervention: client's perception of body image, weight loss, knowledge of heart-healthy eating practices, percent of budget spent on food, and duration of breastfeeding.

Once variables are defined and their means of measurement determined, detailed procedures must be outlined to guide data collection and assure consistency by all those involved throughout the entire study.

Experimental Design

The classic design for evaluation is the experimental model. Study subjects are randomly drawn from the target population and randomly assigned to either the group that gets the program (the experimental group) or to a control group that does not receive any intervention or receives an alternative or placebo intervention. The program is followed according to a definite protocol, and after a relevant period of time outcomes are measured. Differences between groups are computed, and the program is deemed successful if the experimental group has more of the measured outcome than the control group. Statistical techniques are usually applied to determine the statistical significance of the differences.

The classic experimental model is considered the gold standard of effectiveness evaluation; however, it is often difficult to execute. The program may serve most who are eligible, and nonparticipants are likely to be different from participants in lifestyle, age, interests, knowledge, or income and thus are not appropriate comparisons. Professional ethics also may prohibit withholding an intervention from people who need it. Another drawback of using the experimental model is its high cost.

There are ways to overcome these difficulties. When resources are scarce and some people must do without, it is possible to randomize people to either the program or to the control (no service) group. Also when new programs are introduced over time, the delayed receivers can be the controls for those who get the program early. Demonstration projects can be designed to have participants randomly assigned to the program or a control group and thus facilitate use of the experimental design for effectiveness evaluation.

Quasi-Experimental Designs

Quasi-experimental designs are those that do not meet the strict requirements of the classic experimental model but can produce valid results. Cook and Campbell indicate that the most basic criteria for such designs is the extent to which they protect against the effect of extraneous variables on the outcome measures.[4] The best designs are those that control relevant outside factors and lead to valid inferences about the effects of the program.

Time Series

The time series design involves a series of measurements at periodic intervals before the program begins and after the program ends. The trend of the measured variable (the outcome of interest) over time is examined to see if a noteworthy shift in the data can be attributed to the introduction of the program. For example, in point-of-purchase nutrition education in grocery stores, one could measure the volume of high-fat meats purchased weekly for three month before and three months after the grocery store program. A substantial shift in purchasing patterns could be attributed to the education program with this design.

Multiple Time Series

Multiple time series design increases the validity of the effectiveness study. In this design, data are collected on a similar group or setting as a control for the group or setting where the program is offered. Including the control strengthens the interpretation of the study. An example would be doing the time series study of the grocery store education program by collecting data on meat purchasing patterns over the same period of time in one or more other stores where the education program is not available. This comparison helps to separate out the possible effect of something else in the environment, such as a mass media campaign on lean meats, being responsible for causing purchasing patterns to shift.

Nonequivalent Control Group Design

Probably the most common quasi-experimental design is the nonequivalent control group. In this design there is no random assignment of study participants to groups as there would be in a true experiment. Instead, available individuals, such as clients who are not program participants but who have similar characteristics as program participants, are used as a comparison group. Studies of the WIC program have compared the birth outcomes of pregnant WIC participants with the birth outcomes of other low-income women enrolled in Medicaid but not participating in WIC.

In using nonequivalent groups, the investigator must guard against the possible effect of unobserved characteristics that differentiate between the program group and the comparison group. The problem of selection bias can invalidate the findings. An example of selection bias would be in studying the effect of congregate dining participation on dietary intake: nonparticipants may have physical limitations that both restrict their mobility and ability to attend congregate dining sites and affect their ability to prepare and eat a balanced diet. Differences in dietary intakes between participants may be caused by the differences in physical mobility and not by participation in congregate dining.

Matching. To prevent the problems of selection bias, matching can be used to pair members of the experimental and control or comparison groups on defined characteristics. Matching is frequently done by age, income, knowledge score or educational level, and risk level or disease state. Caution must still be used in interpreting study findings because all variables cannot be controlled unless there is randomization.

Self-selection. Another problem in selecting a comparison group for effectiveness studies is self-selection. People who choose to enter a program are likely to be different from those who do not participate. This can be overcome by using only volunteers for both experimental or program and control or comparison groups. To do this, randomly assign those who express interest in participating to the program being studied and to an alternative condition. For example, to evaluate the effectiveness of an education module regarding nutrition for toddlers, parents could be recruited for a community-based program on raising young children. Volunteers could be randomized to enter the nutrition education group or the alternative parenting skills group. The outcome, defined as increasing the variety of foods in young children's diets, would be assessed in both groups. The difference would indicate the effect of the nutrition module. Following the evaluation, the parenting skills group could be given the nutrition information.

Nonexperimental Designs

Sometimes it is impossible to use even a quasi-experimental design. The evaluator then has to resort to one of the three common nonexperimental designs: (1) a "before and after" study of one or more participants, (2) and "after only" study of a group of program participants, and (3) an "after only" study of participants and nonrandom controls. The weakness of all these designs is that they fail to control for many of the threats to validity. With these designs it is highly possible that some other cause could be responsible for an outcome observed in the studied individuals. However, when data on carefully selected process and outcome variables are systematically collected and summarized with care, these designs can provide valuable insights. Some information is better than no feedback at all. Nonexperimental designs do,

however, leave considerable room for differing interpretations of how much change occurred and how much of the observed change was caused by the operation of the program.

Nonexperimental designs provide preliminary data about the possible effects of the program. If, for example, a carefully planned before-and-after study, with all the contamination of outside events, maturation, testing, and so on, finds little change in the participants, the program as it was delivered is probably having little effect. It may not be worthwhile to invest in more rigorous effectiveness evaluation until the program is modified. At this point it may be most productive to direct attention to process evaluation or review of state-of-the-art delivery methods used by other successful programs.

Threats to Internal Validity

The reason so much attention is given to evaluation design is to assure that any conclusion of effect is truly a result of the nutrition program, service, or intervention and not caused by something else. Threats to validity are a series of eight alternative explanations for any observed effects.

1. *History:* Events in addition to the intervention that take place between the pretest and the posttest may provide an explanation of the effects. For example, parents may be taking their child to a physician for a growth problem at the same time they are participating in a nutrition class. If a change is observed in the child's eating patterns, it will be impossible to know if it was caused by the nutrition class, the physician's intervention, or both.

2. *Maturation:* Changes in the study participant, such as growing older, wiser, and more experienced, may modify the observed effect. Maturation is an important threat in studies in which weight and height are the outcome of interest. A pregnant adolescent may be gaining body weight apart from the additional weight needed to support the fetus. Young children may grow out of their baby fat. Nutrition counseling by the nutri-

tionist may not be the primary cause of these changes.

3. *Testing:* The effect of the pretest on the posttest may affect the outcome. For example, subjects in a study might actually enhance their level of nutrition knowledge by simply taking the pretest, or they may become more proficient in test taking and score higher on the posttest even without real learning during the program.

4. *Instrumentation:* A change in measuring instrument or its use between the pretest and the posttest may affect the outcome. This happens when those administering the test or measurement device become more skilled at posttest or when the instrument changes, such as a scale that has not been calibrated properly.

5. *Statistical regression:* The natural tendency is for very high or very low scorers to be measured closer to the mean on a subsequent test.

6. *Selection:* The effect may be due to differences in kinds of people in the experimental group versus the control or comparison group, as discussed in the section on quasi-experimental designs.

7. *Mortality or attrition:* The differential loss of study participants from a particular group may affect the kinds of people left in the groups for final comparisons.

8. *Interaction:* A combination of maturation, history, or instrumentation with selection produces forces that spuriously appear as effects of the intervention.

Awareness of these threats to internal validity alerts the dietitian and nutritionist to exercise caution in making claims about the effectiveness of nutrition programs and services when the programs or specific services have not been adequately evaluated with sound evaluation designs.

COST-EFFECTIVENESS AND COST-BENEFIT STUDIES

Cost-effectiveness and cost-benefit studies go beyond the assessment of effectiveness to relate outcomes to costs. These economic assessments help to address whether the degree of effect or benefit (outcome) is worth the investment of resources necessary to make it happen. In addition to carefully measuring outcomes, economic assessments require investigators to carefully assess the costs or resource requirements for delivery of nutrition services and, in the case of cost-benefit studies, to estimate a value for the results achieved. Cost-effectiveness studies report cost per unit of result. For example, Stunkard and associates compared the cost per 1% decrease in percentage overweight for seven weight loss programs.[25] The highest cost ($108.67) was in a university clinic, followed by a worksite program delivered by professional leaders ($33.61), a clinic using very-low-calorie diets ($28.00), a clinic using behavior therapy ($19.62), a worksite program delivered by lay leaders ($11.10), a commercial program ($7.31), and a worksite program designed by the investigators ($0.92).

Cost-benefit studies convert outcomes into a dollar value so that both costs and outcomes (benefits) are expressed in monetary units. Then conclusions are reported as either a cost-benefit ratio or as net benefits (total monetary benefits minus total monetary costs, including negative outcomes that add future costs). An example of a cost-benefit study is the Brauer and associates study of nutrition counseling for patients with Crohn's disease.[2] The investigators reported a net savings to society of $164 per person during the study year for patients who received six monthly nutrition counseling sessions compared to patients who did not receive nutrition counseling. The economic benefits came from reduced medication use, fewer hosptial days, and fewer days lost from work in the counseled group.

The next section presents the background for cost-effectiveness and cost-benefit analysis in the general context of economic evaluation.

ECONOMIC EVALUATION

Definition and Principles

Economic evaluation has been defined by Stoddart as the comparative analysis of alternative courses of action in terms of both their costs and consequences.[24] Economic evaluation has two essential characteristics: it is concerned with explicit choices between alternative uses of scarce resources, and it structures comparisons of both inputs (costs) and outputs (which are labeled benefits, consequences, effects, or outcomes in various applications) between alternative programs or interventions.[9] The major foci of economic analysis are input "costs" and output "benefits" or "effects." These terms require definition. *Costs* refers to that which is given up to obtain something else (also called *opportunity costs* in the economic lexicon). When resources are allocated to one program or activity, those resources are no longer free to be directed to an alternative use. Resource requirements (inputs) are measured in monetary units as dollar "costs," representing the value forgone by committing the resources to the designated activity.

Consequences or outputs of the activity are often referred to as *effects* or *benefits*. However, these terms have distinct meanings in economic evaluation. *Effects* usually refers to the programmatic objectives of the alternative (e.g., reduced incidence of anemia or an increased nutrition knowledge score), measured in natural units (e.g., number of new cases or standardized knowledge score). The term *benefits* is usually reserved for outputs valued in monetary units (e.g., dollars of medical services avoided). Use of the term *benefits* also covers the fact that consequences can be negative as well as positive. *Outcomes* defined as anticipated and unanticipated consequences of the program and its processes seems to be a more inclusive term for outputs and is used throughout this section. The meanings of these terms are elaborated in a later section describing the cost and outcome framework.

The following outline represents a synthesis of the principles and process of economic analysis:

1. Define the problem
   a. Specify the desired goal to be achieved
   b. Differentiate the perspective for analysis
   c. Identify the alternative means of reaching a goal; these are the alternatives to be compared

2. Structure the costs and outcomes framework
   a. Specify the costs and outcomes to be included in analysis
   b. Determine cost and outcomes using the best available data
   c. Value costs and outcomes according to perspective
   d. Perform discounting
   e. Summarize assumptions, calculations, and conclusions using indexes or an array

3. Interpret the results
   a. Conduct sensitivity analysis
   b. Address ethical issues
   c. Report results with discussion

Stoddart differentiates between "theoretical" and "practical" economic analysis.[24] Theoretical economic analysis is based in the theory of welfare economics and has as its aim the selection of alternatives that maximize utility (benefit) from a societal point of view. Practical economic analysis is based in decision theory and has as its primary purpose the construction of a framework for processing information on costs and outcomes of alternatives for decision making.

This differentiation parallels the identification of the perspective for analysis, which is one of the first steps in economic analysis. The societal perspective includes all costs and outcomes of a program, no matter to whom they accrue, over as long a time as is pertinent and reasonable. In contrast, practical economic analysis takes an institutional or organizational perspective and is interested in maximizing effectiveness in terms of a specific outcome while minimizing costs to the organization.

Stoddart noted that the practical, decision-making approach enables the decision maker "to construct a framwork for processing information on the cost and consequences of alternatives in the belief that a systematic display and examination of information will improve the quality of decision making."[24] A discussion of the framework follows.

Cost and Outcome Framework

The basic framework used in economic analysis evolves from production theory and provides a structure for specifying, measuring or estimating,

Costs	Outcomes

I. Organizing and operating costs within the organization or health sector (e.g., health professionals' time, supplies, equipment, administration and capital costs) *(direct costs)*
II. Costs borne by patients and their families *(patient/indirect costs)*
  • Out-of-pocket expenses
  • Patient and family input into treatment
  • Time lost from work and leisure
III. Psychic costs *(intangible costs)*
  • Grief, pain, suffering
IV. Costs borne externally to the health sector, patients, and their families *(external costs)*
	I. Changes in physical, social, and emotional functioning *(effects)*
	  • Disease-specific indicators
	  • General health status
	  • Patient satisfaction
	  • Sick days
	  • Changes in knowledge, attitude, behavior
	II. Changes in resource use *(benefits)*
	  A. For organizing and operating services within the organization or health sector
	    • For the original condition
	    • For unrelated conditions *(direct benefits)*
	  B. Relating to activities of patients and their families
	    • Savings in expenditure of leisure time input
	    • Savings in lost work time *(indirect benefits)*
	III. Changes in the quality of life of patients and their families *(utility)*

Figure 18-4. A framework for selecting types of costs and outcomes for economic analysis. Adapted from Drummond MF, Stoddart GL, Torrance GW: *Methods for economic evaluation of health care programmes*, New York, 1987, Oxford University Press.

and valuing inputs and outputs of a program or intervention. The input side accounts for resources required to produce the program. Inputs are referred to as *costs*. The output side includes all positive gains or negative losses that result from the activity. These are referred to as *outcomes*. Figure 18-4 outlines the types of costs and outcomes commonly used in economic evaluations of health care programs.

There is no one "correct" way to structure an economic analysis. The goal and perspective for analysis—institutional or societal—determines which costs and outcomes should be included and how each is valued.

Costs

Costs are defined in three categories: direct (organization and operating costs), indirect (out-of-

pocket expenses borne by the participant and family, such as medication, travel, and forgone earnings), and intangible (grief, pain, and suffering). Cost-benefit analysis may also consider external effects experienced by other sectors of the economy.

Outcomes

Whereas inputs are almost always valued in dollars, outcomes can be measured in three basic ways: (1) units natural to the program objectives measured with ad hoc numerical scales (e.g., gain in knowledge scores, pounds of weight loss, or number of cases prevented), (2) economic benefits associated with the health improvements valued in monetary terms as direct (health care resources savings or losses) or indirect (out-of-pocket costs experienced by the patient, losses or gains, which may include improved productivity) and often including intangible quality-of-life factors, and (3) the subjective value or utility of health improvements, as the patient, family, expert, or society perceives them, measured in universal units such as quality adjusted life years (QALY). Issues in the evaluation of effectiveness are discussed elsewhere in this chapter.

Cost-Benefit Versus Cost-Effectiveness Analysis

The valuation step is where cost-effectiveness analysis and cost-benefit analysis are differentiated. When outcomes are expressed in units natural to the objectives of the program or intervention strategy, the method is labeled *cost-effectiveness analysis*. When outcomes are valued in monetary terms, the method is called *cost-benefit analysis*.

The difficulty of measuring and valuing *all* the costs and outcomes associated with the alternatives is widely recognized; however, each analyst must specify a framework that identifies the relevant, important costs and outcomes, given the purpose and perspective of the analysis, and then apply it consistently to the assessment and valuation of all compared alternatives. Stoddart and others who write about economic evaluation indicate that in many applications, particularly in the practical, decision-making approach, it is appropriate to use a restricted model that relies on the best data and involves minimal estimation and valuation, that is, direct cost and direct outcome.[24]

Evaluation of Outcomes

Economic evaluation requires sound estimation of the effectiveness of the compared alternatives.[20] There is considerable concern that many program evaluations, even published studies, do not meet the standards of rigorous evaluation design.[22]

The outcomes selected as indicators of effectiveness must be clearly linked (theoretically and empirically) to the interventions (programs or activities), they must be evaluated in a time frame that has a realistic relationship to the proposed intervention, and they must be evaluated in such a way as to control for other factors that could influence outcomes.[17] Effectiveness data may come from previous epidemiological and clinical studies, or a specific evaluation may be planned as a step in the economic analysis using experimental or quasi-experimental designs.

Experimental designs control for spurious effects and give the best support for *efficacy* (Can it work under ideal conditions of use?); however, the selective admission criteria and controlled conditions of the experiment may limit the generalizability of results to real-world situations. *Effectiveness* evaluation verifies that the alternative produces desired results in routine settings (Does it work under average conditions of use?) and is preferred for interventions that are in wide use.

Many cost-effectiveness and cost-benefit analysis reports rely on estimates of effectiveness derived from previous evaluations. Whether effectiveness evaluation is carried out as part of a cost-effectiveness study or previously collected data are used, the analyst must verify the quality of the methods used to determine effectiveness results.

Cost-Benefit and Cost-Effectiveness Indexes

Two indexes are commonly used in the application of economic analysis. The first is the cost-benefit (effectiveness) ratio, in which alternatives are compared on the basis of expected cost per unit of outcome (benefit or effect). Using cost-benefit (effectiveness) ratios, the alternative with the smallest ratio of costs to benefits (effects) is preferred. The second index is based on net benefits (with outcomes valued in monetary units). Using the net benefit index, alternatives are compared on the basis of excess benefits over costs.

Weinstein and Stason, who defined the foundations of cost-effectiveness analysis for health care and medical practices, recommend a net cost calculation in which the immediate and long-term financial requirements of the alternative are represented by direct health care costs, plus health care costs related to side effects of treatment, plus other health care costs incurred because of added life, minus direct costs averted (benefits due to reduced need for medical care, rehabilitation and other services).[27] This calculation moves benefits forgone to the cost side of the framework. The net cost is then related to a uniform unit of outcome, such as quality adjusted life years (QALY), discussed previously. The net cost approach recognizes that in many health care interventions, benefits do not exceed resource costs. It also has the advantage of allowing comparison between programs and strategies with different objectives, as long as the outcomes can be translated into the universal unit of QALY.

Limitations of Economic Evaluation

Limitations of economic evaluation analytical techniques include uncertainty, discounting, aggregation of data, and equity. Uncertainty about costs and outcomes predicted to occur at some point in the future as a result of the intervention is unavoidable. Sensitivity analysis, which tests whether variations in assumptions affect the conclusions of an analysis, is recommended to assess the robustness of conclusions under differing assumptions. Sensitivity analysis is accepted as a necessary step in economic analyses.

When costs and outcomes are experienced at different points in time, it is necessary to reduce them to present value or a common base year by discounting.[9] Failure to discount leads to serious overestimation of program outcomes, costs, or both that are experienced in the distant future. Further, the results of the analysis may be sensitive to the discount rate (interest rate) used. Cost-effectiveness and cost-benefit analyses of prevention most often use a discount rate of 5%.

The aggregation of complex sets of calculations into an index ratio has problems. Many methodological limitations can be hidden in the "numerical bottom line" of the cost-benefit ratio. Many experts suggest that all the elements that are included in or would be affected by a decision should be explicitly listed or reported in an array (i.e., listed in a table). Presentation of results in an array allows assumptions and underlying values to be challenged. Further, nonquantifiable (intangible) factors can be included. The disadvantage of an array approach is that decision makers have a greater number of elements to consider; however, an advantage is that important intangible or nonquantifiable factors are more likely be taken into consideration.

Social values and equity are frequently concerns of the decision maker but may elude the cost-effectiveness analyst. Using only an efficiency criterion, decision makers may lose sight of other criteria such as equitable allocation of costs and outcomes among members of society. Therefore, addressing ethical issues is included as a specific step in the process of economic evaluation.

Despite these limitations, cost-effectiveness analysis can play an important role in comparing alternatives to deal with priority problems. By forcing articulation of assumptions, by carrying out a sensitivity analysis to explore implications of changing those assumptions, by arraying all elements for review by others, and by considering the ethical implications of conclusions, cost-effectiveness analysis can affect decisions, policies, and resource allocation.

Using Cost-Effectiveness and Cost-Benefit Analysis

Cost-effectiveness and cost-benefit analyses are useful for setting priorities and choosing between different alternatives for achieving health goals. They provide a valuable structuring process for identifying the least costly and most effective alternative. Care must be exercised to structure the cost and outcome framework according to the defined perspective and the analytical goals of the study. The presentation of data in an array allows for review of assumptions and calculations by others. Sensitivity analysis, discounting, and ethical issues must be addressed. Disclosure of the perspective, assumptions, measurement, and valuation will allow decision makers to make best use of the results.

According to Oster,[16] cost-effectiveness analysis has relevance in patient care decision making where there is a choice between different alternatives or interventions for accomplishing a given clinical goal, such as diagnosing a disease, treating an illness, or delivering a service. The choice generally represents competing and mutually exclusive alternatives; the comparisons involve a simultaneous consideration of the costs of different interventions and their associated health outcomes.

Then, on the basis of cost and outcome considerations, most analyses attempt to identify those interventions that are efficient or provide value for money, that is, yield the greatest payoff to health for a given resource cost. Thus cost-effectiveness analyses reframe clinical problems in terms of the trade-offs between costs and outcomes that are embodied in the most efficient ways of accomplishing a given clinical goal.

Economic Analysis in Nutrition

Before 1979, economic analyses were rare in the nutrition literature. At that time the American Dietetic Association proposed a model for estimating the economic benefits of nutrition.[14] Relationships were suggested linking nutrition education and counseling to diet changes, diet changes to health risk factor changes, and risk factor changes to reduced health care costs and other economic benefits. The model, which provides a sound base for considering legitimate linkages of inputs to outcomes, is shown in Figure 18-5. The 1979 publication indicated the need for empirical research to further delineate and verify the predicted relationships. Ten years later, Disbrow reviewed the emerging literature on the costs and benefits of

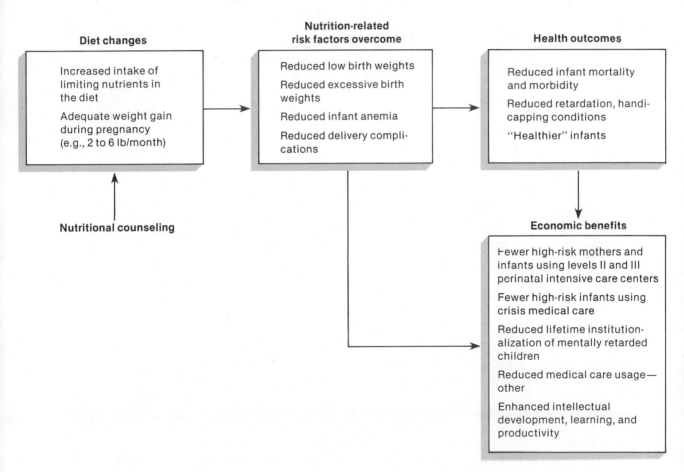

Figure 18-5. Potential economic benefits of nutritional counseling in pregnancy.
Redrawn from *Costs and benefits of nutritional care phase 1, Chicago*, 1979, American Dietetic Association. Copyright The American Dietetic Association. Reprinted by permission.

nutrition care.[8] She identified a total of 35 cost analyses, 164 reports of health outcomes, and only 25 economic analyses in 14 areas of nutrition care. The comprehensive review summarizes data on costs, health status and economic benefits, and results of economic analysis; however, no attempt was made to critique the research methodology used in studies. Following a critical analysis of existing studies in four areas of practice, the American Dietetic Association published summary documents that justify a rational basis for nutrition care in terms of its intermediate-term cost savings and economic gains.[22] Trouba presents a summary document of nutrition intervention in prenatal care.[26]

Community nutrition programs can benefit from the application of cost-effectiveness and cost-benefit analysis to evaluation, planning, justification of specific programs and services. Such studies must be based on valid measurement of outcomes and careful calculation of costs that come from carefully designed evaluations.

PRODUCTIVITY

Economic analysis uses the concept of productivity or efficiency as a foundation. This section explores this concept and shows how productivity measurement is used in the control function.

Productivity is a measure of efficiency. It summarizes the number of units produced (output) relative to the level of resources (inputs) used to produce it. Productivity is always expressed by the formula:

$$\text{Productivity} = \frac{\text{output}}{\text{input}}$$

Output is an expression of the actual result of the production process. Typical output measures are client visits, meals served, and classes presented.

Outcomes are also outputs, but they are more difficult to define and quantify. For example, the output of a grocery store education program could be the exposure of 3500 customers to the message of "eat five fruits and vegetables a day." The desired output may be change in knowledge, fruit and vegetable purchasing or other consumption be-

havior, or, in the long term, prevention of colon cancer. Outcomes like these are difficult to track for community-based interventions. Other evaluation techniques can be planned to examine important but difficult-to-assess outcomes.

Input is the effort or resources used to produce the output. Inputs may be expressed in many ways, for example, staff time, number of full-time equivalent employees (FTEs), clinic sessions, or dollars. The basis for input is the capital and monetary resources of an organization, including human resources and their expertise, supplies and equipment, and facilities.

The aim of management for productivity is to maximize output while minimizing inputs. This is also called *efficiency*, and the terms are used interchangeably. Productivity implies reducing or maintaining the costs of production, increasing services and goal achievement, or both.

Productivity can be improved by changing operations so that the quantity or cost of inputs is reduced. This could be done by substitution (replacing public health nutritionists with dietetic technicians for routine nutrition education activities) or by using existing resources more proficiently (using existing computer hardware and software to streamline client record keeping). Producitivty can also be improved by "working smarter, not harder." For example, by modifying procedures and activities such as adjusting scheduling and clinic flow (and not using additional resources), more clients could be enrolled or those served could achieve a higher level of success.

Productivity Measurement

The challenge of productivity measurement is to create a balance between the need for data to aid decision making and the generation of more information than the organization can use. Productivity measurement should be geared toward measurement of progress toward organizational goals. Common productivity measures in community nutrition include number of patients per clinic session or per clinic hour, monthly meal count per congregate dining site, hours consultation per facility, number of recipe cards picked up (or other means of counting participants) per grocery store food demonstration (or other education event), and number of patients seen per number scheduled (show rate).

Productivity ratios are increasingly being used as performance standards. In ambulatory health care, productivity ratios expressed as number of patients per primary health care provider are used to assess performance and are linked to ability to generate income from third-party payers for reimbursable services. WIC certifications per nutrition professional are used to plan and secure WIC funding. Labor productivity, which relates outputs to personnel costs, is commonly used in measuring and improving productivity. Productivity ratios can be used to compare nutritionist to nutritionist, clinic to clinic, or past period to current period. People involved should have knowledge of productivity measures and results. All staff should know why and how productivity is measured.

Recall that guidelines for personnel in public health nutrition, included in Chapter 17 suggest staffing ratios related to the population of the community. These can serve as standards for staffing and productivity measurement.

McEwan and Messersmith spell out six steps of developing and using a productivity measurement system.[15] This process involves setting performance measures that are meaningful to nutrition staff, measuring performance, comparing actual practice to expected performance standards, determining need for action, and documenting actions taken.

Step 1: Identify activities and tasks and services and outcomes produced. Identify specific activities and tasks that nutrition personnel produce. These can come from job specifications and program goals and objectives. The services and outcomes should correlate to the activities and tasks.

Step 2: Identify resources utilized or necessary to carry out the activities. Identify resources assigned to activities and the services and outcomes that result. This step helps to relate the adequacy and availability of resources to the accomplishment of the activity and the production of desired services and outcomes. Often performance problems relate to inappro-

priate allocation of resources rather than problems with individuals' execution of activities and tasks.

Step 3: Develop ratios and collect data. The ratios are performance measures and should be developed by the individuals using them. The inputs and outputs of ratios should be selected to give quantifiable information about important areas of performance related to accomplishment of program goals and objectives. Measures should not duplicate information available from another source (such as accounting or human resources departments), but available data such as labor costs and work hours may be incorporated into nutrition staff performance ratios.

New recording forms may need to be developed for recording activities, services, and outcomes on a regular basis. Figure 18-6 on p. 512, developed by San Bernadino County, California, allows professional nutrition staff to document time (hours) and units of service (unit) completed in major activity categories. Activity forms should be developed to meet the unique needs of the agency and the performance measures that are to be assessed. All staff should be trained in the use of the recording procedures.

Step 4: Evaluate ratios and analyze performance. Ratios are meaningless unless results are compared with desired performance (standards) and past performance. Documentation and evaluation of performance over time serves as a basis for future comparisons. Table 18-2 on p. 513 provides examples of productivity ratios related to activities and tasks and the resources needed.

Step 5: Implement plan of action for improvement. Once productivity ratios have been obtained and compared with standards and past performance, a course of action can be planned on the basis of whether productivity has increased, decreased, or stayed the same. When specific activities and tasks, resources allocated to the activities, and service and outcome indicators are linked, nutrition program

Name _____

Dates __/__/P.P. _____

Week _____

Program code _____

Program code	600 Administrative supervision (hr)	654 Consultation (hr / unit)	656 Nutrition counseling (hr / unit)	658 High risk nutrition counseling (hr / unit)	660 General nutrition programming (hr)	661 Nutrition implementation (hr / unit)	662 Nutrition education program & resource development (hr / unit)	663 Nutrition screening/assessment (hr / unit)	664 Protocols & quality assurance (hr / unit)	665 Computer nutritional analysis (hr / unit)	666 Mean writing (hr)	667 Therapeutic mean writing (hr)	900 Recruiting, interviewing & orienting (hr)	910 In-service (hr)	950 Meetings (hr)	980 Travel time (hr)
Sat																
Sun																
Mon																
Tue																
Wed																
Thu																
Fri																
Total																

	10 Regular	43 Vacation	44 Holiday	46 Sick leave	79 A.W.O.P.

Employee's signature _____

Supervisor _____

Figure 18-6. Nutrition program time and activity records.

Table 18-2. Productivity measurement in a nutrition program

Tasks/duties	Resources allocated	Productivity (P) measurement	Evaluation	
			Previous period productivity values	Present period productivity values
1. Education of diabetic patients	Dietitian, health care facility, salary	$P = \dfrac{\text{no of patients (pt)}}{\text{no of working hr}}$ $P = \dfrac{\text{no of revisits by pt}}{\text{no of pt visits}}$	$\dfrac{8\ \text{pt}}{8\ \text{hr}} = 1.0$ $\dfrac{2\ \text{revisits}}{8\ \text{pt visits}} = 0.25$	$\dfrac{5\ \text{pt}}{8\ \text{hr}} = 0.625$ $\dfrac{4\ \text{revisits}}{8\ \text{pt visits}} = 0.5$
2. Obtain funding for development of prenatal nutrition classes for low-income families	Dietitian, clerical staff, hours spent	$P = \dfrac{\text{no of grant proposals submitted}}{\text{no of grants}}$ $P = \dfrac{\text{no of grants}}{\text{no of grant awarded}}$	$\dfrac{6\ \text{grants}}{5\ \text{grants submitted}} = 1.2$ $\dfrac{6\ \text{grants}}{4\ \text{grants awarded}} = 1.5$	$\dfrac{6\ \text{grants}}{2\ \text{grants submitted}} = 3$ $\dfrac{6\ \text{grants}}{1\ \text{grant awarded}} = 6$
3. Continue to update professional skills	Professional journals, time, cost, workshop/seminars	$P = \dfrac{\text{no of CE hours}}{\text{no of CE hours completed/mo}}$	$\dfrac{75\ \text{CE hr}}{15\ \text{hr/mo}} = 5.0$	$\dfrac{75\ \text{CE hr}}{10\ \text{CE hr/mo}} = 7.5$

From McEwan CW, Messersmith AM. *J Am Diet Assoc* 87:5, 1987.

managers and staff are better able to identify opportunities for corrective action.

Step 6: Continue the productivity management process. The previous steps relate directly to the control process of defining standards, measuring performance, comparing actual with desired, and taking action as shown in Figure 18-1. McEwan and Messersmith use former performance as the standard or benchmark for future performance.[15] In most situations dietitians and nutritionists would also specify a performance standard for comparison. The standard can be modified over time as actual data on performance are available. Step 6 expresses management commitment to productivity and links productivity assessment with continuous quality management. This step includes revising performance measures, documentation procedures, and forms as needed or as program objectives and activities change.

BUDGETING AND FINANCIAL CONTROL OF NUTRITION PROGRAMS

Budgeting

Budgeting is the systematic, cumulative process through which budgets are created. The budgeting process is used to plan an organization or program's finances in terms of predictions of where the money will come from and how the money will be spent to accomplish specific purposes. Thus budgeting goes hand in hand with program planning and organizing and becomes an important tool of the control function of management.

The Budgeting Process

The budgeting process begins with systematic projections of resource needs (for personnel, supplies and equipment, facilities, travel, contractual services, and administrative overhead costs) and revenue sources. Projections should consider minimum versus ideal levels, strengths and weaknesses of alternative resource allocation plans against projected revenues, prioritizing for resource allocation, and balancing planned expenditures with estimated revenues. This leads to the preparation of

a formal budget document, which is submitted for administrator or funder review. Discussion, negotiation, and compromise may follow. Finally, the approved budget is used as a management tool to guide implementation and control of ongoing nutrition programs and services.

Conventional Zero-Based Budgeting

There are two ways to approach budgeting: make incremental adjustments to the previous year's budget (historical or conventional approach) or start with a clear slate (zero-based budgeting).

The tendency to let historical patterns drive the budgeting process favors existing programs. In the conventional approach the manager focuses on justifying additional funding. However, a historical approach where activities are supported at about the same level as the previous year's may not lead to efficient use of resources or to achievement of program goals and objectives unless direct attention is given to shifting needs and measures of productivity or effectiveness. With reliance on historical trends, it may be difficult to secure dollars for development and pilot testing of innovations in service delivery, and it may be even more difficult to get dollars for implementation of a completely new program.

Figure 18-7 demonstrates how funding levels change over the life span of a program or project. Initially, funds are needed for market research, development, and pilot testing of new program ideas. Following successful development, additional resources must usually be invested to gear up for full implementation, which could include recruitment

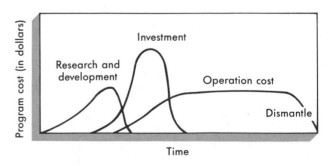

Figure 18-7. Costs over the life span of a program.

or training, specialized equipment such as computers, opening new sites, and securing stocks of supplies. Once the program is implemented, funding needs stabilize until such a time as the program becomes obsolete or low priority. Then the program should be dismantled and resources reallocated to other programs.

In zero-based budgeting, there is no assumption that future needs match those of the past. The entire budget, not just increases, must be justified. Nutrition unit activities are broken down into program "decision packages" consisting of a set of activities for which specific costs and outcomes (benefits) can be outlined and the consequences considered if the decision package is not approved. The decision packages are then ranked in order of importance by using cost and outcome (benefit) projections. Finally, available funds are allocated to decision packages based on relative rank. Lower-ranking decision packages may be dropped or only partially funded. Zero-based budgeting is closely aligned with cost-benefit analysis. The advantage of zero-based budgeting is that it stimulates regular assessment and questioning of existing programs along with consideration of the development of new ideas.

Budget

A budget is the formal statement of proposed expenditures and anticipated resources (revenues) for a specified future period of time. The budget is the backbone of a comprehensive plan of operation for an organization and its programs and services. It expresses plans in monetary terms. The budget communicates organizational and program goals and objectives for a forthcoming period and the allocation of resources to achieve those goals and objectives. Further, the budget, by providing a basis for the analysis of costs and activities, serves as a primary basis for control within the organization and program. Appendix 18-2 illustrates a budget proposal for a complex nutrition unit at the state level. Once the budget is created and approved, regular financial reports enable assessment of program activities against expenditure and revenue projections. In this way the budget becomes a management tool for monitoring and evaluating program performance.

Types of Budgets

The most common budget is the operating budget. It is used to express monetary requirements for planned activities for a specific time period, usually a year or a contractual period. Personnel budgets may be separate or part of the operating budget. Personnel budgets itemize staffing needs by position, full-time equivalents (FTEs), wage or salary rate, fringe benefits, coverage for vacation and sick leaves, and anticipated overtime. Because personnel costs commonly consume the largest percentage of nutrition program funds, personnel budgets merit special care and detail. Capital budgets estimate expenditures for improvements in fixed assets (e.g., buildings) and sources of funds to finance them. Capital budgets outline planned capital expenditures for the long term (i.e., more than 1 budget year). Nutrition program budgeting is infrequently involved in capital budgeting. However, creative programming to achieve education and behavior change goals may require new or remodeled facilities that are specifically designed to meet special needs of nutrition programs (e.g., major remodeling or securing facilities for cooking demonstrations that meet state codes for public food preparation and service); goals to reach isolated target audiences may require new clinic locations for delivery of services.

Parts of a Budget

A budget consists of three parts: (1) a narrative section describing what the program is and what services it provides, (2) the dollars needed to carry out the program, and (3) the statistics that will measure the outputs and outcomes of the program or services. Look for these parts in the budget proposal in Appendix 18-2.

Budgets begin with a concise narrative that generally includes the mission of the organization or sponsoring program; statement of philosophy of the program and major program directions; target population expected to be served, including eligibility criteria and mandated and optional client numbers;

goals and objectives for the budget period, including goals for downsizing, expansion, or reaching new target groups; and workload expectations. The narrative establishes a clear rationale for the allocation of resources and communicates the plan for effective resource utilization. The budget narrative provides assurance that worthwhile activities will be delivered in a well-managed, responsible fashion.

The dollars section generally includes a line-item summary of proposed expenditures by program or cost center, with previous year's actuals, the current year's actual to date and budgeted, and next year's estimated expenditures for comparison; line-item justification (i.e., how the amount was estimated and the basis for allocation to the program or cost center); explanation of administrative overhead costs; determination of projected unit costs; and a complete listing of revenue sources and amounts anticipated. Line-item categories are shown on Figure 18-8.

The statistics section defines the significant data that will be collected to manage and evaluate the program. These statistics, called *outputs*, *outcomes*, or *indicators*, should be related to the objectives of the program or service and have a relationship to organizational and program goals. Examples include number of clients served, units of service delivered, before-and-after rates of anemia, and low birth rate.

Responsible budgeting implies the submission of a budget that accurately reflects resource requirements for accomplishing specific goals and objectives through nutrition programs and services. Inclusion of the previous three parts in the formal budget statement or proposal helps those who must review and approve the budget to understand resource requirements and thereby support the allocation of adequate resources for development and ongoing operation of nutrition programs and services.

The Budget as a Tool for Nutrition Program Management

An accurate budget is an essential ingredient in successful management. The budget is a primary tool for matching resources with identified program priorities. It provides a financial guide to program operations. Dietitians and nutritionists should seek involvement in the budgeting process. It leads to greater understanding of the political nature of resource allocation and the necessity of soundly justified program priorities and estimates of resource needs. With involvement, nutrition program managers gain skill in accurately estimating and convincingly communicating resource needs. As an informed participant in the organization's budgeting process, the nutrition program manager has a better chance of securing sufficient support for the nutrition services that is necessary to meet priority needs.

Budgeting as a Political Process

Budgeting is not merely accounting and allocating; it is also a political process. Budgets can be viewed as an instrument of policy in that allocation of resources is the ultimate expression of priorities. Program and service activities, outcomes, and accomplishment of goals and objectives should follow the allocation of resources. Political pressures influence the determination of priorities, resource allocation, and the budget approval process. Clearly, sound documentation of nutrition needs, along with good communication and visibility of needs and their potential solutions, is necessary to build political support for the allocation of dollars to nutrition services and programs. Building political support is particularly challenging for new initiatives and innovative program ideas that may compete for support, not only with existing nutrition programs that are mandated or expected by various constituencies, but also with other nonnutrition priorities, such as AIDS and other emerging problems. Results of evaluation can be used to leverage political support. In times of scarce resources, which is the case throughout the public as well as private sectors at this time, cost-benefit and cost-effectiveness analysis can be used as a tool to aid resource allocation decisions. Results of cost-benefit and cost-effectiveness studies carry a lot of weight in political decisions.

LINKING PRODUCTIVITY AND BUDGET PROPOSALS

The realities of a recessionary economy and conservative political leadership seriously constrain the funds available for public programs. In times of tight resources, the budgeting process frequently requires identifying programmatic areas that can be cut. Or, more optimistically, a plan for the future should identify funds that can be redirected for productivity improvement or to other initiatives that more effectively and efficiently achieve overall goals and objectives. Although the immediate and long-term goal may be to reduce costs, quality must not be sacrificed. Assurance must be given that changes will not compromise the quality of care as is currently defined by professional practice and is perceived by clients; also, effectiveness in terms of achieving program outcomes must not be compromised.

When new initiatives or ideas for change are proposed, sources for additional resource requirements must be identified. They could be internal reallocation from other programs or departments, increased funding from state and federal contracts and grants, or new outside funding from government agencies or foundations, but very often resources must be freed up from within the existing nutrition unit budget. External sources of funding are addressed in the following Revenue section of this chapter.

Funds for productivity improvement projects must be justified in terms of the necessity and benefits of instituting the proposed changes. A proposal should include presentation of evaluation criteria and current performance, specific plans for change along with the costs and benefits of the change, and methods to be used to document and assess the results of the change that are specific, quantifiable, and valid.

Major initiatives for change, whether productivity or quality improvement projects, program expansion, or the more difficult change of program reduction, require well-thought-out and soundly justified plans. The following criteria should be applied in all situations of major change. When these criteria are met, the nutrition program manager is prepared for the planning, proposing, advocating, negotiating, and compromising that will undoubtedly follow.

These criteria are also a foundation for cutting programs in times of budget cuts and reallocation, organizational restructuring, and labor force reductions. Prioritization as discussed in Chapter 14 is especially relevant to making difficult decisions about what to cut and how. Data from productivity measures and evaluation studies help the nutrition program manager identify the most productive and effective programmatic areas and the highest-performing employees.

1. All initiatives must be central to the mission and goals of the organization and program. In community health and human services programs, this means that the possible impact of the change on the health and nutritional well-being of the community must be considered.

2. Essential programs and services must continue to be appropriate, acceptable, and accessible to the target population.

3. The needs of employees for job security, personal and professional development, reassignment, and retraining, if necessary, must be included in the plan.

4. Cost and benefits of the plan in the immediate and future budget years must be estimated as carefully as possible. Financial implications of staff or service reductions (or expansions) must be calculated. Freed (or required) monetary or personnel resources must be clearly identified. In expansion projects, be sure all internal resources are used at maximum efficiency. Show internal reallocation of resources to indicate serious commitment to balance efficiency aims with program expansion.

5. Develop a flexible plan with actual or projected data as supportive evidence for the change. Identify evaluation procedures to be used to assess the implementation of the plan.

6. Good communication is essential throughout the process. Administration should be in-

Nutrition Unit or Program _____ Budget Report Date _____

Budget for FY 19__	1 FY 19__ Year Before Last	2 FY 19__ Last Year	3 FY 19__ Last Year to This Point	4 FY 19__ This Year to Date	5 FY 19__ This Year	6 Proposed Budget Next Year
	Actual	Actual	Actual	Actual	Budgeted	Estimated
REVENUE/INCOME						
Direct allocation of state or local funds						
Grants or contracts (list)						
Fees collected						
Fund raising/donations						

EXPENSES						
Salaries						
Fringe benefits						
Office supplies/services						
Equipment						
Education materials						
Travel						
Staff development/ continuing ed.						
Contractual services (specify)						
Overhead space						
Administrative services						

Figure 18-8. Sample budget form.

volved early in the process of formulating changes. Regular informational and problem-solving sessions must be held with staff and subordinates, as well as with collaborators and affected clients.

Productivity management means concentrating resources available where the greatest potential for results is. The nutrition program manager must be prepared to tackle some difficult challenges in allocating scarce resources to nutrition programs and activities that meet the needs of the community.

SOURCES OF FUNDS FOR NUTRITION PROGRAMS AND SERVICES—REVENUE

Financing nutrition programs and services involves creatively obtaining and utilizing public and private funding sources, including grants, contracts, third-party reimbursement, and payment for services and products.

The most frequently used sources for funding state and local nutrition programs are the federal block grants to states, WIC, and state revenues. Increasingly, local public health agencies are seeking reimbursement of personal health services through Medicaid and private insurers. Some federal discretionary grants, particularly from agencies of the U.S. Departments of Health and Human Services (DHHS), Agriculture (USDA), and Education (DOE), are available.

The Maternal and Child Health (MCH) Block Grant pays for numerous state and local nutritionist positions. MCH Block Grant funds are supporting nutritionists to work in programs serving children with special health care needs. The Preventive Health and Health Services Block Grant has funded nutritionist positions as part of health promotion programs. Several states have programs that focus on cardiovascular risk reduction, diabetes, or both. The Primary Care Block Grant provides full or partial funding for some nutritionist positions in community health and migrant health centers. Other funding opportunities exist for dietitians and nutritionists involved in programs supported by the Community Services Block Grant, which funds community food and nutrition programs directed to emergency feeding and commodity distribution

programs. Often these programs are operated at the local level through community action agencies rather than health departments.

WIC is the major funder of nutritionist positions in state and local health departments. In fact, WIC funds make up the largest revenue source for most state health departments. The largest portion of funds, however, goes directly to pay for WIC foods.

Several positions in state departments of education are funded by the USDA Child Nutrition Program to oversee and operate the National School Lunch, School Breakfast, Child Care Food, Special Milk, and Summer Food Service Programs. Opportunities exist for state and local public health nutritionists to collaborate with personnel in these programs as they attempt to reach the Healthy People 2000 objectives of bringing these food programs in alignment with the Dietary Guidelines.

Another major funder of nutrition programs is the Administration on Aging's Nutrition Program for Older Americans. Congregate dining and home-delivered meals programs are important access sites for reaching the elderly population.

Nutrition counseling of low-income women in child-bearing years can be provided through the Title X Family Planning Program. Nutrition counseling of the elderly is reimbursable through Medicare Part B if provided under the supervision of the physician. Nutrition services can also be funded with in-home health agencies as a part of the agencies' administrative costs.[10]

The recent emphasis on early identification of children with special needs increases opportunities for funding dietitian or nutritionist positions or reimbursement of services provided. Funds for contractual services may be secured through the Early Intervention Program (0-2) of DOE or the Head Start Program of DHHS. Reimbursement for nutrition screening, assessment, and counseling of low-income children up to age 21 is available through Medicaid, especially within the Early and Periodic Screening, Diagnosis, and Treatment (EPSDT) program.[10]

General tax revenues in many states and local communities fund nutrition programs or nutritionist positions. The state of New York, for example, has funded a large program to reduce hunger, and Montana recently passed legislation enabling support for nutrition initiatives. Other state and local health agencies make internal decisions to allocate a portion of their state or local funding to dietitian or nutritionist positions or activities.

Contractual services offer the greatest opportunity for creative planning and negotiation for support of nutrition programs. Packaged programs may be offered to businesses and corporations as part of workplace health promotion activities. They often include employee screening, counseling, and education, as well as cafeteria programs designed to alter the type of food available to employees.

Other programs such as weight-control programs or heart-healthy cooking classes may be offered to members of the community for a fee.

Innovative programs designed to meet important needs in the community or needs experienced by a special segment of the population could be proposed to private foundations for grants. Private foundations represent a flexible source of funding. The requirement is a good idea and a well-written proposal. Similar to all funding sources, the competition is stiff. Credibility in the community and a good track record with previous nutrition programs increase the chances of securing foundation grants.

A local source of small grants for special projects or special equipment needs are voluntary health organizations such as state affiliates of the American Heart Association or the March of Dimes Birth Defects Foundation and civic organizations and clubs. Local civic organizations routinely support activities that benefit the community. They may be pleased to be asked to support or become involved in nutrition-related activities.

The essential ingredients for securing any source of financial support are a good plan for nutrition programs and services, knowledge about what works, and a commitment to serve the client with high-quality services designed to meet their needs. Most potential funders, whether in government agencies or the private sector, can recognize these ingredients. They have a review and approval process in place to assure that their limited funds go to organizations and programs where the resources will have the greatest payoff in terms of a positive impact on important community health problems.

SUMMARY

The dietitian and nutritionist must carry out all functions of the management process: planning, organizing, directing, and controlling. Attention must be given to the control function to assess the process and outcome of nutrition programs and to adjust plans so that the stated goals and objectives of community nutrition programs and activities are achieved. Using feedforward and feedback loops, the control process enables the nutrition program manager to assure the efficiency and effectiveness of programs throughout all stages of their life span. Budgeting and financial control are important tools for allocating resources for greatest productivity. Productivity and efficiency are important, but effectiveness is crucial. More complex effectiveness and economic evaluations can be used to evaluate nutrition programs.

Control and evaluation require an inquisitive mind, the ability to formulate questions, the discipline to plan and follow through in a consistent manner, and the objectivity and courage to act on the findings. These abilities enable the dietitian and nutritionist to utilize the control process for continuous quality and productivity improvement.

REFERENCES

1. Albrecht K: *Service America: doing business in the new economy*, Homewood, Ill, 1985, Jones-Irwin.
2. Brauer PM, Ines S, Thompson BR: Economic impact of nutrition counselling in patients with Crohn's disease in Canada, *J Can Diet Assoc* 49:236, 1988.
3. Bruce L, Tchabo JG: Nutrition intervention program in a prenatal clinic, *Obstet Gynecol* 74:310, 1989.
4. Cook TD, Campbell DT: *Quasi-experimentation: design and analysis issues for field settings*, Boston, 1979, Houghton Mifflin.
5. Reference deleted in proof.
6. Crosby PB: *Quality is free*, New York, 1979, McGraw-Hill.
7. Deming E: *Quality, productivity, and competitive position*, Cambridge, 1982, Massachusetts Institute of Technology Center for Advanced Engineering Study.
8. Disbrow DD: The costs and benefits of nutrition services: a literature review, *J Am Diet Assoc*, 84(4):S3, 1989.

9. Drummond MF, Stoddart GL, Torrance GW: *Methods for economic evaluation of health care programmes*, New York, 1987, Oxford University Press.

10. Fox MK, editor: *Reimbursement and insurance coverage for nutrition services*, Chicago, 1991, American Dietetic Association.

11. Griffin RW: *Management,* ed 3, Boston, 1990, Houghton Mifflin.

12. Joint Commission on Accreditation of Healthcare Organizations: Characteristics of clinical indicators, *QRB* 50(7):330, 1989.

13. Juran JM, Gryne FM: *Quality planning and analysis,* New York, 1980, McGraw-Hill.

14. Mason M, editor: *Costs and benefits of nutrition care: phase 1,* Chicago, 1979, American Dietetic Association.

15. McEwan CW, Messersmith AM: Productivity management: applying it personally and professionally, *J Am Diet Assoc* 87:581, 1987.

16. Oster G: Economic aspects of clinical decision making: applications in medical care, *Am J Hosp Pharm* 45:543, 1988.

17. Rossi P, Freeman H: Evaluation: a systematic approach, Newbury Park, ed 4, Calif, 1989, Sage.

18. Scholtes PR: *The team handbook,* Madison, Wisc, 1988, Joiner Associates.

19. Scriven M: *Goal-free evaluation.* In E House, editor: *School evaluation,* Berkeley, Calif, 1970, McCutchan.

20. Simko M, Conklin MT: Focusing on the effectiveness side of the cost-effectiveness equation, *J Am Diet Assoc* 89:485, 1989.

21. Splett PL: Assessing effectiveness of nutrition care: prerequisite for cost-effectiveness analysis, *Top Clin Nutr* 5:26, 1990.

22. Splett PL: Effectiveness and cost effectiveness of nutrition care: a critical analysis with recommendations, *J Am Diet Assoc* 91(Suppl)S7, 1991.

23. Splett PL, Russo PM: *Documenting the quality and effectiveness of nutrition care.* In Fox MK, editor: *Reimbursement and insurance coverage for nutrition services,* Chicago, 1991, American Dietetic Association.

24. Stoddart GL: Economic evaluation methods and health policy, *Evaluation and the Health Professionals* 5:393, 1982.

25. Stunkard AJ, Cohen AY, Felix MR: Weight loss competitions at the worksite: how they work and how well, *Prev Med* 18:460, 1989.

26. Trouba PH, Okereke N, Splett PL: Summary document of nutrition intervention in prenatal care, *J Am Diet Assoc* 91(Suppl):524, 1991.

27. Weinstein, MC, Stason WB: Foundations of cost-effectiveness analysis for health and medical practices, *N Eng J Med* 296:716, 1977.

APPENDIX 18-1

WIC Nutrition Services Standards*

The WIC Nutrition Services Standards (NSS) were established for two reasons:

1. To provide state WIC directors and nutritionists with a method for evaluating the quality of nutrition services in their program

2. To encourage states to use their evaluation information to improve nutrition services in their programs

The 12 standards apply to these nutrition services components:

Nutrition/health assessment
Nutrition services plan

Nutrition education
Qualifications and roles of nutritionists
Nutrition staff training
Food packages

The standards do not repeat federal regulations. The regulations prescribe nutrition services to be offered, but do not describe the quality of those services or how they are to be evaluated.

The NSS describe quality nutrition services, not the level of services currently being provided by the states. By using the standards to evaluate their nutrition services, state directors and nutritionists can decide which components of their nutrition services program need improvement. They can plan for change and work toward meeting the stan-

*Adapted from *WIC Nutrition Services Standards*, National Association of WIC Directors, Washington, DC.

dards over time. Because each is at a different starting point, states are not expected to meet all standards by a specific time.

The Food and Nutrition Service (FNS) of the USDA and the National Association of WIC Directors (NAWD) will help states work toward meeting the Nutrition Services Standards. They will provide opportunities at national and regional WIC conferences for states to share information about NSS and other initiatives.

Regional FNS offices will also be available to help states improve their nutrition services. Regional nutritionists will provide guidance and technical assistance in nutrition services and specifically in developing the state nutrition education plan.

State directors and nutritionists are responsible for working toward and meeting standards, for example, by helping local agencies improve their services. (In these standards, *local agency* means an agency providing direct WIC services.)

FNS and NAWD will determine when to revise the standards. Revisions will reflect changes in federal regulations or funding and in nutrition research findings that indicate revision is needed.

WIC NUTRITION SERVICE STANDARDS

Standard 1: Nutrition and Health Assessment

The state agency has documented nutrition risk criteria referenced as necessary by current scientific research, which are applied consistently by all local agencies in the state.*

Assessment of Standard 1

The state agency has nutrition risk criteria for eligibility that:

- Are based on current authoritative references from scientific literature
- Are documented when atypical nutrition risk criteria or nutrition risk levels are used
- Demonstrate coordination with other health programs and private medical practice

*Guidelines for assessment of standards are included for standards 1, 2 and 3 to illustrate how achievement standards are evaluated. All standards have assessment guidelines, but for brevity they are not included.

- Use objective clinical indicators (e.g., laboratory values)
- Indicate priority level

The state agency establishes statewide service high-risk criteria to identify high-risk participants, including:

- Participant category and type
- Qualifying medical or nutritional risk

The state agency establishes policies for the use of "regression" as a nutrition risk, including:

- A requirement for a nutritional assessment to rule out the existence of current risk factors before basing eligibility on regression
- A requirement for written identification of the risk factor to which the participant may regress
- A list of risk factors and priority levels for which eligibility based on regression can be applied
- A limit on the number of times regression can be consecutively applied
- An evaluation of the use of regression as part of local agency monitoring

The state agency includes alcohol intake, drug use, and nicotine use as nutrition risk criteria assuring that:

- The level of use considered a risk is established in accordance with current medical and health authorities and research
- Standard procedures are utilized in local agencies in assessing alcohol, drug, and nicotine use
- Procedures are in place for referral for substance abuse services when these services are available in the service area.

The state agency provides local agencies with written procedures for documenting the nutrition risk assessment in the participant file.

Standard 2: Nutrition and Health Assessment

The state agency has standardized dietary assessment procedures based on current practice, which are utilized consistently by all local agencies in the state.

Assessment of Standard 2

The state agency assures that for determining dietary risk for all participants local agencies use a uniform statewide dietary assessment tool that includes:

- Food frequency when dietary risk is the only eligibility factor
- Analysis of diet based on professionally recognized guidelines (e.g., RDA, AAP, and U.S. Dietary Guidelines for Americans)
- Specific statewide criteria for evaluating dietary adequacy to determine eligibility

The state agency documents the rationale for dietary adequacy standards.

The state agency has standardized procedures for documenting the dietary risk assessment in the participant file.

The state agency approves or provides training for local agency staff on collecting, analyzing, and documenting dietary assessment data.

Standard 3: Nutrition and Health Assessment

The state agency has standardized anthropometric and biochemical assessment procedures based on current practice that are utilized consistently by all local agencies in the state.

Assessment of Standard 3

The state agency approves or provides criteria to local agencies on all equipment used for anthropometric measurements and biochemical analyses.

The state agency establishes standards and frequency of calibration and certification of anthropometric and hematological equipment in local agencies and monitors for compliance.

The state agency approves or provides competency-based training for local agency staff in collecting, reading, interpreting, and documenting anthropometric and biochemical data.

Standard 4: Nutrition Education

The state agency has standard policies for all nutrition education contacts, which include types and number of contracts appropriate for participants' risk status.

Standard 5: Nutrition Education

The state agency has standard evaluation procedures for monitoring the nutrition education provided in local WIC agencies.

Standard 6: Nutrition Education

The state agency promotes the use of appropriate, high-quality, and accurate nutrition education materials.

Standard 7: Nutrition Services Plan

The state agency develops and updates annually a WIC nutrition services plan that includes a needs assessment, long-term and short-term goals and objectives, and an evaluation component as part of the state plan.

Standard 8: Nutrition Services Plan

The state agency assures that local agencies develop an annual nutrition education plan to include a needs assessment, goals, objectives, action plans, and an evaluation component.

Standard 9: Qualifications and Role of the Nutritionist

The state agency assures that a qualified nutritionist provides WIC services and that the role of the WIC nutritionist is defined.

Standard 10: Nutrition Staff Training

The state agency assures through training that competent staff perform certification procedures and provide nutrition education.

Standard 11: Food Packaging

The state agency has uniform policies and guidelines for food package tailoring in accordance with current authoritative medical and health information.

Standard 12: Food Packaging

The state agency has policies and procedures for authorizing WIC foods, which are based on cost, availability, nutritional value, and participant acceptance.

APPENDIX 18-2

Budget proposal

NARRATIVE DESCRIPTION
Agency: Department of Health Services
Program: Bureau of Nutrition Services
Program Description
Plans, develops, and implements nutrition services. Priority for services is placed on the following high-risk groups: women in childbearing years, 0- to 5-year-olds, schoolchildren, adults (parents of children), and the elderly. Services are delivered through five systems—screening, referral, monitoring, aide development, and food delivery—to decrease undernutrition and overnutrition. The bureau administers the special Supplemental Food Program For Women, Infants, and Children (WIC), which reaches 60% of the high-risk population; provides training in nutrition to community health workers, allied health personnel, group care facilities, educational institutions, and the public; and formalizes training through community colleges and universities to develop indigenous nutrition manpower.

Program Goal
To develop and provide high-quality nutrition services as an integral component of health care, thereby improving nutrition and health in the population with a reduction in the number of people requiring sick care services and a decrease in health care costs.

Program Plans
1. To deliver nutrition and supplemental food services to 36,200 individuals and their families, including 1000 older adults, to reduce the prevalence of malnutrition (undernutrition and overnutrition) by 30% in 1 year.
2. To implement the statewide nutrition surveillance system by June 1992 for use by local health-related agencies as a tool for monitoring, program planning, and evaluation.
3. Training in nutrition: (a) 90% of community nutrition workers will be able to develop, implement, and evaluate the client nutrition education plan within 7 months of employment; (b) 60% of nutritionists and dietitians and 3% of other health personnel will participate in at least one training session with evaluation mechanism; (c) 90% of the management personnel in aged, day-care, and other group care facilities referred for nutritional care and/or food service assistance will be followed up to bring at least one previously deficient factor to standard; (d) 75% of those in educational facilities will implement one or more follow-up sessions in which nutrition is related to one or more existing disciplines in the curriculum; (e) 7% of the public will receive nutrition information to improve their diets and/or learn of other sources of help through consultation, group sessions, and mass media.
4. To develop a career ladder for community nutrition workers by December 1992.

Outputs/Outcomes
1. *Screening.* Screened 30,230 people in 14 counties and 9 Indian tribes. Screening revealed that 58% of the population had high serum cholesterol, 13% were anemic, 16.9% were short for their age, 5.2% were underweight, and 14.6% were overweight.
2. *Monitoring.* Follow-up of those at risk resulted in 41.4% of the population decreasing their high serum cholesterol level, 65% of the population overcoming anemia, 44% making improvements in their height measurements, 51% overcoming underweight, and 22% reducing overweight. A

survey on outcome of pregnancy in three projects showed that 92% to 100% of WIC mothers delivered full-term mature infants. A computer system to facilitate program evaluation was designed and piloted and will be implemented statewide December 1992.

3. *Referral.* Approximately 4500 referrals were made to and from the nutrition program, utilizing over 100 different agencies.

4. *Supplemental Food and Nutrition Instruction* was provided to 46,400 WIC recipients— 12,280 infants, 11,800 pregnant and lactating women, and 22,320 children.

5. *Training.* Trained 132 (100%) community nutrition workers; 7 (100%) EPSDT) health assistants; 198 (62%) nutritionists and dietitians; 271 (1.5%) other health personnel; 161 (11.5%) of the personnel in aged and group care facilities; 1061(0.1%) of those in educational facilities; 455,733 (20%) of the public through 49 workshops, 84 on-the-job in-service programs, 72,099 individual consultation sessions, 3 seminars, and 31 mass media presentations. A curriculum was designed for the education of community nutrition workers to improve job skills and mobility; 27 (25%) community nutrition workers are enrolled at a community college in a pilot for evaluation.

PERSONNEL JUSTIFICATION

At A and B level funding: Funds would be insufficient to cover merit increases. Continued lack of opportunity for advancement may result in high staff turnover, especially in the field of nutrition, where nationwide salaries are more competitive.

At C level funding: Five nutrition personnel (4.75 FTEs) will be funded to complete the following duties related to program planning, implementation, and evaluation of nutrition services for 34,795 individuals.

Public Health Nutrition Director

1. Responsible for program planning, direction, and evaluation for delivery of nutrition services to 34,795 clients, which is a 27% increase in the aging and non-WIC-eligible segment of the population over the period between 1989 and 1990.

2. Responsible for directing and implementing the hypothetical state's role in national nutrition surveillance and state-based data collection and analysis for use by local health-related agencies. Responsible for collection and evaluation of data on nutritional care services for older adults. Overall direction of $10 million federally funded Supplementtal Food Program for high-risk pregnant women and children, serving 27,500 clients.

Public Health Nutrition Consultant (Training Coordinator)

1. Responsible for coordination of statewide training activities through the identification of need, cataloging of resources, planning of programs, and establishment of evaluation tools to provide training in nutrition for the following:

   a. 90% of community nutrition workers will be trained so that they will be able to develop, implement, and evaluate nutrition education plan within 7 months of employment.

   b. 60% of nutritionists and dietitians and 3% of other health personnel should participate in at least one training session with an evaluation mechanism.

   c. 90% of the management personnel in aged, day-care, and other group care facilities referred for nutritional care and other group care facilities referred for nutritional care and/or food service assistance will be followed up so that at least one previously deficient factor is brought to standard.

   d. 75% of those in educational facilities will implement one or more follow-up sessions in which nutrition is related to one or more existing disciplines in the curriculum.

   e. 7% of the public will receive nutrition information through consultation, group sessions, and mass media.

2. Service as liaison between Bureau of Nutrition Services and other Department of Health service bureaus, local health departments, and other health agencies in the areas of training statewide.

Table 18-A. State summary of expenditures and budget requests (in thousands)

Expenditure classification	Acutal expenditures 1990	Estimated expenditures 1991	Increase or decrease requested			Request 1992	Recommended 1992
			A	B	C		
FTE No	4.8	4.8				4.8	
Personal services	139.5	155.0	0.7	0.6	6.2	162.5	
Employee related	8.8	11.6	0.1	0.1	−0.4	11.4	
Professional services	1.9	16.6	0.3	0.5		17.4	
Travel	6.6	7.2	0.1	0.2		7.5	
Other operating expenditures	13.6	26.5	2.9	2.6		31.2	
Equipment		1.3	2.9			0.9	
OPERATIONS SUBTOTAL	175.2	223.0	7.0	4.0	5.8	235.7	
Other	128.8	152.3				213.5	
Total appropriated	304.0	375.3	64.1	4.0	5.8	449.2	
Add federal funds							
Add other funds							
TOTAL PROGRAM—SUM OF STATE, FEDERAL, AND OTHER							

3. Responsible for the development and implementation of a career ladeer for community nutrition workers in conjunction with the local community college.

Public Health Nutrition Consultant (75% FTE)

1. Provides technical assistance in public health nutrition for persons 55 years of age and older with services to 1000 aging individuals statewide. Promotes, conducts, and assists in conducting training programs in nutritional care and food services with an evaluation mechanism for 10% of the personnel in aged and group care facilities in 14 counties.
2. Provides information or counseling in nutrition to the public and other agencies statewide.
3. Participates in coordinating field experience throughout the state for master's students, dietetic trainees, and others from 12 university settings in the United States.

Public Health Nutrition Consultant (Funded by Maternal and Child Health, Assigned to Nutrition)

1. Integrates and coordinates Special Supplemental Food Program (WIC) with existing health department programs of MCH and nutrition in seven counties.
2. Analyzes nutrition surveillance data for seven counties for program planning, evaluation, and contractual compliance.

Secretary III

1. Provides administrative support and prepares a variety of involved statistical and fiscal reports for Public Health Nutrition Director.
2. Maintains correspondence with subvention contractors, other bureaus, and outside agencies and people; maintains filing system for the bureau.
3. Arranges travel schedules, conferences, and presentations for Director.

Clerk Typist II

1. Types reports and correspondence for one nutrition specialist.
2. Other responsibilities include answering telephone, greeting visitors, explaining rules and regulations to public, and making appointments.

ACTIVITY JUSTIFICATION

At B level funding: An additional 2061 cholesterol determinations at $0.78.4 per test* would be completed for $1616. This is the estimated number of tests necessary to screen and follow up the clients to be served at this funding level (34,700 clients). An additional $663 is needed for educational materials.

At C level funding: A total of 34,795 clients would be screened. The additional cholesterol tests would cost $119.

*Cost per test includes standards and controls.

Appendixes

APPENDIX A

Healthy Communities 2000 Model Standards: Guidelines for Community Attainment of the Year 2000 National Health Objectives

NUTRITION

Model Standards Goal:

Community residents will achieve optimal nutritional status that will reduce premature death and disability.

Model Standards Note: *Healthy People 2000 Objectives* are national in scope and are provided as a guide for action by state and local communities. As such, they have been restated in their entirety without change. The target for each of these objectives has been repeated verbatim as a reference for community use. However, communities are encouraged to establish targets based on their own situations and where possible establish targets that are more ambitious than the national reference.

Model Standards Note: In this edition the word "other" has been added to each *Healthy People 2000 Objective* which contains a Special Population Target. The use of the word "other" is meant to suggest that communities may wish to develop special population targets for community-specific subpopulations, for example, for selected age, race, sex, income, and/or other high-risk groups.

How to Use Model Standards

Communities are encouraged to use the objectives spelled out in *Healthy People 2000* as a guide for action by state and local communities. At the same time, this third edition recognizes the need for communities to select and develop objectives and individual targets based on their own situations. *Healthy Communities 2000: Model Standards* serves as a guidebook and a process for planning community public health services.

Model Standards Principles

- Emphasis on health outcomes
- Flexibility

From *Healthy Communities 2000: Model Standards*, ed 3, Copyright 1991 by the American Public Health Association. Reprinted with permission.

- Focus upon the entire community
- Government as residual guarantor
- The importance of negotiation
- Standards and guidelines
- Accessibility of services
- Emphasis on programs

Steps for Putting Standards to Use

A series of steps or activities are outlined below to assist health agencies in implementing Model Standards.* Model standards can be used in combination with one or more planning tools as mentioned below; however, communities are encouraged to adapt this process to their specific needs and to use local discretion in deciding how to make the best use of this guidebook.

Activities for Implementation

- Assess and determine the role of one's health agency.
- Assess the lead health agency's organizational capacity.
- Develop an agency plan to build the necessary organizational capacity.
- Assess the community's organizational and power structures.
- Organize the community to build a stronger constituency for public health and establish a partnership for public health.
- Assess the health needs and available community resources.
- Determine local priorities.
- Select outcome and process objectives that are compatible with local priorities and the *Healthy People 2000* objectives.

*These steps are adapted from a list of activities for ensuring the achievement of the year 2000 national health objectives discussed at a Centers for Disease Control meeting, August 21, 1990.

- Develop communitywide intervention strategies.
- Develop and implement a plan of action.
- Monitor and evaluate the effort on a continuing basis.

Community Implementation

In preparing this section of the model standards two vital needs were identified: to establish a visible governmental presence at the local level and to define its essential role as the guarantor of the public's health. To accomplish this, this section describes activities essential to implementing the standards, the infrastructure resources that must be maintained, and administrative requirements for the official governmental health agency responsible at the local level. The Institute of Medicine's (IOM) report on the *Future of Public Health* stressed, "No citizen from any community no matter how small or remote should be without identifiable and realistic access to the benefits of public health protection, which is possible only through a local component of the public health delivery system."

The editorial framework used reflects the recommendation of this IOM report that government's essential functions should be assessment, policy development, and assurance.

Objectives related to assessment:
1. Community health assessment
2. Health statistical and epidemiologic consultation and capacity
3. Quality laboratory services
4. Identification of underserved populations
5. Assessment, monitoring, and evaluation of programs

Policy development

Every official health agency should exercise responsibility to serve the public interest in the development of comprehensive public health policies by promoting use of the scientific knowledge base in decision making and by leading in developing public health policy. The accomplishment of these objectives should assure residents that the community has a process for developing health policy which, in fact, protects health.

Assurances

Assuring that vital services are provided in all communities is an indispensable role of govern-

ment. The community needs to identify its own process by which it assures itself of services necessary to achieve agreed-upon goals.

Nutrition Health Status Objectives

Model standards outline specific health status objectives in terms of nutrition-related disorders, deaths from coronary heart disease, cancer deaths, prevalence of overweight, low birth weight, weight gain during pregnancy, and growth retardation among low-income children as seen in the following table that indicates the focus, objective, and indicator.

The following specific risk reduction objectives continue in the nutrition section of model standards:

Dietary fat and saturated fat intake
Consumption of complex carbohydrates and fiber-containing foods
Practices to attain appropriate body weight
Consumption of calcium-rich foods
Salt and sodium intake
Iron deficiency
Breast feeding
Prevention of baby bottle tooth decay
Food labels

The following specific services and protection objectives continue in the nutrition section of model standards:

Comprehensive nutrition plan
Community nutrition education program
Nutrition services for at-risk populations
Nutrition labeling
Availability of processed foods reduced in fat and saturated fat
Nutrition information in grocery stores
Food choices in restaurants and foodservice operations
Home-delivered meals for older adults
Nutrition education in schools
Nutrition education in work sites
Nutrition assessment and counseling
Nutrition services
Breastfeeding promotion programs
Hospital policies
Nutrition monitoring

Nutrition model standard goal: community residents will achieve optimal nutritional status that will reduce premature death and disability

Focus	Objective	Indicator
Health status objectives		
Nutrition-related disorders	1. By ____ the prevalence of ___*___ nutrition-related disorders will be reduced to ____ among target population.	Prevalence of specific nutrition-related disorders
Deaths from coronary heart disease	2. By ____ (2000) reduce coronary heart disease deaths to no more than ____ (100) per 100,000 people. (Age-adjusted baseline: 135 per 100,000 in 1987) *Special Population Target* **Coronary Deaths (per 100,000)** **1987 Baseline** **2000 Target** a. Blacks 163 ____ (115) b. Other ____	Coronary heart disease death rate
Cancer deaths	3. By ____ (2000) reverse the rise in cancer deaths to achieve a rate of no more than ____ (130) per 100,000 people. (Age-adjusted baseline: 133 per 100,000 in 1987) *(Note: In its publications, the National Cancer Institute age-adjusts cancer death rates to the 1970 U.S. population. Using the 1970 standard, the equivalent baseline and target values for this objective would be 171 and 175 per 100,000, respectively.)*	Nutritionally related cancer deaths (i.e., breast, colorectal)
Prevalence of overweight	4. By ____ (2000) reduce overweight to a prevalence of no more than ____ (20) percent among people aged 20 and older and no more than 15 percent among adolescents aged 12 through 19. (Baseline: 26 percent for people aged 20 through 74 in 1976-80, 24 percent for men and 27 percent for women; 15 percent for adolescents aged 12 through 19 in 1976-80)	Percent overweight

Special population targets

Overweight Prevalence	1976-80 Baseline†	2000 Target
a. Low-income women aged 20 and older	37%	— (25%)
b. Black women aged 20 and older	44%	— (30%)
c. Hispanic women aged 20 and older		— (25%)
Mexican-American women	39%‡	
Cuban women	34%‡	
Puerto Rican women	37%‡	
d. American Indians/ Alaska Natives	29-75%§	— (30%)
e. People with disabil- ities	36%‖	— (25%)
f. Women with high blood pressure	50%	— (41%)
g. Men with high blood pressure	39%	— (35%)
h. Other	—	

* Insert specific nutrition-related disorder, e.g., obesity, anemia, retarded growth, elevated serum cholesterol, coronary artery disease, colon cancer, hypertension, and osteoporosis.
† Baseline for people aged 20-74.
‡ 1982-84 baseline for Hispanics aged 20-74.
§ 1984-88 estimates for different tribes.
‖ 1985 Baseline for people aged 20-74 who report any limitation in activity due to chronic conditions.

Continued.

Nutrition model standard goal: community residents will achieve optimal nutritional status that will reduce premature death and disability—cont'd

Focus	Objective	Indicator
	(Note: For people aged 20 and older, overweight is defined as body mass index (BMI) equal to or greater than 27.8 for men and 27.3 for women. For adolescents, overweight is defined as BMI equal to or greater than 23 for males aged 12 through 14, 24.3 for males aged 15 through 17, 25.8 for males aged 18 through 19, 23.4 for females aged 12 through 14, 24.8 for females aged 15 through 17, and 25.7 for females aged 18 through 19. The values for adolescents are the age- and gender-specific 85th percentile values of the 1976-80 National Health and Nutrition Examination Survey (NHANES II), corrected for sample variation. BMI is calculated by dividing weight in kilograms by the square of height in meters. The cut-points used to define overweight approximate the 120 percent of desirable body weight definition used in the 1990 objectives.	
Low birth weight	5. Reduce low birth weight to an incidence of no more than — percent of live births. (Model standards note: The community may wish to develop special population targets, for example, by age, race, sex, income, handicapping conditions, etc., for community relevant subpopulations.)	Incidence of low and very low birth weights
Weight gain during pregnancy	6. Increase to at least — percent the proportion of mothers who achieve the minimum recommended weight gain during their pregnancies. (Model standards note: All pregnancy weight gain should be adjusted for weight status prior to pregnancy. Recommended weight gain is defined as recommended in the 1990 report by the National Academy of Science, *Nutrition during Pregnancy.*	Percent achieving appropriate weight gain
Growth retardation among low-income children	7. By ____ (2000) reduce growth retardation among low-income children aged 5 and younger to less than — (10) percent. (Baseline: Up to 16 percent among low-income children in 1988, depending on age and race/ethnicity)	Prevalence of growth retardation

Special population targets

Prevalence of Short Stature	1988 Baseline	2000 Target
a. Low-income black children < age 1	15%	—(10%)
b. Low-income Hispanic children < age 1	13%	—(10%)
c. Low-income Hispanic children age 1	16%	—(10%)
d. Low-income Asian/ Pacific Islander children age 1	14%	—(10%)
e. Low-income Asian/ Pacific Islander children aged 2-4	16%	—(10%)
f. Other	—	

(Note: Growth retardation is defined as height for age below the fifth percentile of children in the National Center for Health Statistics' reference population.

APPENDIX B

The Future of Public Health: Summary and Recommendations

Institute of Medicine Report:

National Academy of Sciences*

WHY STUDY PUBLIC HEALTH

Many of the major improvements in the health of the American people have been accomplished through public health measures. Control of epidemic diseases, safe food and water, and maternal and child health services are only a few of the public health achievements that have prevented countless deaths and improved the quality of American life. But the public has come to take the success of public health for granted. Health officials have difficulty communicating a sense of urgency about the need to maintain current preventive efforts and to sustain the capability to meet future threats to the public's health.

This study was undertaken to address a growing perception among the Institute of Medicine membership and others concerned with the health of the public that this nation has lost sight of its public health goals and has allowed the system of public health activities to fall into disarray. Public health is what we, as a society, do collectively to assure the conditions in which people can be healthy. This requires that continuing and emerging threats to the health of the public be successfully countered. These threats include immediate crises, such as the AIDS epidemic; enduring problems, such as injuries and chronic illness; and impending crises foreshadowed by such developments as the toxic by-products of a modern economy.

These and many other problems demonstrate the need to protect the nation's health through effective, organized, and sustained efforts by the public sector. Unfortunately, the findings of this

*Washington, DC, 1988, National Academy Press, adapted.

committee confirm the concerns that led to the study. The current state of our abilities for effective public health action, as documented in this volume, is cause for national concern and for the development of a plan of action for needed improvements. In the committee's view, we have slackened our public health vigilance nationally, and the health of the public is unnecessarily threatened as a result.

An impossible responsibility has been placed on America's public health agencies: to serve as stewards of the basic health needs of entire populations, but at the same time avert impending disasters and provide personal health care to those rejected by the rest of the health system. The wonder is not that American public health has problems, but that so much has been done so well, and with so little.

The Committee for the Study of the Future of Public Health is keenly aware of the public health system's many achievements and of the dedication and sustained efforts of public health workers across the country. The committee's purpose, however, is to bring the difficulties of public health to the attention of the nation in order to mobilize action to strengthen public health. Successes as great as those of the past are still possible, but not without public concern and concerted action to restore America's public health capacity.

This volume envisions the future of public health, analyzes the current situation and how it developed, and presents a plan of action that will, in the committee's judgment, provide a solid foundation for a strong public health capability throughout the nation.

THE APPROACH

During the past 2 years, the committee has studied America's public health system in detail. It has attempted to see public health in action, as revealed by data and as perceived by those involved in it, both inside and outside public health agencies. It has examined demographic and epidemiologic statistics, agency budgets, organization charts, program plans, statutes, and regulations. It has visited localities in six states and spoken with more than 350 people: state and local health officers, public health nurses, sanitarians, legislators, citizen activists, public administrators, voluntary agency personnel, private physicians, and many others. In addition, public meetings were held in Boston, Chicago, New Orleans, and Las Vegas, as well as a conference in Houston on public health education attended by public health educators and practitioners. Finally, the committee reviewed the history of American public health and visited with health officials in Toronto to glimpse the enterprise as practiced in another country, where universal entitlement to medical care is part of the context for that practice.

THE STATE OF U.S. PUBLIC HEALTH

Throughout the history of public health, two major factors have determined how problems were solved: the level of scientific and technical knowledge, and the content of public values and popular opinions. Over time, public health measures have changed with important advances in understanding the causes and control of disease. In addition, practice was affected by popular beliefs about illness and by public views on appropriate governmental action. As poverty and disease came to be seen as societal as well as personal problems, and as governmental involvement in societal concerns increased, collective action against disease was gradually accepted. Health became a social as well as individual responsibility. At the same time, advances such as the discovery of bacteria and identification of better ways to control and prevent communicable disease made possible effective community action under the auspices of increasingly professional public health agencies.

The Public Health Mission

Knowledge and values today remain decisive elements in the shaping of public health practice. But they blend less harmoniously than they once did.

On the surface there appears to be widespread agreement on the overall mission of public health, as reflected in such comments to the committee as "public health does things that benefit everybody," or "public health prevents illness and educates the population." But when it comes to translating broad statements into effective action, little consensus can be found. Neither among the providers nor the beneficiaries of public health programs is there a shared sense of what the citizenry should expect in the way of services, and both the mix and the intensity of services vary widely from place to place.

In one state the committee visited, the state health department was a major provider of prenatal care for poor women; in other places, women who could not pay got no care. Some state health departments are active and well equipped, while others perform fewer functions and get by on relatively meager resources. Localities vary even more widely: in some places, the local health departments are larger and more sophisticated technically than many state health departments. But in too many localities, there is no health department. Perhaps the area is visited occasionally by a "circuit-riding" public health nurse—and perhaps not.

Lack of agreement about the public health mission is also reflected in the diversion in some states of traditional public health functions, such as water and air pollution control, to separate departments of environmental services, where the health effects of pollutants often receive less notice.

In some states, mental health is seen as a public health responsibility, but in many the two are organizationally distinct, making it difficult to coordinate services to multiproblem clients. Some health departments are part of larger departments of "social and health services," where public health scientists find their approaches, which benefit society as a whole, stamped with a negative welfare label.

Such extreme variety of available services and organizational arrangements suggests that contemporary public health is defined less by what public health professionals know how to do than by what the political system in a given area decides is appropriate or feasible.

The Knowledge Base and Its Application

This summary of the state of U.S. public health began with the observation that both technical knowledge and public values determine how public health is practiced. Clearly, the current impact of public values is troublesome, as political dilemmas attest. But there are also problems on the knowledge front.

Effective public health action must be based on accurate knowledge of the causes and distribution of health problems and of effective interventions. Despite much progress, there are still significant knowledge gaps for many public health problems, for example, the health risks of long-term exposure to certain toxic chemicals or the role of stress in disease.

Because public health is an applied activity, operating under fiscal constraints, it is often difficult to mobilize and sustain necessary research. In our site visits, we found that only one of six states had made a substantial investment in research. Similarly, technical expertise is unevenly distributed: public health employees in some larger states have a considerable skill level, but many others do not. The problem is exacerbated by a shortage of epidemiologists and other trained experts. In many jurisdictions low salary structures and unrewarding professional environments may further inhibit the acquisition of expertise.

In addition, there has been little attention in public health to management as a technical skill in its own right. Management of a public health agency is a demanding, high-visibility assignment requiring, in addition to technical and political acumen, the ability to motivate and lead personnel, to plan and allocate agency resources, and to sense and deal with changes in the agency's environment and to relate the agency to the larger community. Progress in public health in the United States has been greatly advanced throughout its history by outstanding individuals who fortuitously combined all these qualities. Today, the need for leaders is too great to leave their emergence to chance. Yet there is little specific focus in public health education on leadership development, and low salaries and a low public image make it difficult to attract

outstanding people into the profession and to retain them until they are ready for top posts.

THE FUTURE OF PUBLIC HEALTH: RECOMMENDATIONS

In conducting this study, the committee has sought to take a fresh look at public health—its mission, its current state, and the barriers to improvement. The committee has concluded that effective public health activities are essential to the health and well-being of the American people, now and in the future. But public health is currently in disarray. Some of the frequently heard criticisms of public health are deserved, but this society has contributed to the disarray by lack of clarity and agreement about the mission of public health, the role of government, and the specific means necessary to accomplish public health objectives. To provide a set of directions for public health that can attract the support of the total society, the committee has made three basic recommendations dealing with:

- The mission of public health,
- The governmental role in fulfilling the mission, and
- The responsibilities unique to each level of government

The rest of the recommendations are instrumental in implementing the basic recommendations for the future of public health. These instrumental recommendations fall into the following categories: statutory framework; structural and organizational steps; strategies to build the fundamental capacities of public health agencies—technical, political, managerial, programmatic, and fiscal; and education for public health.

THE PUBLIC HEALTH MISSION, GOVERNMENTAL ROLE, AND LEVELS OF RESPONSIBILITY

Mission

The committee defines the mission of public health as fulfilling society's interest in assuring conditions in which people can be healthy. Its aim is to generate organized community effort to address the public interest in health by applying scientific and technical knowledge to prevent disease and promote health. The mission of public health is addressed by private organizations and individuals as well as by public agencies. But the governmental public health agency has a unique function: to see to it that vital elements are in place and that the mission is adequately addressed.

The Governmental Role in Public Health

The committee finds that the core functions of public health agencies at all levels of government are assessment, policy development, and assurance.

Assessment

The committee recommends that every public health agency regularly and systematically collect, assemble, analyze, and make available information on the health of the community, including statistics on health status, community health needs, and epidemiologic and other studies of health problems. Not every agency is large enough to conduct these activities directly; intergovernmental and interagency cooperation is essential. Nevertheless, each agency bears the responsibility for seeing that the assessment function is fulfilled. This basic function of public health cannot be delegated.

Policy Development

The committee recommends that every public health agency exercise its responsibility to serve the public interest in the development of comprehensive public health policies by promoting use of the scientific knowledge base in decision-making about public health and by leading in developing public health policy. Agencies must take a strategic approach, developed on the basis of a positive appreciation for the democratic political process.

Assurance

The committee recommends that public health agencies assure their constituents that services necessary to achieve agreed-upon goals are provided, either by encouraging actions by other entities (private or public sector), by requiring such action through regulation, or by providing services directly.

The committee recommends that each public

health agency involve key policymakers and the general public in determining a set of high-priority personal and communitywide health services that governments will guarantee to every community member. This guarantee should include subsidization or direct provision of high-priority personal health services for those unable to afford them.

Levels of Responsibility

In addition to these functions, which are common to federal, state, and local governments, each level of government has unique responsibilities.

States

The committee believes that states are and must be the central force in public health. They bear primary public sector responsibility for health.

The committee recommends that the public health duties of states should include the following:

- Assessment of health needs in the state based on statewide data collection
- Assurance of an adequate statutory base for health activities in the state
- Establishment of statewide health objectives, delegating power to localities as appropriate and holding them accountable
- Assurance of appropriate organized statewide effort to develop and maintain essential personal, educational, and environmental health services; provision of access to necessary services; and solution of problems inimical to health
- Guarantee of a minimum set of essential health services
- Support of local service capacity, especially when disparities in local ability to raise revenue and/or administer programs require subsidies, technical assistance, or direct action by the state to achieve adequate service levels.

Federal

The committee recommends the following as federal public health obligations:

- Support of knowledge development and dissemination through data gathering, research, and information exchange

- Establishment of nationwide health objectives and priorities, and stimulation of debate on interstate and national public health issues
- Provision of technical assistance to help states and localities determine their own objectives and to carry out action on national and regional objectives;
- Provision of funds to states to strengthen state capacity for services, especially to achieve an adequate minimum capacity, and to achieve national objectives
- Assurance of actions and services that are in the public interest of the entire nation such as control of AIDS and similar communicable diseases, interstate environmental actions, and food and drug inspection

Localities

Because of great diversity in size, powers, and capacities of local governments, generalizations must be made with caution. Nevertheless, no citizen from any community, no matter how small or remote, should be without identifiable and realistic access to the benefits of public health protection, which is possible only through a local component of the public health delivery system.

The committee recommends the following functions for local public health units:

- Assessment, monitoring, and surveillance of local health problems and needs and of resources for dealing with them;
- Policy development and leadership that foster local involvement and a sense of ownership, that emphasize local needs, and that advocate equitable distribution of public resources and complementary private activities commensurate with community needs
- Assurance that high-quality services, including personal health services, needed for the protection of public health in the community are available and accessible to all persons; that the community receives proper consideration in the allocation of federal and state as well as local resources for public health; and that the community is informed about how to obtain public health, including personal health, ser-

vices, or how to comply with public health requirements.

Education for Public Health

Many educational paths can lead to careers in public health. However, the most direct educational path to a career in public health is to obtain a degree from a school of public health. Many of the 25 schools of public health are located in research universities and thus have a dual responsibility to develop knowledge and to produce well-trained professional practitioners. These dual roles are not always easy to balance.

Many observers feel that some schools have become somewhat isolated from public health practice and therefore no longer place a sufficiently high value on the training of professionals to work in health agencies. The dearth of professional agency leadership noted by the committee during the study may lend support to this view. The observed variations in agency practice, inadequate salaries, and frequently negative image of public health practice may partly account for any less-than-desirable responses by the educational institutions to the needs of practice.

In addition, most public health workers have no formal training in public health, and their need for basic grounding may not be appropriately met by the degree programs appropriate to prepare people for middle- and upper-level positions. To these ends the committee recommends:

- Schools of public health should establish firm practice links with state and/or local public health agencies so that significantly more faculty members may undertake professional responsibilities in these agencies, conduct research there, and train students in such practice situations. Recruitment of faculty and admission of students should give appropriate weight to prior public health experience as well as to academic qualifications.
- Schools of public health should fulfill their potential role as significant resources to government at all levels in the development of public health policy.
- Schools of public health should provide stu-

dents an opportunity to learn the entire scope of public health practice, including environmental, educational, and personal health approaches to the solution of public health problems; the basic epidemiological and biostatistical techniques for analysis of those problems; and the political and management skills needed for leadership in public health.

- Research in schools of public health should range from basic research in fields related to public health, through applied research and development, to program evaluation and implementation research. The unique research mission of the schools of public health is to select research opportunities on the basis of their likely relevance to the solution of real public health problems and to test such applications in real life settings.

- Schools of public health should take maximum advantage of training resources in their universities, for example, faculty and courses in schools of business administration, and departments of physical, biological, and social sciences. The hazards of developing independent faculty resources isolated from the main disciplinary departments on the campus are real, and links between faculty in schools of public health and their parent disciplines should be sought and maintained.

- Because large numbers of persons being educated in other parts of the university will assume responsibilities in life that impact significantly on the public's health, e.g., involvement in production of hazardous goods or the enactment and enforcement of public health laws, schools of public health should extend their expertise to advise and assist with the health content of the educational programs of other schools and departments of the university.

- In view of the large numbers of personnel now engaged in public health without adequate preparation for their positions, the schools of public health should undertake an expanded program of short courses to help upgrade the competence of these personnel. In addition, short course offerings should provide opportunities for previously trained public health professionals, especially health officers, to keep up with advances in knowledge and practice.

- Because the schools of public health are not, and probably should not try to be, able to train the vast numbers of personnel needed for public health work, the schools of public health should encourage and assist other institutions to prepare appropriate, qualified public health personnel for positions in the field. When educational institutions other than schools of public health undertake to train personnel for work in the field, careful attention to the scope and capacity of the educational program is essential. This may be achieved in part by links with nearby schools of public health.

- Schools of public health should strengthen their response to the needs for qualified personnel for important, but often neglected, aspects of public health such as the health of minority groups and international health.

- Schools of public health should help develop, or offer directly in their own universities, effective courses that expose undergraduates to concepts, history, current context, and techniques of public health to assist in the recruitment of able future leaders into the field. The committee did not conclude whether undergraduate degrees in public health are useful.

- Education programs for public health professionals should be informed by comprehensive and current data on public health personnel and their employment opportunities and needs.

CONCLUDING REMARKS

This report conveys an urgent message to the American people. Public health is a vital function that is in trouble. Immediate public concern and support are called for in order to fulfill society's interest in assuring the conditions in which people can be healthy. History teaches us that an organized community effort to prevent disease and promote health is both valuable and effective. Yet public health in the United States has been taken for granted, many public health issues have become inappropriately politicized, and public health responsibilities have become so fragmented that deliberate action is often difficult if not impossible.

Restoring an effective public health system neither can nor should be achieved by public health professionals alone. Americans must be concerned that there are adequate public health services in their communities, and must let their elected representatives know of their concern. The specific actions appropriate to strengthen public health will vary from area to area and must blend professional knowledge with community values. The committee intends not to prescribe one best way of rescuing public health, but to admonish the readers to get involved in their own communities in order to address present dangers, now and for the sake of future generations.

APPENDIX C

Graduate Programs in Public Health Nutrition*

Case Western Reserve University
Department of Nutrition
10900 Euclid Avenue
Cleveland, OH 44106-4906
(216)368-2440
FAX: (216)368-6644

Columbia University Teachers College
Dept of Nutrition Education
Box 137
New York, NY 10027
(212)678-3950

Cornell University
Assistant Professor
Division of Nutritional Sciences
Martha Van Rensselear
Ithaca, NY 14853
(607)255-2141

Eastern Kentucky University
Community Nutrition Program
Department of Home Economics

Richmond, KY 40475
(606)622-1175

Loma Linda University
Nutrition Program
Nichol Hall, Room 1102
Dept of Public Health & Preventive Medicine
School of Medicine
Loma Linda, CA 92350
(714)824-4657

New York Medical College
Director, Nutrition Program & Professor
Dept of Community & Preventive Medicine
Munger Pavilion
Valhalla, NY 10595
(914)993-4257

Pennsylvania State University
Nutrition in Public Health
College of Human Development
216 Henderson Human Development Bldg
University Park, PA 16802
(814)863-2920

*Active university membership, revised 5/91.

Southern Illinois University
Department of Animal Sciences, Food &
    Nutrition
School of Agriculture
Carbondale, IL 62901
(618)453-5193

Tufts University
Frances Stern Nutrition Center
Tufts University Medical School
New England Medical Center Hospital, Box 783
750 Washington Street
Boston, MA 02111
(617)956-5273
FAX: (617)350-8325

Tulane University
Nutrition Program Director
Tulane University School of Public Health &
    Tropical Medicine
New Orleans, LA 70112
(504)588-5371

University of California, Berkeley
Public Health Nutrition Program
School of Public Health
Berkeley, CA 94720
(415)642-4252

University of Hawaii
Public Health Nutrition Program
Dept of Public Health Sciences
School of Public Health
1960 East West Road D140F
Honolulu, HI 96822

University of Michigan
Program in Public Health Nutrition
School of Public Health
1420 Washington Heights
Ann Arbor, MI 48109
(313)764-3307
FAX· (313)763-5455

University of Minnesota
Public Health Nutrition
School of Public Health
Box 197 Mayo
D355 Mayo Memorial Bldg.
420 Delaware Street SE
Minneapolis, MN 55455
(612)625-4100

University of North Carolina
Dept of Nutrition
School of Public Health
McGavvan-Greenberg Bldg.
CB #7400
Chapel Hill, NC 27599-7400
(919)966-7229
FAX: (919)966-7216

University of Puerto Rico
Coordinator, Nutrition Program
Graduate School of Public Health
Medical Sciences Campus
GPO Box 5067
San Juan, Puerto Rico 00936
(809)758-2525, Ext. 1433 or 1460

University of Tennessee
Dept of Nutrition & Food Science
229 Jessie Harris Bldg.
1215 Cumberland Avenue
Knoxville, TN 37996-1900
(615)974-6267
FAX: (615)974-8546

University of Toronto
Dept of Nutrition Sciences
Faculty of Medicine
Fitzgerald Bldg.
150 College Street
Toronto, Ontario, Canada M5S 1A8

APPENDIX D

The Association of State and Territorial Public Health Nutrition Directors

MISSION

The mission of the Association of State and Territorial Public Health Nutrition Directors (ASTPHND) is to promote achievement of optimal nutritional status for all sectors of the American population. ASTPHND provides leadership for national and state food and nutrition policy, programs, and services from the state health agency perspective through communication, education, research, and advocacy.

FUNCTIONS

- To serve as an official body with whom other professional groups in public health and related fields can work on nutrition programs and problems of mutual concern
- To advise the Association of State and Territorial Health Officials (ASTHO) and other organizations on legislation and public policy related to food and nutrition issues and concerns and to advocate for implementation
- To serve as a channel through which directors of public health nutrition programs of the states, territories, commonwealths, districts, and possessions of the United States may exchange information for the enrichment and improvement of public health nutrition programs
- To foster and recommend standards for the education of practitioners in the field of public health nutrition

MEMBERSHIP

The Association of State and Territorial Public Health Nutrition Directors (ASTPHND) is composed of nutrition directors of the departments of health of the states, territories, commonwealths, districts, and possessions of the United States who have been appointed to membership by the health agency chief official.

ASTPHND membership includes 56 nutrition directors: the 50 states, the District of Columbia, American Samoa, Guam, Mariana Islands, Puerto Rico, and the Virgin Islands.

For a free booklet listing all of the nutrition directors and their affiliations, write to:

ASTPHND Association Office
415 Second Street, NE #200
Washington, DC 20002
(202)546-6963
(202)544-9349 (FAX)

Membership services of the association include an annual educational meeting, a quarterly newsletter, a membership handbook, representation in related conferences, and membership in coalitions interested in promoting good nutrition health.

APPENDIX E

Newsletters Related to Diet and Health

	Publisher/Subscription Address	Editor Subscription Rates/Frequency	Directed to
Advocacy Update	Public Voice for Food and Health Suite 522 1001 Connecticut Avenue NW Washington, DC 20036	Free of charge Monthly	Consumer organizations
Calorie Control Commentary	Calorie Control Council 5775 Peachtree-Dunwoody Rd. Atlanta, GA 30342	Free of charge 2/3 Issues/year	Professionals
Cholesterol and Coronary Disease . . . Reducing the Risk	Science & Medicine 79 Madison Avenue New York, NY 10016	Editorial board Free of charge 6 Issues/year	Professionals
Cholesterol & Blood Pressure Update	Citizens for Public Action on Blood Pressure & Cholesterol Suite 1002 7200 Wisconsin Avenue Bethesda, MD 20814	$9/Year Quarterly	Public
The Consumer Affairs Letter	George Idelson PO Box 65313 Washington, DC 20035	$99-195/year Monthly	Public
Consumer Magazines Digest: Nutrition & Health Related Food Topics	Consumer Choices Unlimited, Inc. PO Box 1985 Evanston, IL 60204	$67-97/year Monthly	Public and professionals
Contemporary Nutrition	General Mills, Inc. PO Box 5588 Stacy, MN 55079	Free of charge in US 10 Issues/year	Professionals
Dairy Council Digest	National Dairy Council 6300 N. River Road Rosemont, IL 60018	$4.50/Year/US $5.50/Year/foreign Bimonthly	Professionals
Dietetic Currents	Ross Laboratories 625 Cleveland Avenue Columbus, OH 43216	$20.00/Year	Professionals
FDA Consumer	FDA, UPHS, DHHS 5600 Fishers Lane Rockville, MD 20857	$12/$15/year 10 Issues/year	Public and professionals
Food & Nutrition News	National Live Stock and Meat Board 444 N. Michigan Ave. Chicago, IL 60611	Free of charge 5 Issues/year	Professionals

Adapted from *Nutrition Notes*, Bethesda, Md, December 1991, American Institute of Nutrition.

	Publisher/Subscription Address	Editor Subscription Rates/Frequency	Directed to
Food Insight	International Food Information Council Suite 430 1100 Connecticut Ave, NW Washington, DC 20036	Free of charge Quarterly	Professionals
Food News for Consumers	USDA, Food Safety & Inspection Service FSIS/ILA, Rm 1165, So Washington, DC 20250	$5.00/Year Quarterly	Public and professionals
Environmental Nutrition	Environmental Nutrition, Inc. 2112 Broadway New York, NY 10073	$36.00/Year Quarterly	Public and professionals
Food Protection Report	Charles Felix Associates PO Box 1581 Leesburg, VA 22075	$125/Year Monthly	Professionals
FYI	Vitamin Nutrition Information Service Hoffman-LaRoche, Inc. Nutley, NJ 07110	Free of charge	Professionals
Guide to Healthy Eating	Physicians Committee for Responsible Medicine PO Box 6322 Washington, DC 20015	$14.95/Year 6 Issues/year	Public
Heart News Digest	National Center for Cardiac Information 9606 Blincoe Court Burke, VA 22015	$25/Year Quarterly	Public and professionals
NCL Bulletin	National Consumers League 815 15th Street, NW Suite 928 Washington, DC 20005	$20/Year Bimonthly	Public
Nutrition Close-up	Egg Nutrition Center 2301 M Street, NW, S 405 Washington, DC 20037	Free of charge 4 Issues/year	Professionals
Nutrition News	National Dairy Council 6300 N. River Road Rosemont, IL 60018	$4.00/Year/US $5.00/Year/foreign 3 Issues/year	Professionals
Nutrition Research Newsletter	Lyda Associates, Inc. PO Box 700 Palisades, NY 10964	$96-$106/Year Monthly	Professionals
Obesity & Health	Healthy Living Institute 402 S. 14th Street Hettinger, ND 58639	$79/Year Monthly	Professionals
Obesity Update	Special Projects Network 6900 Grove Road Thorofare, NJ 08086	Free of charge to physicians 6 Issues/year	Physicians

	Publisher/Subscription Address	Editor Subscription Rates/Frequency	Directed to
On Your Mark	The Sugar Association 1101 15th Street, NW Washington, DC 20005	Free of charge Quarterly	Professionals
Supermarket Savvy	Leni Reed Associates, Inc. PO Box 7069 Reston, VA 22091	$68/Year Bimonthly	Professionals
Tufts University Diet & Nutrition Letter	White Publications 53 Park Place New York, NY 10007	$20/Year Monthly	Public
University of California, Berkeley, Wellness Letter	Health Letter Associates 5 Water Oak Fernandina Beach, FL 32034	$20-$29/Year Monthly	Public

Index

Tables are indicated by *t*; figures are indicated by *f*.

549